SOMATOSTATIN

ADVANCES IN EXPERIMENTAL MEDICINE AND BIOLOGY

Recent Volumes in this Series

Volume 182
GENE EXPRESSION IN MUSCLE
Edited by Richard C. Strohman and Stewart Wolf

Volume 183
DRUGS AFFECTING LIPID METABOLISM VIII
Edited by David Kritchevsky, William L. Holmes, and Rodolfo Paoletti

Volume 184
MECHANISMS OF CELL-MEDIATED CYTOTOXICITY II
Edited by Pierre Henkart and Eric Martz

Volume 185
IMMUNOBIOLOGY OF PROTEINS AND PEPTIDES III: VIRAL AND BACTERIAL ANTIGENS
Edited by M. Z. Atassi and Howard L. Bachrach

Volume 186
MICROENVIRONMENTS IN THE LYMPHOID SYSTEM
Edited by G. G. B. Klaus

Volume 187
AIDS-ASSOCIATED SYNDROMES
Edited by Sudhir Gupta

Volume 188
SOMATOSTATIN
Edited by Yogesh C. Patel and Gloria S. Tannenbaum

SOMATOSTATIN

Edited by

Yogesh C. Patel

McGill University
and Royal Victoria Hospital
Montreal, Quebec, Canada

and

Gloria S. Tannenbaum

McGill University and
McGill University-Montreal Children's Hospital Research Institute
Montreal, Quebec, Canada

SPRINGER SCIENCE+BUSINESS MEDIA, LLC

Library of Congress Cataloging in Publication Data

Main entry under title:

Somatostatin.

(Advances in experimental medicine and biology; v. 188)
"Proceedings of a satellite symposium of the Seventh International Congress of Endocrinology, entitled Somatostatin, held June 29-30, 1984, in Montreal, Quebec, Canada"—T.p. verso.
Includes bibliographies and index.
1. Somatostatin—Congresses. I. Patel, Yogesh C. II. Tannenbaum, Gloria S. III. International Congress of Endocrinology (7th: 1984: Québec, Québec,) IV. Series.
[DNLM: 1. Somatostatin—congresses. W1 AD559 v.88/WK 515 S693 1984]
QP572.S59S66 1985 574.19'2456 85-9441
ISBN 978-1-4615-7888-8 ISBN 978-1-4615-7886-4 (eBook)
DOI 10.1007/978-1-4615-7886-4

Proceedings of a satellite symposium of the Seventh International Congress of Endocrinology, entitled Somatostatin, held June 29-30, 1984, in Montreal, Quebec, Canada

Originally published by Plenum Press New York in 1985
Softcover reprint of the hardcover 1st edition 1985

PREFACE

Montreal has had a longstanding interest in somatostatin. Two years ago when the final planning began for the International Congress of Endocrinology in Quebec City in July 1984, we seized the opportunity for having a separate Satellite Symposium on somatostatin here in Montreal. We felt that after a decade of uniformly vigorous growth in somatostatin research, the opportune moment had arrived for a review of the most significant past developments and for setting the directions for the future. Knowing the futility of trying to cover every aspect of the burgeoning somatostatin field in a two day scientific program, we opted for a detailed analysis of selected areas which were reasonably mature and of areas of greatest new activity. To attain these objectives, 27 leading international experts actively involved in their fields were invited to present an indepth review of their work in one of five major categories of somatostatin research. Thirty minutes at the end of each session were assigned for a three way, comprehensive discussion of some of the core concepts between the session moderators, the panellists and the audience. The feedback that we have received from the participants leaves little doubt that the meeting was a scientific and social success.

This book fulfills our final commitment towards the Meeting which was to record the proceedings in a timely publication. Chapters were received from all but one of the invited speakers and have been carefully edited to ensure uniformity of presentation and nomenclature. Transcripts of the panel discussions required extensive editing to transform the frequently unstructured spoken word into lucid prose. The resultant product, we believe, qualifies as a state of the art monograph on somatostatin research which should excite all scholars in the field and be of value to anyone interested in the biology of neuropeptide systems.

Montreal, 1984

Yogesh C. Patel
Gloria S. Tannenbaum

ACKNOWLEDGEMENTS

The success of the Somatostatin Symposium and the timely publication of this volume were made possible by the generous contributions of a large number of individuals and organizations. C. Srikant played a dominant role at all stages of this undertaking. We acknowledge with gratitude the organizational help provided by Doris Ruggere in particular, and additionally by Nicoletta Jacovidou, Anoop Brar, Hans Zingg, David Dunn, Irene Pierzchala, Jean-Claude Painson, Wendy Gurd and Sylvie Barrett. Both C. Srikant and Hans Zingg shared some of the burden of editing and proofreading. Special thanks are due to Maria Correia for her indispensible contributions as secretary throughout this entire venture, and to Lucy Felicissmo for undertaking the mammoth task of retyping the book. We are grateful to John Matzka and Pat Vann of Plenum Press for their unfailing cooperation at all times. We express our warm appreciation to our generous financial sponsors, in particular McGill University, The Medical Research Council of Canada, Fonds de la Recherche en Sante du Quebec, Montreal Children's Hospital Research Institute and the various pharmaceutical and other companies. Lastly we extend our sincere thanks to all the contributors to the volume for the outstanding quality of their chapters and for their promptness.

Y.C.P.
G.S.T.

NOTE ON NOMENCLATURE

Beginning with a solitary tetradecapeptide substance, the steady proliferation of other somatostatin peptides has left in its wake a great deal of nomenclatural confusion. As far as possible throughout the present text we have shown a preference for the use of 'somatostatin' as a general term and of S as its abbreviation. The specific molecular forms somatostatin-14, somatostatin-28, prosomatostatin, preprosomatostatin are designated as S-14, S-28, pro-S, prepro-S, and somatostatin-like immunoreactivity or immunoreactive somatostatin as SLI or IRS respectively. In deference to the large number of authors who prefer the more catchy SS abbreviation for somatostatin, we have retained in this book the SS format as well, although its use becomes somewhat cumbersome for such terms as SSLI and IRSS. Abbreviations such as SRIF, SST, SOM, IMRS serve little additional purpose and have been dropped from the text.

CONTENTS

CONTRIBUTORS

Yves Agid
Laboratoire de Medecine
Experimentale de la Pitie
Paris, France

Philip C. Andrews
Department of Biochemistry
Purdue University
West Lafayette, Indiana, U.S.A.

Andrew Baird
Laboratories for Neuroendo-
crinology
The Salk Institute
San Diego, Ca., U.S.A.

Charles Bakhit
BCR-1, Research Institute
Scripps Clinic
La Jolla, CA., U.S.A.

Robert Benoit
Montreal General Hospital
Research Institute
McGill University
Montreal, Canada

Michael Berelowitz
Div. of Endocrinology and Met.
University of Cincinnati
College of Medicine
Cincinnati, OH., U.S.A.

Floyd E. Bloom
BCR-1, Research Institute
Scripps Clinic
La Jolla, CA., U.S.A.

Peter Böhlen
Laboratories for Neuroendo-
crinology
The Salk Institute
San Diego, CA., U.S.A.

Susan Bonner-Weir
Department of Internal Medicine
Medical College of Virginia
Richmond, VA., U.S.A.

Paul Brazeau
Centre de Recherche
Hopital Notre Dame
Montreal, Canada

Marvin R. Brown
Peptide Biology Laboratory
The Salk Institute
La Jolla, CA., U.S.A.

Paul Cohen
Groupe de Neurobiochimie
Cellulaire et Moleculaire
Universite Pierre et Marie Curie
Unite Associee au CNRS No. 554
Paris, France

David H. Coy
Section of Endocrinology and
Metabolism
Department of Medicine
Tulane University
School of Medicine
New Orleans, LA., U.S.A.

Kiertisin Dharmsathaphorn
Division of Gastroenterology
Department of Medicine
University of California
San Diego Medical Center
San Diego, CA., U.S.A.

Jack E. Dixon
Department of Biochemistry
Purdue University
West Lafayette, IN., U.S.A.

Laneta J. Dorflinger
Laboratory of Toxicology
Harvard School of Public Health
Boston, MA., U.S.A.

Robert Elde
Department of Anatomy
University of Minnesota
Minneapolis, MN., U.S.A.

Alain Enjalbert
Unite 159, INSERM
Paris, France

John W. Ensinck
University of Washington
Department of Medicine RC-14
Seattle, WA., U.S.A.

Jacques Epelbaum
Unite 159, INSERM
Paris, France

Frederick Esch
Laboratories for Neuroendo-crinology
The Salk Institute
San Diego, CA., U.S.A.

Laurel A. Fisher
Peptide Biology Laboratory
La Jolla, CA., U.S.A.

John E. Gerich
Diabetes and Metabolism Research Laboratory
Mayo Clinic
Rochester, MN., U.S.A.

Pablo Gluschankof
Groupe de Neurobiochimie Cellulaire et Moleculaire
Universite Pierre et Marie Curie
Unite Associee au CNRS No. 554
Paris, France

Sophie Gomez
Groupe de Neurobiochimie Cellulaire et Moleculaire
Universite Pierre et Marie Curie
Unite Associee au CNRS No. 554
Paris, France

Richard H. Goodman
Division of Endocrinology
Tufts New England Medical Center
Boston, MA., U.S.A.

Reza F. Green
Departments of Anatomy and Developmental Biology and Cancer
Albert Einstein College of Medicine
Bronx, N.Y., U.S.A.

Roger H. Guillemin
Laboratories for Neuroendo-crinology
The Salk Institute
San Diego, CA., U.S.A.

Joel F. Habener
Laboratory of Molecular Endo-crinology
Massachusetts General Hospital and the Howard Hughes Medical Institute
Harvard Medical School
Boston, MA., U.S.A.

Michel Hamon
Unite 114, INSERM
Paris, France

Andrea A. Heldsinger
Dept. of Surgery and Internal Med
University of Michigan Medical School
Ann Arbor, MI., U.S.A.

Simon J. Hocart
Section of Endocrinology and Metabolism
Department of Medicine
Tulane University School of Medicine
New Orleans, LA., U.S.A.

Tomas Hökfelt
Department of Histology
Karolinska Institute
Stockholm, Sweden

France Javoy-Agid
Laboratoire de Medecine Experimentale de la Pitie
Paris, France

Olle Johansson
Department of Histology
Karolinska Institute
Stockholm, Sweden

Howard M. Katzen
Merck Institute for Therapeutic Research
Rahway, N.J., U.S.A.

Bruce D. Koch
Laboratory of Toxicology
Harvard School of Public Health
Boston, MA., U.S.A.

Leonard Koda
BCR-1, Research Institute
Scripps Clinic
La Jolla, CA., U.S.A.

Claude Kordon
Unite 159, INSERM
Paris, France

Y. Lamour
Unite 159, INSERM
Paris, France

Valentine A. Lance
Section of Endocrinology and Metabolism
Department of Medicine
Tulane University
School of Medicine
New Orleans, LA., U.S.A.

Lars-Inge Larsson
Unit of Histochemistry
University Institute of Pathology
Copenhagen, Denmark

Nicholas Ling
Laboratories for Neuroendocrinology
The Salk Institute
San Diego, CA., U.S.A.

Malcolm J. Low
Division of Endocrinology
Tufts New England Medical Center
Boston, MA., U.S.A.

Peter Marbach
Preclinical and Clinical Research Department
Sandoz Limited
Basle, Switzerland

Irme Mezo
Section of Endocrinology and Metabolism
Department of Medicine
Tulane University
School of Medicine
New Orleans, LA., U.S.A.

Marc R. Montminy
Division of Endocrinology
Tufts New England Medical Center
Boston, MA., U.S.A.

Alain Morel
Groupe de Neurobiochimie Cellulaire et Moleculaire
Universite Pierre et Marie Curie
Unite Associee au CNRS No. 554
Paris, France

John H. Morrison
BCR-1, Research Institute
Scripps Clinic
La Jolla, CA., U.S.A.

Emmanuel Moyse
Unite 159, INSERM
Paris, France

William A. Murphy
Section of Endocrinology and Metabolism
Department of Medicine
Tulane University
School of Medicine
New Orleans, LA., U.S.A.

Michael Neufeld
Preclinical & Clinical Research Department
Sandoz Limited
Basle, Switzerland

Pierre Nicolas
Groupe de Neurobiochimie
Cellulaire et Moleculaire
Universite Pierre et Marie Curie
Unite Associee au CNRS No. 554
Paris, France

Bryan Noe
Department of Anatomy
Emory University
School of Medicine
Atlanta, GA., U.S.A.

Ruth F. Nutt
Merck Institute for Therapeutic Research
Rahway, N.J., U.S.A.

Yogesh C. Patel
Fraser Laboratories
McGill University
Department of Medicine and
Neurology and Neurosurgery
Royal Victoria Hospital
Montreal, Canada

Robert A. Peterfreund
Peptide Biology Laboratory
The Salk Institute for
Biological Studies
San Diego, CA., U.S.A.

Gary L. Pittenger
Department of Surgery and
Internal Medicine
University of Michigan Medical
Department of Surgery and
School
Ann Arbor, MI., U.S.A.

Janos Pless
Preclinical and Clinical
Research Department
Sandoz Limited
Basle, Switzerland

Richard Robbins
Neuroendocrine Section
Endocrinology Division
University of Colorado
Health Sciences Center
Denver, CO., U.S.A.

Richard Saperstein
Merck Institute for Therapeutic Research
Rahway, N.J., U.S.A.

Agnes Schonbrunn
Laboratory of Toxicology
Harvard School of Public Health
Boston, MA., U.S.A.

Volker Schusdziarra
Department of Internal Medicine
University of Ulm
Steinhovelstrasse, Germany

Susumo Seino
Department of Surgery and
Internal Medicine
University of Michigan
Medical School
Ann Arbor, MI., U.S.A.

Dennis Shields
Departments of Anatomy and
Developmental Biology and Cancer
Albert Einstein College of
Medicine
Bronx, N.Y., U.S.A.

Eve E. Slater
Merck Institute for Therapeutic
Research
Rahway, N.J., U.S.A.

Joachim Spiess
Peptide Biology Laboratory
The Salk Institute
La Jolla, CA., U.S.A.

Coimbatore B. Srikant
Fraser Laboratories
McGill University
Department of Medicine
Royal Victoria Hospital
Montreal, Canada

Sanford L. Steelman
Merck Institute for Therapeutic
Research
Rahway, N.J., U.S.A.

Javier Sueiras-Diaz
Section of Endocrinology and
Metabolism
Department of Medicine
Tulane University
School of Medicine
New Orleans, LA., U.S.A.

Gloria S. Tannenbaum
Departments of Pediatrics and
Neurology and Neurosurgery
McGill University and the
Montreal Children's Hospital
Montreal, Canada

Wylie W. Vale
Peptide Biology Laboratory
The Salk Institute for
Biological Studies
San Diego, CA., U.S.A.

Aaron I. Vinik
Department of Surgery and
Internal Medicine
University of Michigan
Medical School
Ann Arbor, MI., U.S.A.

Thomas G. Warren
Departments of Anatomy and
Developmental Biology and Cancer
Albert Einstein College of
Medicine
Bronx, N.Y., U.S.A.

William B. Wehrenberg
Laboratories for Neuroendo-
crinology
The Salk Institute
San Diego, CA., U.S.A.

Gordon C. Weir
Department of Internal Medicine
Medical College of Virginia
Richmond, VA., U.S.A.

Shao Y. Ying
Laboratories for Neuroendo-
crinology
The Salk Institute
San Diego, CA., U.S.A.

Hans H. Zingg
Laboratory of Molecular
Endocrinology
McGill University
Department of Medicine
Royal Victoria Hospital
Montreal, Canada

I

BIOSYNTHESIS OF SOMATOSTATIN

1

EXPRESSION OF ANGLERFISH PREPROSOMATOSTATIN GENES IN MAMMALIAN CELLS: STUDIES ON THE SYNTHESIS AND POST-TRANSLATIONAL PROCESSING OF SOMATOSTATIN PRECURSORS

DENNIS SHIELDS, THOMAS G. WARREN AND REZA F. GREEN

Departments of Anatomy & Developmental Biology & Cancer
Albert Einstein College of Medicine
Bronx, NY 10461

INTRODUCTION

The major form of somatostatin (SS) is a 14 amino acid peptide (SS-14, SRIF) that inhibits the secretion of other peptide hormones including growth hormone, insulin and glucagon. It is synthesized in several tissues including brain, hypothalamus and pancreatic islets and its amino acid sequence is highly conserved in most species (1). Biosynthetic studies (2, 3) have demonstrated the existence of another somatostatin, SS-28, which is the SS-14 containing an additional 14 amino acids localized at the amino terminus; this peptide has also been isolated directly from several tissues (4-7). It is now well established that SS-14 is synthesized as part of a larger precursor, preprosomatostatin (prepro-SS), which is about eight times larger than the mature hormone (8).

In recent years the primary amino acid sequence of several prepro-SS molecules has been deduced from cloned cDNAs generated from a number of species including fish pancreatic islets (9-11), a rat thyroid medullary carcinoma (12, 13), and a human somatostatinoma (14). Rat and human prepro-SS are virtually identical in amino acid sequence differing in only four residues, two in the signal peptide and two in the propeptide. Two forms of prepro-SS, designated I and II (9), are present in anglerfish islets; prepro-SS I encodes a 121 amino acid precursor whereas prepro-SS II encodes a 124 residue precursor. In contrast to the rat and human precursors, anglerfish prepro-SS I and II share little homology in either their signal peptides or the prohormone region and have little homology to the mammalian precursors (38%). Catfish islets also have two SS precursors one which contains SS-14 and a second SS-22 that has only 50% homology with SS-14 (10, 11); surprisingly there is only 42%

amino acid sequence homology in the signal and propeptide between the anglerfish and catfish SS-14 precursors.

In all these species the overall organization of the prepro-SS molecule is highly conserved in that it consists of a hydrophobic signal peptide of 23 to 25 amino acids (8, 12, 15) followed by a proregion of 90-100 residues. The mature hormone is located at the carboxyl terminus of the proregion and is preceded by pairs of basic amino acids: Arg-Lys. Paired basic amino acids are characteristic of proteolytic processing sites for excision of many polypeptide hormones from their precursors (16). Furthermore these basic residues are part of a subset of six amino acids (Ala-Pro-Arg-Glu-Arg-Lys) which are present in all SS-14 precursors and SS-28 molecules sequenced to date. With the exception of anglerfish preprosomatostatin II, all the precursors contain only a single set of paired basic amino acids suggesting that additional cryptic bioactive peptides are absent. This contrasts with other hormone precursors, many of which are polyproteins containing several hormones (16). Hence prepro-SS may be one of the simplest precursor polypeptide hormones.

The hexapeptide domain containing the paired basic amino acids is located upstream from and immediately adjacent to the mature hormone (Fig. 1) in all preprosomatostatins except catfish SS-22. The conservation of this peptide, in contrast to other regions of the propeptide suggests it may have functional significance. Furthermore, despite differences in primary amino acid sequence between the fish and mammalian species, comparison of hydrophobic and hydrophilic residues (see below) as well as secondary structure predictions (17) suggests that the same structural domains are highly conserved in all species of SS precursor, implying that such regions may be functionally important. It is possible that the conserved domains could function in (a) providing the correct protein conformation to facilitate processing of SS-14 or SS-28; (b) in intracellular transport and targetting of pro-SS from the ER through organelles of the secretory apparatus where prohormone processing occurs. To test these hypotheses we have used both gene transfer experiments as well as <u>in vitro</u> reconstitution experiments using cell-free systems supplemented with microsomal membranes. The aim of these studies is to investigate processing and intracellular transport of preprosomatostatins by identifying functionally important domains in the precursors.

As a first step towards understanding the function of such domains we have introduced anglerfish prepro-SS cDNA into mammalian cells (COS) by using an SV-40 expression vector. By employing recombinant DNA and gene transfer techniques we have an advantage over classical pulse-chase experiments in that the experimental substrate i.e., prepro-SS can be manipulated prior to introduction into the recipient cells. Thus we can directly test the functional

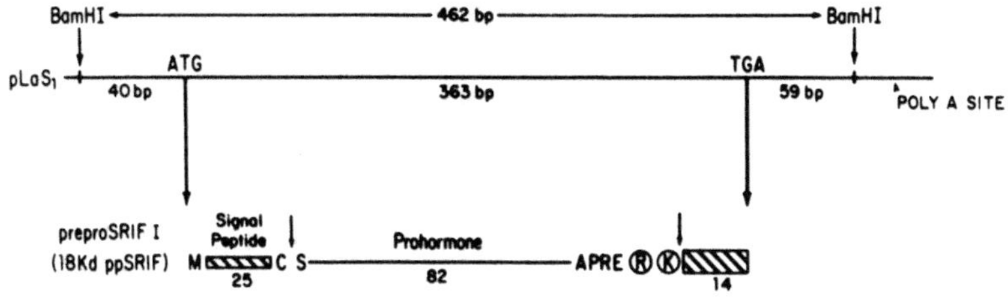

Fig. 1. Diagram of anglerfish prepro-SS I. The upper line represents prepro-SS (preproSRIF) cDNA, the Bam H1 restriction sites encompassing the coding region of the precursor are indicated; this DNA fragment was cloned into the Bam HI site of pJC119 (see Fig. 4). The lower line shows the organization and partial amino acid sequence of the precursor polypeptide: the site of the signal peptide cleavage is indicated between residues Cys and Ser, the hexapeptide is indicated APRERK, mature SS-14 is located at the carboxyl terminus of the precursor. The one letter amino acid code is: C=Cys; S=Ser; A=Ala; P=Pro; R=Arg; E=Glu; K=Lys. Based on data from Hobart et al. (9) and Warren and Shields (15).

importance of various parts of the precursor molecule. Our results suggest that COS cells, which do not normally secrete polypeptide hormones, contain the necessary proteolytic enzymes for converting prepro-SS to the mature hormone and also possess the apparatus to secrete it from the cell.

RESULTS

Structural Features of Prepro-SS

With the determination of the complete amino acid sequences of several preprosomatostatins, it was apparent that the human and rat precursors are virtually identical. However, there is considerable variation in the signal peptides and propeptides of the different forms of fish prepro-SS. When the amino acid sequences of the fish preprosomatostatins are compared to the rat and human precursors the most highly conserved regions of the polypeptide are the mature hormone and a six amino acid sequence located at the amino terminus of the hormone.

To determine if this region might constitute a common domain in all the precursors, we used a series of computer programs to predict the hydrophilicity (Fig. 2) and hydrophobicity (Fig. 3) of each of the preprosomatostatins. To assess the overall hydrophilicity, the algorithm of Hopp and Woods (18) was used. Rather surprisingly,

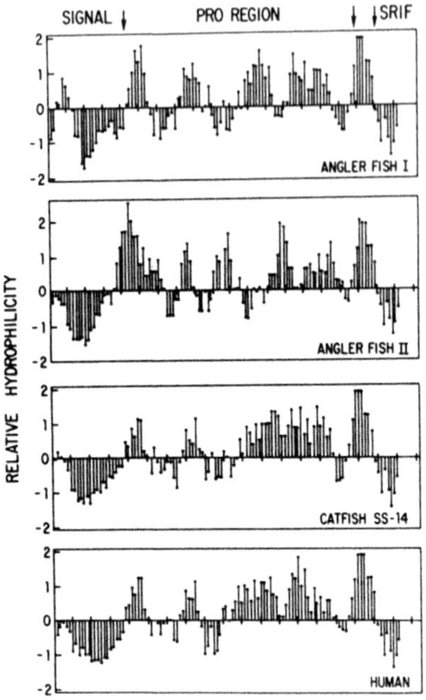

Fig. 2. Hydrophilicity profile of anglerfish prepro-SS I and II, catfish prepro-SS-14 and human prepro-SS using the algorithm of Hopp and Woods (18). The profile of the rat prepro-SS is identical to the human precursor. Arrows indicate the actual or proposed site of signal peptide cleavage and the hexapeptide (APRERK) respectively.

there is significant conservation of hydrophilic regions in each precursor which appear to be located in potentially important processing sites. The hydrophobic signal peptide is followed by a hydrophilic region; similarly the conserved hexapeptide, indicated by the arrows, preceding mature SS-14 represents the most intensely hydrophilic domain of the precursor. This type of analysis suggests that both these domains are located on the surface of the molecule and hence would be accessible to proteolytic digestion. These results i.e. the relative hydrophilicity of the region following the signal sequence, are consistent with the known site of signal peptide cleavage of anglerfish preprosomatostatins by signal peptidase (15). Furthermore since the hexapeptide domain is also the most hydrophilic, and contains the paired basic amino acids Arg-Lys, the data are also consistent with the proposal that this region represents the cleavage site for excision of the mature hormone SS-14 from its precursors (19).

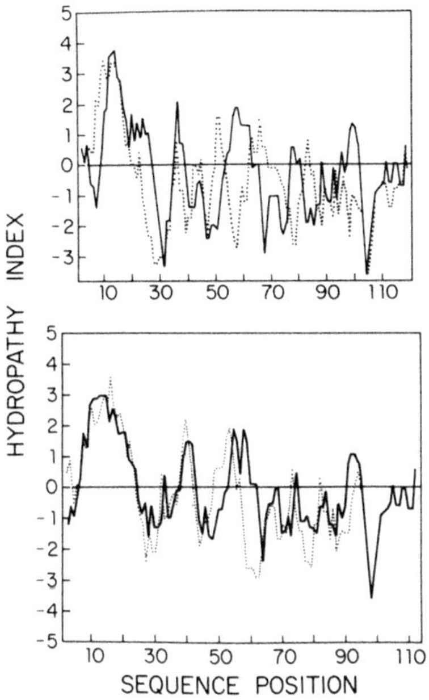

Fig. 3. Hydropathy index of anglerfish prepro-SS I (——) and II, (....) [upper panel]. Catfish prepro-SS-14 (——) and human prepro-SS (....) [lower panel] using the hydropathy scale of Kyte and Doolittle (20).

To assess the validity of this type of analysis, we also employed another quite different algorithm (20) based on the intrinsic hydrophobicity of each amino acid. The data are expressed as a hydropathy index, with hydrophobic domains having a negative value (Fig. 3). Consistent with the above data, this analysis predicts exactly the same overall conservation of hydrophobicity as the Hopp and Wood algorithm. Identical domains are predicted to be highly conserved even though completely different parameter values are used in performing these two methods of analysis. Since the hexapeptide has the greatest negative hydropathy, it is most likely to be located on the surface of the molecule. Our results are analogous to those of Argos et al. (17) who also assessed the potential helical domains in these prepro-SS molecules. Based on these analyses we feel that the domain structure of preprosomatostatins may have functional significance particularly with respect to post-translational processing of the precursor. To test this hypothesis we have used gene transfer experiments to insert prepro-SS and mutated forms of the precursor into cells which do not normally synthesize the hormone.

Expression of Prepro-SS cDNA

To obtain expression of anglerfish prepro-SS DNA in cells that do not normally synthesize the hormone, an SV-40-pBR322 expression vector pJC119 was used. This vector has previously been used in studies on the expression of several membrane proteins (21). During construction of pJC119, most of the coding region of the SV-40 late gene, VP-1, including its initiation codon was deleted. The remainder of the late region is intact including the sites for transcription initiation and polyadenylation. pJC119 contains several convenient cloning sites near the VP-1 promoter, in particular a Bam H1 site. Also during construction of pJC119 the large T antigen of the SV-40 early region was inactivated. This is normally required for viral gene expression. We therefore used COS cells, which are constitutive for this early gene function, to obtain expression of the prepro-SS cDNA which was cloned into pJC119. The anglerfish cDNA clone used in these experiments was pLAS-1 (9) which contains the complete prepro-SS I cDNA cloned into the Pst-I site of pBR322, and encodes a prepro-SS that migrates with an apparent Mr = 18,000 upon sodium dodecyl sulphate-polyacrylamide gel electrophoresis (SDS-PAGE) (15). Cleavage of pLAS-1 with Bam HI results in a DNA fragment which encompasses about 40 nucleotides upstream from the initiator Met to the beginning of the poly A addition site i.e., the complete coding region of prepro-SS I (Fig. 1). The Bam HI fragment was ligated into a synthetic Bam HI-site in the promoter region of the VP-1 late gene (Fig. 4). The resulting plasmid was designated pSVppS18.

COS cells were transfected with pSVppS18 (22) and at various times following transfection, aliquots of the culture medium were

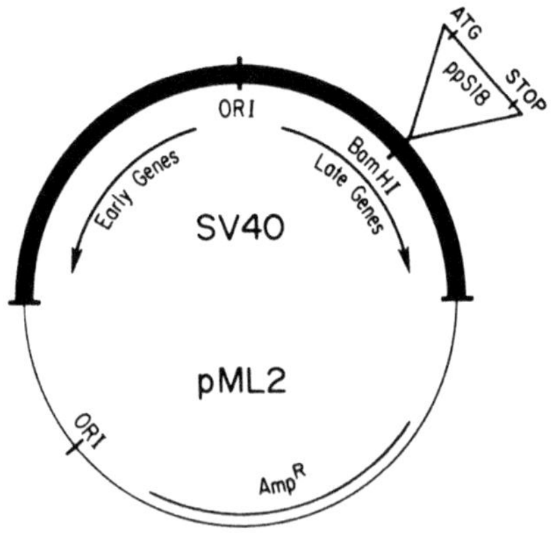

Fig. 4. Construction of pSVppS18 expression into a synthetic Bam HI fragment of pLAS-1 encoding the complete sequence of anglerfish prepro-SS I, including the initiator Met (ATG) was ligated into the late promoter of the SV-40 VP-1 gene in the expression vector pJC119.

assayed for somatostatin immunoreactivity using a highly sensitive radioimmunoassay (23). Two days following transfection, immunoreactive SS-14 was present in the culture medium and significant levels were found three days after transfection (Table 1). In contrast, SS-14 immunoreactivity was not detected in medium obtained from cells transfected with the vector pJC119, or with a vector designated pSVI-40, in which the prepro-SS cDNA was inserted into the VP-1 gene in the incorrect orientation with respect to the SV40 late promoter.

Translation of Anglerfish Prepro-SS mRNA in COS Cells

Having shown that cells transfected with plasmid pSVppS18 synthesized and secreted SS-14 immunoreactive material into the tissue culture medium, we wanted to determine the molecular basis of this immunoreactivity. It is possible that it resulted from synthesis and secretion of either pro-SS or the mature hormone. We therefore analyzed both the intracellular and extracellular SS-immunoreactive material using several different techniques. Cells transfected with plasmids pSVppS18, pSVI-40 or pJC119 were labelled with [^{35}S] Met and following incubation were lysed and treated with either non-immune or rabbit anti-SS-14 antiserum; the resulting immunoprecipitates were resolved by SDS-PAGE (Fig. 5). Only cells transfected with pSVppS18 had detectable immunoreactive SS-14 and this polypeptide

Table 1

		SS-14 immunoreactivity (pg/10^6 cells)		
		Days after transfection		
Experiment	Plasmid	1	2	3
A	pJC119	0	ND	0
	pSVI-40	0	ND	0
	pSVppS18	0	ND	1488
B	pSVppS18	0	279	809
C	pSVppS18	0	272	955

COS-7 cells were transfected with the indicated plasmid and at 1, 2 and 3 days after transfection, aliquots of the culture medium were removed and the amount of SS-14 immunoreactive material determined by radioimmunoassay (23) using rabbit anti-SS-14 serum, RSS1 (15).

comigrated exactly with the Mr = 17,000 pro-SS synthesized in the *in vitro* system supplemented with microsomal membranes (compare lanes 1 and 5), a result suggesting that the COS cell signal peptidase cleaved the nascent signal peptide correctly. COS cells transfected with either pJC119 or pSVI-40 or untreated cells had no detectable pro-SS polypeptides (lanes 3,7 & 9).

To determine that the putative Mr = 17,000 pro-SS synthesized in COS cells resulted from correct cleavage of the signal peptide, we determined the partial NH_2-terminus of this polypeptide. Previously, we have shown (8, 15) that the Mr = 17,000 pro-SS synthesized *in vitro* in the presence of microsomal membranes is derived from the Mr = 18,000 prepro-SS by cleavage of the signal peptide at residue 25 (Cys). Consequently, if the COS cells synthesized authentic pro-SS by cleaving the nascent signal peptide correctly, then from the predicted amino acid sequence of the precursor, leucine residues should be detected at positions 10, 12, 13, 14 and

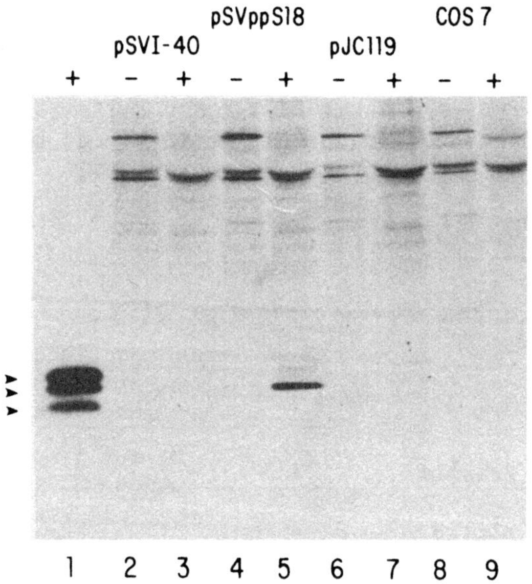

Fig. 5. Expression of anglerfish prepro-SS in COS 7 cells; analysis of intracellular SS-14-immunoreactive polypeptides. The cell lysate was treated with rabbit anti-SS-14 serum RSS-1, (+) or non-immune serum (-) and the immunoprecipitates resolved by SDS-PAGE. Lane 1: Translation products of anglerfish prepro-SS mRNA synthesized *in vitro* in the presence of microsomal membranes. Arrows indicate the migration of Mr = 18,000 prepro-SS I, Mr = 17,000 prepro-SS I and prepro-SS II, respectively. Lanes 2-9: products synthesized *in vivo* by COS 7 cell following transfection with plasmid DNA.

19 and methionine at residue 26 of pro-SS (9). Transfected COS cells were labelled with [^{3}H] Leu, and [^{35}S] Met, treated with anti-SS-14 antisera and the immunoprecipitates resolved by SDS-PAGE. The putative pro-SS was excised from the gel and subjected to 30 cycles of automatic Edman degradation (Fig. 6). As predicted, leucine residues were detected at positions 10, 12, 13, 14 and 19 and methionine at 26, demonstrating not only correct cleavage of the signal peptide by the COS cells but also that the Mr = 17,000 polypeptide was indeed authentic pro-SS.

Identification of SS Immunoreactive Polypeptides

Since appropriately transfected COS cells synthesize authentic pro-SS we wanted to determine the nature of the immunoreactive somatostatins present in the tissue culture medium (Table 1). This material could be due to secretion of pro-SS or could result from proteolytic processing of the propeptide to the mature hormone followed by its secretion. During the course of our experiments, we observed that with increasing periods of chase of up to 3 hours, labelled pro-SS disappeared from cell lysates. Furthermore, we were

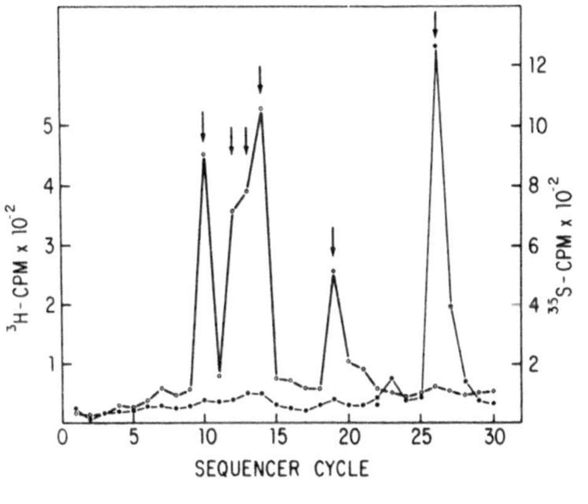

Fig. 6. Partial NH_2-terminal sequence of anglerfish pro-SS I synthesized by COS 7 cells. Following transfection with pSVppS18 DNA, cells were labelled with [^{35}S] Met and [^{3}H] Leu, harvested, washed, lysed and the cell lysate treated with RSS1 anti-SS-14 serum. The immunoprecipitates were resolved by SDS-PAGE. The radiolabelled pro-SS polypeptide was located by autoradiography and excised from the dried gel. The eluted polypeptide was then subjected to 30 cycles of automated Edman degradation (15, 24) and the radioactivity in each cycle determined by scintillation counting.
S Met: •——•; H Leu: o——o.

unable to detect pro-SS in the chase medium of appropriately transfected COS cells at any time following a pulse of [^{35}S]Cys. This implied either (i) that the COS cells were converting pro-SS to the mature hormone and secreting it into the culture medium and we were unable to resolve such a small polypeptide upon our SDS-PAGE system or (ii) that pro-SS was secreted into the medium and degraded by extracellular proteases. To distinguish between these possibilities, we performed a series of pulse-chase experiments and analyzed the SS-14-immunoreactive material, present in the culture, by high performance liquid chromatography (HPLC). COS cells were transfected with either pSVppS18 or pSVI-40 and labelled with both [^{35}S] Cys and [^{3}H]Phe, which are present in mature SS-14, for 3 hours. At the end of the incubation, aliquots of the culture medium were treated with anti-SS-14 antiserum. The resulting antibody antigen complexes were dissociated and the SS-14 immunoreactive material analyzed by HPLC (Fig. 7). A major peak of [^{3}H] and [^{35}S]

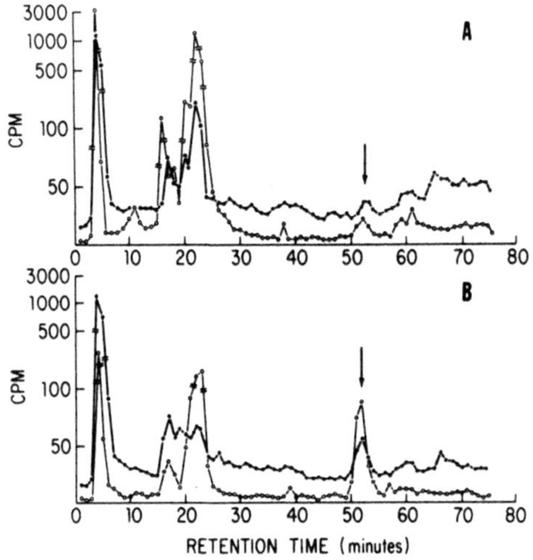

Fig. 7. Characterization of somatostatin immunoreactive material secreted by COS 7 cells transfected with pSVppS18 or pSVI-40: Analysis by HPLC. COS 7 cells transfected with pSVI-40 (Panel A) or pSVppS18 (Panel B) were incubated with [^{35}S] Cys and [^{3}H] Phe. The medium was collected and treated with RSS 1 anti-SS-14 serum. The immunoprecipitates were washed extensively, dissociated by incubation in 2N acetic acid and applied directly to a Waters μ Bondapak C_{18} reverse phase column. The column was eluted with a gradient of acetonitrile in 0.1% trifluoroacetic acid(15). Gradient fractions, corresponding to 30 sec, were collected, dried and counted directly. The arrow indicates the elution of native SS-14.
[^{35}S]Cys: ●——●; [^{3}H]Phe: o——o.

radioactivity was found which coeluted exactly with native mature somatostatin, retention time 52 min (Fig. 7B). Furthermore this material was totally absent from cells transfected with pSVI-40 (Fig. 7A) suggesting that it derived from the presence of the pre-pro-SS cDNA. A major peak of radioactive material eluting with a retention time of 23 min was seen in cells transfected with pSVI-40 (Fig. 7A) and this was also present at a much lower level, in cells transfected with pSVppS18. The nature of this material is unknown at present.

These data strongly suggest that COS cells were able to proteolytically process pro-SS correctly and secrete the mature hormone into the tissue culture medium.

DISCUSSION

It is now well established that most small polypeptide hormones are synthesized as part of larger precursors, termed prohormones, many of which are polyproteins containing the sequence of several differerent hormones usually flanked by pairs of basic amino acids (16). These prohormones may have several functions including correct folding of the precursor molecule to facilitate proteolytic cleavage and/or post-translational modification and in intracellular transport to ensure that the precursor is sorted to the correct organelle. In recent years, gene transfer experiments have been used to investigate the biosynthesis and intracellular transport of a number of integral membrane proteins (22, 25-28). These experiments have defined important cytoplasmic and membrane domains which may play a role in regulating the sorting of integral membrane glycoproteins prior to insertion into the plasma membrane. To investigate the role of propeptides in precursor polypeptide hormone synthesis and post-translational proteolytic processing, we have used a similar approach to that used for studies on membrane biosynthesis. The rationale for these experiments was to identify functional domains that may be involved in generating the mature hormone from its precursor.

We have chosen the somatostatin precursor as a model for these studies because: (i) the complete amino acid sequence of prepro-somatostatin has been deduced in several species including anglerfish, catfish, rats and humans; (ii) the primary events in cotranslational processing of the nascent prepro-SS have been elucidated (8, 12, 15, 29) as well as distal processing steps (3, 30), and (iii) the organization of the precursor is identical in all species, i.e., the mature hormone resides at the carboxyl terminus of pre-pro-SS and is preceded by a pair of basic amino acids: Arg-Lys (Fig. 1). These residues are a subset of six amino acids, Ala-Pro-Arg-Glu-Arg-Lys, that are highly conserved in most somatostatin precursors. The conservation of this hexapeptide suggests that it may have functional significance, and since it contains a pair of basic amino acids, it is most likely the site of proteolytic cleavage of the mature hormone. Furthermore in all preprosomatostatins examined to date, there is considerable conservation of hydrophobic and hydrophilic domains (Figs. 2 and 3) as well as the potential for formation of helical domains (17). The conservation of these structural domains is surprising since the fish and mammalian precursors, for example, share only about 40% amino acid sequence homology in their signal peptides and proregions. Finally, prepro-SS may represent the simplest of the known peptide hormone precursors because in most species they have only a single set of basic amino acids and hence most likely encode only a single bioactive peptide. This contrasts significantly with preproenkephalins (31), prepro-opiomelanocortin (32) or prepro egg laying hormone (33) for example. The conservation of domains as well as the proteolytic processing site suggests that structural features of the precursor may be important for generating the mature hormone. It is possible that the conserved structural domains may also function in the intracellular targeting of the nascent prohormone through the organelles of the secretory apparatus in order to facilitate post-translational modification.

As a first step towards decoding the structural information in pro-SS, we introduced anglerfish prepro-SS I cDNA into mammalian cells to examine the synthesis, proteolytic processing and secretion of mature somatostatin. The data demonstrate that the SRIF cDNA was transcribed from the SV-40 late gene VP-1 promoter into a functionally active mRNA that was significantly larger than the "wild type" mRNA (data not shown). Translation of this mRNA in a cell-free system yielded products that were indistinguishable from those obtained with natural mRNA (data not shown). Translation of this anglerfish prepro-SS mRNA in vivo in COS cells resulted in synthesis of pro-SS since the nascent signal peptide had been cotranslationally cleaved correctly yielding the authentic pro-hormone. By analogy to earlier in vitro reconstitution experiments (24) such a result was not expected. However, the finding that COS cells could process pro-SS to the mature hormone and secrete it was rather unexpected and implies that these cells have the enzymes and secretory apparatus necessary to fulfill this function. This result contrasts with data from CV-1 and AGMK (African Green Monkey Kidney) cells which are closely related to COS cells; these cells were unable to process influenza hemagglutinating protein into HA_1 and HA_2, a reaction which involves cleavage at a set of tetrabasic residues (25). Similarly, Gruss and Khoury (34) found that proinsulin rather than insulin was secreted from AGMK cells transfected with SV-40 containing the rat-preproinsulin gene. However in contrast to pro-SS cleavage, cleavage of proinsulin to insulin is more complex and involves proteolysis at two separate pairs of basic amino acids located on both the amino and carboxyl sides of the connecting peptides (16). It might be argued therefore that COS cells lack the required enzymes to carry out these reactions. Recently Moore et al. (35) demonstrated that mouse ATt-20 cells but not L cells were able to process proinsulin to mature insulin suggesting the same enzymatic machinery may be involved in processing proinsulin and proopiomelanocortin.

The reason why we have observed proteolytic processing of pro-SS to SS-14 in these experiments whereas other precursors do not appear to be processed, may be related to the methods used to detect the mature hormone. In all previous studies the cleavage products were analysed by SDS-PAGE followed by autoradiography. In these experiments we used HPLC followed by direct liquid scintillation counting of the eluted fractions to identify SS-14. Because this is a more sensitive detection method than autoradiography, we may have identified a low level of proteolytic processing which would not be seen when autoradiographic methods were employed. Although we have not quantitated the level of SS-14 secreted during pulse-chase experiments nor the efficiency of the COS processing system, our data show relatively low level of SS-14 secreted compared to pro-insulin secretion in ATt-20 cells (35). Nevertheless our results do strongly suggest that propeptide protease(s) are present in COS cells and perhaps all cells, albeit at a rather low level. In this context it is noteworthy that we did not observe cleavage of pro-SS to SS-28 whose sequence is also encoded within prepro-SS I. Since anglerfish SS-28 was shown to be derived only from prepro-SS II (3, 36), which was absent in these transfected COS cells, this suggests that the COS cell processing does reflect the true physiological processing of prepro-SS I. It would therefore be of interest to investigate the cleavage products of pro-SS in ATt-20 cells to investigate precursor processing and secretion in both the "constitutive" and "regulated" secretory pathways (37).

It might be argued that cleavage of the pro-SS by COS cells was an extracellular event and occurred due to the presence of proteases either secreted by the cells or present in the culture medium. However several lines of evidence argue against this. Firstly, incubation of COS cells or medium alone with pro-SS (synthesized in vitro in the presence of microsomal membranes) did not generate somatostatin peptides which coeluted with SS-14 on HPLC. Furthermore, it is unlikely that contaminating proteases would generate only SS-14 from pro-SS but rather a series of somatostatin peptides containing extra amino acids. We would also expect much of the SS-14 itself to be degraded into separate peptides since the hormone contains two Lys residues. Since we did not observe non-specific proteolysis under the conditions used in these experiments, we conclude that the pro-SS was cleaved intracellulary into the mature hormone.

Having successfully introduced prepro-SS DNA into COS cells, we are currently generating deletion mutants as well as using site-specific mutagenesis to change single amino acids in the hydrophobic and hexapeptide domains of the molecule. These mutants should be particularly useful to determine if unprocessed pro-SS can be secreted, as well as the role of the dibasic amino acids in processing of pro-SS and indeed if structural domains are necessary for prohormone processing.

ACKNOWLEDGMENT

We thank Mr. M. Brenner for excellent technical assistance, Ms. E. Horowitz and C. Hubertus for typing the manuscript and Ms. Etta Eskdrige for the computer analysis. This work was supported by NIH grant AM21860. DS is the recipient of a Research Career Development Award AM01208 and an Irma T. Hirschl Salary Award. T.W. was supported by training grant 2T32 AM07329.

REFERENCES

1. Reichlin, S 1983 Somatostatin, New Engl J Med 309:1495.
2. Noe BD, Fletcher DJ, Spiess J 1979 Evidence for the existence of a biosynthetic precursor for somatostatin. Diabetes 28:724.
3. Noe BD, Spiess J 1983 Evidence for biosynthesis and differential post-translational proteolytic processing of different (pre)prosomatostatins in pancreactic islets. J Biol Chem 258:1121.
4. Esch F, Böhlen P, Ling N, Benoit R, Brazeau P, Guillemin R 1980 Primary structure of ovine hypothalamic somatostatin-28 and somatostatin-25. Proc Natl Acad Sci (USA) 77:6827.
5. Pradayrol L, Jørnvall H, Mutt V, Ribert A 1980 N-terminally extended somatostatin: the primary structure of somatostatin-28. FEBS Letters 109:55.
6. Schally AV, Huang W-Y, Chang RCC, Arimura A, Redding TW, Millar RP, Hunkapiller MW, Hood LE 1980 Isolation and structure of pro-somatostatin: A putative somatostatin precursor from pig hypothalamus. Proc Natl Acad Sci (USA) 77:4489.
7. Spiess J, Vale W 1980 Multiple forms of somatostatin-like activity in rat hypothalamus. Biochemistry 19:2861.
8. Shields, D 1980 In vitro biosynthesis of fish islet preprosomatostatin: Evidence of processing and segregation of a high molecular weight precursor. Proc Natl Acad Sci (USA) 77:4074.
9. Hobart P, Crawford R, Shen L-P, Raymond P, Rutter WJ 1980 Cloning and sequence analysis of cDNAs encoding two distinct somatostatin precursors found in the endocrine pancreas of anglerfish. Nature 288:137.
10. Minth CD, Taylor WL, Magazin M, Tavianini MA, Collier K, Weith HL, Dixon JE 1982 The structure of cloned DNA complementary to catfish pancreatic somatostatin-14 messenger RNA. J Biol Chem 257:10372.

11. Magazin M, Minth CD, Funckes CL, Dechenes R, Tavianini MA, Dixon JE 1982 Sequence of a cDNA encoding pancreatic preprosomatostatin-22. Proc Natl Acad Sci (USA) 79:5152.
12. Goodman RH, Aron DC, Roos BA 1983 Rat pre-prosomatostatin. J Biol Chem 258:5570.
13. Funckes CL, Minth CD, Deschenes R, Magazin M, Tavianini MA, Sheets M, Collier K, Weith HL, Aron DC, Roos BA, Dixon JE 1983 Cloning and characterization of a mRNA encoding rat preprosomatostatin. J Biol Chem 258:8781.
14. Shen L-P, Pictet RL, Rutter WJ 1982 Human somatostatin I: Sequence of the cDNA. Proc Natl Acad Sci (USA) 79:4575.
15. Warren TG, Shields D 1984 Cell-free biosynthesis of multiple preprosomatostatins: Characterization by hybrid selection and amino-terminal sequencing. Biochemistry 23:2684.
16. Steiner DF, Quinn PS, Chan SJ, Makh J, Tager HS 1980 Processing mechanisms in the biosynthesis of proteins. Ann NY Acad Sci 343:1.
17. Argos P, Taylor WL, Minth CD, Dixon JE 1983 Nucleotide and amino acid sequence comparisons of preprosomatostatins. J Biol Chem 258:8788.
18. Hopp TP, Woods KR 1981 Prediction of protein antigenic determinants from amino acid sequences. Proc Natl Acad Sci (USA) 78:3824.
19. Shields D, Warren TG, Green RF, Roth SE, Brenner WM 1981 The primary events in the biosynthesis and post-translational processing of different precursors to somatostatin. In: Rich DH, Gross E (eds) Peptides: Synthesis-Structure-Function. Pierce Chemical Company.
20. Kyte J, Doolittle RF 1982 A simple method for displaying the hydropathic character of a protein. J Mol Biol 157:105.
21. Sprague J, Condra JH, Arnhetter H, Lazzarini RA 1983 Expression of a recombinant DNA gene coding for the vesicular stomatitis virus nucleocapsid protein. J Virol 45:773.
22. Rose JK, Bergmann JE 1982 Expression from cloned cDNA of cell-surface and secreted forms of glycoprotein of vesicular stomatitis virus in eukaryotic cells. Cell 30:753.
23. Green R, Shields D 1984 Sodium butyrate stimulates somatostatin production by cultured cells. Endocrinology 114:1990.
24. Shields D, Blobel G 1977 Cell-free synthesis of fish preproinsulin, and processing by heterologous mammalian microsomal membranes. Proc Natl Acad Sci (USA) 74:2059.
25. Gething M-J, Sambrook J 1981 Cell-surface expression of influenza haemagglutinin from a coned DNA copy of the RNA gene. Nature 293:620.
26. Sveda MM, Lai C-J 1981 Functional expression in primate cells of cloned DNA coding for the hemagglutinin surface glycoprotein of influenza virus. Proc Natl Acad Sci (USA) 78:5488.
27. Davis AR, Bos TJ, Nayak DP 1983 Active influenza virus neuraminidase is expressed in monkey cells from cDNA cloned in simian virus 40 vectors. Proc Natl Acad Sci (USA) 80:3976.

28. Yost CS, Hedgpeth J, Lingappa VR 1983 A stop transfer sequence confers predictable transmembrane orientation to a previously secreted protein in cell-free systems. Cell 34:759.
29. Warren TG, Shields D 1982 Cell-free biosynthesis of somatostatin precursors: Evidence for multiple forms of preprosomatostatin. Proc Natl Acad Sci (USA) 79:3729.
30. Fletcher DJ, Noe BD, Bauer GE, Quigley JP 1980 Characterization of the conversion of a somatostatin precursor to somatostatin by islet secretory granules. Diabetes 29:593.
31. Comb M, Seeburg PH, Adelman J, Eiden L, Herbert E 1982 Primary structure of the human Met- and Leu-enkephalin precursor and its mRNA. Nature 295:663.
32. Nakanishi S, Inoue A, Kita T, Nakamura M, Chang ACY, Cohen SN, Numa S 1979 Nucleotide sequence of cloned cDNA for bovine corticotropin- -lipotropin precursor. Nature 278:423.
33. Scheller RH, Jackson JF, McAllister LB, Rothman BS, Mayer E, Axel R 1983 A single gene encodes multiple neuropeptides mediating a stereotyped behavior. Cell 32:7.
34. Gruss P, Khoury G 1981 Expression of simian virus 40-rat preproinsulin RNA processing signals. Proc Natl Acad Sci (USA) 78:113.
35. Moore H-P H, Walker MD, Lee F, Kelly RG 1983 Expressing a human proinsulin cDNA in a mouse ACTH-secreting cell. Intracellular storage, proteolytic processing, and secretion on stimulation. Cell 35:531.
36. Noe BD 1981 Synthesis of one form of pancreatic islet somatostatin predominates. J Biol Chem 256:9397.
37. Gumbiner B, Kelly RB 1982 Two distinct intracellular pathways transport secretory and membrane glycoproteins to the surface of pituitary tumor cells. Cell 28:51.

2

SOMATOSTATINS OF THE CHANNEL CATFISH

JACK E. DIXON AND P. C. ANDREWS

Department of Biochemistry
Purdue University
West Lafayette, Indiana 47907

ABSTRACT

Pancreatic tissue of the channel catfish (Ictalurus punctatus) contains two somatostatins. The amino acid sequence of a 14-residue containing peptide (SS-14) is identical in sequence and has the same mass ion by fast atom bombardment mass spectrometry as mammalian SS-14. A 22-residue somatostatin (SS-22) has also been isolated and its amino acid sequence determined. The amino acid sequence differs from that reported by Oyama et al. (J Biol Chem 255:2251, 1980) in two of the 22-residues (positions 5 and 19). Somatostatin-22 is a glycoprotein, with carbohydrate attached at Thr-5. Several 22-residue peptides have been purified and all of them have identical amino acid compositions and different carbohydrate structure and/or composition. SS-22 has 7 amino acid residues which are identical to those observed in SS-14. The nucleotide sequence of the two cDNAs coding for SS-14 and SS-22 have been determined. The mRNAs encode precursors to SS-14 and SS-22 of 114 and 105 residues, respectively. The two precursors also have different amino acid sequence at the site of prohormone proteolytic processing. Analysis of genomic DNA reveals that SS-14 and SS-22 sequences are present on different restriction fragments and thus are encoded by separate genes.

INTRODUCTION

Somatostatin was first isolated from ovine hypothalamic fragments using the inhibition of growth hormone release as an assay (1). Subsequently, somatostatin has been found in a number of other tissues and has been demonstrated to display a variety of physiological functions (2-5). Generally, the function of somatostatin is to inhibit the release of certain biologically active substances: growth hormone in the pituitary (1), glucagon and insulin in the pancreas (2), and secretin, gastrin, and cholecystokinin in specific epithelial cells of the gastrointestinal tract (3-5).

Studies of the biosynthesis of somatostatin have demonstrated the presence of larger "precursor" forms of the hormones (1-6). Both the anglerfish pancreas (1) and rat pancreatic islets (6) synthesize precursors to somatostatin which ultimately result in a hormone of 14 amino acid residues (SS-14). In the pancreas of the channel catfish, there are two predicted somatostatin precursors (12, 13). One of the precursors gives rise to SS-14 (12), while the other precursor appears to generate somatostatin-22 (SS-22) (13).

In this paper we shall review progress on the isolation and characterization of the peptides and mRNAs corresponding to catfish somatostatin-14 and -22.

RESULTS AND DISCUSSION

The pancreas of birds and mammals consists largely of exocrine tissue with only a small amount of endocrine tissue. In contrast, the pancreas of certain teleost fish contain increased ratios of endocrine to exocrine tissues. This phenomenon is illustrated in Figs. 1A and B, which compare the relative concentrations of endocrine and exocrine cells in typical avian and teleost pancreas. The teleost pancreas contains an increased proportion of endocrine cells making this an attractive tissue for studies on the biosynthesis, expression, and physiology of pancreatic hormones. The anglerfish, *Lophius americanus* and the channel catfish, *Ictalurus punctata* are the two teleosts most frequently utilized for this purpose.

Isolation, Characterization and Amino Acid Sequence of Catfish SS-14 and SS-22

The 14-residue somatostatin from catfish was purified by Andrews and Dixon (14) and shown to be identical to SS-14 from several other sources by amino acid composition and Edman degradation. In order to verify the structure of SS-14 we have utilized a new mass spectrometric technique that allows one to determine the molecular weight of relatively large molecules such as peptides (17). The sample containing the peptide is dissolved in an acid-glycerol solution and then bombarded with a beam of xenon atoms using a few kilovolts of kinetic energy. This technique has been referred to as fast atom bombardment-mass spectrometry. Protonated peptides and/or fragments of the peptides are analyzed by the mass spectrometer. The molecular ion of catfish pancreatic SS-14 determined by FAB/MS is identical to that for synthetic SS-14 (Fig. 2), further illustrating the identity of their structures. The

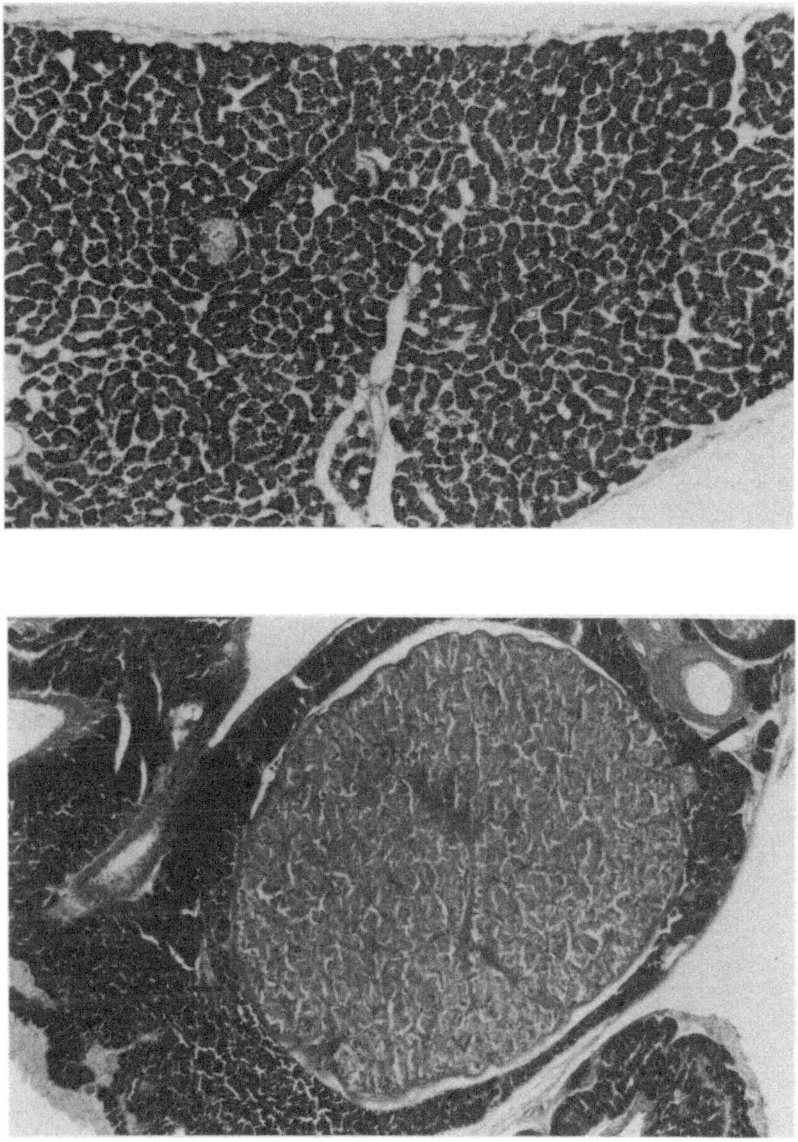

A

B

Fig. 1. Light microscopic sections of: (A) avian pancreas (x 6 magnification); and (B) catfish pancreas (Ictalurus punctatus). Arrows indicate the endocrine tissue (x 6).

additional peaks surrounding the average molecular ion [1639 (M/Z)] result from the isotope distribution of carbon, nitrogen etc. found in the molecule.

Another somatostatin having 22 residues was isolated from the catfish endocrine pancreas and its amino acid sequence determined (15). The concentration of SS-22 in the catfish pancreas is 93 nmol/g tissue, as compared with 63 nmol/g tissue for SS-14 (14). Following the purification of SS-22 reported by Oyama et al. (15, 16) Andrews and co-workers (17) developed an improved purification procedure for this peptide and demonstrated that there were several forms of SS-22, all having identical amino acid compositions. The major 22-residue peptide isolated from the catfish pancreas has been referred to as SS-22a (17). The amino acid sequence of SS-22a determined by this laboratory (17) is shown in Table 1. All cycles of Edman degradation resulted in PTH amino acids which were identified by high performance liquid chromatography except cycle 5 (Table I) where no amino acid was observed. The absence of an amino acid in cycle 5 suggests that the residue normally found in this position was modified, resulting in a chlorobutane-insoluble phenylthiohydantoin derivative.

Careful examination of the data obtained from our amino acid analysis revealed the presence of an amino sugar in each hydrolysate of the various forms of SS-22. This observation suggested that all forms of SS-22 examined were glycopeptides. The alditol acetates derived from SS-22 were analyzed and the results demonstrated that 1 mole of galactose and 1 mole of N-acetyl-galactosamine were present per mole of peptide (Table II). Some of the minor forms of

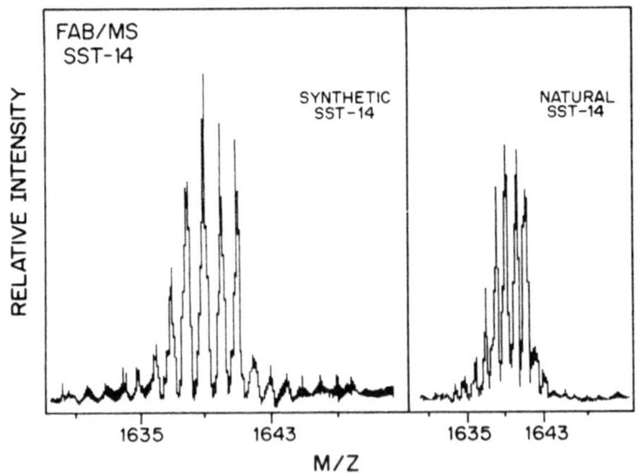

Fig. 2. Mass spectrum of SS-14 (shown as SST-14). Fast atom bombardment-mass spectrometry was carried out as described by Andrews et al. (17) FAB/MS of SS-14 and synthetic SS-14. Both show a mass ion of 1639 ± 1 (M/Z).

SS-22 also contained sialic acid in addition to the two carbohydrate residues noted above.

The residue not detected in the amino acid sequence at cycle 5, but suggested on the basis of the cDNA sequence of SS-22 and by subtractive amino acid analysis, is threonine. In order to establish that the carbohydrate was attached to a Thr residue in cycle 5, we have developed a novel method to identify the site of O-glycosylation (17). Somatostatin-22a was treated with base under conditions to effect β-elimination of the carbohydrate and the resulting intermediate "trapped" with [^{35}S]-2-mercaptoethanol. Automated Edman degradation of the radiolabeled material (Fig. 3) indicated that the label was incorporated only into residues 5 and 11. The label

Table I.

Cycle	Amino acid	nmoles	Sequence predicted from cDNA (13)
1	Asp	41.4	Asp
2	Asn	66.6	Asn
3	Thr	35.1	Thr
4	Val	78.6	Val
5	-	-	Thr
6	Ser	11.7	Ser
7	Lys	133	Lys
8	Pro	26	Pro
9	Leu	60	Leu
10	Asn	37.1	Asn
11	PECys	44.6	Cys
12	Met	47.7	Met
13	Asn	37.1	Asn
14	Tyr	36.9	Tyr
15	Phe	34.9	Phe
16	Trp	45.1	Trp
17	Lys	60.3	Lys
18	Ser	7.4	Ser
19	Arg	18.9	Arg
20	Thr	6.0	Thr
21	Ala	18.3	Ala
22	PECys	4.9	Cys

Automated Edman degradation of SS-22a. Somatostatin-22a was reduced and pyridylethylatd as described for SS-14 (14). Excess reagents were removed by passage over a Biogel P-2 column equilibrated with 1 N formic acid. The pyridylethylated SS-22a was sequenced by automated Edman degradation (17). PECys is S-pyridylethylcysteine.

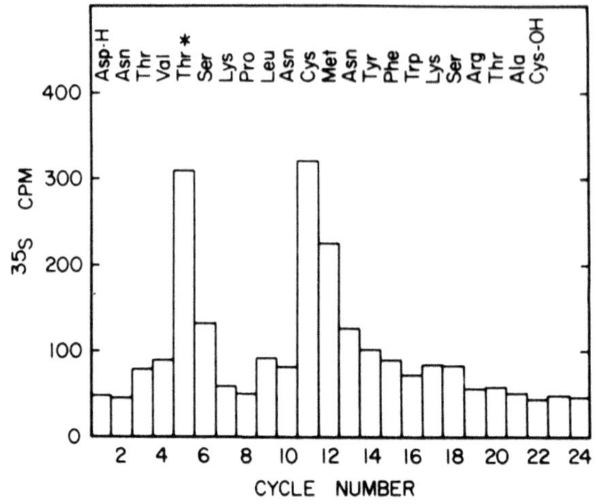

Fig. 3. Location of O-linked carbohydrate. Automated Edman degradation of base-eliminated, [^{35}S]-labeled SS-22a. The asterisk indicates site of glycosylation.

incorporated into residue 5 indicated the site of O-glycosylation was at Thr-5. Radiolabeled material is also seen in cycle 11 where a Cys residue has been identified by Edman degradation. Cystine is also known to undergo β-elimination under these conditions and thus radiolabeled material should be seen in both residues 11 and 22. The absence of appreciable radioactivity in the last cycle of the sequence (Cys-22) most likely reflects loss of material from the sequenator. The adduct formed using 2-mercaptoethanol is more efficiently washed from the sequencing cup.

We have also determined the average molecular ion of SS-22a by FAM/MS to be 2,943 ± 1 (M/Z) (Fig. 4). This mass is consistent with the data described above as well as the sequence data deduced from the cDNA with the addition of one residue of galactose and one residue of N-acetylgalactosamine (Mass = 2,943). The amino acid

Table II. Carbohydrate Composition of Somatostatin-22a

	Peptide	Galactose	N-Acetylgalactosamine
nmol	450	535	495
molar ratio	1.0	1.2	1.1

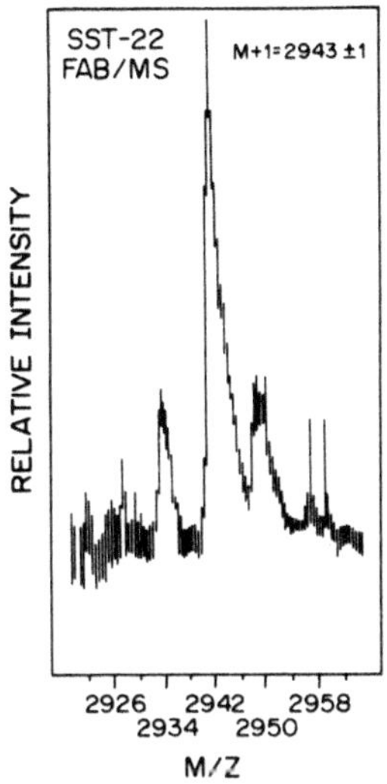

Fig. 4. Mass spectrum of SS-22a (shown as SS-22). FAB/MS shows an average molecular ion of 2,943 ± 1 (M/Z).

sequence of SS-14 and SS-22 are shown in Fig. 5. Identical amino acid residues found in both peptides are enclosed. It is of interest to note that both the positions of the two Cys residues as well as the biologically important Phe.Trp.Lys sequences have been conserved.

Biological Activities of SS-14 and SS-22

The biological activity of SS-22 appears to be 10- to 100-fold less potent than SS-14 in the inhibition of growth hormone release from rat pituitary cells and in insulin and glucagon release from rat pancreas (18). Similar potencies were observed on inhibition of growth hormone release from rat GH-3 cells (Hinkle PM et al., unpublished observations). However, these heterologous assay systems do not allow firm conclusions to be drawn regarding the function or relative potencies of these two hormones in catfish. The production of two different somatostatins in similar quantities by the same tissue suggests that the two peptides may have different physiological roles.

Immunoreactive SS-22 has also been reported in catfish brain and intestine, although the levels are well below those seen in the catfish pancreas (19). Very low levels of SS-22 immunoreactivity were found in anglerfish islets. Attempts to isolate and characterize SS-22 from the anglerfish islet have proven unsuccessful (20). A survey for immunoreactive SS-22 in the islets of a number

H·Asp·Asn·Thr·Val·Thr*·Ser·Lys·Pro·Leu·Asn·Cys·Met·Asn·Tyr·Phe·Trp·Lys·Ser·Arg·Thr·Ala·Cys·OH [a]

H·Ala·Gly·Cys·Lys·Asn·Phe·Phe·Trp·Lys·Thr·Phe·Thr·Ser·Cys·OH [b]

Fig. 5. Amino acid sequences of catfish SS-22(a) and SS-14(b). Amino acid residues common to both peptides are enclosed within a box.

of other salt-water teleosts also failed to detect significant levels of catfish SS-22 immunoreactivity (20), although low levels of immunoreactive SS-22 could be detected in a human insulinoma (21). It remains to be seen if this unusual peptide found in high levels in the catfish pancreas is also present in a number of other pancreatic tissues obtained from several species. Most evidence supports the idea that abundant immunoreactive SS-22 is not present in a number of other pancreatic tissues obtained from several species (19-21).

Cloning and Sequencing of the cDNAs Corresponding to SS-14 and SS-22

The first evidence that SS-14 was also present in catfish pancreas was based upon results obtained from the cDNA sequence studies carried out by Taylor et al. (12). The initial studies used the synthetic oligonucleotide primer, d(T-T-C-C-A-G-A-A-G-A-A), the sequence of which was deduced from the amino acid sequence Phe-Phe-Trp-Lys present in SS-14. The cDNA transcripts resulting from reverse transcription of poly(A)-mRNA from catfish pancreas using 5' end-labeled primer were resolved by gel electrophoresis. The major transcript was eluted and sequenced. This sequence was shown to be complementary to a mRNA coding for SS-14.

Following the successful cloning of the mRNA isolated from the catfish pancreas by Minth et al. (23) several clones were selected, characterized and sequenced. The cDNAs corresponding to SS-14 and SS-22 (13) are shown in Figs. 6 and 7 along with the deduced amino acid sequences of preprosomatostatin-14 and -22. The cDNA corresponding to preprosomatostatin-14 contains 350 nucleotides in the 3' noncoding region, 345 nucleotides in the coding region, and 104 nucleotides in the 5'-untranslated region. The mRNA codes for a precursor to somatostatin-14 which is 114 amino acids (Mr = 12,386) in length. Preprosomatostatin-14 has a sequence of hydrophobic amino acids at the NH_2-terminus, followed by a connecting peptide of approximately 75 amino acids. The sequence Arg-Lys precedes somatostatin-14. The nucleotide sequence of a precursor to somatostatin-22 encodes a precursor that is 105 amino acids (Mr = 11,500). Preprosomatostatin-22 cDNA consists of 36 nucleotides in the 5' untranslated region, 315 nucleotides that code for the precursor to

```
                                                                                                   Met Pro Ser Thr
AGAAGUCGCCCCAAAAACUACAGCAGUAAGAACUGACGUUUCGGUGUUUUUUGCCCUCCCUCCACCAAUUUUUCCACCAAAUCCAGCUUUAUUUCUUUUUGAAG AUG CCC UCC ACG

Arg Ile Gln Cys Ala Leu Ala Leu Leu Ala Val Ala Leu Ser Val Cys Ser Val Ser Gly Ala Pro Ser Asp Ala Lys Leu Arg Gln Phe
CGG AUC CAG UGC GCC CUG GCU CUC CUG GCC GUC GCG CUC UCC GUC UGC AGC GUC UCA GGC GCG CCG UCU GAU GCC AAA CUG CGC CAG UUC

Leu Gln Arg Ser Ile Leu Ala Pro Ser Val Lys Gln Glu Leu Thr Arg Tyr Thr Leu Ala Glu Leu Leu Ala Glu Leu Ala Gln Ala Glu
CUC CAG AGG UCG AUU CUU GCA CCG UCU GUA AAA CAG GAG CUC ACC AGG UAC ACG CUC GCA GAG CUG CUC GCA GAG CUC GCG GAA GCC GAA

Asn Glu Val Leu Asp Ser Asp Glu Val Ser Arg Ala Ala Glu Ser Glu Gly Ala Arg Leu Glu Met Glu Arg Ala Ala Gly Pro Met Leu
AAC GAG GUG CUG GAC UCG GAC GAG GUG UCU CGC GCC GCG GAA AGC GAG GGC GCG CGC CUG GAG AUG GAG CGA GCC GCC GGU CCC AUG CUG

                 **  **
Ala Pro Arg Glu Arg Lys Ala Gly Cys Lys Asn Phe Phe Trp Lys Thr Phe Thr Ser Cys  *
GCU CCC CGC GAG CGC AAA GCC GGC UGC AAG AAU UUC UUC UGG AAA ACU UUC ACG UCG UGU UAAUCGUUUAGUCGAAAUACUUUCCUCAUAGUCUAUAAAU

AUCUAUCUAUUUUUCCCUUCCCUCCCCCCACACAUACAUAUACAUGUAUACAAUUUGUUUCUUUCUUUAGUUUUCAAGCUCACAUCAUGAUGUCUGCAUAAAAUGUAAAUAAAAUAAUA

AUAAUAAUAAUAAUUUAAAAAAAGAUGUUCCAUUUAUUAAGUGUUAUCAAUUUACGGUUCUAUGAAGGAAUGUUUUAUGGAUGUAUGGAAAUUCUGUUAGAGAUCUGUACUUUAGAUGGA

AAUAUUUAACAAAAACAAAUAUUUUUAAUUGUUUGAAUAAAAUAUAUGUUUCACAGCC(A)15
```

Fig. 6. The nucleotide sequence of a cDNA corresponding to SS-14. The corresponding amino acid sequence for the preprohormone is written above the nucleotide sequence. The mature hormone is underlined and follows the two adjacent basic residues which are recognition sites for cleavage of SS-14.

somatostatin-22, and 269 nucleotides in the 3' untranslated region. The putative preprohormone contains a sequence of hydrophobic amino acids at the amino terminus that has the properties of a "signal" peptide. A connecting sequence of approximately 57 amino acids is followed by a single Arg-Arg sequence, which immediately precedes the hormone. Hybridization selection of mRNA, followed by translation of the mRNA in a wheat germ cell-free system resulted in the

```
                                  -83
                                  Met Ser Ser Ser Pro Leu Arg Leu Ala Leu Ala Leu Met Cys Leu Val
CCGCCCAGCUCGAAAUCUUCACCAGCUACCAAGAAG AUG UCG UCU UCA CCA CUC CGU CUC GCU CUU GCC CUC AUG UGC CUG GUC

Ser Ala Val Gly Val Ile Ser Cys Gly Arg Pro His Val Val Leu Asn Ser Ala Leu Glu Glu Ala Arg Asn Val
UCA GCC GUC GGU GUC AUA UCG UGC GGC CGG CCU CAU GUG GUU UUG AAU UCG GCU CUG GAA GAG GCU CGC AAC GUG

Pro Phe Gly Glu Glu Val Pro Glu Arg Leu Thr Leu Pro Glu Leu Gln Trp Met Leu Ser Asn Asn Glu Leu Thr
CCG UUU GGA GAA GAG GUA CCA GAG AGA CUC ACU CUU CCU GAG CUC CAG UGG AUG CUC AGU AAC AAC GAG CUC ACG
                                                              *   *  1
Pro Val Gln Val Glu Glu Ala Pro Arg Ser Arg Leu Glu Leu Val Arg Arg Asp Asn Thr Val Thr Ser Lys Pro
CCC GUU CAG GUG GAA GAA GCC CCU CGC AGC AGG CUG GAG CUG GUC AGG AGA GAC AAC ACG GUG ACG AGC AAA CCA
                                                 22
Leu Asn Cys Met Asn Tyr Phe Trp Lys Ser Arg Thr Ala Cys  *
CUC AAC UGC AUG AAC UAC UUC UGG AAG UCC AGG ACA GCA UGC UGAGCUCAUUUCGACCCACGAGCCAGAGCCGGGGCACCGUUC

AGGCCCGUUAACAUGCUGCGAAUCACUCACCAUUUCCCUCCCCUUCAGCGUACACCUCUGAGACAAGCAGACAUGCUCGUUCUCUGGCUUCCAGCACAC

CAGAGCCUCGGUUAAUUAUUUUUAAUUUUAGCAGCUGUAGGAAUUGUAGAACAUGUACCAAUAUUGGGUGCCAAUUUUAUCCUGCUCUGAAGCACAAAC

GCUCUGAAAUAAACAAUACAGCAUUAAC(A)24
```

Fig. 7. Nucleotide sequence of the insertions in somatostatin-22 clones. The mRNA sequence and predicted amino acids for preprosomatostatin are given. Amino acids are numbered beginning with the first residue of somatostatin-22. The presumed initiator methionine is at position-83.

synthesis of a single polypeptide having a molecular weight of approximately 10,000 as estimated on sodium dodecyl sulfate/polyacrylamide gels.

Analysis of genomic DNA from the channel catfish reveals that somatostatin-14 and somatostatin-22 are present on different restriction fragments, confirming that these two hormones are encoded by different genes.

ACKNOWLEDGMENT

We would like to thank a number of people who have contributed results presented in this review: W.L. Taylor, H.L. Weith, K. Collier, C. Funckes, M. Magazin, Carolyn Minth, Robert Deschenes, Marie Tavianini, Charles Heinrickson, Dean Fetterolf, Bradley Sheares, and Mark Hermodson.

REFERENCES

1. Brazeau P, Vale W, Burgus R, Ling N, Butcher M, Rivier J, Guillemin R 1973 Hypothalamic polypeptide that inhibits the secretion of immunoreactive pituitary growth hormone. Science 179:77.
2. Koerker D, Ruth W, Chideckel E, Palmer J, Goodner CJ, Ensinck J, Gale CG 1974 Somatostatin: Hypothalamic inhibitor of the endocrine pancreas. Science 184:482.
3. Polak J, Pearse AGE, Grimelius L, Bloom SR, Arimura A 1975 Growth-hormone release-inhibiting hormone in gastrointestinal and pancreatic D cells. Lancet 1:1220.
4. Bloom SR, Thorner MO, Mortimer CH, Besser GM, Hall R, Gomez-Pan A, Roy VM, Russell RCG, Coy DH, Kastin AJ, Schally AV 1975 Inhibition of gastrin and gastric-acid secretion by growth-hormone release-inhibiting hormone. Lancet 2:1106.
5. Konturek SJ, Tasler J, Obtulowicz W, Coy DH, Schally AV 1976 Effect of growth hormone-release inhibiting hormone on hormones stimulating exocrine pancreatic secretion. J Clin Invest 58:1.
6. Patzelt C, Tager HS, Carroll RJ, Steiner DF 1980 Identification of prosomatostatin in pancreatic islets. Proc Natl Acad Sci (USA) 77:2410.
7. Goodman RH, Lund PJ, Jacobs JW, Habener JF 1980 Preprosomatostatins: products of cell-free translations of messenger RNAs from anglerfish islets. J Biol Chem 255:6549.
8. Shields D 1980 In vitro biosynthesis of fish islet preprosomatostatin: Evidence of processing and segregation of a high molecular weight precursor. Proc Natl Acad Sci (USA) 76:4074.

9. Lauber M, Camier M, Cohen P 1979 Higher molecular weight forms of immunoreactive somatostatin in mouse hypothalamic extracts: Evidence of processing in vitro. Proc Natl Acad Sci (USA) 76:6004.
10. Noe BD, Fletcher DJ, Bauer GE, Weir GC, Patel Y 1978 Somatostatin biosynthesis occurs in pancreatic islets. Endocrinology 102:1675.
11. Noe BD 1981 Synthesis of one form of pancreatic islet somatostatin predominates. J Biol Chem 256:937.
12. Taylor WL, Collier KJ, Deschenes RJ, Weith HL, Dixon JE 1981 Sequence analysis of a cDNA coding for a pancreatic precursor to somatostatin. Proc Natl Acad Sci (USA) 78:6694.
13. Magazin M, Minth CD, Funckes CL, Deschenes RJ, Tavianini MA, Dixon JE 1982 Sequence of a cDNA encoding pancreatic preprosomatostatin-22. Proc Natl Acad Sci (USA) 79:5152.
14. Andrews PC, Dixon JE 1981 Isolation and structure of a peptide hormone predicted from a mRNA sequence: a second somatostatin from the catfish pancreas. J Biol Chem 256:8267.
15. Oyama H, Bradshaw RA, Bates OJ, Permutt A 1980 Amino acid sequence of catfish pancreatic somatostatin I. J Biol Chem 255:2251.
16. Oyama H, Hirsch HJ, Gabbay KH, Permutt A 1980 Isolation and characterization of immunoreactive somatostatin from fish pancreatic islets. J Clin Invest 65:993.
17. Andrews PC, Pubols MH, Hermodson MA, Sheares BM, Dixon JE 1984 Structure of the 22-residue somatostatin from catfish: an O-glycosylated peptide having multiple forms. J Biol Chem 259:13267.
18. Oyama H, Martin J, Sussman K, Weir GL, Permutt A 1981 The biological activity of catfish pancreatic somatostatin. Regulatory Peptides 1:387.
19. Fletcher DJ, Trent DF, Weir GC 1983 Catfish somatostatin is unique to piscine tissues. Regulatory Peptides 5:181.
20. Andrews PC, Pubols MH, Dixon JE unpublished results.
21. Oyama H, Gabbay K, Loo SW, Hirsch H, Greider M, Permutt A 1982 Radioimmunoassay for pancreatic somatostatin with an antibody to catfish pancreatic somatostatin. Regulatory Peptides 3:383.
22. Minth CD, Taylor WL, Magazin M, Tavianini M, Collier K, Weith HL, Dixon JE 1982 The structure of cloned DNA complementary to catfish pancreatic somatostatin-14 messenger RNA. J Biol Chem 257:10372.

3

BIOSYNTHESIS OF RAT PREPROSOMATOSTATIN

RICHARD H. GOODMAN, MARC R. MONTMINY, MALCOLM J. LOW AND JOEL F. HABENER*

Division of Endocrinology, Tufts New England Medical Center and *Laboratory of Molecular Endocrinology, Howard Hughes Medical Institute, Massachusetts General Hospital, Boston, Mass. 02111

ABSTRACT

The biologically active forms of somatostatin, somatostatin-14 (SS-14) and somatostatin-28 (SS-28) arise by post-translational cleavage of prosomatostatin. Prosomatostatin in turn is derived from a larger precursor, preprosomatostatin. We have previously reported the structure of a complementary DNA moelcule encoding rat preprosomatostatin. The nucleotide sequence of this cDNA indicated that SS-14 and SS-28 are located at the carboxy-terminus of a 116 amino acid precursor. At the amino-terminus of the precursor is a hydrophobic region characteristic of a leader or pre-sequence. Sequential Edman degradations of cell-free translation products synthesized in the presence of microsomal membranes indicate that preprosomatostatin is cleaved within the endoplasmic reticulum to form prosomatostatin, a precursor of 92 amino acids. To begin to elucidate the factors which regulate the expression of the rat somatostatin gene, we have determined the sequence of the gene isolated from recombinant bacteriophage libraries. The gene spans 1.2 kilobases in length and is interrupted within the coding sequence of prosomatostatin by a single intron of 630 bases. A variant of the Goldberg-Hogness promotor, TTTAAA, is located 31 bases upstream from the transcriptional start point. A repetitive sequence was identified in the 5' region of the gene within 650 bases of the promoter. The nucleotide sequence of this region reveals an alternating GT sequence 42 bases in length characteristic of DNA with Z-forming potential. Such sequences are thought to influence the expression of other eukaryotic genes.

Although a great deal has been learned about the physiology of somatostatin, relatively little is known about the factors which regulate its biosynthesis. In part, this lack of understanding is due to problems inherent in studying small peptides in complex tissue preparations. Recombinant DNA technology has provided a means to address some of these problems and may soon allow our understanding of somatostastin biosynthesis to equal our knowledge of the hormone's physiology.

Like other regulatory peptides, somatostatin is synthesized as a larger precursor. The existence of high molecular weight forms of somatostatin was first suggested by Arimura et al. using antibodies to the tetradecapeptide form of SS-14 which cross-react with larger species (1). These larger forms, detected initially in porcine hypothalamus and stomach, were postulated to represent precursor forms of SS-14 (2).

Subsequent structural studies confirmed the hypothesis that the somatostatin sequence could be found within that of a larger molecule. Pradayrol et al. isolated and sequenced an amino-terminally extended form of somatostatin derived from porcine intestine (3). This larger form, which contains the sequence of SS-14 with an additional 14 amino acid extension, has been designated SS-28. SS-28 was later identified in extracts of porcine (4) and ovine (5) hypothalamus. Because a dibasic sequence, Arg-Lys, lies adjacent to the sequence of SS-14, it has been suggested that SS-28 may serve as an intermediate in the formation of the tetradecapeptide. Similar dibasic sequences have been found to act as prohormone cleavage sites in other hormone precursors (6).

In addition to serving as an intermediate in the biosynthesis of SS-14, SS-28 has been shown to possess its own biological activity. The relative potency of SS-28 compared to SS-14 has not been tested in all systems, but several studies have indicated that the two forms may differ in their potency and biological activity (7-12).

Studies using heterologous cell-free translational systems have determined that hormone precursors, like other secretory proteins, are synthesized as prehormones, or pre-prohormones in some instances (6). The pre-regions of such precursors refer to the hydrophobic portions at the amino-termini which are involved in transport through the endoplasmic reticulum. The pro-regions designate the additional peptide sequences which remain after the removal of the hydrophobic leader sequence. To be consistent with this nomenclature, SS-28 is not a true prohormone, although it may still be a precursor of SS-14. In general, the pro-regions are cleaved at sequences of dibasic amino acids. There are several exceptions to this rule, however. Prohormone cleavage can occur after single amino acids and after non-basic amino acids. The lack of proteolytic processing at dibasic sequences within a number of hormones including parathyroid hormone, the alpha subunit of glycoprotein hormones, and vasoactive intestinal peptide indicates that such sequences are clearly not sufficient for cleavage. It is likely that additional features of prohormones, including tertiary structure or other post-translational modifications, may influence whether a particular dibasic sequence is used for cleavage.

Forms of somatostatin larger than SS-28 have been isolated from a number of tissues including hypothalamus, cerebral cortex, and jejunum (2, 13-17). These larger forms appear to have molecular weights between 11,000-15,000 and may therefore represent true prohormones. In one instance, this larger form appeared to have biological activity (18). Most studies have suggested that the prohormonal form of somatostatin makes up only a small portion of the total radioimmunoreactive hormone in tissue extracts, cultured cells, or culture media. These studies are complicated, however, by the difficulty in extrapolating radioimmunoassay results to different molecular forms of the ligand.

Regardless of the absolute amount of prohormone present in tissue, it does seem fairly certain that the 11,000-15,000 mol wt forms serve as precursors for SS-14 and SS-28. Pulse and pulse-chase studies have demonstrated a transfer of radioactivity from these forms to SS-14 and SS-28 indicating that the high molecular weight forms are, in fact, precursors of the smaller peptides (17, 19).

Immunoprecipitation analysis of cell-free translation products derived from mRNAs from a variety of tissues have confirmed the hypothesis that somatostatin is initially synthesized as a 14,000-16,000 molecular weight precursor (20-24). Our laboratory showed that polyadenylated RNA from anglerfish islets directed the synthesis of two discrete somatostatin-related products of Mr = 16,000 and Mr = 14,000 which represented the pre-prohormonal forms of somatostatin in this species (20). When the cell-free translations were performed in the presence of microsomal membranes, which have the ability to remove the hydrophobic leader sequences, smaller somatostatin-related products of Mr = 14,5000 and Mr = 13,500 were identified. These smaller products represent the somatostatin prohormones. Using similar techniques, Shields et al. have observed as many as nine separate somatostatin-related cell-free translation products (25). Subsequent studies by Hobart et al. (26) established the amino acid sequences of two of the anglerfish preprosomatostatins (pre-pro-SSI and pre-pro-SSII) using recombinant DNA techniques.

The low sensitivity of the immunoprecipitation technique prevented us from being able to identify preprosomatostatin in cell-free translations of mammalian mRNAs. The structural similarity of the anglerfish somatostatin I cDNA to related sequences in mammalian cDNA libraries made this identification possible, however. For these studies, we used the anglerfish cDNA (27) to screen a cDNA library prepared from a transplantable rat medullary thyroid carcinoma (28-30).

The nucleotide and corresponding amino acid sequence of the rat preprosomatostatin cDNA is depicted in Fig. 1. These sequences predict a 116 amino acid protein of molecular weight 12,737, similar in size to the forms identified by cell-free translations. An identical sequence has been reported by Funckes et al. (31). The coding sequence of SS-14 is found at the carboxy-terminus of the precursor, preceded by an Arg-Lys sequence and followed by a stop codon. This structure had been predicted previously by Patzelt et al. (17) using pulse-chase studies. Adjacent to the SS-14 sequence is a region corresponding to $SS\text{-}28_{[1-12]}$, the amino-terminal portion of SS-28 (32). The sequence of rat SS-28 is identical to that found in porcine and ovine tissues (3-5).

RAT PRE-PROSOMATOSTATIN

TGCGGACCTGCGTCTAGACTGACCCACCGCGCTCAAGCTCGGCTGTCTGAGGCAGGGGAG

ATG CTG TCC TGC CGT CTC CAG TGC GCG CTG GCC GCG CTC TGC ATC
Met Leu Ser Cys Arg Leu Gln Cys Ala Leu Ala Ala Leu Cys Ile 15

GTC CTG GCT TTG GGC GGT GTC ACC GGG GCG CCC TCG GAC CCC AGA
Val Leu Ala Leu Gly Gly Val Thr Gly Ala Pro Ser Asp Pro Arg 30

CTC CGT CAG TTT CTG CAG AAG TCT CTG GCG GCT GCC ACC GGG AAA
Leu Arg Gln Phe Leu Gln Lys Ser Leu Ala Ala Ala Thr Gly Lys 45

CAG GAA CTG GCC AAG TAC TTC TTG GCA GAA CTG CTG TCT GAG CCC
Gln Glu Leu Ala Lys Tyr Phe Leu Ala Glu Leu Leu Ser Glu Pro 60

AAC CAG ACA GAG AAC GAT GCC CTG GAG CCT GAG GAT TTG CCC CAG
Asn Gln Thr Glu Asn Asp Ala Leu Glu Pro Glu Asp Leu Pro Gln 75

GCA GCT GAG CAG GAC GAG ATG AGG CTG GAG CTG CAG AGG TCT GCC
Ala Ala Glu Gln Asp Glu Met Arg Leu Glu Leu Gln Arg Ser Ala 90

AAC TCG AAC CCA GCC ATG GCA CCC CGG GAA CGC AAA | GCT GGC TGC
Asn Ser Asn Pro Ala Met Ala Pro Arg Glu Arg Lys | *Ala Gly Cys* 105

AAG AAC TTC TTC TGG AAG ACA TTC ACA TCC TGT | TAG CTTTAATATT
Lys Asn Phe Phe Trp Lys Thr Phe Thr Ser Cys | *Stop* 116

GTTGTCTCAGCCAGACCTCTGATCCCTCTCCTCCAAATCCCATATCTCTTCCTTAACTCC

CAGCCCCCCCCCCAATGCTCAACTAGACCCTGCGTTAGAAATTGAAGACTGTAAATACAA

AATAAAATTATGGTGAAATTATGpoly(A)

Fig. 1. Structure of the preprosomatostatin cDNA derived from a rat medullary thyroid carcinoma. Underlined sequences include the leader region, the potential N-glycosylation site, and the biologically active SS-28 and SS-14 peptides.

Adjacent to the SS-28 sequence is a single Arg residue which appears to serve as a prohormone cleavage site. Although single basic amino acid residues are not classical cleavage sites, similar processing sites have been identified in precursors of other neuropeptides (6). It is possible, however, that the sequence depicted in Fig. 1 represents the precursor of SS-14 and that a separate gene with a clasical dibasic region flanking SS-28 (1-12) exists as a precursor for SS-28. To date, there is no evidence for such a separate gene. It is perhaps noteworthy that a single nucleotide change would convert the Gln residue at position 87 to Lys, forming the expected Lys Arg cleavage site. Whether the Gln-Arg sequence evolved from a classical Lys-Arg cleavage site is unknown. The significance for processing of the single Arg residue separating SS-28 from the remainder of the prohormone is also unknown.

At the amino-terminus of the precursor lies a region of hydrophobic amino acids characteristic of a leader sequence. Consideration of the nature of the amino acids adjacent to this region has allowed Argos et al. to predict the probable cleavage site of the leader sequence from prosomatostatin (33). To examine this issue directly, we have performed sequential Edman degradations on prosomatostatin generated in cell-free translations supplemented with microsomal membranes (30).

Translations performed in the presence of microsomal membranes were carried out with [^{3}H]-Phe and [^{3}H]-Pro, amino acids which are not found within the putative leader sequence. The prosomatostatin form was immunoprecipitated using antisera to SS-14 and was microsequenced using an automated Beckman sequencer. Because the structure of the precursor was known from the cDNA sequence, we could determine the cleavage site of the leader region from the positions of the radiolabeled Phe and Pro residues. This site occurs between the Gly and Ala residues at positions 24-25. This particular cleavage site, following the small neutral amino acid glycine, is typical of the signal processing sites used in other presecretory proteins (34).

Following removal of the leader sequence, a 92 amino acid prosomatostatin form of molecular weight 10,389 is formed. This 92 amino acid prohormone presumably corresponds to the largest form of somatostatin isolated from tissue extracts. Within the pre-region (amino acid residues 61-63) is the sequence Asn-Gln-Thr which represents a potential N-glycosylation site. The possibility that prosomatostatin may be glycosylated has been raised by several investigators (17, 35) but definitive evidence for this modification is lacking. In our cell-free translations, microsomal membranes do not appear to glycosylate the precursor (30). Nonetheless, it is possible that prosomatostatin is glycosylated _in vivo_ in some tissues.

The biological function of the pro-region of somatostatin, like that of many other regulatory hormone precursors, is unknown. This region may function simply as a "spacer" to allow the nascent peptide to be transported through the cellular processing machinery. Alternatively, the pro-region may provide some tertiary structure necessary for processing or may contain additional signals important for intracellular transport. Finally, the pro-region may be further processed to generate other biologically active peptides.

One strong argument in favor of a specific biological function for the pro-region of the somatostatin precursor is the degree of conservation of this region between different species. Comparison of the rat somatostatin precursor with anglerfish preprosomatostatin I reveals a considerable degree of homology (30). Over 30% of the amino acid positions are strictly conserved and many of the amino acid substitutions are conservative in nature. As expected from this high degree of relatedness, the tertiary structures of the precursors estimated by calculations of hydrophobicity, β-helix, and α-turn are quite similar. Anglerfish preprosomatostatin II appears to be considerably divergent within the pro-region (26).

The human preprosomatostatin sequence, determined by Shen et al. (36), is remarkably homologous to the rat precursor. Within the two 116 amino acid precursors, there are only four amino acid substitutions. Two of these substitutions occur within the leader sequence and presumably do not alter the hydrophobic nature of this region. The other two substitutions, a Thr for Ala at position 43 and a Pro for Ser at position 74, occur within the pro-region of the precursors. This high degree of conservation suggests that the pro-region does not function simply as a "spacer."

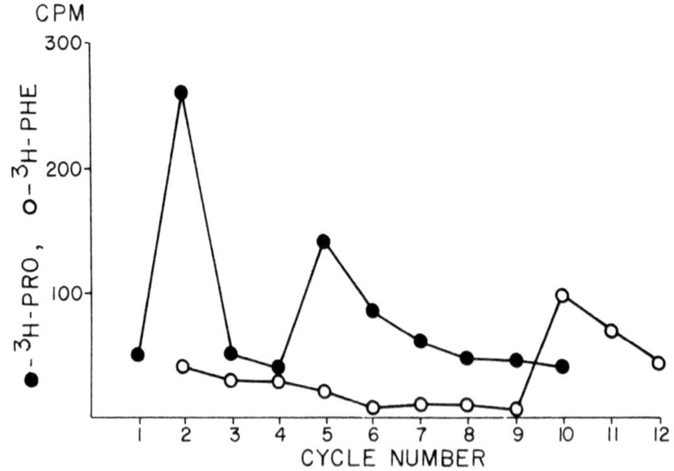

Fig. 2. Sequential Edman degradations of rat prosomatostatin labeled with [^{3}H]-Phe and [^{3}H]- Pro.

In an effort to determine the biologic fate and function of the pre-region of the rat somatostatin precursor, we have raised an antiserum to a synthetic peptide corresponding to the midportion of the precursor (Fig. 3). This region (designated rat somatostatin cryptic peptide, RSCP) was chosen because it represents the most hydrophilic segment of the precursor and was therefore thought likely to be exposed as an antigenic site. Antiserum to the 15-amino acid synthetic peptide was initially used to immunoprecipitate prosomatostatin and preprosomatostatin generated in cell-free translation reactions. Having demonstrated that the antiserum recognized high molecular weight forms of the somatostatin precursor, we then used it to localize the RSCP antigen in rat brain (37).

By immunocytochemical analysis, the RSCP-reaction product could be seen in cell bodies, axons, and axon terminals in all regions of the brain where immunoreactive SS-14 could be found. In particular, staining could be visualized in somatostatin-containing cell bodies in the paraventricular and periventricular nuclei in the anterior hypothalamus with projections to the terminal fields in the exterior zone of the median eminence (Fig. 4, 5). These studies indicate that at least a portion of the pro-region of the somatostatin precursor is transported from neuronal cell bodies to axon terminals where it potentially could be secreted. RSCP-immunoreactive material has also been identified in other somatostatin-containing tissues including spinal cord and endocrine pancreas (37, and unpublished data).

The molecular form of the RSCP-immunoreactive material has not been definitely determined. In preliminary studies, we have used gel filtration chromatography to characterize the RSCP-immunoreactive material (38). Extracts of rat median eminence and periventricular nuclei were eluted from a Sephadex G-50 (superfine) column with 1% formic acid and were analyzed using a RSCP radioimmunoassay. Four main peaks of RSCP-immunoreactivity could be discerned in both tissues. Peak I was in the void volume. Peak II had an approximate molecular weight of 9,000-11,000 compatible in size with the intact prohormone. Peak III was approximately 6,000-7,000 molecular weight, and peak IV was 4,000-5,000. Peaks I, II, and III also contain somatostatin-immunoreactivity. These data are most consistent with a proteolytic cleavage site near the amino-

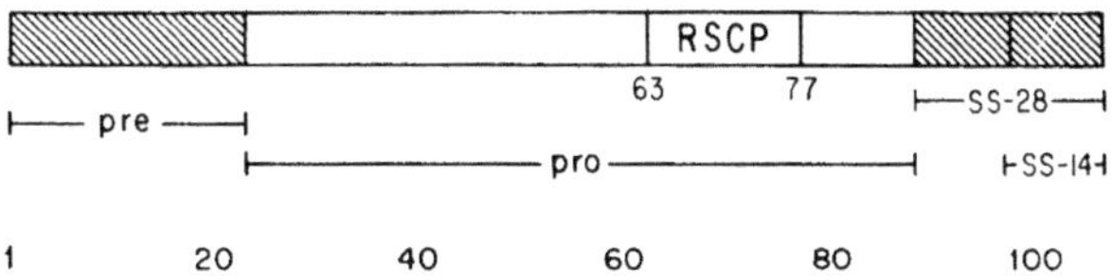

Fig. 3. Position of rat somatostatin cryptic peptide (RSCP) within the somatostatin precursor.

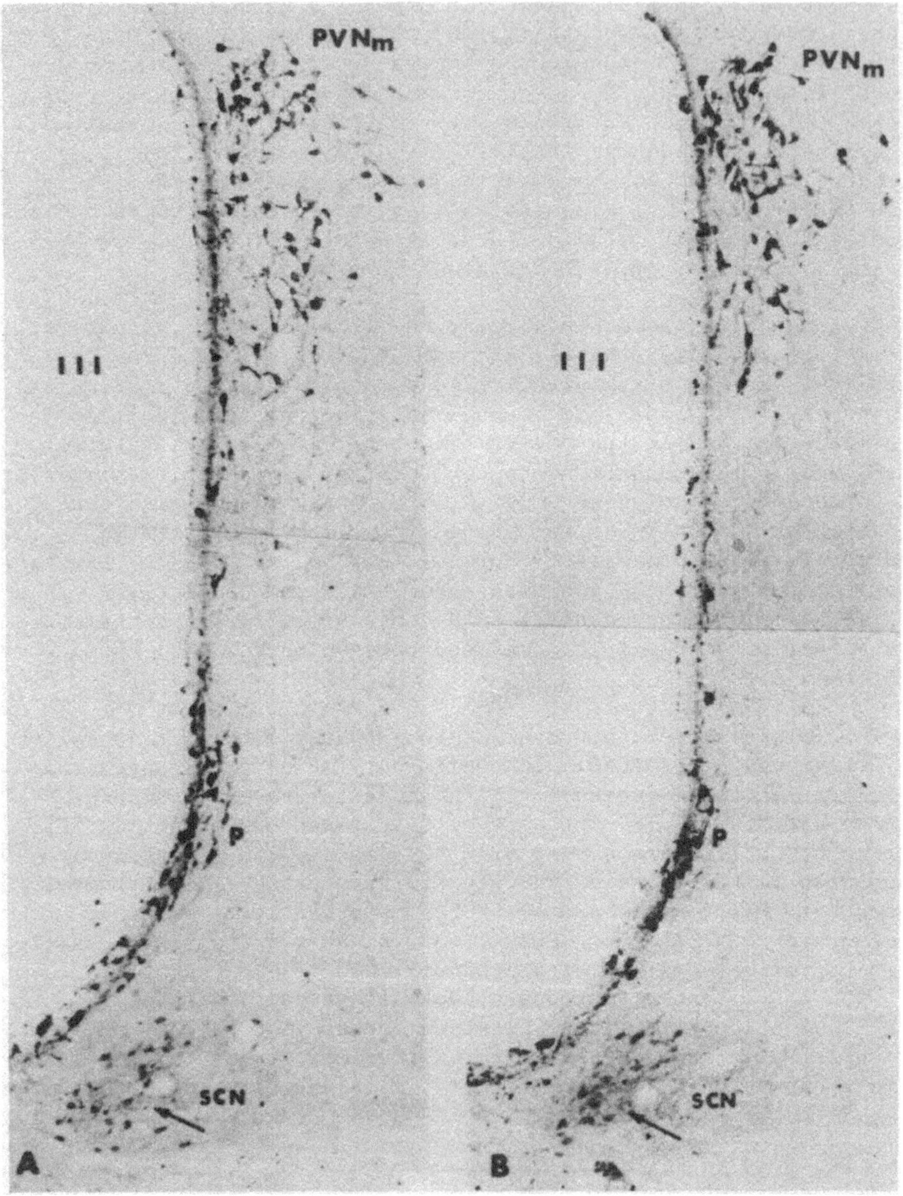

Fig. 4. Serial sections through the rat anterior hypothalamus stained with antiserum to RSCP (left) and SS-14 (right). Paraventricular nucleus (PVN_m), periventricular nucleus (P), and suprachiasmatic nucleus (SCN) are delineated.

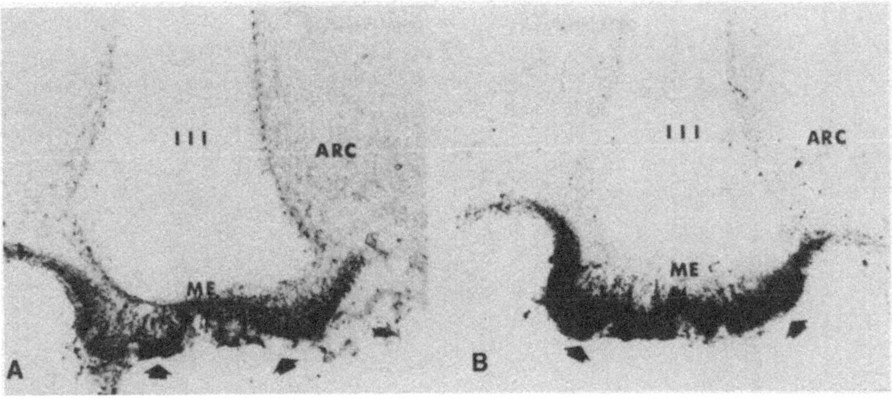

Fig. 5. Immunoreactivity RSCP (left) and SS-14 (right) in the terminal fields of the median eminence (ME).

terminus of the pro-region. Benoit et al. have recently characterized a prosomatostatin-related peptide which appears to be generated by proteolytic cleavage between the Leu-Leu bond at positions 56-57 (39). Processing at this side would generate fragments which correspond to those seen in our gel chromatographic analysis. Interestingly, this cleavage site is within a region which is relatively highly conserved between the rat and anglerfish somatostatin I precursors.

As discussed above, the tissue-specific processing of prosomatostatin could be due to expression of separate somatostatin genes or to cellular specificity of processing enzymes. In the case of some regulatory peptides, such as pro-opiomelanocortin, differential processing appears to be due to cell-specific factors (40). Other peptides, including anglerfish prosomatostatin I and II, may contain information for differential processing within their separate primary structures (41).

To establish the number of somatostatin-related sequences in the rat genome, we performed Southern blot hybridizations of DNA isolated from rat spleen (Fig. 6). This analysis suggested that there is a unique somatostatin gene in the rat, with a single intervening sequence separating the region encoding the leader sequence from the SS-28 and SS-14 sequences. Longer exposures of the blots revealed additional weakly hybridizing bands however, indicative of distantly related sequences. Although most consistent with the existence of a single somatostatin gene, these studies do not rule out the existence of a multigene family of somatostatin-related peptides as found in lower species.

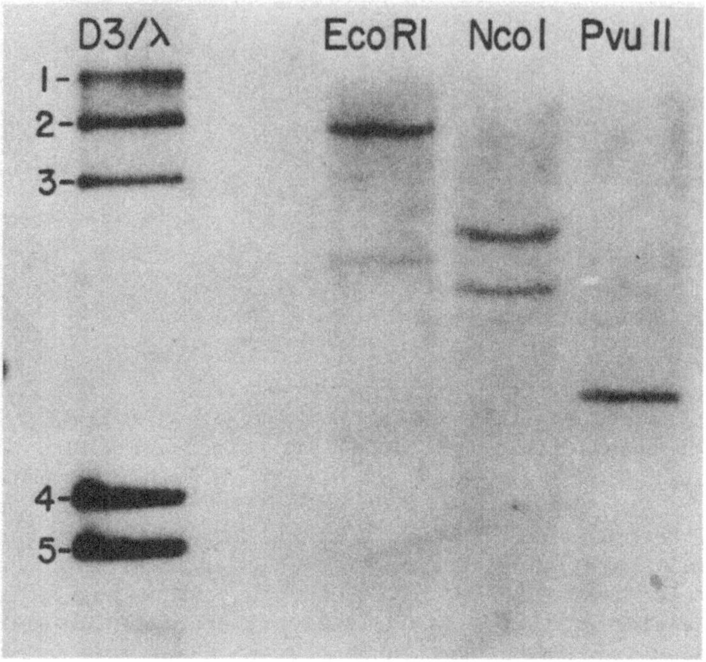

Fig. 6. Southern blot hybridization of restriction enzyme digests of rat spleen DNA. DNA was digested with the restriction enzymes Eco R1, Nco 1, or Pvu 2, electrophoresed through an 0.8% agarose gel, and transferred to nitrocellulose. The blot was hybridized to a ^{32}P labeled cDNA fragment encoding rat preprosomatostatin. Lane D3/λ represents size markers (labeled 1-5): 23, 9.4, 6.7, 2.3, and 2.0 kilobase pairs. An 0.6 kilobase Pvu 2 hybridizing band is not shown.

To facilitate the identification of factors that regulate somatostatin gene expression, we have used the somatostatin cDNA as a hybridization probe to screen rat genomic libraries cloned in Charon 4A bacteriophages (42). One library, prepared from a partial EcoR1 digest of rat liver genomic DNA, contained a recombinant bacteriophage which encoded the 5' exon of the somatostatin gene and extended 15 kilobases in the 5' direction. A second bacteriophage, isolated from a partial Hae III genomic library, contained sequences which overlapped with the first bacteriophage and extended 10 kilobases in the 3' direction (43). The restriction maps of the two recombinant bacteriophages isolated corresponds to that seen in digests of genomic DNA, indicating that there has been no rearrangement during construction of the libraries.

Fragments of the bacteriophage inserts were subcloned into the plasmid pBR322 and subjected to nucleotide sequencing. A schematic illustration of the rat somatostatin gene is depicted in Fig. 7.

The somatostatin gene is interrupted by a single intervening sequence of 630 bases. Characteristic GT/AG donor-acceptor sites are present at the ends of the intervening sequence. The intervening sequence, as predicted by Southern blotting experiments, occurs near the midportion of the precursor between the Gln and Glu codons at positions 46-47. Unlike some other regulatory peptide genes, the rat somatostatin gene does not appear to be divided into functional domains by the intervening sequence. The intervening sequence occurs in the same position in the human gene where it is somewhat longer (36). This difference in length is due primarily to the presence of a repetitive sequence within the human gene.

The transcriptional initiation point of the rat somatostatin gene was determined by S-1 nuclease mapping. The length of the 5' untranslated region determined by this technique is 102 bases. Thirty-one bases upstream from the transcriptional initiation point is an atypical Goldberg-Hogness promoter, TTTAAA. Comparison of the rat and human somatostatin gene promoter regions (Fig. 8) reveals an extraordinarily high level of nucleotide sequence conservation. The similarity in sequence between the two species suggests that this entire region may be particularly important for gene regulation.

A repetitive sequence was identified in the 5' region of the rat somatostatin gene within 650 bases of the promotor. This repetitive element, a portion of which is shown in Fig. 9, was found to occur at a frequency of approximately 10,000 copies per genome. As shown in Fig. 9, the sequence contains a long region of alternating purine and pyrimidine bases. This sequence is significant because of its potential for adopting the Z-configuration.

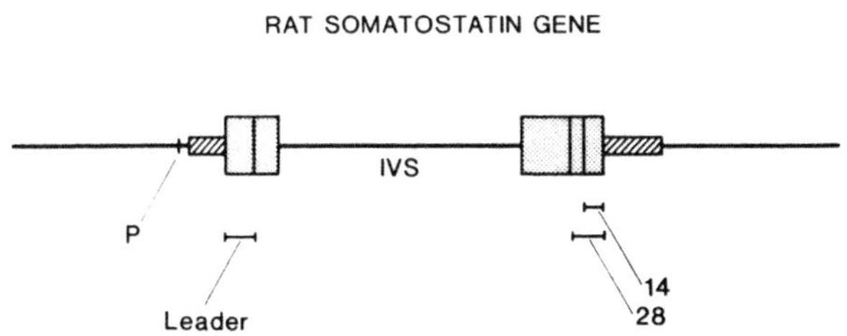

Fig. 7. Schematic depiction of the rat somatostatin gene. P refers to promoter region, IVS to intervening sequence, 28 and 14 to SS-28 and SS-14 regions. Coding sequence is shown by dotted boxes, untranslated regions by hatched areas.

```
          -260
HUMAN     AATGTGTATGCTCATAG-CACTGAGTGAAAATAAAAGATTGTATAAATCGTGGGCATGTGGAATTGTGTGTGCCTGTGCGTGTG
             *  *****    * * *********  **    ****** * *     *** ***  *  *****    ********** * ***
RAT       ATGGGATATGCATGTCGACACTGAGTG--AAGGCAAGATTATTTGGTCTGTGTGGCGTGGAGAATTTCATGTGCCTGTGTGGGTG

          -180
HUMAN     CAGTATTTTTTTTTTTTTAAGTAA----------GCCACTTTAGATCTTGTCACCTCCCCTGTCTTCTGT-GATT-GATTTTGCG
          ***  *** ***** ** **  **          ************ **** ********  ***** * **** *********
RAT       CAGGCTTTCTTTTTCTTCAAAAAAAAAAAAAATAAACCACTTTAGATCGTGTCGCCTCCCCTCACTTCTTTTGATTTGATTTTGCG

          -100                                                                      -31
HUMAN     AGGCTAATGGTGCGTAAAAGGGCTGGTGAGATCTGGGGGCGCCTCCTAGCCTGACGTCAGAGAGAGAGTTTAAAACAGAGGGAGA
          ********************  ************************* * ***********************    ******
RAT       AGGCTAATGGTGCGTAAAAGCACTGGTGAGATCTGGGGGCGCCTCCTTGGCTGACGTCAGAGAGAGAGTTTAAAAA--GGGGAGA

          -10     +
HUMAN     CGGTTGAGAGCACACAAGCCGCTTTAGGAGCGAGGTTCGGAGCCATCG .......
          * ** ****** *    ** ***  *****        **** * **
RAT       CCGTGGAGAGCTCGATAGCGGCTGAAGGAGACGCTACTGGAGTCGTCT .......
                           +
```

Fig. 8. Comparison of rat and human somatostatin gene 5' flanking sequences. Atypical Goldberg-Hogness promoter (TATA box) is underlined and + indicates transcription initiation point. Gaps are introduced to maintain homology.

The existence of a DNA configuration other than the B or right-handed helical form was first demonstrated by Wand and co-workers (44) in 1979. Using x-ray crystallography, they observed that poly $(dG\text{-}dC)_3$ crystals formed left-handed helical structures. This configuration was termed Z-DNA because of the zig-zagging nature of the phosphate backbone. The Z-configuration preserves base pairing but requires high cation (2.7 M NaCl) concentrations in solution to prevent conversion to the B DNA form. In an effort to find conditions which would stabilize the Z configuration, Behe and Felsenfeld (45) found that methylation of the cytosine residues shifted the equilibrium significantly towards the Z form. This finding, coupled with evidence that cytosine methylation may be important in gene regulation, aroused speculation on the existence and significance of Z DNA in biological systems.

Researchers have recently obtained more specific structural information on the localization of Z-forming sequences in eukaryotic chromosomes. To characterize areas in mammalian genomes with Z-forming potential, Hamada et al. (46) used poly (dG-dC) and poly (dT-dG) oligonucleotides to probe Southern blots of mammalian genomic DNAs. They observed a dark smear of hybridization in every species tested. This indicated that Z-forming areas were represented with high frequency, random dispersion, and considerable evolutionary conservation. Plaque hybridizations of genomic libraries established that each genome contains approximately 20,000 copies of the alternating purine-pyrimidine sequences with an

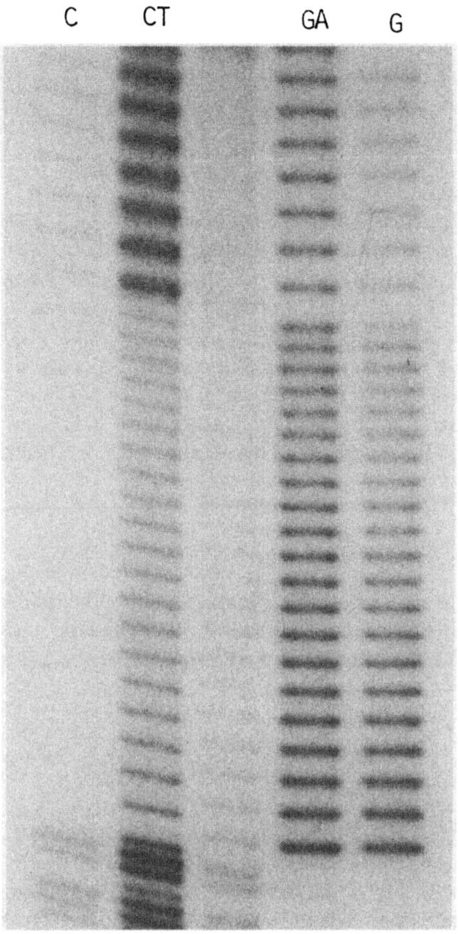

Fig. 9. Nucleotide sequence of a portion of the repetitive element in the 5' flanking region of the rat somatostatin gene.

average length of 50 bases. These observations are consistent with our results concerning the nature and frequency of the somatostatin repetitive element.

Specific examples of long, tandemly-repeated, purine-pyrimidine stretches have been reported for a few other eukaryotic genes in addition to rat somatostatin. Miesfeld et al. (47) found a stretch of 17 dT-dG dinucleotides 1.5 kilobases upstream from the beta-globin gene. Nishioka and Leder (48) observed 31 dC-dA doublets 300 bases downstream from the human K2-V region immunoglobulin gene. A $(dT\text{-}dG)_{25}$ stretch is also present in the intron of the cardiac muscle actin gene (49) and a similar sequence has been found within the IVS of the human somatostatin gene (36). The positioning of the Z element relative to the promoter region in these genes does not appear favorable for transcriptional regulation however. The rat somatostatin gene may therefore provide a model system for establishing a causal link between Z-DNA switching and the functional state of a gene.

In summary, recombinant DNA technology has elucidated the structure of the somatostatin precursor and gene and has provided antibodies and cDNA probes for analysis of the biosynthesis and processing of the precursor. Among the questions which remain are 1) is somatostastin synthesis regulated and, if so, how does this regulation occur, 2) what is the function of the pro-region, and 3) how is the processing of prosomatostatin to SS-14 and/or SS-28 controlled. Further technological advances within the next few years will undoubtedly provide the answers to these questions.

ACKNOWLEDGMENT

This work was supported by grant AM31400 and AM25532 from the NIH. We thank Dr. Ronald Lechan for performing the immunocytochemical studies and Ms. Elinor Triggs for excellent secretarial help.

REFERENCES

1. Arimura A, Sato H, Coy D, Schally AV 1975 Radioimmunoassay for GH-release inhibiting hormone. Proc Soc Exp Biol Med 148:784.
2. Spiess J, Vale W 1978 Investigation of larger forms of somatostatin in pigeon pancreas and rat brain. Metab 27 (Suppl. I): 1175.
3. Pradayrol L, Jørnvall H, Mutt V, Ribet A 1980 N-terminally extended somatostatin: The primary structure of somatostatin-28. FEBS Lett 109:55.
4. Schally AV, Huang W, Chang LL, Arimura A, Redding TW, Millar RP, Hunkapiller MW, Hood LE 1980 Isolation and structure of pro-somatostatin: a putative precursor from pig hypothalamus. Proc Natl Acad Sci (USA) 77:4489.
5. Esch F, Böhlen P, Ling N, Benoit R, Brazeau P, Guillemin R 1980 Primary structure of ovine hypothalamic somatostatin-28 and somatostatin-25. Proc Natl Acad Sci (USA) 77:6827.
6. Loh YP, Brownstein MJ, Gainer H 1984 Proteolysis in neuropeptide procesing and other neural functions. Ann Rev Neurosci 7:189.
7. Mandarino L, Stenner D, Blanchard W, Nissen S, Gerich J, Ling N, Brazeau P, Böhlen P, Esch F, Guillemin R 1981 Selective effects of somatostatin-14, -25, and -28 on in vitro insulin and glucagon secretion. Nature 291:76.

8. Brown M, Rivier J, Vale W 1981 Somatostatin 28: selective action on the pancreatic B-cell and brain. Endocrinology 108:2391.
9. Konturek SJ, Tasler J, Jaworek J, Pawlik W, Walus KM, Schusdziarra V, Meyers CA, Coy DH, Schally AV 1981 Gastrointestinal, secretory, motor, circulatory, and metabolic effects of prosomatostatin. Proc Natl Acad Sci (USA) 78:1967.
10. Brazeau P, Ling N, Esch F, Böhlen P, Benoit R, Guillemin R 1981 High biological activites of the synthetic replicates of somatostatin-28 and -25. Regul Peptides 1:255.
11. Susini C, Esteve JP, Vayesse N, Pradayrol L, Ribet A 1980 Somatostatin-28: effect on exocrine pancreatic secretion in conscious dogs. Gastroenterology 79:720.
12. Meyers CA, Murphy WA, Redding TW, Coy DH, Schally AV 1980 Synthesis and biological actions of prosomatostatin. Proc Natl Acad Sci (USA) 77:6171.
13. Schally AV, Dupont A, Arimura A, Redding TW, Nishi N, Linthicum GL, Schlesinger DH 1976 Isolation and structure of growth hormone-release inhibiting hormone from porcine hypothalami. Biochemistry 15:509.
14. Arimura A, Sato H, Dupont A, Nishi N, Schally AV 1975 Somatostatin: abundance of immunoreactive hormone in rat stomach and pancreas. Science 189:1007.
15. Lauber M, Camier M, Cohen P 1979 Higher molecular weight forms of immunoreactive somatostatin in mouse hypothalamic extracts: evidence of processing in vitro. Proc Natl Acad Sci (USA) 76:6004.
16. Trent DF, Weir GG 1981 Heterogeneity of somatostatin-like peptides in rat brain, pancreas, and gastrointestinal tract. Endocrinology 108:2033.
17. Patzelt C, Tager HS, Carroll RJ, Steiner DF 1980 Identification of prosomatostatin in pancreatic islets. Proc Natl Acad Sci (USA) 77:2410.
18. Rorstad OP, Epelbaum J, Brazeau P, Martin JB 1979 Chromatographic and biological properties of immunoreactive somatostatin in hypothalamic and extrahypothalamic brain regions of the rat. Endocrinology 105:1083.
19. Fletcher DJ, Noe BD, Bauer GE, Quigley JP 1980 Characterization of the conversion of a somatostatin precursor to somatostatin by islet secretory granules. Diabetes 29:593.
20. Goodman RH, Lund PK, Jacobs JW, Habener JF 1980 Pre-prosomatostatins: products of cell-free translations of messenger RNAs from anglerfish islets. J Biol Chem 255:6549.
21. Goodman RH, Lund PK, Barnett FH, Habener JF 1981 Intestinal pre-prosomatostatin: identification of mRNA coding for a precursor by cell-free translations and hybridization with a cloned islet cDNA. J Biol Chem 256:1499.
22. Joseph-Bravo P, Charli JL, Sherman T, Boyer H, Bolivar F, McKelvy JF 1980 Identification of a putative hypothalamic mRNA coding for somatostatin and of its product in cell-free translation. Biochem Biophys Res Commun 94:1004.

23. Shields D 1980 In vitro biosynthesis of somatostatin. J Biol Chem 255:11625.
24. Oyama H, O'Connell K, Permutt 1980 Cell-free synthesis of somatostatin. Endocrinology 107:845.
25. Warren TG, Shields D 1982 Cell-free biosynthesis of somatostatin precursors: evidence for multiple forms of pre-prosomatostatin. Proc Natl Acad Sci (USA) 77:4074.
26. Hobart P, Crawford R, Shen L, Pictet R, Rutter W 1980 Cloning and sequence analysis of cDNA encoding two distinct somatostatin precursors found in endocrine pancreas of anglerfish. Nature 288:137.
27. Goodman RH, Jacobs JW, Chin WW, Lund PK, Dee PC, Habener JF 1980 Nucleotide sequence of a cloned structural gene coding for a precursor of pancreatic somatostatin. Proc Natl Acad Sci (USA) 77:5869.
28. Jacobs JW, Goodman RH, Chin WW, Dee PC, Habener JF, Bell NH, Potts JT Jr 1981 Calcitonin structure gene codes for multiple polypeptides. Science 213:457.
29. Goodman RH, Jacobs JW, Dee PC, Habener JF 1982 Somatostatin-28 encoded in a cloned cDNA obtained from a rat medullary thyroid carcinoma. J Biol Chem 257:1156.
30. Goodman RH, Aron DC, Roos BA 1983 Rat pre-prosomatostatin: structure and processing by microsomal membranes. J Biol Chem 257:1156.
31. Funckes M, Minth D, Deschenes R, Magazin M, Tavianini MA, Sheets M, Collier M, Weith HL, Aron DC, Roos BA, Dixon J 1983 Cloning and charcterization of a mRNA-encoding rat preprosomatostatin. J Biol Chem 258:8781.
32. Benoit R, Böhlen P, Ling N, Briskin A, Esch F, Brazeau P, Ying SY, Guillemin R 1982 Presence of somatostatin-28 (1-12) in hypothalamus and pancreas. Proc Natl Acad Sci (USA) 79:917.
33. Argos P, Taylor WL, Minth CD, Dixon JE 1983 Nucleotide and amino acid sequence comparisons of pre-prosomatostatins. J Biol Chem 258:8799.
34. Von Heijne G 1983 Patterns of amino acids near signal-sequence cleavage sites. Eur J Biochem 133:17.
35. Aron DC, O'Neil J, Birnbaum RS, Muszynski M, Sabo SW, Fleming AA, Roos BA, Somatostatin-producing rat medullary thyroid carcinoma - identification and preliminary characterization of high molecular weight forms of somatostatin. Program of the 69th Annual Meeting of the Endocrine Society, San Francisco, June 1982, (Abstract 246).
36. Shen L-P, Pictet RC, Rutter WJ 1982 Human somatostatin I:sequence of the cDNA. Proc Natl Acad Sci (USA) 79:4575.
37. Lechan RM, Goodman RH, Rosenblatt M, Reichlin S, Habener JF 1983 Pro-somatostastin-specific antigen in rat brain: Localization by immunocytochemical staining with an antiserum to a synthetic sequence of pre-prosomatostatin. Proc Natl Acad Sci (USA) 80:2780.

38. Low MJ, Lechan RM, Rosenblatt M, Goodman RH, Distribution and content of prosomatostatin-specific antigen in rat brain. Program of the 65th Annual Meeting of the Endocrine Society, San Antonio, June 1983 (Abstract 281).
39. Benoit R, Böhlen P, Esch R, Ling N, Alford B, Isolation and characterization of two peptides derived from prosomatostatin in rat brain. Program of the 13th Annual Meeting of the Neurosciences Society, Boston 1983 (Abstract 219:13).
40. Uhler M, Herbert E, D'Eustachio P, Ruddle FD 1983 The mouse genome contains two nonallelic pro-opiomelanocortin genes. J Biol Chem 258:9444.
41. Noe BD, Spiess J, Identification, isolation and characterization of a primary cleavage product of (pre) prosomatostatin II in pancreatic islets. Program of the 65th Annual Meeting of the Endocrine Society, San Antonio, June 1983 (Abstract 17).
42. Sargent TD, Wu JZ, Sala-Trepst TM, Wallace RG, Reyes AA, Bonne J 1979 The rat serum albumen gene: analysis of cloned sequences. Proc Natl Acad Sci (USA) 76:3256.
43. Montminy M, Goodman RH, Horovitch S, Habener JF 1984 Primary structure of the gene encoding rat pre-prosomatostatin. Proc Natl Acad Sci (USA) 81:3337.
44. Wang A, Quigley GJ, Koplack FJ, Crawford JL, van Boom JH, Vander Marel G, Rich A 1979 Molecular structure of a left-handed double helical DNA fragment at atomic resolution. Nature 282:680.
45. Behe M, Felsenfeld G 1981 Effects of methylation on a synthetic polynucleotide: the B-Z transition in poly (dG-m^{5}dC). Proc Natl Acad Sci (USA) 78:1619.
46. Hamada H, Petrino MG, Kakunga T 1982 A novel repeated element with Z-DNA forming potential is found in evolutionarily diverse eukaryotic genomes. Proc Natl Acad Sci (USA) 79:6465.
47. Miesfeld R, Krystal M, Arnheim M 1981 A member of a new repeated sequence family which is conserved throughout eukarytic evolution is found between the human S and B globin genes. Nucl Acids Res 9:5931.
48. Nishioka Y, Leder P 1980 Organization and complete sequence of identical embryonic and plasmacytoma K V-region genes. J Biol Chem 255:3691.
49. Hamada H, Petrino M, Kakunaga T 1982 Molecular structure and evolutionary origin of human cardiac actin gene. Proc Natl Acad Sci (USA) 79:5901.

4

APPROACHES TO THE STUDY OF SOMATOSTATIN BIOSYNTHESIS

HANS H. ZINGG*, JOEL F. HABENER** AND Y.C. PATEL***

*Laboratory of Molecular Endocrinology, McGill University, Department of Medicine, Royal Victoria Hospital, Montreal, Quebec H3A 1A1, Canada

**Laboratory of Molecular Endocrinology, Massachusetts General Hospital, and the Howard Hughes Medical Institute, Harvard Medical School, Boston, Massachusetts 02114, U.S.A.

***Fraser Laboratories, McGill University, Departments of Medicine, Neurology and Neurosurgery, Royal Victoria Hospital & Montreal Neurological Institute, Montreal, Quebec H3A 1A1, Canada

ABSTRACT

Our current knowledge of the processes regulating somatostatin biosynthesis is still scarce. Approaches used for the direct investigation of somatostatin biosynthesis in different tissues include 1) analysis of incorporation of labeled amino acids into somatostatin-like immunoreactivity (SLI), 2) cell-free translation of mRNA isolated from SLI producing tissues and 3) analysis of mRNA coding for somatostatin by cDNA blot hybridization.

Amino acid incorporation into SLI has been studied in a variety of systems, including anglerfish and rat pancreas, frog retina, rat dorsal root ganglia, cerebral cortex and hypothalamus. We have studied the neuronal biosynthesis of somatostatin using monolayer cultures of neonatal rat hypothalamic cells. Following pulse labeling with [^{3}H]phenylalanine, the cellular extracts contained material that bound specifically to an immobilized anti-somatostatin antibody. Analysis of the bound label by gel chromatography and HPLC provided evidence for the presence of labeled somatostatin-14 (S-14), somatostatin-28 (S-28) and a precursor molecule of Mr 15,000 (15 K SLI). Pulse-chase experiments demonstrated a transfer of label from 15K SLI to material corresponding to S-28 and S-14.

Using cloned cDNAs complementary to somatostatin mRNA, the presence of somatostatin mRNA has been demonstrated in anglerfish pancreas and intestine, rat hypothalamus and antrum, as well as in a rat medullary thyroid carcinoma and a rat pancreatic cell line. We have recently studied the developmental regulation of somatostatin gene expression in the rat brain and stomach. Messenger RNA hybridizing specifically to a rat somatostatin cDNA probe was already clearly detectable in tissue extracts derived from brains of one week old rat fetuses. A marked increase of somatostatin mRNA occured between day 14 and day 21 of embryonic life. By contrast, in tissue extracts derived from stomach, somatostatin mRNA remained undetectable until shortly before birth. These marked differences in the tissue specific regulation of somatostatin gene expression during ontogenesis may reflect basic differences in the developmental regulation of somatostatin gene expression in neural vs. nonneural tissues or may be related to the onset of functional activity in the organs studied.

INTRODUCTION

In contrast to the detailed structural information available on the anglerfish, catfish, rat and human somatostatins and their precursors (1-4), our current knowledge of the processes controlling the biosynthesis of these molecules is relatively scarce. Although the regulation of the amounts of somatostatin-like peptides stored in and released from different tissues has been the subject of extensive investigations, these data do not give direct information on the regulation of somatostatin biosynthesis *per se*. Approaches used for direct investigations of somatostatin biosynthesis include 1) analysis of incorporation of labeled amino acids into somatostatin-like peptides *in vivo* and *in vitro*, 2) cell free translation of mRNA isolated from somatostatin producing tissues followed by immunological identification of the translation products, and 3) direct measurement and quantitation of mRNA coding for somatostatin by cDNA blot hybridization. In this chapter some aspects of the contributions made by these different approaches will be reviewed.

RESULTS AND DISCUSSION

Incorporation of Labeled Amino Acids

The first investigations on the mode of somatostatin biosynthesis were performed using the anglerfish pancreatic islets. Noe et al. (5, 6) showed that fish islets *in vitro* incorporated labeled amino acids into a large form of SLI of Mr = 8,000-15,000. During a subsequent chase period, label was transferred from the larger precursor peptides to a smaller form corresponding to S-14. Label incorporation into the S-14 like form increased with the length of the chase period. On the other hand, label incorporation was inhibited by cycloheximide. These experiments were the first to demonstrate that in the pancreas, somatostatin biosynthesis occurs in situ via ribosomal synthesis of precursor forms which are subsequently processed to S-14 (5). The role of the larger form of labeled SLI as a biosynthethic precursor of S-14 was further established by showing that incubation of this form with cell-free supernate from islet tissue, or with trypsin, yielded a labeled peptide that was immunologically and biochemically indistinguishable from synthetic S-14 (6).

Similar experiments performed in rat islets by Patzelt and coworkers (7) showed label incorporation into a 12.5 kilodalton precursor protein which was processed during a subsequent chase period to S-14. This transfer of label occured without any apparent involvement of a major intermediate form.

Demonstration of somatostatin biosynthesis in neurons proved to be a more difficult task. A major reason for the increased difficulties encountered in this experimental approach consists in the marked cellular heterogeneity which is characteristic of neural tissues. Using the frog retina, Yamada and Basinger (8) showed incorporation of [^{35}S]cysteine into material which bound specifically to immobilized antisomatostatin antibody. Chromatography of the labeled retinal SLI revealed four peaks. One coeluted with S-14 whereas the other three represented forms of SLI of a higher molecular weight. None of these latter forms coeluted, however, with S-28.

For the investigation of neuronal somatostatin biosynthesis in mammals, the rat dorsal root ganglia, cerebral cortex and hypothalamus have been used as model systems. Freshly dissected dorsal root ganglia were shown to incorporate [^{3}H]phenylalanine into S-14 and S-28 as characterized by immunoprecipitation and HPLC (9). Robbins and Reichlin utilized dispersed telencephalic cells kept in culture to show incorporation of [^{3}H]phenylalanine into somatostatin-like material comigrating with S-14, S-28 as well as an 11.5K precursor form (10).

In view of the high concentration of somatostatin in the hypothalamus, where SLI is localized in parvicellular neurons in the periventricular area, we chose to investigate the neuronal biosynthesis of somatostatin in an in vitro system consisting of monolayer cultures of neonatal rat hypothalamic cells kept in culture for up to 6 weeks (11). Specific somatostatin-positive neurons were identified in the cultures by immunocytochemistry in a subpopulation of cultured hypothalamic neurons. These neurons comprised a small proportion (1%) of the total population of nerve cells, a finding compatible with the density of somatostatin positive neurons observed in sections of rat hypothalamus. Two separate lines of evidence attested to the biosynthesis of SLI in these neuronal cultures: Firstly, time course studies indicated that, after an initial decline, the cellular content increased progressively to reach a maximum value of 381 fmol/dish at day 46 (11). Characterization of the newly synthesized SLI by gel chromatography and RIA showed three peaks of immunoreactivity corresponding to 15,000 mol wt SLI, S-28 and S-14, suggesting that all three known tissue forms of SLI have been synthesized by the cultured somatostatin cells. Secondly, pulse-labeling studies showed that after incubation of the cells with [^{3}H]phenylalanine, the cellular extracts, purified by adsorption to C_{18} silica, contained material that bound specifically to immobilized antisomatostatin antibody. Analysis by gel chromatography and HPLC of the specifically bound label provided evidence for the presence of labeled S-14, S-28 and the 15,000 mol wt molecule (Fig. 1). Results from the pulse-chase experiments suggest that after a short pulse period, label is preferentially incorporated into a form corresponding in its elution position on gel chromatography to 15,000 mol wt SLI, whereas during the following chase period, transfer of label is observed from the 15,000 mol wt region to peaks eluting in the position of S-14 and S-28 (Fig. 2). These studies demonstrate that cultured hypothalamic neurons are capable of synthesizing three somatostatin-like peptides, one of which (15,000 mol wt SLI) serves as a biosynthetic precursor for both, S-28 and S-14.

The _in vivo_ incorporation of labeled amino acid precursors into S-14 and S-28 has been studied by Fernstrom and coworkers (12-14). Following [^{35}S]cysteine injection into the third ventricle of rats,

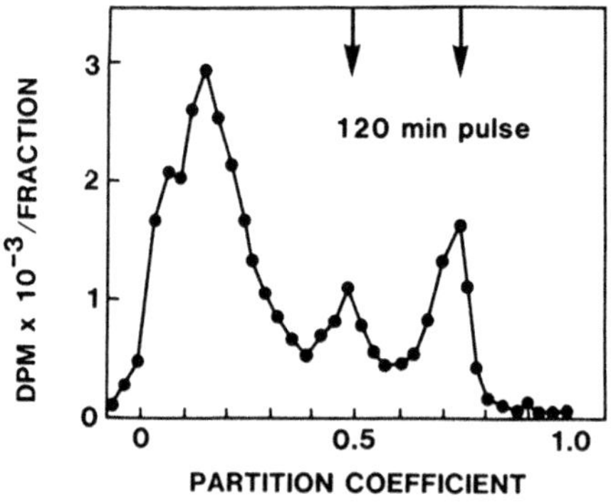

Fig. 1. Elution profile of [^{3}H]labeled SLI, purified from cell extracts of 40 culture dishes incubated for 2 h in the presence of [^{3}H]phenylalanine. Following purification by adsorption to C_{18} silica and affinity chromatography, the SLI eluted from the affinity column was fractionated on a Sephadex G-50 column. The two arrows indicate the elution position of S-28 (left arrow) and S-14 (right arrow).

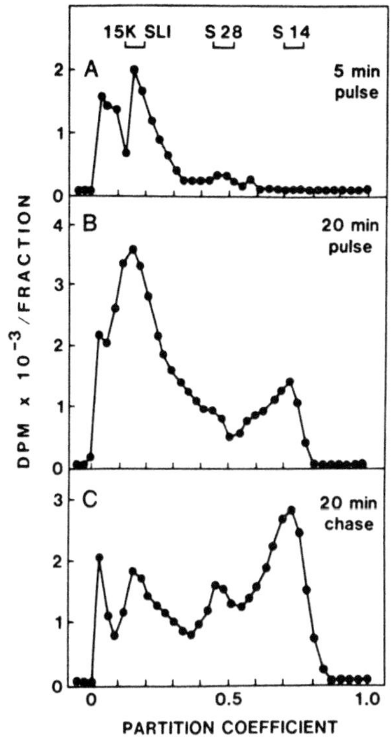

Fig. 2. Elution profile on Sephadex G-50 of labelled SLI purified from cell extracts. Twenty dishes were incubated for either 5 min (A) or 20 min (B and C) in the presence of [^{3}H]phenylalanine. In "C" the pulse period was followed by a 20 min chase period.

the authors demonstrated label incorporation into forms which corresponded, after two successive HPLC separations, to S-14 and S-28 (12). Hypophysectomy diminished label incorporation into both peptides by more than 50% suggesting a possible growth hormone feedback mechanism influencing hypothalamic somatostatin biosynthesis. In addition, label incorporation into S-14 or S-28 was shown to be independent of the state of hydration of the animal (14).

Taken together, the incorporation studies clearly establish that S-14 and S-28 are synthesized ribosomally as parts of larger precursor forms. In contrast to the fish, this process appears to involve in mammals only one major precursor form.

Cell Free Translation

An alternative approach to the study of somatostatin biosynthesis is to isolate mRNA from somatostatin producing tissues and to translate it into protein using a cell free translation system. This approach offers the advantage that it allows the identification of intact precursor forms which still contain an uncleaved signal sequence. Translation of anglerfish islet mRNA in a wheat germ protein synthesizing system yielded two major immunoprecipitable somatostatin-like peptides which differed in their apparent size by 1 kilodalton (15, 16). More recently, Warren and Shields identified a total of 9 distinct forms of somatostatin immunoreactive peptides resulting from cell free translation of anglerfish islet mRNA (17). Their studies suggest that these translation products are each encoded by a different mRNA species. In mammals, the translation products of rat and bovine hypothalamic mRNA have been analyzed and, in both cases, a single somatostatin-like protein of Mr = 15 kilodaltons was identified (18, 19). These studies confirm that, in contrast to the fish pancreas, there is no evidence for plurality of somatostatin precursors in the mammalian hypothalamus.

Identification of Somatostatin mRNA by cDNA Hybridization

Using cloned cDNAs complementary to somatostatin mRNA, the presence of somatostatin mRNA has been demonstrated by blot hybridization in anglerfish pancreas and intestine, rat hypothalamus and antrum as well as in a rat medullary thyroid carcinoma and a rat pancreatic tumor cell line (1, 2, 4, 18, 20-23). Whereas two species of mRNA were detected in the anglerfish, only one species of somatostatin mRNA has been detected so far in the mammalian tissues examined. Green and Shields showed recently that treatment of cultured rat pancreatic tumor cells by sodium butyrate led to a twelve fold increase in cellular levels of somatostatin mRNA (22). Although sodium butyrate is known to stimulate gene transcription by its inhibitory action on histone deacetylases, it remains to be investigated if the observed effect on somatostatin mRNA levels are due to a specific increase in somatostatin gene transcription, an inhibition of somatostatin mRNA degradation or both.

We have recently studied the developmental regulation of somatostatin gene expression in the rat. We chose to focus these studies on two tissues in which somatostatin is relatively abundant: brain, where somatostatin is present in neurons, and stomach, where somatostatin containing D cells are present in the antral region. Tissue extracts from rat brain and stomach, as well as from pancreas and duodenum, contained only one species of mRNA which hybridized specifically to a rat somatostatin cDNA probe (3) (Fig. 3). Thus it appears that in the rat, only a single somatostatin gene is expressed in both neural and non neural tissues. In addition, the size of the somatostatin mRNA appeared to be identical in both tissues. Using RNA and DNA size markers, the length of the somatostatin mRNA was estimated at 650 ± 20 bases.

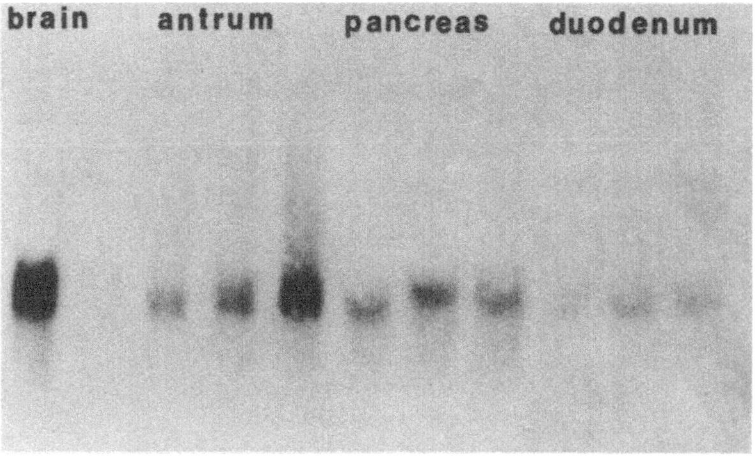

Fig. 3. Autoradiograph of blot of preprosomatostatin mRNA extracted from neuronal and intestinal tissues. RNA extracted from adult brain (24 µg), antrum (6, 12 and 24 µg), pancreas (6, 12 and 24 µg) and duodenum (6, 12 and 24 µg) was electrophoresed in 1.5% agarose, transferred to a nylon membrane and hybridized to a labelled preprosomatostatin cDNA probe.

To determine the levels of somatostatin mRNA in neural and non-neural tissues during development, a quantitative radiodensitometric hybridization assay was developed (23). Messenger RNA hybridizing specifically to a rat somatostatin cDNA probe, was already clearly detectable in tissue extracts derived from the brain of one week old fetuses (5 mm crown-rump length) (Fig. 4). A marked increase in the concentration of somatostatin mRNA occured between day 14 and 21 of embryonic life. No further increase in tissue concentrations of somatostatin mRNA was noted from this point onwards until adult life. Birth especially does not seem to be associated with any further increase in brain somatostatin mRNA levels. By contrat, in tissue extracts derived from stomach (or upper abdomen for 1 and 2 week old fetuses), somatostatin mRNA remained undetectable until shortly before birth. A first sharp rise in gastric somatostatin mRNA concentration occured immediately following birth. This was followed by a more gradual rise during the first weeks of postnatal life and this rise continued until adult age (Fig. 4). This difference in the developmental regulation of somatostatin gene expression may also be linked to the activity of the organs expressing the gene. The analysis of the ontogenesis of additional genes in the two tissues studied as well as the study of the ontogenesis of somatostatin gene expression in additional neural and gut-endocrine tissues will help to clarify these issues. In view of its widespread distribution, the somatostatin system should provide an

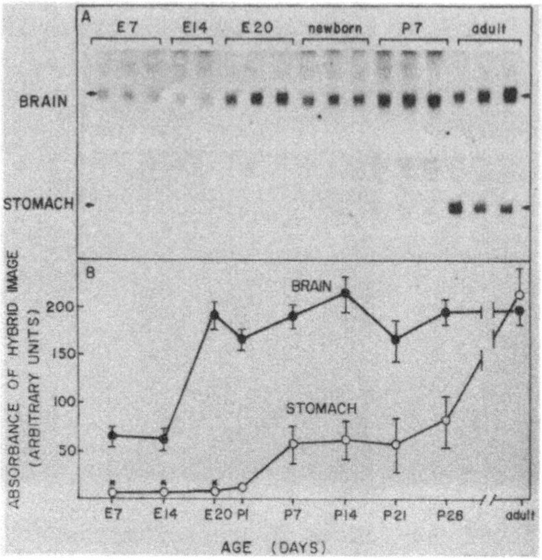

Fig. 4. (A) Preprosomatostatin mRNA in the developing rat brain and stomach determined by RNA blot hybridization. 48 μg RNA extracted from brain (upper row) and stomach (lower row) of rats of the indicated ages was electrophoresed in each lane and hybridized to a labeled preprosomatostatin cDNA probe.
(B) Plot of preprosomatostatin mRNA concentrations in rat brain and stomach as a function of age. The blot illustrated in "A" as well as two additional blots were quantitatively analyzed by densitometric scanning and the averaged data were plotted. Each point, therefore, represents the mean ± SE of 3-6 independent measurements.
Asterisks denote levels of mRNA which were below the detection limits of the assay used.

interesting model system for further studies on the developmental regulation of gene expression.

REFERENCES

1. Hobart P, Crawford R, Shen L-P, Pictet R, Rutter WJ 1980 Cloning and sequence analysis of cDNAs encoding two distinct somatostatin precursors found in the endocrine pancreas of anglerfish. Nature 288:137.
2. Taylor WL, Collier KJ, Deschenes RJ, Weith HL, Dixon JE 1981 Sequence analysis of a cDNA coding for a pancreatic precursor to somatostatin. Proc Natl Acad Sci (USA) 78:6694.

3. Goodman RH, Jacobs JW, Dee PC, Habener JF 1981 Somatostatin-28 encoded in a cloned cDNA obtained from a rat medullary thyroid carcinoma. J Biol Chem 257:1156.
4. Shen L-P, Pictet RL, Rutter WJ 1982 Human somatostatin I: sequence of the cDNA. Proc Natl Acad Sci (USA) 79:4575.
5. Noe BD, Fletcher DJ, Bauer GE, Weir GC, Patel YC 1978 Somatostatin biosynthesis occurs in pancreatic islets. Endocrinology 102:1675.
6. Noe BD, Fletcher DJ, Spiess J 1979 Evidence for the existence of a biosynthetic precursor for somatostatin. Diabetes 28:724.
7. Patzelt C, Tager HS, Carroll RJ, Steiner D 1980 Identification of prosomatostatin in pancreatic islets. Proc Natl Acad Sci (USA) 77:2410.
8. Yamada T, Basinger S 1982 Biosynthesis of somatostatin-like immunoreactivity by frog retinas in vitro. J Neurochem 39:1539.
9. Harmar A, Ivell R, Keen P 1982 The de novo biosynthesis of somatostatin and a related peptide in isolated rat dorsal root ganglia. Brain Res 242:365.
10. Robbins RJ, Reichlin S 1983 Somatostatin biosynthesis by cerebral cortical cells in monolayer culture. Endocrinology 113:574.
11. Zingg HH, Patel YC 1982 Biosynthesis of immunoreactive somatostatin by hypothalamic neurons in culture. J Clin Invest 70:1101.
12. Franco-Bourland RE, Fernstrom JD 1981 In vivo biosynthesis of L-[^{35}S]Cys-Arginine vasopressin, -oxytocin, and -somatostatin: rapid estimation using reversed phase high pressure liquid chromatography. Endocrinology 109:1097.
13. Van Itallie CM, Fernstrom JD 1983 In vivo studies of somatostatin-14 and somatostatin-28 biosynthesis in rat hypothalamus. Endocrinology 113:1210.
14. Van Itallie CM, Fernstrom JD 1982 Hypothalamic somatostatin-14 and -28 biosynthesis: effects of anesthetics and hypophysectomy. Brain Res 249:177.
15. Shields D 1980 In vitro biosynthesis of fish islet preprosomatostatin: evidence of processing and segregation of a high molecular weight precursor. Proc Natl Acad Sci (USA) 77:4074.
16. Goodman RH, Lund PK, Jacobs JW, Habener JF 1980 Preprosomatostatins. J Biol Chem 255:6549.
17. Warren TG, Shields D 1982 Cell-free biosynthesis of somatostatin precursor: Evidence for multiple forms of preprosomatostatin. Proc Natl Acad Sci (USA) 79:3729.
18. Joseph-Bravo P, Charli JL, Sherman T, Boyer H, Bolivar F, McKelvy JF 1980 Identification of a putative hypothalamic mRNA coding for somatostatin and of its product in cell-free translation. Biochem Biophys Res Commun 94:1004.
19. Ivell R, Richter D 1982 In vitro messenger ribonucleic acid directed synthesis and processing of an immunologically identified precursor to tetradecapeptide somatostatin from bovine hypothalamus. Biochemistry 21:1204.

20. Goodman RH, Lund PK, Barnett FH, Habener JF 1981 Intestinal preprosomatostatin. J Biol Chem 256:1499.
21. Funckes CL, Minth CD, Deschenes MM, Tavianini MA, Sheets M, Collier K, Weith HL, Aron DC, Roos BA, Dixon JE 1983 Cloning and characterization of a mRNA-encoding rat preprosomatostatin.
22. Green R, Shields D 1984 Sodium butyrate stimulates somatostatin production by cultured cells. Endocrinology 114:1990.
23. Zingg HH, Goodman RH, Habener JF 1984 Developmental expression of the rat somatostatin gene. Endocrinology 115:90.

BIOSYNTHESIS OF SOMATOSTATIN

PANEL DISCUSSION

MODERATOR: J. HABENER

DR. J. HABENER (Boston): I have a couple of comments of a general nature aimed at providing a summary of what we have heard this morning which might point out some of the areas that I am sure all of you are thinking about. Starting with the gene, some of the questions are (1) why are there so many somatostatin genes and why aren't they carried through in evolution? In the fish it appears that there are at least 3 genes. In the mammal, all indications are that there is only one, although Bill Rutter mentioned that this may not necessarily prove to be true. What's happened to the fish genes in the course of evolution and why are they in the fish and not in higher mammals? (2) The second question concerns the regulation region. In addition to the canonical regulators, TATA and CAT we've got tissue specific regulator-enhancers, -and then metabolic regulators that are specific for the expression of specific genes. How does the somatostatin gene fit into this picture with this nicely conserved sequence very closely located upstream from the TATA sequence? Interestingly, notably absent in the somatostatin gene expression appears to be splicing variations of the transcript which we have seen in a number of neuropeptide encoding genes. Why is this the case? It seems to be a fairly simple gene with one intervening sequence which notably does not divide the bioactive peptides, somatostatin-28 and somatostatin-14. (3) Getting to the level of translational and posttranslational processing, we ask why are there two forms of somatostatin, somatostatin-14 and -28? Why is there a long N-terminal peptide, the propeptide? Does it have any function? Does the somewhat surprising conservation in this sequence between fish and mammals mean anything? And now the more interesting aspect that Jack Dixon has brought up, the glycosylation, at least of the catfish somatostatin-22 molecule. What is the significance of this event? What I would like to do now is open the discussion to the audience. We can take questions either directed specifically to a given speaker or any general questions, and we will try to answer them.

DR. R. BENOIT (Montreal): Dr. Rutter, what will be the criteria if a second somatostatin gene was found in the human or in the rat for determining whether it is indeed a second somatostatin gene and not just a member of a family of genes coding for different peptides? What is not clear in my mind is where do we draw the line between a second gene for somatostatin and, for example, in terms of peptides that are very close together like VIP, glucagon, and other peptides, when we can be sure that we are really dealing with a second gene.

DR. W. RUTTER (San Francisco): I assume that question is directed to me. Well, at the trivial level, a second gene means a second gene, right? But at a rather more meaningful level, there is a continuum, isn't there? - between a gene that has exactly the same function and presumably operates with the same receptor, and another set of genes that have different functions, and different receptors that are easily distinguishable. Now the point that I was trying to make with respect to the two kinds of somatostatins in anglerfish - is, at least by that one assay using a human system, that it appeared that the receptors for the two cell types for glucagon and insulin respectively saw those two molecules differently, even though they are quite homologous structurally. It suggested that because they had different functional attributes, they should be recognized as a separate gene. Now if you talk about a gene family, one can think of a gene family in terms of a whole set of genes having identical functions: for example, we know that in the rat, there are a total of nine different amylase genes having exactly the same function, and 4 of those operate out of the salivary gland and liver, and three of them from the pancreas, but there is no difference functionally between those genes, etc. That's part of an amylase family. On the other hand, there is a broader family of genes which have completely different functions and include a lot of those subsets. For example, if you take the serine-proteinase family, the trypsin-like family, as you know there are now at least ten different specialized forms of those genes. So, if you just generalize that concept and apply it to hormones, then I would be presenting a case that there is a good physiological reason for more than one type of somatostatin, because of its manifold physiological purposes. It is for sure that there is more than one kind of gene in the fish and we would love to see rather more specific physiological data to support the genetic data on that. In the case of higher organisms, as everybody says, we draw a blank, and we draw a blank either because there is only a single gene that does the job or we draw a blank because we don't have yet the right probes to select the other gene in the family which have different functions. We simply don't know the answer to that.

DR. J. ENSINCK (Seattle): I was fascinated by the evidence that Jack Dixon had on glycosylation of the peptides. Is there any evidence that (a) this is a rate limiting phenomenon? (b), is there any variation in the biological activity as you glycosylate the peptide?

DR. J. DIXON (West Lafayette): There really are two questions here. We would think that on the basis of the fact that we have actually never seen, or should say, we have not isolated any non-glycosylated forms of somatostatin-22, that glycosylation certainly would not be a rate limiting step. To say that another way, there appears to be a spectrum of these molecules, some of which contain the two sugars that I mentioned, and at least two others that contain sialic acid that are linked in different ways, so I would think that if the glycosylation appeared to be a rate-determining step, we would find appreciable concentrations of maybe the non-glycosylated forms. In regards to their biological activities, I can only give you an answer that really comes from some preliminary results that we have done as well as some results from Alan Permutt's lab. As you may remember, he isolated somatostatin-22, and indeed tested it in a similar way to that which Bill Rutter mentioned, i.e. using a rat pancreatic cell culture system to look at the activities of somatostatin-22. In that situation it is at least a 100-fold less efficient than the corresponding 14 (S-14) in eliciting the spectrum of biological activities. In collaboration with Patti Hinkle we have also looked at this in the GH_3 cell system for growth hormone modulation and again find that catfish somatostatin-22 is far less active. Now, if I was to speculate on actually what I think is going on here, I think this is related to the first question in part. I think what we are actually seeing is another somatostatin whose function we clearly haven't defined yet. I draw the analogy between the sequences of CCK and gastrin where there are substantial overlaps in certain parts of the amino acid sequence and where the physiology clearly indicates that they perform two similar but distinct functions and I would suspect that would be the case for 22 and 14, but we don't have any evidence for that specifically.

DR. J. HABENER: I would like to expand on that just a moment. I gather this is O-linked sugar, since it's on threonine. Do you know if anybody has looked at the posttranslational processing in cell free systems by translation of the somatostatin-22 message to see if it is actually glycosylated by microsomes?

DR. J. DIXON: The answer to that question is no.

DR. R. ROBBINS (Denver): I have a question directed to both Goodman and Shields in regard to their very elegant demonstrations that a gene can express somatostatin in cells that don't ordinarily express it. The question is related to the biological expression of a peptide in regard to the proteases that process the prohormone. We found in our secretion studies that in general, the kinds of peptides that a cell secretes is closely related to the kinds of peptides that are found intracellularly. And we have always had the bias that what is inside of a cell is generally the kind of peptide that is going to be secreted for instance, from the hypothalamus or from the gut whether it is S-14 or S-28. Since these two forms deliver slightly different biological messages to the target cell, we are wondering whether it is in the proteases that process the prohormone that the signal for a particular cleavage lies, or whether it is the kind of secretagogue that determines which peptide comes out. So my question to Dick and to Dennis is whether or not the proteases that can process prosomatostatin to S-14 or S-28 are present in all cells and whether or not this is a nonspecific level of enzymatic processing or whether these types of enzymes are specific to certain kinds of cells and convey a biologically important message.

DR. D. SHIELDS (New York): Okay, if I could address at least one or two aspects of that. We were surprised when we put the anglerfish preprosomatostatin into the COS cells (if I didn't point out, these are originally derived from African green monkey kidney cells or derivative of that line) to see that in fact the prosomatostatin was converted to the mature hormone. This is because in transfection experiments where other genes have been put into these cells, for example, hemagglutinating protein which is cleaved into two subunits at tetrabasic amino acids, this cleavage doesn't occur. In the case of somatostatin though, we have seen cleavage, of the anglerfish prosomatostatin I down to S-14 on many different occasions, so we believe it's not nonspecific. This suggests that there may be a very low level of processing enzyme activity in all cells. In cells specialized for producing large amounts of peptide hormones, perhaps we see just an enhancement of what may be an endogenous low level in all cells. I should point out that we only see somatostatin-14 produced off the preprosomatostatin-I and that is quite consistent with Bryan Noe's finding that, in fact the anglerfish preprosomatostatin-I gives rise to S-14, whereas preprosomatostatin-II gives rise to anglerfish S-28. We haven't seen any anglerfish S-28 in these transfected cells, so I think whatever processing we are seeing, is specific.

DR. R. GOODMAN (Boston): Our results are consistent with what Dennis was talking about. In the pituitary cells which are making somatostatin, and these again appear to be entirely or almost entirely gonadotrophs, there is processing to both S-28 and S-14. In addition, there is very clearly a difference between the processing patterns between these pituitary cells, and say, liver or kidneys, or other cells that we have looked at. So, it does seem as though there is some specificity in terms of cell type for which cells have the ability to process completely, and that the pituitary has absolutely none of the large forms of somatostatin. The other thing which is peculiar to me is that luteinizing hormone which is clearly made by the gonadotrophs as well, isn't cleaved at those basic sequences. We just haven't worked out what the meaning of all this is. We are in the process of trying to demonstrate whether the somatostatin is actually in the same secretory granules as LH is, indicating that it would be exposed to the same enzymes. We really don't have that information yet.

DR. W. RUTTER: Maybe I can make a comment about that as well, not from studies of somatostatin but from studies with the insulin gene. There, Laub and others in my laboratory have done rather extensive studies in COS cells of expression of the insulin gene, and there we see very little if any processing of the insulin gene, the removal of the connecting peptide, etc. On the other hand, if one uses that same system in the ACTH-producing AtT-20 cells, as Moore and Kelly have done with the system we provided them, one gets precise processing and gets only the production of insulin. Now the COS cell is derived from the kidney cell which is in fact a secretory cell, as you well know, and it's not surprising that such a secretory cell would have some amount of a cleavage enzyme that is there. Unfortunately though, the complicating aspect about SV 40 is that under the usual circumstances and, this is an indirect question to Dennis, under the usual circumstances, the cells at high levels of expression begin to lyse so that any trypsin-like molecule found in the medium could adventitiously lyse the product such that you would get that product.

DR. D. SHIELDS: I actually had anticipated that somebody like Bill would ask me that question. What you say is quite true, that the cells can lyse and therefore one can be looking at a non-specific proteolytic event. We have done a number of controls which suggest that at least in the time courses that we are using for these experiments, that in fact is not the case. If we synthesize prosomatostatin in a cell-free system by adding microsomal membranes and then take that material and add it to the culture medium containing COS cells and then take that material and analyse it by HPLC we see only prosomatostatin; we don't see conversion to the mature hormone over the time course of these experiments. Over very long time courses, far longer than what we have been using, there is a little bit of degradation, but then the degradation we see is entirely non-specific and we see a whole random selection of peptides. We don't see any peptides which coelute with somatostatin- 14. So, I think that what we are seeing is specific but I should point out, and, as Bill mentioned, it's a relatively inefficient processing in COS cells and certainly far less efficient than seen by R. Kelly in AtT-20 cells.

DR. Y.C. PATEL (Montreal): I want to pursue the catfish somatostatin story a little bit further with Jack Dixon. It seems to me that the catfish somatostatin-22 molecule is a crucial intermediate in the evolutionary development of S-28, the mammalian form as we know it. This molecule is present in large amounts in the catfish pancreas. It seems to be structurally very different from the mammalian 28 variety. We have heard that in the anglerfish pancreas, the mature product of the second prosomatostatin is a 28 amino acid peptide (anglerfish S-28) which is more closely related in structure to the mammalian S-28 molecule. Like its mammalian counterpart, anglerfish S-28 appears to have strong insulin-selective inhibitory effects in the pancreas based on the data that Bill Rutter has just presented. And yet the mammalian pancreas is remarkable for its very low levels of S-28. There are only small quantities of S-28 present in this tissue, so understanding the biological activity of catfish S-22 should provide us with some insights into the potential functional role of S-28 in the human or mammalian pancreas. The reported bioassay data on catfish S-22 shows that it does not have much activity. However, it is not clear whether the earlier bioassays were carried out with natural catfish S-22 or with synthetic material based on the Oyama sequence which we now know to be incorrect. My questions are as follows: (1) have you tested your catfish S-22 molecule for such biological activities as insulin suppression and (2) do you find using immunocytochemical localization studies against catfish S-22 that you can identify different subsets of islet cells containing either the 14 form or the 22 form?

DR. J. DIXON: Let me begin by saying that although the original report regarding the sequence was in fact incorrect in two of the residues, there is absolutely no doubt in my mind that the peptide that Bradshaw, Permutt, Oyama, and colleagues characterized, was in fact the same molecule that we have dealt with, which reflects on your question, have people really tested the biological activity? I think, in fact, the materials that have been used are the naturally occurring glycosylated forms of somatostatin and not a synthetic peptide. My personal bias is that that group had in fact a glycosylated somatostatin as we do. The other thing I want to mention is that we have reasonable quantities of most of the somatostatin- 22s that I mentioned, in various glycosylated forms. Our lab is not really a physiology lab but we would be happy to make these materials available to anyone that would like to test them. The material that we sent to Patti Hinkle was in fact the glycosylated material and it has biological activities that are at least 100 times lower than those of S-14. In regards to the immunochemical localization experiments, we have carried out some studies with Al Floyds who is down at I.U. Medical School. I think those are very interesting because they clearly point out two or three important things. (1) Somatostatin-14 and somatostatin-22 are present in very distinctly different types of cells. (2) Somatostatin-22 is almost always found in cells that one can find descriptions of in the literature as so-called "poorly fixed" cells or "vacuolated cells." I can show you some slides later of these if you'd like. (3) A reasonably large percentage of the time, one sees somatostatin-22 and somatostatin-14 cells in juxtaposition to one another.

DR. J. HABENER: We need some volunteer physiologist from the audience to take Jack up on his offer to find out what is the real target cell of somatostatin-22, the correct glycosylated form.

DR. G. WEIR (Richmond): I wanted to ask Dr. Goodman a question. I was fascinated in the demonstration that the somatostatin gene could be introduced into the ovum and then be expressed in rats after they'd grown up and I was curious as to what these rats were like. They seem to reproduce reasonably well, which is impressive. Did they have high somatostatin levels? Did you look at the function of the endocrine pancreas? Did you look at other pituitary functions? How heavy were they, etc?

DR. R. GOODMAN: The fact that these mice were of normal size, could be categorized, I think, as a moderately disappointing result. The reason for that may be because the somatostatin receptor, as I understand it, is fairly sensitive to downregulation, and it may be that continued high levels of production of somatostatin from the time of conception basically throughout development may in fact downregulate those receptors. We haven't really looked at that directly, although it would be possible to do it. In terms of other endocrine testing, we haven't done that either. The serum levels of somatostatin in these animals are extraordinarily high; they are as high as in patients with somatostatinomas but the molecular form of the somatostatin in the plasma is predominantly a 7000 dalton form. The biological activity of this form isn't really clear. The fact that the gonadotrophs make authentic (on the basis of HPLC analysis), somatostatin-14 and 28, and presumably secrete the same two molecuels in the vicinity of growth hormone producing cells, and other pituitary cells, at least makes you think about the possibility of a biologically active form of somatostatin that we made as being present in an important area. The other puzzling aspect is that the gonadotroph cells, which seem to be uniformly expressing the somatostatin gene, are apparently normal in that these animals reproduce normally. Our initial thought the first time we saw staining in the gonadotrophs was that we had integrated into a transcriptional unit in these particular cells either in the LH gene or in some other transcriptional unit in these cells; but the fact that we see this over and over gain indicates that's probably not true; that maybe it's something related to the metallothionine promoter or possibly the DNA flanking regions which are responsible for the particular production in those cells.

DR. J. HABENER: I just might add to something that Dick said. The blood levels of somatostatin in the third generation transgenic mice were something like 1000 times the normal levels. Given that at least 1% is somatostatin-14, the levels are still 10 times the normal level and the animals have absolutely no observable phenotypic abnormalities. They're reproducing, growing, eating, etc.

DR. W. VALE (La Jolla): Can you regulate the production of this somatostatin by GnRH or sex steroids? Since LH and FSH can be dissociated at various times, can you dissociate this regulation of somatostatin secretion by the gonadotrophs?

DR. R. GOODMAN: Actually the regulation of somatostatin in these animals is by zinc or cadmium. Whether or not the regulation of production or the secretion can be modified with GnRH, I would guess would really depend on whether we find on the basis of the EM studies if LH and FSH are localized in the same secretory granules or not. If they are then I would guess that we probably could, but we haven't done those studies. It does appear as though most of the correlation, at least in our hands, for FSH staining isn't really all that good. That is, there appear to be a population of cells which are staining for LH alone but we are really not sure of that.

DR. D. SHIELDS: I would just like to ask Dick one question also on the transgenic mice in relation to processing. You said, I think if I understood it correctly, that the somatostatin that was in the liver of these transgenic mice remained as the high molecular weight prosomatostatin form and that you didn't see S-14 or S-28, is that right?

DR. R. GOODMAN: The predominant form was a 7000 dalton form but there was clearly some somatostatin-14 and somatostatin-28 made. Now the overall levels of hormone are by far the greatest in the liver. The slide which I showed was expressed on a ng/mg protein basis, so that overall most of the somatostatin made in the animals is made in the liver; but on a concentration basis the pituitary makes several orders of magnitude more. I suspect that the material which is in the plasma is predominantly originating from the liver and there are clearly all three forms there.

DR. J. HABENER: Thank you Dick. I would like to ask Hans Zingg a question, two questions actually. The first concerns the rather marked expression of the somatostatin gene in the gut at the time of birth. Is that true for the other islet hormones and GI hormones, that there is a delayed expression until birth? The second question is about the message, the hybridization band. Could you comment on the width of the hybridization band seen in the hypothalamus compared to the one observed in the intestine.

DR. H. ZINGG (Montreal): In respect to your second question we have tried to further dissociate and identify several bands within this relatively broad band of brain messenger RNA, as well as intestinal RNA. It appears on that slide that I have shown that the brain messenger RNA produces a slightly broader band than say the message isolated from the antrum. Although we have never been able to separate clearly two different bands of brain messenger RNA, my hunch would be that it is rather a continuum of probably different lengths of messenger RNA which could be due to heterogeneity in the poly A tail rather than two distinct populations of messenger RNA. As to your first question, I think that as far as I am aware, insulin has been detected within the pancreas before birth in embryonic animals. It is also interesting to compare the data of messenger RNA with the data on somatostatin-like immunoreactivity which indicates that already at day seven, messenger RNA has been detected at an age when the peptide hasn't been detected yet; so there might be a nonparallelism between the appearance of the messenger RNA and the peptide which would imply that there might be additional steps, not only transcriptional steps that regulate the developmental expression of somatostatin as well as of insulin and glucagon.

DR. J. HABENER: One possible explanation for the apparent heterogeneity in the message might be multiple transcriptional initiation sites, given the peculiar nature of the promoter region. Bill, would you have something you might add?

DR. W. RUTTER: I had a similar reaction due to the data of Dr. Zingg, and because of the relative importance of the possibility of multiple species in the brain it seems to me it would be very useful to carry out primary extension experiments where the precise 5' terminus could be located and quantified.

DR. H. ZINGG: I would just like to add a provocative question to the data that Dick Goodman showed us with his very high levels of somatostatin, even if only a small percentage of that somatostatin is biologically active. If he had done the same experiment say with glucagon or with insulin I think these animals would have been in such a shape that he would have had to be very quick in his experiments in order to get some tissues out of the living animal. Dick Goodman's experiments then lead us to the somewhat provocative conclusion that at least circulating somatostatin is perhaps not as important as we thought initially. Furthermore, is somatostatin in itself a hormone necessary for survival?

DR. J. HABENER: Which points to perhaps its major role as being an intercellular regulator and perhaps also a lumone?

II

BIOSYNTHESIS AND PROCESSING OF SOMATOSTATIN

5

SOMATOSTATIN-14 LIKE IMMUNOREACTIVE FORMS IN THE RAT: CHARACTERIZATION, DISTRIBUTION AND BIOSYNTHESIS

YOGESH C. PATEL, HANS H. ZINGG AND C. B. SRIKANT

Fraser Laboratories, McGill Univ. Depts. of Medicine, and Neurology and Neurosurgery, Royal Victoria Hospital

Montreal Neurological Inst., Montreal, Quebec, Canada

Tetradecapeptide somatostatin (S-14) was the original form of somatostatin to be isolated (1). The majority of antisera raised against this molecule are directed against the central and C-terminal segments (2) and detect, in addition to S-14, higher mol wt N-terminally extended forms, of which the two principal ones correspond to somatostatin-28 (S-28) and prosomatostatin (pro-S) (Fig. 1). Somatostatin forms detected as S-14 like immunoreactivity (S-14 LI) in mammalian tissues consist of S-14, S-28, pro-S, [des Ala^1]S-14 (S-13, the principal biologically active circulating metabolite of S-14), and somatostatin-25. The latter species was isolated from ovine hypothalamus along with S-28 but is now generally believed to be a degradation product rather than a naturally occurring somatostatin peptide.

Based on structural studies of the isolated peptide or cDNA sequence analyses, the exact sequence of S-14 is now known to occur in ovine, porcine, bovine and rat hypothalamus, in rat, human, pigeon, chicken and fish pancreas, and in the rat thyroid (1, 3-12). The S-28 structure has been shown to be common to ovine, porcine and bovine hypothalamus, porcine gut, human pancreas, and rat thyroid (4, 7, 11-16). The exact mammalian S-28 structure has not been confirmed in lower species. Two closely related 28 amino acid peptides, however, have recently been isolated from chicken hypothalamus and anglerfish pancreas respectively (10, 17). The avian form differs in only one amino acid from mammalian S-28 (leucine substituting for methionine), whereas the fish peptide differs by 9 amino acids. At the present time, little is known about the immunoreactivity of these two new molecules in S-14 LI RIA systems, although theoretically the Leu form of S-28 should exhibit the same reactivity

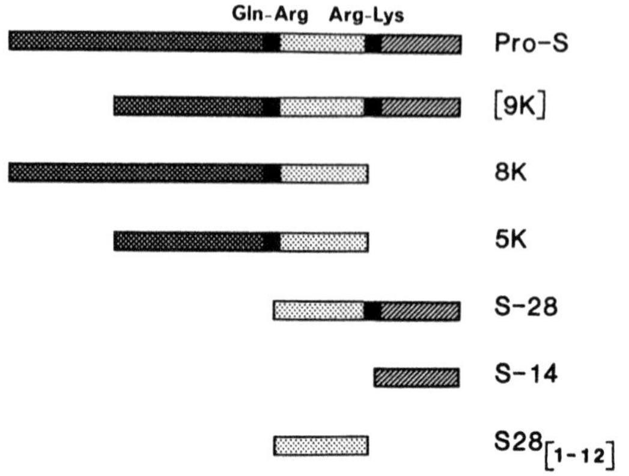

Fig. 1. Mammalian prosomatostatin and its cleavage products.

as the mammalian [Met] S-28 form. Further comparative animal studies need to be undertaken to establish the precise time of evolution of the mammalian form of S-28. Although the occurrence of S-14 LI in invertebrate species has been increasingly reported (18), the molecular nature of this material has not been adequately characterized.

Molecular Heterogeneity of Tissue Pro-S

In recent studies, we have shown that the very high mol wt form of S-14 LI corresponding to pro-S is heterogeneous, consisting of two forms of approximate mol wt 12,000 (12K) and 9,000 (9K) which can be readily separated on Sephadex G-75 columns. This heterogeneity is best exemplified by the hypothalamus as illustrated in Fig. 2 which is an HPLC chromatogram of the molecular forms of S-14 LI in an acetic acid extract of 10 freshly obtained rat hypothalami. S-14 LI was determined by RIA of the eluting fractions. Four peaks were identified, two of which correspond to synthetic S-14 and S-28. The remaining two peaks which together comprised ∿5% of the total hypothalamic S-14 LI, were found on rechromatography on Sephadex G-75 columns to have mol wts of 12,000 and 9,000 respectively. When assayed in serial dilutions, immunorectivity from the two peaks exhibited parallelism of the dose response curves with synthetic S-14. For convenience, the two forms will be referred to as pro-S (A) the 12K form, and pro-S (B) the 9K form. Heterogeneity of the pro-S related immunoreactivity in gel filtration studies has been previously observed by other investigators as well, but not fully characterized. Lauber et al. (19) reported the presence of 15,000 and 10,000 mol wt forms of S-14 LI in HCl-urea extracts of mouse hypothalami. Robbins and Reichlin observed similar heterogeneity of very high mol wt (>10,000) S-14 LI in tissue and media from cultured cerebrocortical cells (20).

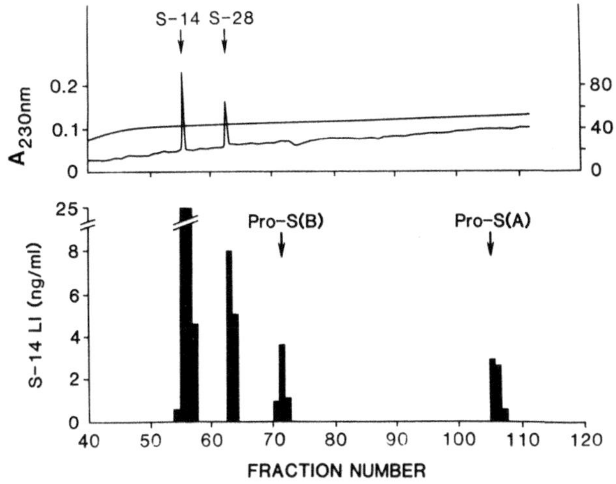

Fig. 2. HPLC chromatogram of S-14 LI forms in rat hypothalamic extracts. A C-18 reverse phase column was eluted with 8-50% acetonitrile - 0.2% HFBA gradient. Fractions were monitored for S-14 LI by RIA. The upper panel shows the elution position of synthetic S-14 and S-28 detected spectrophotometrically.

Since the rat pro-S sequence contains a typical glycosylation site at residues 37-39, we wondered whether N-linked glycosylation could explain the size difference between pro-S (A) and pro-S (B). To investigate this, 6-12 pmol of HPLC purified pro-S (A) and pro-S (B) were reacted with a Concanavilin A-Sepharose column specifically eluted with a gradient of α-D-methylmannoside (0-0.5 M). Neither form exhibited specific binding to Concanavilin A-Sepharose thus excluding N-glycosidic linkage of an oligosaccharide chain to the asparagine residue at position 37 of pro-S. Similar absence of glycosylation of bovine hypothalamic pro-S and mouse hypothalamic pro-S has been previously observed (21, 22).

To determine whether pro-S (B) is a product of the enzymatic cleavage of pro-S (A) the processing of pro-S (A) by hypothalamic enzymes was investigated. HPLC purified pro-S (A) material was incubated at 37 C, pH 7.4 with a hypothalamic extract from which endogenous S-14 LI had been removed by affinity chromatography. Analysis of the incubation mixture on Sephadex G-75 columns showed a progressive, time-dependent conversion of pro-S (A) (KD 0.23) to pro-S (B) (KD 0.35). This suggests that pro-S (B) is derived by enzymatic cleavage of pro-S (A) and probably represents an N-terminally shortened form of pro-S (A).

Biological Activity of Prosomatostatin

The potential biological activity of the two pro- forms was explored using a radioreceptor assay. In this assay, the ability of the two pro-S fractions to interact with brain membrane S-14 receptors was examined and compared with the binding potencies of the S-28 peak from HPLC and synthetic S-14 standards. HPLC purified hypothalamic S-28 material showed a reduced binding potency compared to S-14 as also previously demonstrated for synthetic S-28 in this radioreceptor assay system (23). Both pro-S forms exhibited dose-dependent inhibition of radioligand binding to membrane S-14 receptors. The dilution slope of pro-S (B) was parallel to that of S-14 and S-28. Its binding potency was 7% of that of S-14 and 12% of that of S-28. Pro-S (A) appeared to interact more strongly than pro-S (B) with S-14 receptors but its inhibition curve was non-parallel with that of S-14. These data coupled with the published findings of Spiess and Vale (24) who demonstrated that a 12,000 mol wt form of S-14 LI is capable of inhibiting GH secretion with a potency approximately a third that of S-14, clearly suggest that these high mol wt forms of S-14 LI are biologically active. Whether pro-S (B) is a degradation product of pro-S (A) remains to be determined. If pro-S (B) is a naturally occurring form then the biosynthetic relationships between pro-S (A) and pro-S (B) and their biological functions other than as precursors need to be elucidated.

Tissue Distribution of S-14 LI Forms

S-14 LI in acetic acid extracts of rat tissues elutes from Sephadex G-50 columns as 3 peaks corresponding to S-14, S-28, and a 12K form (referred to as pro-S). This material is heterogeneous as indicated above but the two forms, pro-S (A) and pro-S (B) cannot be readily resolved by G-50 chromatography. As depicted in Fig. 3, S-14 is a predominant form in all neural tissues and virtually the exclusive form in the retina and peripheral nerves. The relative abundance of S-14, S-28 and pro-S material in the whole brain and spinal cord, expressed as a percent of total S-14 LI, is respectively 67%, 25% and 7% (25).

A more detailed study of the regional brain distribution of the three S-14 LI forms has been carried out by Gomez et al. (26). Although S-14 was the predominant molecular species in the hypothalamus, cortex, brain stem, cerebellum, amygdala, and neurohypophysis, highly variable quantities of S-28 (5%-41%) and pro-S (3-20%) were found.

In the pancreas and stomach, S-14 accounts for 95% of total S-14 LI. Very small quantities of S-28 and pro-S are found in these tissues under a variety of physiological and experimental conditions (adult tissues, neonatal tissues, cultured islet and antral cells). On the other hand, the gut tissues distal to the stomach are rich in

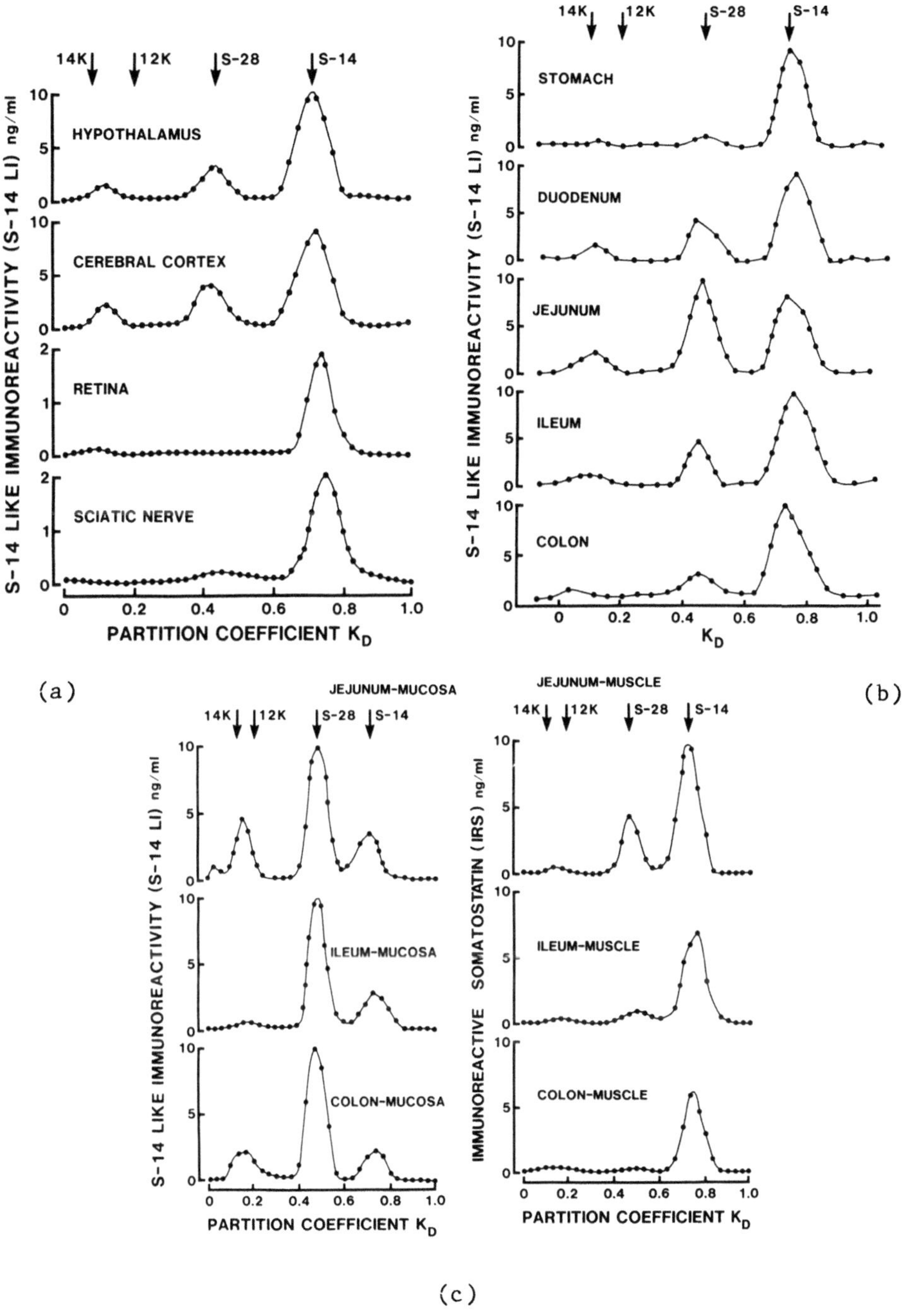

Fig. 3. Comparison of the relative abundance of immunoreactivity corresponding to pro-S, S-28 and S-14 in rat tissues (Sephadex G-50 chromatography in 6 M urea).

high mol wt forms. Within the gut, somatostatin cells are distributed either as mucosal D cells or as enteric neurons in the submucous and myenteric plexuses. Separate chromatographic analyses of the mucosa and muscle layers shows that S-28 and not S-14 is a predominant form in the mucosal D cells whereas in the enteric plexuses S-14 is the main immunoreactive species. The intestinal mucosa represents the sole rat tissue with a preponderance of S-28 relative to S-14. Only two other tissues similarly richer in S-28 than S-14 have been described. These include the guinea pig retina and some instances of human somatostatin producing tumors (27, 28).

The quantitative data to show the relative abundance of the three main forms of S-14 LI in the entire brain, gut and pancreas of the rat is summarized in Table 1. The total content of S-14 in these three organs which represent the main somatostatin containing tissues in the rat, is 1659 pmol. This value accounts for 71% of the S-14 in these tissues compared to 526 pmol or 23% for S-28 and 140 pmol or 6% for pro-S.

Secretion

All 3 forms of S-14 LI appear to be secreted *in vivo* and *in vitro* from somatostatin-producing tissues. The relative amounts of the 3 forms released acutely, in general, reflect their intracellular concentrations. In peripheral plasma and in static *in vitro* incubation systems, however, there may be a preferential accumulation of pro-S and S-28 compared to S-14 due to differential degradation of S-14 relative to the higher mol wt forms (25, 29). Immunoreactivity equivalent to S-14, S-28 and possibly pro-S has been identified in hypophyseal portal blood (30). Abdominal portal vein likewise contains each of the 3 forms in concentrations which are proportional to the relative abundance of the 3 forms in the pancreas and gut (25). The *in vitro* release of the 3 forms has been

Table 1. Relative Amounts of Total S-14 LI and of Pro-S, S-28 and S-14 SLI in Brain, Gut, Pancreas (pmol)

Organ	Total S-14 LI	Pro-S	S-28	S-14
Brain	643	45	161	437
Gut	1568	99	362	1107
Pancreas	120	2.4	2.4	115
Total (brain, gut and pancreas)	2331	146 (6%)	526 (23%)	1659 (71%)

clearly documented from fragments of median eminence and of neurohypophysis subjected to K+ stimulation, and from cultured hypothalamic and cerebrocortical cells under basal, and a variety of stimulated conditions (30, 31-33).

As expected, S-14 is virtually the exclusive form to be released from the pancreas and stomach. This has been shown using the isolated perfused pancreas, cultured islet cells, and cultured antral cells (34-37). No data are currently available on the direct assessment of the molecular forms of S-14 LI released from the intestine which abounds in S-28 and higher mol wt S-14 LI. That these forms are readily released needs to be documented.

Biosynthesis

In the fish pancreas, where much of the work on somatostatin biosynthesis has been carried out, four separate preprosomatostatins have been identified, two each in the anglerfish and catfish islets respectively (38-40). These four precursors represent products of four separate somatostatin genes. Somatostatin-14 and anglerfish S-28 are the two separate and independent products of anglerfish pro-S I and anglerfish pro-S II respectively (9, 17). The catfish precursors yield S-14 and a 22 amino acid peptide (catfish S-22) respectively as their mature products (39, 40). Recent immunocytochemical data indicate that the two anglerfish and catfish products are localized in two distinct populations of islet D cells, suggesting that each of the two anglerfish and catfish genes is expressed in separate cells (17, 41).

This situation is very different to that which pertains in mammals. All evidence so far points to a single mammalian prepro-S, which in the rat, at least, appears to be the product of a single somatostatin gene (42). The finding of distinctive patterns of tissue distribution of the S-14 LI molecular forms in the rat suggests differential processing of the single rat pro-S to S-14 and S-28 in a tissue-specific manner. It raised the possibility of several biosynthetic pathways for S-14 and S-28 synthesis as follows:

(i) pro-S → S-28 → S-14 + S-28[1-12]
(ii) pro-S → S-14
(iii) pro-S → S-28

We reasoned that pro-S could undergo sequential breakdown to S-28 and then to S-14 and the S-28[1-12] fragment. A second possibility was direct processing of S-14 from pro-S, and the third possibility was cleavage of pro-S to S-28 without further breakdown to S-14.

To investigate these different possibilities, pulse-chase studies were carried out to examine the incorporation of [^{3}H] phenylalanine into S-14 LI forms by 2 separate in vitro somatostatin-containing systems, cultured hypothalamic neurons and cultured islet cells. Dispersed neonatal rat hypothalamic cells or islet cells were cultured in monolayers and used at 2 weeks (hypothalamus), or 5-7 days (islets). An identical experimental protocol was used for both systems. Following short pulse and chase incubations, with [^{3}H]Phe, the cultured cells were scraped, extracted in acetic acid and the labelled peptides purified by adsorption to C_{18} silica cartridges. Labelled S-14 LI was isolated by affinity chromatography and the individual immunoreactive components separated on Sephadex G-50 columns in 6 M urea (43).

The results of the [^{3}H]Phe incorporation studies with the hypothalamus are depicted in Fig. 4. Following a 5 min pulse incubation, labelled S-14 LI consisted entirely of high mol wt material eluting in the position of pro-S. A more prolonged 20 min pulse incubation already showed transfer of radioactivity from the pro-S peak region to S-14 without the formation of S-28. During a 20 min chase period, further transfer of radioactivity to S-14 occurred concomitant with the appearance of a small peak corresponding to S-28.

In the case of islet cells, almost identical findings were elicited. After a 30 min pulse incubation, [^{3}H]Phe S-14 LI was resolved into 3 peaks corresponding to pro-S, S-28, and S-14 (ratio 75:5:20) consistent with the early synthesis of S-14. During subsequent chase (30 min) the ratio altered to 30:5:65 due to transfer of the radioactivity from the high mol wt pro-S region. A small peak co-chromatographing with S-28 was seen early as well but its size remained unaltered during chase.

These findings in the hypothalamus and pancreas illustrate two important points. First, that S-14 can be processed directly from pro-S in both the hypothalamus and islets and that this pathway may be the main route for S-14 synthesis in these two tissues, and second that there does not appear to be any precursor-product relationship between S-28 and S-14. Indeed, the two peptides appear to be synthesized independently. Similar conclusions have been reached by Robbins et al. (44) and by Van Itallie and Fernstrom (45). In the former study, cultured rat cerebrocortical cells were shown to synthesize S-14 almost entirely from a 11,500 mol wt precursor (pro-S), and not via S-28. The latter group investigated the in vivo biosynthesis of S-14 and S-28 in the rat hypothalamus after injection of [^{35}S]cysteine into the 3rd ventricle. The time course of incorporation of the radioactivity into S-14 and S-28 reached a maximum simultaneously, once again excluding a clear precursor-product relationship between them and suggesting independent synthesis of the two peptides.

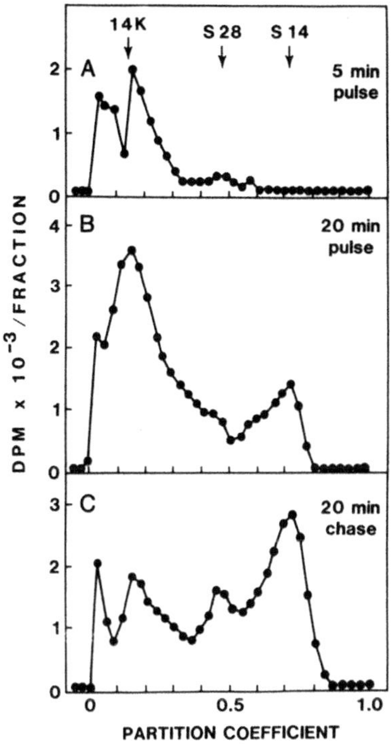

Fig. 4. Elution profile on Sephadex G-50 of labelled S-14 LI purified from hypothalamic cell extracts following pulse-chase studies. 20 dishes were incubated with [^{3}H]phenylalanine for either 5 min (A) or 20 min (B and C). In C, the pulse period was followed by a 20 min chase period. Pro-S elutes from this column close to the void volume at a position ($K_D = 0.15$) corresponding to Mr = 14,000 (14K SLI).

If direct processing is important it should theoretically generate a molecule equivalent to pro-S without the S-14 sequence. In an attempt to identify such a molecule, we analysed by gel chromatography, acetic acid extracts of hypothalamus and pancreas for S-28[1-12]like immunoreactive forms using a radioimmunoassay directed towards the 1-12 region of the S-28[1-12] sequence. This assay detects S-28[1-12], S-28, and pro-S and should theoretically recognize our postulated high mol wt forms bearing the S-28[1-12]but not the S-14 sequence (2) (Figs. 1, 5A). On Sephadex G-75 columns (data not shown), two high mol wt peaks of S-28[1-12]LI were identified in hypothalamic extracts eluting at $K_D = 0.23$ (M_r = 12,000), and $K_D = 0.35$ (M_r = 9,000). These 2 peaks comprised respectively 20% and 4% of the total immunoreactivity. The remaining immunoreactivity eluted as a broad peak from K_D 0.5 to K_D 0.8 which was heterogeneous and overlapped the elution positions of S-28 and S-28[1-12].

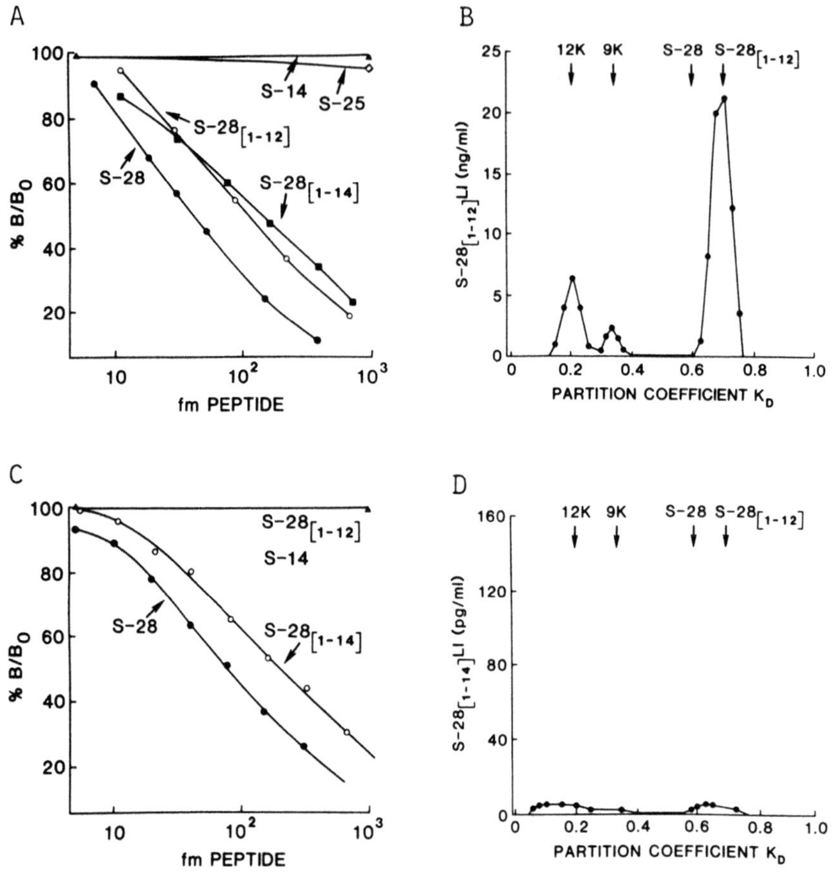

Fig. 5. Elution profiles of S-28[1-12] LI (panel B) and S-28[1-14] LI (panel D) in hypothalamic extracts after removal of S-14 LI by affinity chromatography. Three peaks of S-28[1-12] LI were present corresponding to Mr = 12,000 (12K), Mr = 9,000 (9K) and synthetic S-28[1-12]. The 12K and 9K forms were unreactive as S-28[1-14]LI suggesting that they contained the S-28[1-12] sequence but were devoid of the S-28[13-14] and S-14 sequence. A Sephadex G-75 column was eluted with 6 M urea. Panels A and C illustrate the properties of the RIAs for S-28[1-12]LI (panel A) and S-28[1-14]LI (panel C) used for monitoring column fractions in B and D respectively.

Although the two high mol wt peaks (K_D = 0.23, K_D = 0.35) eluted in the identical positions of pro-S (A) and pro-S (B) and thus could not be distinguished from them, simultaneous measurements of immunoreactivity in these two peaks both as S-28[1-12]LI and as S-14 LI showed that the amount of S-28[1-12]LI in these peaks was greatly in excess of that which could be accounted for by coeluting pro-S (A) and pro-S (B). In order to analyse this material further, and show that it is distinct from pro-S (A) and pro-S (B), S-28[1-12]LI in hypothalamic extracts was characterized following initial removal of all S-14 LI (i.e. pro-S (A), pro-S (B), S-28, S-14) from the extracts by affinity chromatography using S-14 LI antibodies immobilized on an Affigel-10 column. The elution pattern on Sephadex G-75 column of hypothalamic S-28[1-12]LI after removal of S-14 LI is depicted in Fig. 5B. Three peaks of immunoreactivity were identified eluting at K_D = 0.23, K_D = 0.35, and K_D = 0.8 corresponding to the two previously identified 12,000 and 9,000 mol wt peptides, and synthetic S-28[1-12]. For additional characterization, the affinity purified S-28[1-12] fractions in Fig. 5B were assayed using a separate radioimmunoassay directed against S-28[1-14]. This assay (Fig. 5C) does not recognize S-28[1-12] and thus requires the dibasic amino acid Arg-Lys hinge in S-28 to be intact. As expected, it will detect pro-S. A comparison of the 2 profiles shows that the 2 high mol wt forms are detected only as S-28[1-12]LI (Fig. 5B) and not as S-28[1-12]LI (Fig. 5D) providing strong immunochemical evidence that these two high mol wt forms are devoid of the -Arg-Lys-S-14 sequence. Both forms were found in high concentrations in the pancreas as well (46). Our present speculation is that they represent end products resulting from the direct processing of the two pro-S forms to S-14. Benoit et al. have recently reported in preliminary form the isolation and sequencing of 2 novel S-28[1-12] containing peptides from the rat hypothalamus (47). The larger of these two molecules is a 76 amino acid peptide (8K peptide) which represents the whole pro-S sequence without -Arg-Lys-S-14. The smaller of the two molecules contains 44 amino acids and has the S-28[1-12] sequence at its C-terminus. It represents the 8K form from which a 32 amino acid N-terminal segment has been removed by cleavage at a Leu-Leu bond. These findings shed some light on the possible nature of the pro-S (B) molecule identified in our studies. Given the size difference between pro-S (A) and pro-S (B), the latter molecule most likely represents the full prosomatostatin molecule without the N-terminal 32 amino acid segment cleaved at the Leu-Leu bond. Verification of this will require additional N-terminal sequence analysis of pro-S (B).

If direct processing of pro-S → S-14 is the main pathway for S-14 synthesis, it leaves unexplained the finding of high concentrations of the S-28[1-12] fragment in the pancreas and hypothalamus recently reported by Benoit and others, which could be argued as providing evidence for cleavage of S-28 → S-14 + S-28[1-12] (32, 46, 48). On the other hand, it is conceivable that S-28[1-12]

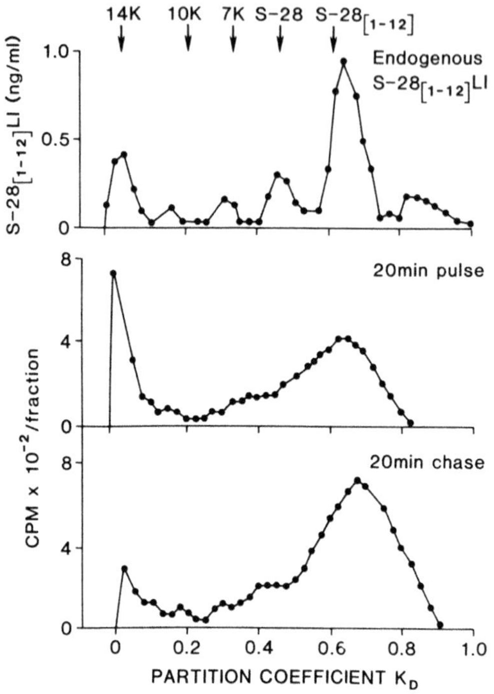

Fig. 6. Elution profile on Sephadex G-50 of [^{35}S] methionine labelled S-28[1-12]LI purified from hypothalamic cell extracts following pulse-chase studies. 20 dishes were incubated with [^{35}S] methionine for 20 min (pulse, middle panel) followed by a 20 min chase period (lower panel). The upper panel shows for comparison the molecular forms of unlabelled S-28[1-12]LI in hypothalamic extracts measured by RIA.

may be cleaved from the 8K and 5K S-28[1-12]LI form. To investigate these relationships further, pulse-chase studies with [^{35}S] methionine were carried out in the hypothalamus. [^{35}S] labelled S-28[1-12] like forms were isolated by affinity chromatography using antibody R21 (Fig. 5, upper left panel) and characterized on Sephadex G-50 columns. Following a 20 min pulse incubation (Fig. 6, middle panel), radioactivity was incorporated into a high mol wt peak which appeared heterogeneous and probably consisted of a mixture of the two pro-S forms and the 8K and 5K S-28[1-12] like forms which are indistinguishable from pro-S by G-50 chromatography. A peak coeluting with S-28[1-12] was already evident at this time and in fact comprised ∿ 50% of the total counts. During subsequent 20 min chase (Fig. 6, lower panel), this peak increased as a result of transfer of label from the high mol wt forms. A number of intermediate peaks were labelled but there was no convincing S-28 peak. These data are not sufficiently mature to provide a complete understanding of the biosynthetic relationships between the several S-28[1-12] like forms. They do suggest however, that synthesis of S-28[1-12] is rapid, occurring not from S-28, but probably from higher mol wt precursors.

CONCLUSIONS

In view of the recent emergence of several new somatostatin-like peptides, additional pulse-chase type data will be required to define the exact biosynthetic relationships between these forms. As far as the synthesis of S-14 is concerned, two important conclusions can already be drawn:

(i) the finding of large concentrations of high mol wt S-28[1-12] like forms without the S-14 sequence, as well as pulse-chase data, provide strong evidence that S-14 can be synthesized by direct processing of pro-S to S-14. This pathway appears to be an important route for S-14 synthesis in the hypothalamus and the pancreas;

(ii) S-14 could be derived through cleavage of S-28. However, the inability to demonstrate a kinetic precursor-product relationship between S-28 and S-14 suggests that this conversion is either extremely rapid, occurring within 20-30 min, or that it is relatively unimportant.

Like S-14, S-28[1-12] appears to be derived not from S-28, but from higher mol wt precursors. Finally, the question of the synthesis of S-28 remains enigmatic. In particular, whether S-28, like S-14 is an end product of the processing of pro-S needs to be determined.

ACKNOWLEDGMENTS

This work was supported by grants from the Canadian Medical Research Council (MT6196), and the NIH (AM 21373). Dr. Patel is a Scientist of the Canadian Medical Research Council and Drs. Zingg and Srikant are Chercheurs Boursiers of the F.R.S.Q.

REFERENCES

1. Brazeau P, Vale W, Burgus R, Ling N, Butcher M, Rivier J, Guillemin R 1973 Hypothalamic polypeptide that inhibits the secretion of immunoreactive growth hormone. Science 179:77.
2. Patel YC 1984 Radioimmunoassay of somatostatin related peptides. In: Pohl SL, Larner J (eds) Methods in Diabetes Research. John Wiley and Sons, Inc., New York, p 307.

3. Schally AV, Dupont A, Arimura A, Redding TW, Nishi N, Linthicum GL, Schlesinger DH 1976 Isolation and structure of somatostatin from porcine hypothalami. Biochemistry 15:509.
4. Ivell R, Richter D 1982 Fingerprint analysis of bovine hypothalamic preprosomatostatin. Identification of somatostatin-28 at the C terminus. Eur J Biochem 129:81.
5. Böhlen P, Benoit R, Ling N, Guillemin R, Brazeau P 1981 Isolation and characterization of rat hypothalamic somatostatin-14. Endocrinology 108:2008.
6. Benoit R, Böhlen P, Brazeau P, Ling N, Guillemin R 1980 Isolation and characterization of rat pancreatic somatostatin. Endocrinology 197:2127.
7. Shen L-P, Pictet RL, Rutter WJ 1982 Human somatostatin I: Sequence of the cDNA. Proc Natl Acad Sci (USA) 79:4575.
8. Spiess J, Rivier JE, Rodkey JA, Bennett CD, Vale W 1979 Isolation and characterization of somatostatin from pigeon pancreas. Proc Natl Acad Sci (USA) 76:2974.
9. Noe BD, Spiess J, Rivier JE, Vale W 1979 Isolation and characterization of somatostatin from anglerfish pancreatic islets. Endocrinology 105:1410.
10. Hasegawa Y, Miyamoto K, Nomura M, Igurashi IM, Kargawa K, Matsuo H 1984 Isolation and amino acid compositions of four somatostatin-like substances in chicken hypothalamic extract. Endocrinology 115:433.
11. Goodman RH, Aron DC, Roos BA 1982 Rat pre-prosomatostatin: Structure and processing by microsomal membranes. J Biol Chem 258:5570.
12. Funckes CL, Minth CD, Deschenes R, Magazin M, Tavianini MA, Sheets M, Collier K, Weith HL, Aron DC, Roos BA, Dixon JE 1983 Cloning and characterization of a mRNA-encoding rat preprosomatostatin. J Biol Chem 258:8781.
13. Esch F, Böhlen P, Ling N, Benoit R, Brazeau P, Guillemin R 1980 Primary structure of ovine hypothalamic somatostatin-28 and somatostatin-25. Proc Natl Acad Sci (USA) 77:6827.
14. Spiess J, Villarreal J, Vale W 1982 Isolation and sequence analysis of a somatostatin-like polypeptide from ovine hypothalamus. Biochemistry 20:1982.
15. Schally AV, Huang WY, Chang RC, Arimura A, Redding TW, Millar RP, Hunkapiller MW, Hood LE 1980 Isolation and structure of pro-somatostatin: A putative somatostatin precursor from pig hypothalamus. Proc Natl Acad Sci (USA) 77:4489.
16. Pradayrol L, Jørnvall H, Mutt V, Ribet A 1980 N-terminally extended somatostatin: The primary structure of somatostatin-28. FEBS Lett 109:55.
17. Noe BD, Debo G, Spiess J 1984 Comparison of prohormone processing activities in islet microsomes and secretory granules: Evidence for distinct converting enzymes for separate islet prosomatostatins. J Cell Biol 99:578.
18. Reichlin S 1983 Somatostatin. N Engl J Med 309:1495.

19. Lauber M, Camier M, Cohen P 1979 Higher molecular weight forms of immunoreactive somatostatin in mouse hypothalamic extracts: Evidence of processing in vitro. Proc Natl Acad Sci (USA) 76:6004.
20. Robbins RJ, Reichlin S 1983 Somatostatin biosynthesis by cerebral cortical cells in monolayer culture. Endocrinology 113:574.
21. Ivell R, Richter D 1982 In vitro messenger ribonucleic acid directed synthesis and processing of an immunologically identified precursor to tetradecapeptide somatostatin from bovine hypothalamus. Biochemistry 21:1204.
22. Lauber M, Camier M, Cohen P 1979 Immunological and biochemical characterization of distinct high molecular weight forms of neurophysin and somatostatin in mouse hypothalamus extracts. FEBS Lett 97:343.
23. Srikant CB, Patel YC 1981 Receptor binding of somatostatin-28 is tissue specific. Nature 294:259.
24. Spiess J, Vale W 1980 Multiple forms of somatostatin-like activity in rat hypothalamus. Biochemistry 19:2861.
25. Patel YC, Wheatley T, Ning C 1981 Multiple forms of immunoreactive somatostatin: Comparison of distribution in neural and nonneural tissues and portal plasma of the rat. Endocrinology 109:1943.
26. Gomez S, Morel A, Nicolas P, Cohen P 1983 Regional distribution of the Mr 15,000 somatostatin precursor, somatostatin-28 and somatostatin-14 in the rat brain suggests a differential intracellular processing of the high molecular weight species. Biochem Biophys Res Commun 112:297.
27. Spira AW, Shimizu Y, Rorstad OP 1984 Somatostatin-like immunoreactivity in the guinea pig retina: Chromatographic characterization, localization and development. J Steroid Biochem 20:6B, p. 1617 (abstract #26).
28. Patel YC, Ganda O, Benoit R 1983 Pancreatic somatostatinoma: Abundance of somatostatin-28(1-12) like immunoreactivity in tumor and plasma. J Clin Endocrinol Metab 57:1048.
29. Patel YC, Wheatley T, Fitz-Patrick D, Brock G 1980 A sensitive radioimmunoassay for immunoreactive somatostatin in extracted plasma: Measurement and characterization of portal and peripheral plasma in the rat. Endocrinology 107:306.
30. Chihara K, Arimura A, Schally AV 1979 Immunoreactive somatostatin in rat hypophyseal portal blood: effects of anaesthetics. Endocrinology 104:1434.
31. Zingg HH, Patel YC 1979 Somatostatin precursors: Evidence for presence in and release from rat median eminence and neurohypophysis. Biochem Biophys Res Commun 90:466.
32. Charpenet G, Patel YC 1985 Characterization of tissue and releasable molecular forms of somatostatin-28(1-12) like immunoreactivity in rat median eminence. Endocrinology 116: (in press).
33. Peterfreund RA, Vale W 1981 High molecular weight somatostatin secretion by cultured rat brain cells. Brain Res 239:463.

34. Conlon JM, Rouiller D, Boden G, Unger RH 1979 Characterization of immunoreactive components of insulin and somatostatin in canine pancreatic juice. FEBS Lett 105:23.
35. Patel YC, Pierzchala I, Ning C, Wheatley T 1981 Somatostatin-28 is more potent than somatostatin-14 in inhibiting insulin and glucagon secretion from cultured rat islets. Clin & Invest Med 4:14B.
36. Chiba T, Seino Y, Goto Y, Kadowaki S, Taminato T, Abe H, Kato Y, Matsukura S, Nozawa M, Imura H 1978 Somatostatin release from isolated perfused rat stomach. Biochem Biophys Res Commun 82:731.
37. Jacovidou N, Patel YC 1984 Somatostatin secretion from monolayer cultures of rat antral cells. Program 7th International Congress of Endocrinology, Quebec City 1984, Excerpta Medica International Congress Series 652, p. 720 (Abstract #919).
38. Hobart P, Crawford R, Shen L-P, Pictet R, Rutter WJ 1980 Cloning and sequence analysis of cDNAs encoding two distinct somatostatin precursors found in the endocrine pancreas of anglerfish. Nature 288:137.
39. Taylor WL, Collier KJ, Deschenes RJ, Weith HL, Dixon JE 1981 Sequence analysis of a cDNA coding for a pancreatic precursor to somatostatin. Proc Natl Acad Sci (USA) 78:11798.
40. Magazin M, Minth CD, Funckes CL, Deschenes R, Tavianini MA, Dixon JE 1982 Sequence of a cDNA encoding pancreatic preprosomatostatin-22. Proc Natl Acad Sci (USA) 79:5152.
41. Dixon JE, Andrews PC 1985 Somatostatin of the channel catfish. In Somatostatin. Patel YC and Tannenbaum GS (eds), Plenum Press, New York.
42. Montminy MR, Goodman RH, Horovitch SJ, Habener JF 1984 Primary structure of the gene encoding rat preprosomatostatin. Proc Natl Acad Sci (USA) 81:3337.
43. Zingg HH, Patel YC 1982 Biosynthesis of immunoreactive somatostatin by hypothalamic neurons in culture. J Clin Invest 70:1101.
44. Robbins RJ, Mothon S, Reichlin S 1983 Somatostatin-28 is not the precursor of somatostatin-14 in cerebral cortical cells. Program 65th Annual Meeting US Endocrine Society, San Antonio, June 1983 (Abstract #85).
45. Van Itallie CA, Fernstrom JD 1983 In vivo studies of somatostatin-14 and somatostatin-28 biosynthesis in rat hypothalamus. Endocrinology 113:1210.
46. Patel YC 1983 A high molecular weight form of somatostatin-28(1-12) like immunoreactive substance without somatostatin-14 immunoreactivity in the rat pancreas: Evidence that somatostatin-14 synthesis can occur independently of somatostatin-28. J Clin Invest 72:2137.

47. Benoit R, Böhlen P, Esch F, Ling N, Alford B 1983 Isolation and characterization of two peptides derived from prosomatostatin in rat brain. Program of the 13th Annual Meeting of the Society for Neuroscience, Boston, p 748 (Abstract).
48. Benoit R, Ling N, Bakhit C, Morrison JH, Alford B, Guillemin R 1982 Somatostatin-28(1-12) like immunoreactivity in the rat. Endocrinology 111:2149.

6

SOMATOSTATIN-28 [1-12] - LIKE PEPTIDES

R. BENOIT*, P. BOHLEN, N. LING, F. ESCH, A. BAIRD, S.Y. YING, W.B. WEHRENBERG AND R. GUILLEMIN
Laboratories for Neuroendocrinology

J.H. MORRISON**, C. BAKHIT**, L. KODA** AND F.E. BLOOM**
A.V. Davis Center for Behavioral Neurobiology
The Salk Institute, P.O. Box 85800, San Diego, CA 92138

ABSTRACT

The search for a peptide corresponding to the NH_2-terminus of somatostatin-28 (SS-28) in tissues has led to the isolation and characterization of somatostatin-28[1-12] from pancreas and hypothalamus. Somatostatin-28[1-12]-like immunoreactivity [SS-28[1-12]-LI] is widely distributed throughout the central nervous sytem and the digestive system of rodents and primates, reaching levels comparable to those of somatostatin-14 (SS-14). Antibodies directed against the C-terminal end of the dodecapeptide are more specific and constitute excellent markers for the "prosomatostatin" system in mammalian tissues. In rat brain, SS-28[1-12]-LI material is highly concentrated in nerve fibres and terminals, especially in the median eminence, layer I of neocortex, the outer molecular layer of the dentate gyrus and the striatum. Additionally, immunoreactivity is observed in large multipolar or occasionally pyramidal-like neurons of the neocortex. SS-28[1-12] is secreted from hypothalamus and amygdala by a calcium dependent mechanism. No biological role is presently known for the dodecapeptide.

Two other peptides of Mr = 8000 (8K) and Mr = 5000 (5K) which contain SS-28[1-12] at their carboxy-termini are present in acid extracts from rat pancreas, brain and spinal cord. These two

* Present address: Montreal General Hospital Research Institute, 1650 Cedar, Montreal H3G 1A4, CANADA.
**Present address: BCR-1, Research Institute, Scripps Clinic, 10666 N. Torrey Pines Rd, La Jolla, CA 92037

peptides were isolated from an acid extract of rat brains using ion-exchange chromatography, gel permeation chromatography and reverse-phase HPLC. Results from amino acid analysis and partial sequencing were compared to the sequence of the cDNA encoding rat pre-prosomatostatin (prepro-SS) and revealed that the 8K peptide is a 76 amino acid molecule corresponding to prepro-SS[25-100] and that the 5K peptide, which contains 44 amino acids, corresponds to prepro-SS [57-100]. The 5K peptide was generated after cleavage of a Leu-Leu bond at position 56-57 of prepro-SS. The four most predominant peptides of the "prosomatostatin system" presently characterized are: SS-14, SS-28[1-12], SS-28 and prepro-SS[25-100]. Studies on pooled perfusates from rat hypothalamic tissue show that prepro-SS [25-100] is released with SS-28[1-12] _in vitro_ and accounts for 22% of the total SS-28[1-12]-like immunoreactive material released during depolarization. The 5K peptide is apparently not secreted.

The presence of prepro-SS[25-100] in brain implies that, first, prosomatostatin can serve as an immediate precursor for SS-14 without going through SS-28 as an intermediate step and second, other peptides could conceivably be derived from the cryptic portion of the precursor.

INTRODUCTION

The characterization of SS-28 seven years after the identification of SS-14 brings a new dimension to research on somatostatin (1, 2). The same SS-28 structure (see Fig. 1) is present in all mammals studied (3-6) and it is as potent as SS-14 for inhibiting the

SS14 OR SS28(15-28)

H_2N-ALA-GLY-CYS-LYS-ASN-PHE-PHE-TRP-LYS-THR-PHE-THR-SER-CYS-OH

SS28

H_2N-SER-ALA-ASN-SER-ASN-PRO-ALA-MET-ALA-PRO-ARG-GLU-ARG-LYS-
-ALA-GLY-CYS-LYS-ASN-PHE-PHE-TRP-LYS-THR-PHE-THR-SER-CYS-OH

SS28(1-12)

H_2N-SER-ALA-ASN-SER-ASN-PRO-ALA-MET-ALA-PRO-ARG-GLU-OH

Fig. 1. Structures of: the original tetradecapeptide SS-14, the NH_2-terminally extended somatostatin of 28 amino acids (SS-28) and the peptide corresponding to the first 12 amino acids of SS-28, SS-28[1-12].

secretion of several hormones. If SS-28 represents merely another "paninhibitor" like SS-14, then why was its NH_2-terminal sequence preserved from rodents to humans? An interesting possibility is that the addition of the 14 amino acids at the NH_2-terminus could confer more inhibitory properties to the new molecule. Indeed some investigators, comparing biological potencies of SS-28 and SS-14 on glucagon, growth hormone and insulin secretion, concluded that SS-28 is more potent (7-11); but others concluded that it is not (12-13). Somatostatin-28 has no effect in vitro on the secretion of pituitary FSH, LH or ACTH - hormones not affected by SS-14 in normal physiology. Another possibility could be that the NH_2-terminus is endowed with a physiological role different from that of SS-14. Given the presence of a dibasic pair of amino acids in the middle of the octacosapeptide (Fig. 1), we hypothesized that SS-28 could be cleaved into SS-14 and SS-28[1-14] and started to search for the NH_2-terminal segment SS-28[1-14] in tissues.

Isolation and Characterization of SS-28[1-12]

As soon as antibodies against the NH_2-terminus of SS-28 were generated (S298), acid extracts from rat hypothalamic and pancreatic tissues were screened for the presence of SS-28-like immunoreactive peptides. Indeed, immunoreactive material corresponding to the NH_2-terminus of SS-28 was found in these tissue extracts, but the material was not SS-28[1-14]. Rather, rat hypothalamic and pancreatic extracts contained a dodecapeptide (Fig. 1) corresponding to the first 12 amino acids of SS-28 based on amino acid analysis and immunoreactivity of the isolated material. Comparison of retention times on HPLC with synthetic SS-28[1-12]-OH and SS-28[1-12]-NH_2 showed that the peptide was not amidated. Thus, we concluded that the mature NH_2-terminal fragment of SS-28 is SS-28[1-12] with a free COOH-terminus.

The levels of SS-28[1-12] and SS-14 in tissues such as hypothalamus and pancreas were similar; moreover, in a rat medullary thyroid carcinoma of the anaplastic variety where SS-28 was present with no SS-14, no SS-28[1-12] could be detected either (15). Our data were thus compatible with SS-28 being a precursor of both SS-28[1-12] and SS-14.

Production of Specific Antibodies Against SS-28, SS-28[1-12] and SS-14

In order to study the relationship between these three peptides, specific markers were needed for each of them. An antibody specific for SS-14 was generated using [Tyr^{11}] SS-14 conjugated to BSA (S310 in Fig. 2). The production of an antibody specific for SS-28 presented a more demanding task. Immunization of rabbits against SS-28-[Tyr^{29}] conjugated to BSA produced an antibody population (S309, see Fig. 3 upper panel) directed against the first 14 amino

```
S310                      I/////////----------I   SS14

SS9                       I----/////////------I   SS14 or SS28(15-28)

S329   I------------///////////////////-------I   SS28

S309   I///////////////////-------------------I   SS28

S298   I/////////////////---------------------I   SS28

S320   I--------//////////I                       SS28(1-12)
```

Fig. 2. Schematic representation of the recognition sites of antibody populations used in radioimmunoassays and immunohistochemical localization of prosomatostatin derived peptides. Immune plasma S310 recognizes the first 8 amino acids at the NH_2-terminus of SS-14, while immune plasma SS9recognizes the middle portion of SS-14 comprising amino acids 5 to 10. Immune plasma S329 is directed against the central region of SS-28, between amino acids 12 and 24. In contrast, S298 is directed against the NH_2-terminus of SS-28 from amino acid 1 to $\leq$11, thus recognizing both SS-28 and SS-28[1-12]. For details on immune plasma S309 and S320, see Fig. 3.

acids of SS-28 and as a result, this antibody recognizes SS-28 but also shows a 10% cross-reactivity with SS-28[1-12]. Interestingly, S309 could detect larger molecular forms related to somatostatin but due to its characteristics, it was not clear if those molecular forms corresponded to large SS-28 or to large SS-28[1-12]-like peptides. However, when first blocked with synthetic SS-28[1-12], S309 has remained the best available marker for SS-28 in immunohistochemistry (16). For detection by radioimmunoassay of SS-28 and molecular forms larger than SS-28 ("6K" and "9.5K" SS-28-LI), we relied on an antibody population (S329) directed against the central portion of SS-28 (ref. 17). Finally, an immune plasma (S320), which recognizes the last eight amino acids at the COOH-terminus of SS-28[1-12], served as the most specific marker for SS-28[1-12] because cross-reactivity with SS-28 is 0.01% (Fig. 3 lower panel). Using these specific immune plasma, SS-28[1-12], like SS-14, was found to be distributed widely throughout the central nervous system reaching its highest level in hypothalamus and amygdala by radioimmunoassay (Table 1 & Fig. 4). When tissue extracts from various rat brain regions were analyzed for their content of SS-14 using S310, SS-28-like immunoreactivity (SS-28-LI) using S329, and SS-28[1-12]-LI using S320, the levels of SS-28[1-12] LI were found to be similar or slightly higher than those of SS-14 (Fig. 4). However, in the intestine, SS-28-LI clearly predominates (Fig. 5). High levels of

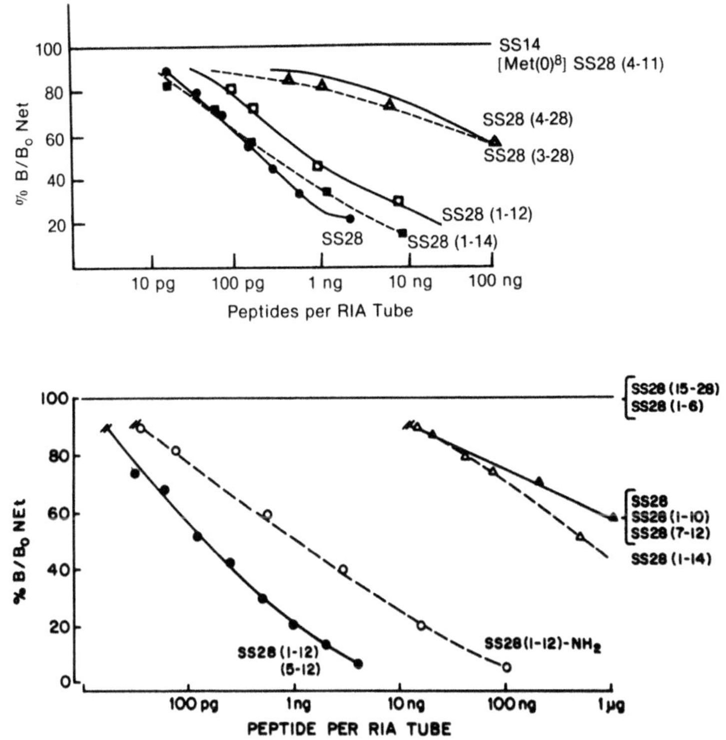

Fig. 3. Cross-reactivity studies comparing 2 antisera raised in rabbits. Upper panel shows displacement curves in the case of S309 which recognizes amino acids 1 to 14 of SS-28. The tracer used is iodinated SS-28-[Tyr^{29}] and the antibody dilution is 1/10,000. Lower panel illustrates results with S320, an immune plasma directed against amino acids 5 to 12 of SS-28[1-12]. The tracer used is iodinated [Tyr]-SS-28[1-12]. Cross-reactivity with SS-28 is <0.01% on a molar basis.

SS28[1-12]LI in the digestive system were found in the stomach (147± 10 pmol/g), in the pancreas (77 ± 15 pmol/g) and in the colon (73 ± 6 pmol/g).

Immunohistochemical Localization of SS-28[1-12] in Brain

Immunohistochemical studies performed in rat archicortex (18) and neocortex (19) showed a preferential distribution of SS-28[1-12]LI in nerve fibres and terminals whereas SS-28-LI was detected mostly in cell bodies. The situation however is different in the hypothalamus where the three peptides SS-14, SS-28 and SS-28[1-12] are highly concentrated in nerve terminals. A "routing

Table 1. Distribution of SS-28[1-12]LI in the Rat Central Nervous System (from ref. 20)

REGIONS (N=6)	Wet Wt MG ± SEM	SS28(1-12)-LI pmol per 100 MG ± SEM	SS28(1-12)-LI pmol per REGION ± SEM
OLFACT BULB	79 ± 5	2.5 ± 0.1	2.0 ± 0.1
NEOCORTEX	481 ± 24	19.8 ± 1.2	94.7 ± 6.3
REMAINING TELENCEPHALON	422 ± 24	21.1 ± 0.8	88.9 ± 5.6
HIPPOCAMPUS	100 ± 11	14.3 ± 1.2	13.9 ± 1.1
HYPOTHALAMUS	40 ± 1	90.8 ± 8.2	35.8 ± 2.4
THALAMUS	86 ± 9	10.9 ± 0.9	9.1 ± 0.8
MESENCEPHALON	142 ± 7	12.1 ± 1.2	17.1 ± 1.9
PONS	121 ± 6	9.7 ± 0.7	11.9 ± 1.0
MEDULLA	53 ± 6	21.7 ± 3.7	10.6 ± 1.0
CEREBELLUM	244 ± 5	2.7 ± 0.2	6.6 ± 0.5
SPINAL CORD	361 ± 5	23.9 ± 2.3	86.4 ± 8.4

mechanism" could possibly operate in the extra-hypothalamic central nervous system where certain prosomatostatin derived peptides would rather be sequestered in cell bodies while others would be transported to different nerve terminals of the same polyvalent neuronal unit. Studies performed in rat brain reveal that the densest terminal plexus of SS-28[1-12] positive fibres are found in the median eminence, layer I of neocortex, striatum and the outer molecular layer of the dentate gyrus (Fig. 6)

At the present time, our observations indicate that prosomatostatin-derived peptides are present in the same set of multipolar or bipolar cells. One rare cell type however stains with antibodies directed against SS-28[1-12]. It is a large multipolar or pyramidal-shaped neuron (cell body 30 μm diameter) with extensive dendritic arborization and radial axonal processes (Fig. 6D). SS-28[1-12]LI is also widely distributed in sheep, monkey and human brain. In these species, the positive terminal fields present in cortex are even denser than in the rat and exhibit a high degree of regional variation (Morrison JH et al., in preparation).

Secretion of SS-28[1-12]Like Immunoreactive Peptides

Previous studies have shown that SS-14 and SS-28 can be released from hypothalamic tissue *in vitro* (20-22). Similarly, Bakhit et al. showed that a SS-28[1-12]like peptide can be released *in vitro* from perfused hypothalamic tissue by a calcium-dependent mechanism (23). More recent work done by Sheward and colleagues

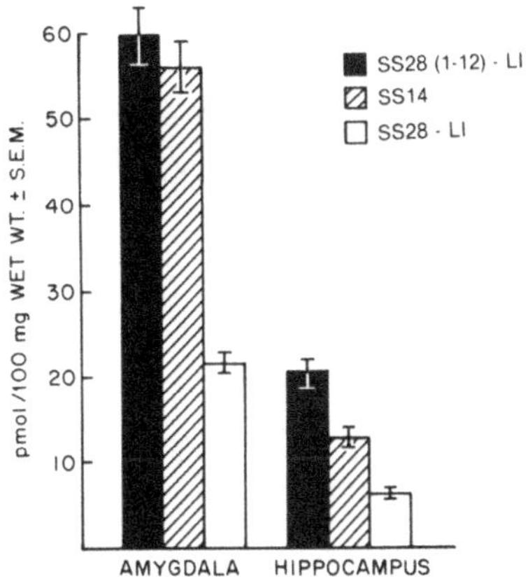

Fig. 4. Distribution of SS-14, SS-28[1-12]LI and SS-28LI in two brain regions using S310, S320 and S329 antibodies respectively.

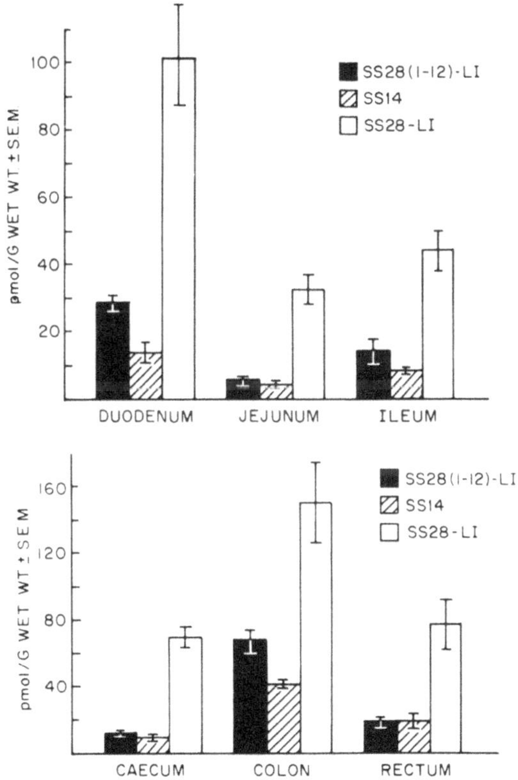

Fig. 5. Distribution of SS-14, SS-28[1-12] LI and of SS-28LI in the small (upper panel) and the large (lower panel) intestine.

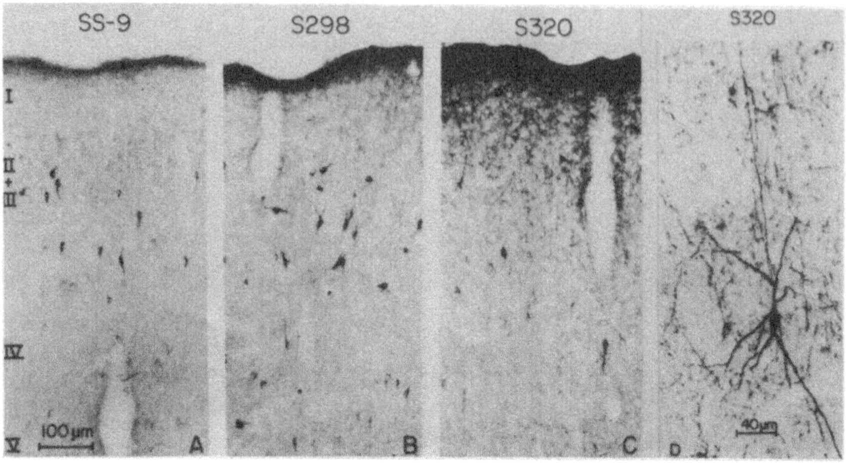

Fig. 6. A, B and C: superficial 700 µm of the dorsolateral cortex of the rat. In A, staining pattern obtained with an antibody population directed against the central portion of SS-14 so that both SS-14 and SS-28 are detected. Note the presence of numerous cell bodies and few fibres. In B, staining pattern obtained with an antibody population (S298) which recognizes SS-28 and SS-28[1-12]. Note that density of labelled cells is similar to that shown in A; however, such an immune plasma labels more dendrites and axonal processes than a SS9 type of antibody. In C, staining pattern obtained with an antibody population (S320) which recognizes SS-28-[1-12], but not SS-28 nor SS-14. Note low density of cell bodies and very high density of fibres particularly in layer I. In D, example of a large, multipolar neuron labelled with S320 in layer V of dorsolateral cortex. Note extensive dendritic processes along with radial axonal processes extending toward the pia. A more common somatostatin type of neuron is present at 40 µm left of the large cell. From ref. 19.

demonstrates that in rats a SS-28[1-12]like peptide is secreted into hypophysial portal blood and that its release increases 4 to 5 fold after electrical stimulation of the median eminence (24).

Biological Activity of SS-28[1-12]

Synthetic SS-28[1-12] at concentrations up to 10^{-7} M does not modify basal or stimulated secretion of FSH, LH, GH and ACTH from rat anterior pituitary cells in monolayer culture. The dodecapeptide does not modify the action of SS-14 or SS-28 on GH secretion. In the rat, SS-28[1-12] has no effect on the high levels of plasma

TSH and prolactin due to primary hypothyroidism, while both SS-14 and SS-28 decrease circulating TSH levels (Fig. 7). Until now, no receptor could be demonstrated for SS-28[1-12] in brain or pituitary when iodinated [Tyr]-SS-28[1-12] was used as the ligand. However, preliminary work done in rats indicates that SS-28[1-12] can depress spontaneous neuronal activity in vivo when applied iontophoretically to neurons of the parietal cortex and hippocampus (25).

Large Forms of SS-28[1-12]Like Material

Fractionation of various tissue extracts (from brain, spinal cord and pancreas) on Sephadex G-75 columns showed that the majority of the SS-28[1-12]-LI corresponds to the dodecapeptide (17, 26). The rest, accounting usually for 30-40% of the immunoreactive material, was composed of two larger peptides of Mr = 5,000 and Mr = 8,000 respectively. Due to the high concentration of SS-28[1-12]LI in layer I of rat neocortex, we first started to purify the large molecular forms of SS-28[1-12] from this tissue (Fig. 8). However, due to the percentage of the large molecular forms being rather low in that brain region (13%-18%), as well as the poor recovery after HPLC, we finally opted for a large-scale isolation program involving whole rat brains without cerebellum (Fig. 9). After homogenization and defatting, the extract was first purified by ion-exchange chromatography (carboxymethyl cellulose, CMC) on a 425 ml bed volume column using stepwise isocratic elution with ammonium acetate (27). Two major SS-28[1-12]-like immunoreactive components eluted from the CMC column, a more acidic component

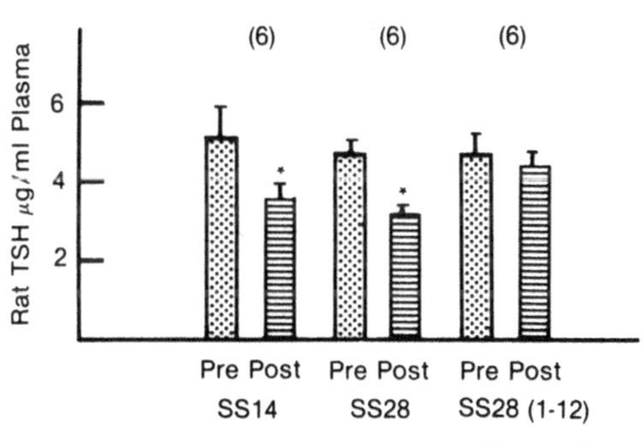

Fig. 7. Effect of SS-14, SS-28 and SS-28[1-12] on plasma TSH levels in thyroidectomized rats (350 g). 10 nmol of each peptide was given 4 times sc every 15 min to 6 hypothyroid rats. Plasma samples were taken under ether anaesthesia immediately before the first injection and 15 min after the last one. Each animal served as its own control. *indicates statistical significance ($p < 0.05$) by the multiple range test of Duncan. There was no statistical difference between the inhibitory effects of SS-28 and SS-14 on plasma TSH levels.

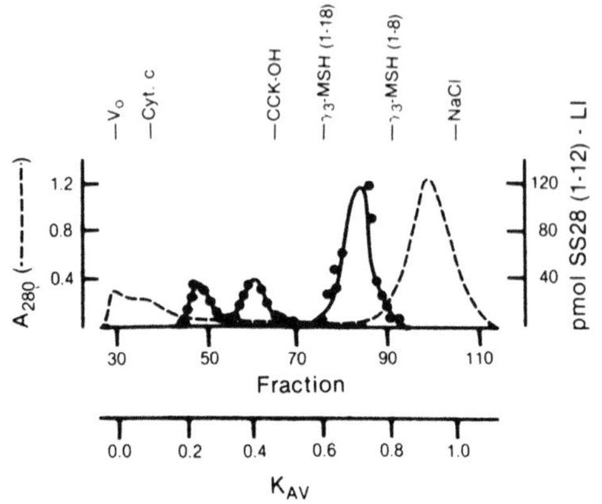

Fig. 8 Sephadex G-75 gel permeation chromatography of an acid extract of 5.9 g rat neocortex (wet wt). Load: 200 mg dry wt. Bed volume of column: 616 ml. Elution with 30% acetic acid (V/V), 6 ml fractions, flow rate of 18 ml per h. The column was calibrated with Cytochrome C: mol wt 12,384, cholecystokinin: mol wt 3834; γ_3-MSH[1-18]: mol wt 2226 and γ_3-MSH[1-8]: mol wt 1094.

(peak I) and a second less acidic component (peak II). These two components accounted for 75% of the total immunoreactivity. A third component (peak III) accounting for only small amounts of immunoreactive material was not purified further.

After gel permeation chromatography on Sephadex G-75, the more acidic component (peak I) eluted as a peptide of about 5,000 daltons. For each 100 g (wet wt) of brain tissue extracted, 1 nmol 5K peptide was obtained after gel filtration. Subsequent purification steps involved DEAE Sephadex A-25 anion-exchange chromatography followed by semi-preparative reverse-phase high-performance liquid chromatography (RPLC) with pyridine formate/n-propanol as the mobile phase (Fig. 10). At each purification step, only one major immunoreactive peak was observed. Finally, a homogeneous material was obtained after analyticaL RPLC performed on octadecylsilyl silica columns using 3 consecutive mobile phases: triethylammonium phosphate/acetonitrile, 0.1% trifluoroacetic acid/acetronitrile and 0.1% heptafluorobutyric acid/acetonitrile. After 6N HCl hydrolysis, the amino acid composition of the 5K peptide was found to consist of: Asx 7.2, Thr 1, Ser 2.5, Glx 11.8, Gly 0.1, Ala 5.8, Val 0.1, Met 1.8, Ile 0.1, Leu 5.2, Tyr, Phe, His, Trp, Lys and Cys 0, Arg 3.1 and Pro 5.1. These results were compatible with a peptide of 44 amino acids. Microsequencing of 1 nmol of the 5K peptide on an Applied Biosystem gas-phase sequencer (28) establised the following NH_2-terminal structure:

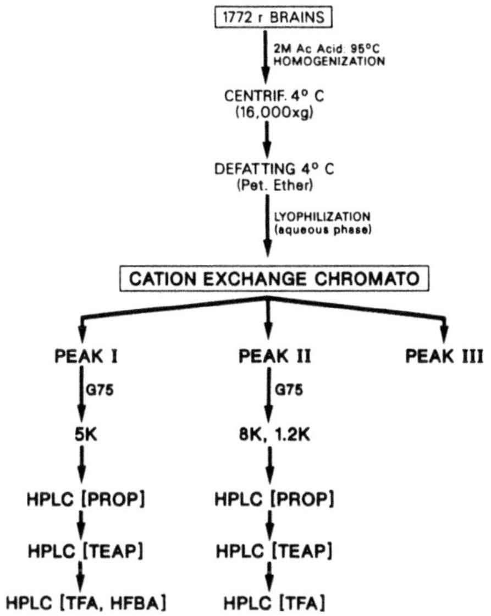

Fig. 9. Diagram summarizing the steps involved in the purification of the 5K and 8K SS-28[1-12]like peptides. Prop = pyridine formate/1-propanol system, TEAP = triethylammonium phosphate with acetonitrile, TFA = trifluoroacetic acid with acetonitrile, HFBA = heptafluorobutyric acid with acetonitrile.

Leu-Ser-Glu-Pro-Asn-Gln-Thr-Glu-Asn-Asp-
Ala-Leu-Glu-Pro-Glu-Asp-Leu-X-Gln-Ala

Fractions corresponding to peak II from CMC chromatography (Fig. 9) were lyophilized and further purified by gel filtration on Sephadex G-75. Three major immunoreactive zones were observed. The major one corresponded to the dodecapeptide SS-28[1-12] and accounted for 62% of the immunoreactivity; a small zone was compatible with a peptide of 3,000 daltons, and finally an immunoreactive peak corresponding to the 8K SS28[1-12]like peptide accounted for 24% of the immunoreactivity. Further purification of the 8K peptide was carried out (Fig. 11) using a similar approach as used for the 5K peptide except that the DEAE anion-exchange step was omitted. Amino acid analysis revealed the amino acid composition as: Asx 7.9,Thr 2, Ser 4.6, Glx 16.7, Gly 1.8, Ala 11.6, Val 0.3, Met 1.9, Ileu 0.1, Leu 11.5, Tyr 1, Phe 1.8, His, Trp and Cys 0, Lys 2.7, Arg 5.4 and Pro 6.7 which is compatible with a 76 amino acid peptide. Gas-phase sequencing establised the NH_2-terminal sequence as:

Ala-Pro-Ser-Asp-Pro-Arg-Leu-Arg-Gln-Phe-X-Gln-Lys

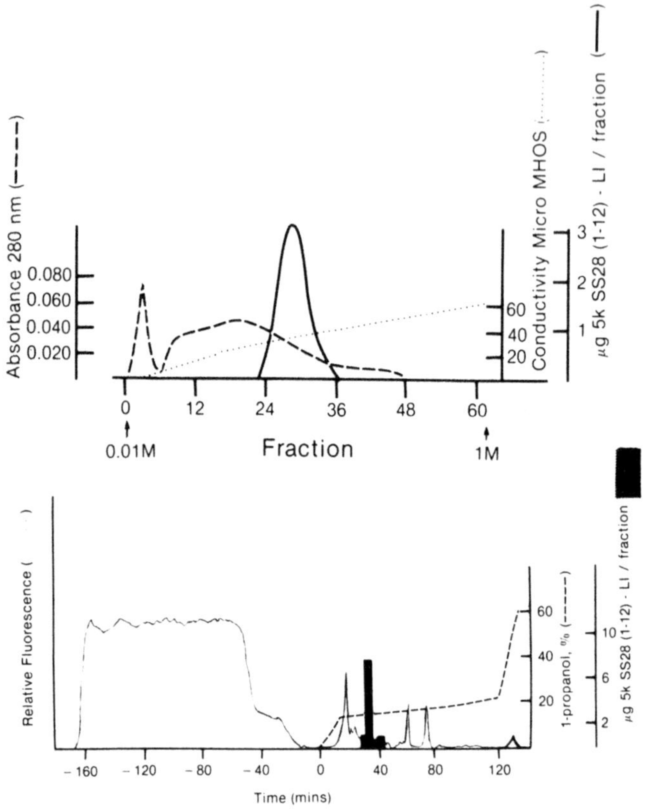

Fig. 10. Upper panel. Purification of the 5K SS-28[1-12]-like peptide on DEAE Sephadex A25 anion-exchange chromatography. Thirty mg material obtained from gel permeation chromatography was dissolved in 10 ml 0.01 M ammonium acetate pH 6.2 and loaded onto a 2x9.5 cm column (bed vol 30 ml). A salt gradient from 0.01 M to 1 M ammonium acetate, pH isocratic at 6.2, was used to elute the column at a flow rate of 230 ml/h at 4C. Fractions of 9 ml size were collected. The immunoreactive material eluted in one peak after 269 ml of buffer (269 ml on a total buffer volume of 515 ml; ratio R = 0.52).
Lower panel. Reverse-phase HPLC of an aliquot from the previous DEAE step (fractions 25 to 34) loaded directly onto a C18 column (4.6 mm X 25 cm) with pyridine formate/ 1-propanol as the mobile phase. Model 332 Altex liquid chromatograph. Flow rate 0.6 ml/min. Fraction size 1.8 ml. The first large peak of fluorescence seen during loading represents the effect of ammonium acetate on the fluorescamine detection system. Out of a load of 18 μg 5K SS-28-[1-12]like peptide, 13.8 μg immunoreactive material eluted from the column mostly in one fraction which was used for further purification.

The same NH_2-terminal sequence was confirmed for both the 5K and the 8K peptides by repeating the whole isolation and characterization procedure.

Goodman et al. (29), Shen et al. (30) and Funckes et al. (31) have recently sequenced two cDNAs encoding rat and human prepro-SS. Based on their work, SS-28 is located at the COOH-terminus of a precursor of 116 amino acids in which only 4 amino acid substitutions took place between rodents and humans (Fig. 12, upper panel). If we compare our data against the sequence of rat prepro-SS, it is obvious that the 8K peptide represents prepro-SS[25-100], (mol wt 8481), and that the 5K peptide corresponds to the last 44 amino acids of the 8K molecule i.e. prepro-SS[57-100], (mol wt 4936). Furthermore, our results are in agreement with those of Goodman et al. (29) who showed that prosomatostatin starts with Ala^{25} and contains 92 amino acids (mol wt 10,386).

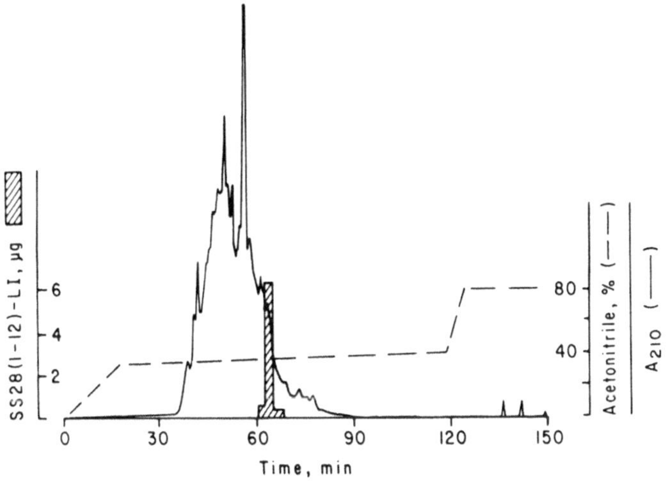

Fig. 11. Purification of the 8K SS-28[1-12]like peptide. The material obtained after semi-preparative HPLC with a pyridine formate/1-propanol solvent system was loaded onto a C18 column (4.6 mm x 25 cm). The column was eluted with a mobile phase of acetonitrile in triethylammonium phosphate buffer using a Model 332 Altex liquid chromatograph. Flow rate was 0.6 ml/min and fraction size 1.8 ml. Most of the immunoreactive material (6 µg) eluted in one fraction which was used for further purification on two consecutive reverse-phase systems employing trifluoroacetic acid/acetonitrile as the mobile phase which yielded a homogeneous material suitable for characterization.

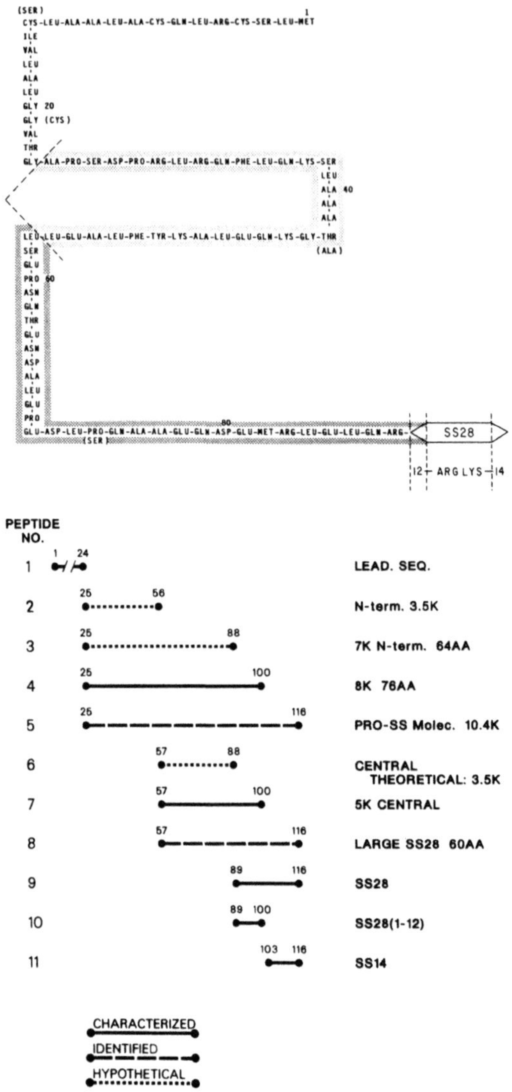

Fig. 12. Upper panel. Schematic representation of mammalian prepro-SS based on data from refs. 29-31 and the present work. The dashed lines indicate the cleavage sites. The amino acids in parenthesis indicate the substitutions occuring in human prepro-SS. The SS-28 sequence (see Fig. 1) occupies the COOH-terminus of the precursor ie. from residue 89 to 116 of prepro-SS. Lower panel. Peptides derived from rat prepro-SS based on data from: (1) SS-14, SS-28 and SS-28[1-12] characterizations, (2) reports on the presence of a 6K SS-28 in brain extracts (17, 35, 36), (3) the present work and (4) data from refs. 29, 31 on the sequence of the cDNA encoding rat prepro-SS from a medullary thyroid carcinoma.

Based on the four cleavage sites identified at positions 24-25, 56-57, 88-89 and 102-103, a total of 11 peptides could be generated from preprosomatostatin (Fig. 12 lower panel). The schematic diagram of Fig. 12 represents a working frame, not a collection of final information. More recent findings indicate that modification of tissue processing and extraction procedure, such as immediate extraction after tissue dissection along with the use of peptidase inhibitors (pepstatin, PMSF and bacitracin) result in 10 times less 5K peptide recovered per brain (4 to 5 pmol vs 50 pmol) after the gel filtration step. We presently cannot exclude the possibility that the 5K peptide corresponds to a fragment generated during tissue processing and/or extraction. Identification of peptides derived from the NH_2-terminal portion of the precursor, along with pulse-chase studies, will determine if the Leu-Leu bond at position 56-57 is a natural cleavage site or not. At present, peptides 4, 9, 10 and 11 in Fig. 12 can be considered as the main peptides derived from prosomatostatin that are presently characterized in brain. It is now clear from our observations that brain SS-14 can be generated directly from prosomatostatin: cleavage of the basic pair Arg-Lys preceding the tetradecapeptide yields SS-14 and prepro-SS[25-100]. The presence of a 8K SS-28[1-12]LI peptide in pancreas as well as observations made by Patzelt and collaborators indicate that such a processing also occurs in pancreas (26, 32). Previous work by Spiess and Vale (5, 33) indicated that a "12K" somatostatin (which in retrospect represented probably the whole 10K prosomatostatin) was more likely a precursor of hypothalamic SS-14, than SS-28. In contrast, Zingg and Patel concluded from their studies (34) that SS-28 can serve as a precursor for SS-14. The relative importance of 10K prosomatostatin vs SS-28 as an immediate precursor of SS-14 remains to be assessed by pulse-chase studies. The same is true for SS-28[1-12] and its relation to prepro-SS[25-100] and SS-28.

Release of Prepro-SS[25-100] from Rat Hypothalamus

In order to establish if the 5K and the 8K SS-28[1-12]-like peptides were released by nervous tissue, we analyzed the molecular forms of the SS-28[1-12]LI present in hypothalamic perfusates obtained during potassium depolarization of rat hypothalamic slices. When these perfusates were fractionated by gel permeation chromatography (Fig. 13), several SS-28[1-12]LI peaks were observed. A major one eluted at a position corresponding to the dodecapeptide SS-28[1-12] and a smaller peak eluted as 8K SS-28[1-12] ie. prepro-SS[25-100]. A third peak appearing in the salt region represented interference by small molecules. No 5K SS-28[1-12]like peptide was detectable in these hypothalamic perfusates. These results indicated that 78% of the SS-28-[1-12]like material released by the hypothalamus correspond to SS-28[1-12] and 22% correspond to prepro-SS[25-100].

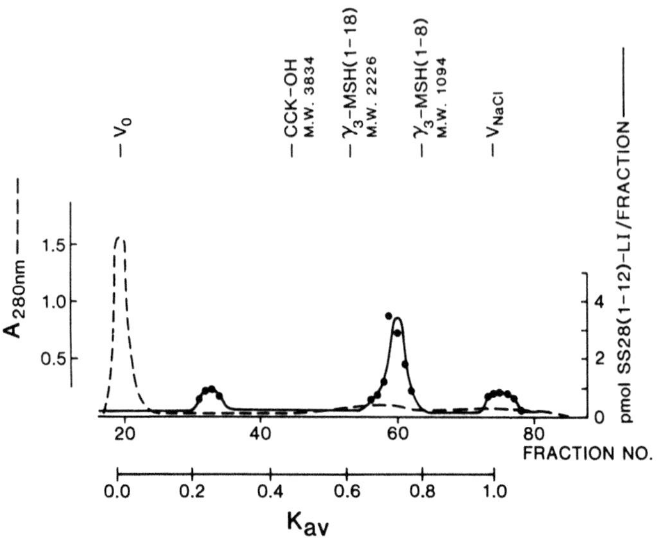

Fig. 13. Sephadex G-75 gel permeation chromatography of pooled perfusates of rat hypothalami. The perfusates were obtained from 12 chambers each containing 5 hypothalami cross-cut at 250 µm intervals and perfused with 50 mM KCl in a Krebs-bicarbonate solution as described by Bakhit et al. (37). Load: 700 mg dissolved in 30% (vol/vol) acetic acid. Column dimensions = 2.7 x 108 cm. Elution with 30% acetic acid. Fraction size 8.5 ml.

As more peptides derived from prosomatostatin are being isolated and characterized, it is important to identify the ones that are present in nerve terminals and secreted. This represents the first step toward the identification of the potentially bioactive candidates.

ACKNOWLEDGMENT

We are grateful to Barbara Alford, Roland Schroeder, Doug Lappi and Fred Castillo for technical assistance. Research supported by NIH grants (HD-09690 and AM-18811) and the Medical Research Council of Canada.

REFERENCES

1. Pradayrol L, Jørnvall H, Mutt V, Ribet A 1980 N-terminally extended somatostatin: the primary structure of somatostatin-28. FEBS Lett 109:55.

2. Brazeau P, Vale W, Burgus R, Ling N, Butcher M, Rivier J, Guillemin R 1973 Hypothalamic polypeptide that inhibits the secretion of immunoreactive pituitary growth hormone. Science 179:77.
3. Schally AV, Huang W-Y, Chang RCC, Arimura A, Redding TW, Millar RP, Hunkapiller MW, Hood LE 1980 Isolation and structure of pro-somatostatin: a putative somatostatin precursor from pig hypothalamus. Proc Natl Acad Sci (USA) 77:4489.
4. Esch F, Böhlen P, Ling N, Benoit R, Brazeau P, Guillemin R 1980 Primary structure of ovine hypothalamic somatostatin-28 and somatostatin-25. Proc Natl Acad Sci (USA) 77:6827.
5. Spiess J, Villareal J, Vale W 1981 Isolation and sequence analysis of a somatostatin-like polypeptide from ovine hypothalamus. Biochemistry 20: 1982-1988.
6. Böhlen P, Brazeau P, Esch F, Ling N, Guillemin R 1981 Isolation and chemical characterization of somatostatin-28 from rat hypothalamus. Regulatory Peptides 2:359.
7. Brazeau P, Ling N, Esch F, Böhlen P, Benoit R, Guillemin R 1981 High biological activity of the synthetic replicates of somatostatin-28 and somatostatin-25. Reguatory Peptides 1:255.
8. Rodriguez-Arnao MD, Rainbow SJ, Comaru-Schally AM, Meyners CA, Gomez-Pan A, Woodhead S, Schally AV, Coy DH, Hall R 1981 Effects of prosomatostatin on growth hormone and prolactin response to arginine in man. Comparison with somatostatin. Lancet 14:353.
9. Meyers CA, Murphy WA, Redding TW, Coy DH, Schally AV 1980 Synthesis and biological actions of prosomatostatin. Proc Natl Acad Sci (USA) 77:6171.
10. Mandarino L, Stenner D, Blanchard W, Nissen S, Gerich J, Ling N, Brazeau P, Böhlen P, Esch F, Guillemin R 1981 Selective effects of somatostatin-14,-25 and -28 on *in vitro* insulin and glucagon secretion. Nature 291:76.
11. Brown M, Rivier J, Vale W 1981 Somatostatin-28: selective action on the pancreatic B-cell and brain. Endocrinology 108:2391.
12. Pradayrol LL, Bommelaer G, Fourmy D, Fagot-Recurat P, Rozental G, Essaid A, Bousson M, Wunsch E, Ribet A 1982 Inhibition de la libération de l'hormone de croissance chez l'homme: effets comparés des somatostatines-14 et -28. Gastroenterol Clin Biol 6:166.
13. Vaysse N, Pradayrol L, Chayvialle JA, Pignal F, Esteve JP, Susini F, Descos F, Ribet A 1981 Effects of somatostatin-14 and somatostatin-28 on bombesin stimulated release of gastrin, insulin and glucagon in the dog. Endocrinology 108:1843.
14. Benoit R, Böhlen P, Ling N, Briskin A, Esch F, Brazeau P, Ying S-Y, Guillemin R 1982 Presence of somatoatin-28(1-12) in hypothalamus and pancreas. Proc Natl Acad Sci (USA) 79:917.
15. Benoit R, Böhlen P, Ling N, Brazeau P, Shibasaki T, Guillemin R, A somatostatin-28-like peptide in rat medullary thyroid carcinoma. Program of the 65th annual meeting of the Fed Amer Soc Exper Biol, Atlanta, GA 1981, p 457 (abstract 1289).

16. Ravazzola M, Benoit R, Ling N, Guillemin R, Orci L 1983 Immunocytochemical localization of prosomatostatin fragments in maturing and mature secretory granules of pancreatic and gastrointestinal D-cells. Proc Natl Acad Sci (USA) 80:215.
17. Benoit R, Ling N, Alford B, Guillemin R 1982 Seven peptides derived from prosomatostatin in rat brain. Biochem Biophys Res Commun 107:944.
18. Morrison JH, Benoit R, Magistretti PJ, Ling N, Bloom FE 1982 Immunohistochemical distribution of pro-somatostatin related peptides in the hippocampus. Neurosci Lett 34:137.
19. Morrison JH, Benoit R, Magistretti PJ, Bloom FE 1983 Immunohistochemical distribution of pro-somatostatin related peptides in cerebral cortex. Brain Res 262:344.
20. Iversen LL, Iversen SD, Bloom F, Douglas C, Brown M, Vale W 1978 Calcium-dependent release of somatostatin and neurotensin from rat brain in vitro. Nature (Lond.) 273:161.
21. Kewley CF, Millar RP, Berman MC, Schally AV 1981 Depolariation and ionophore-induced release of octacosa somatostatin from stalk median eminence synapotosomes. Science 213:913.
22. Peterfreund RA, Vale W 1982 High molecular weight somatostatin secretion by cultured rat brain cells. Brain Res 239:463.
23. Bakhit C, Benoit R, Bloom FE 1983 Release of somatostatin-28-(1-12) from hypothalamus in vitro. Nature (Lond.) 301:524.
24. Sheward WJ, Benoit R, Fink G 1984 Somatostatin-28[1-12] is secreted into hypophysial portal vessel blood in the rat. Neuroendocrinology 38:88.
25. Bloom FE, Aldenhoff J, Bakhit C, Benoit R, French E, Gruol D, Koda L, Morrison J, Siggins G, Gut peptides in the brain: implications for therapeutics. In IInd World Conference on Clinical Pharmacology and Therapeutics. Symposium on Neuropeptides, Washington, 1983.
26. Benoit R, Ling N, Bakhit C, Morrison JH, Alford B, Guillemin R 1982 Somatostatin-28 1-12 -like immunoreactivity in the rat. Endocrinology 111:2149.
27. Benoit R, Böhlen P, Esch F, Ling N 1984 Neuropeptides derived from prosomatostatin that do not contain the somatostatin-14 sequence. Brain Res 311:23.
28. Esch F 1984 Polypeptide microsequence analysis with the commercially available gas-phase sequencer. Anal Biochem 136:39.
29. Goodman RH, Aron DC, Roos BA 1983 Rat pre-prosomatostatin. Structure and processing by microsomal membranes. J Biol Chem 258:5570.
30. Shen L-P, Pictet RL, Rutter WJ 1982 Human somatostatin I: sequence of the cDNA. Proc Natl Acad Sci (USA) 79:4575.
31. Funckes CL, Minth CD, Deschenes R, Magazin M, Tavianini MA, Sheets M, Collier K, Weith HL, Aron DC, Roos BA, Dixon JE 1983 Cloning and characterization of a mRNA-encoding rat preprosomatostatin. J Biol Chem 258:8781.

32. Patzelt C, Tager HS, Carroll RJ, Steiner DF 1980 Identification of prosomatostatin in pancreatic islets. Proc Natl Acad Sci (USA) 77:2410.
33. Spiess J, Vale W 1980 Multiple forms of somatostatin-like activity in the rat hypothalamus. Biochemistry 19:2861.
34. Zingg HH, Patel YC 1982 Processing of synthetic somatostatin-28 and a related endogenous rat hypothalamic somatostatin-like molecule to somatostatin-14 by hypothalamic enzymes. Life Sci 30:525.
35. Sagar SM, Landry D, Millard WJ, Badger TM, Arnold MA, Martin JB 1982 Depletion of somatostatin-like immunoreactivity in the rat central nervous sytem by cysteamine. J Neurosci 2:225.
36. Ackland J, Ratter S, Bourne GL, Rees LH 1983 Characterization of immunoreactive somatostatin in human fetal hypothalamic tissue. Regulatory Peptides 5:95.
37. Bakhit C, Koda L, Benoit R, Morrison JH, Bloom FE 1984 Evidence for selective release of somatostatin-14 and somatostatin-28[1-12] from rat hypothalamus. J Neurosci 4:411.

7

PROTEOLYTIC EVENTS IN THE POST-TRANSLATIONAL PROCESSING OF SOMATOSTATIN PRECURSORS FROM RAT BRAIN CORTEX AND ANGLERFISH PANCREATIC ISLETS

PAUL COHEN, ALAIN MOREL, PABLO GLUSCHANKOF, SOPHIE GOMEZ AND PIERRE NICOLAS

Groupe de Neurobiochimie Cellulaire et Moléculaire
Université Pierre et Marie Curie
Unité Associée au CNRS no 554
96 boulevard Raspail, 75006 Paris, France

ABSTRACT

An Arg-Lys esteropeptidase which converts somatostatin-28 (S-28) into somatostatin-14 (S-14) was detected in rat brain cortical extracts using a synthetic undecapeptide substrate mimicking the octacosapeptide sequence at the restriction site. This enzyme system was unable to release either the octacosapeptide or S-14 from the 15,000 mol wt (15K) rat hypothalamic precursor. This argues in favor of sequential degradation of the precursor into S-14 *via* S-28 as an obligatory intermediate.

Another *in vivo* processing system was analyzed in the anglerfish pancreatic Brockmann organs. Here, cloning of two cDNA corresponding to two mRNA species predicts two distinct somatostatins precursors, called prosomatostatins I and II (Hobart et al., Nature 288:137, 1980). While a single S-14 can be detected in extracts made from this pancreatic tissue, indistinguishable from the mammalian species, two S-28 species could be separated by HPLC. Immunochemical and biochemical evidence indicates that the second species should correspond to anglerfish S-28 (AF S-28), the product of prosomatostatin-II processing *in vivo*. Amino acid analysis, together with the determined complete amino acid sequence of this peptide, demonstrates that this is indeed the case and that AF S-28 contains in its C-terminal half the [Tyr^7,Gly^{10}] derivative of S-14.

These observations give an example of a AFS-28 being a terminal active product of prosomatostatin processing. They suggest that this octacosapeptide, which is potent on the inhibition of growth hormone release by anterior pituitary cells, may play such a role in the gastrointestinal tract of the anglerfish. These results, while not excluding alternative routes, give support to a sequential processing of the 15 K precursor → S-28 → S-14.

INTRODUCTORY REMARKS

Post-translational proteolytic cleavages are believed to occur during the processing of neuropeptide and hormone precursors produced by secretory systems both in the nervous system and peripheral organs. Examination of the now establised structures of a number of large molecular weight proforms indicates that doublets, as well as triplets or double pairs of basic residues (Lys or Arg) may provide recognition signals in the hydrolytic process. In most cases these residues are found either preceding or else flanking the sequence of the so-called "mature" peptide in the primary structure of the precursor.

.....YY-----------------------YY.....

Neuropeptide sequence

Y Lys or Arg residue.

Attempts to characterize these proteolytic systems have been so far unsuccessful mainly because both the products of processing and the mechanism of the hydrolytic reaction(s) could not be properly characterized (1). In both pancreatic (2, 3) and hypothalamic (4, 5) systems, S-28 and S-14 appear to derive biosynthetically from a 15K precursor in which they occupy the C-terminal position (Scheme 1).

In the octacosapeptide S-28, a double Arg^{-2}, Lys^{-1} can be found at position -2, -1 from the N-terminus of the S-14 sequence (6-8). A lone Arg residue at position -15 was determined in the amino acid sequences of all the pancreatic precursors so far sequenced (2, 3).

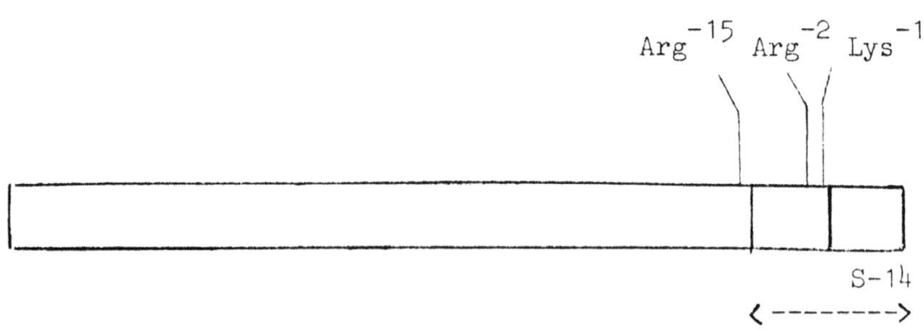

(Scheme 1)

Prosomatostatin. A diagrammatic representation.

Indeed, looking at the sequence from a chemist's point of view, one can reasonably expect that different enzymes might be involved in the conversion of the prohormone into either S-28 or S-14. Therefore the prosomatostatin system is a particularly well-suited one to study the mechanisms by which production of "mature" hormones occurs.

In the present survey, we will firstly analyse the results of efforts we have made to identify one of these enzyme systems in the brain. Secondly, we will describe a particular form of in vivo processing occurring in the pancreatic tissue of a Teleostean fish, Lophius Piscatorius.

Brain Maturases: The Basic Doublet Specific Endoprotease Converting S-28 into S-14

Preliminary observations

Mouse hypothalamic extracts contain a single form of 15,000 mol wt immunoreactive somatostatin which can be purified by repetitive HPLC. This species, with a pI approximating 5.3, is homogenous by isoelectric focusing (9). Exposure of this form to crude hypothalamic extracts (previously freed of somatostatin-like immunoreactivity by affinity chromatography on antisomatostatin-antibodies) leads to smaller molecular weight species unequivocally identified as S-14 and S-28 (9, 10).

This indicates that the predominant 15 K form from the hypothalamus, the product of a single gene, is a common precursor for both S-28 and S-14 (9). It suggests that the hypothalamus contains proteases able to produce the selective endoproteolytic cleavages of the precursor to release the "mature" neuropeptides.

A search for a Arg-Lys esteropeptidase

This was undertaken using a routine enzyme assay with a synthetic substrate consisting of a peptide mimicking the S-28 restricting sequence:

Pro-Arg-Glu-Arg-Lys-Ala-Gly-Ala-Lys-Asn-Tyr (NH_2) (Peptide I)

This substrate was chosen since it possesses the following structural features:

i) it includes the Arg-Lys doublet and mimics the sequence of S-28 situated on both sides of this putative signal;

ii) it also contains solitary Arg and Lys residues which permit the monitoring of possible fragments resulting from secondary cleavage at these loci by trypsin-like activities;

iii) the Phe^6 residue of S-14 is replaced by a Tyr^6 moiety, allowing for ^{125}I-labelling to produce a radiolabelled substrate.

Therefore the following reaction was analyzed:

Pro-Arg-Glu-Arg-Lys-Ala-Gly-Ala-Lys-Asn-Tyr*(NH_2) (Peptide I)

↓ Arg-Lys endopeptidase

?) Pro-Arg-Glu-Arg-Lys + Ala-Gly-Ala-Lys-Asn-Tyr*(NH_2) (Peptide II)

(Scheme 2)

The production of Peptide II was monitored quantitatively by reference to the corresponding synthetic product. Preliminary evaluation of this activity in various regions of the rat brain indicated that it occurred in the neocortex, the hypothalamus and the neurohypophysis. In the molecular sieve fractionation of a crude cortex extract (see Fig. 1) it was found contaminated by a degrading activity defined as producing the fragment Asn-Tyr*(NH_2).

The cortex was chosen as a source for the Arg-Lys peptidase since in this region the contamination by the degrading activity was found to be the lowest (11).

Preliminary purification of the activity was attempted by several techniques including:

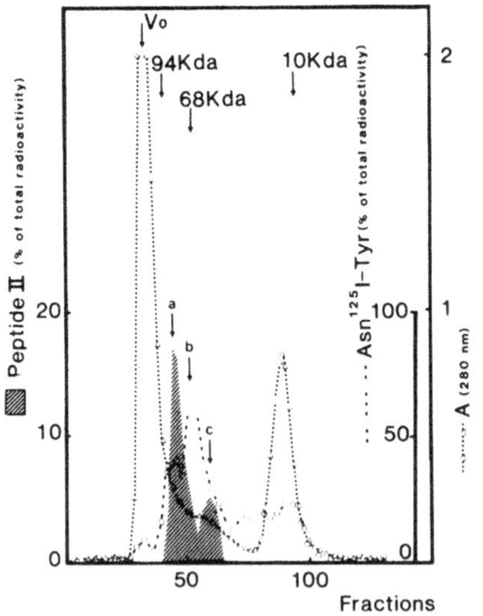

Fig. 1. Fractionation on a Sephadex G-150 column of the Arg-Lys esteropeptidase activity (hatched peaks).

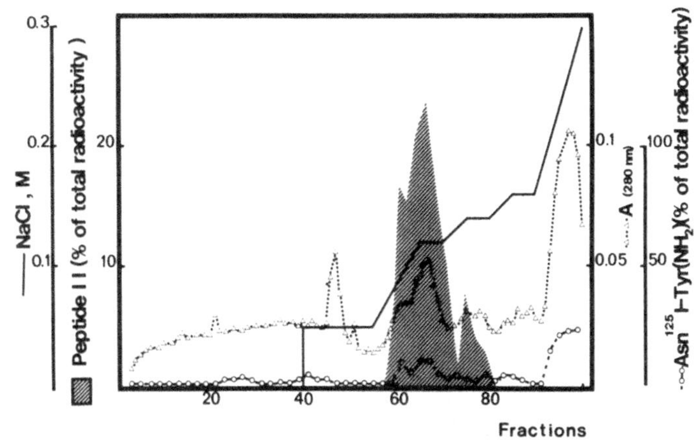

Fig. 2. Further fractionation, on a Mono Q cationic column, of the Arg-Lys esteropeptidase activity. In both experiments the activity was monitored as production of Peptide II (see text) (ref. 11).

i) subsequent ion-exchange chromatography of the previous molecular sieve filtration fraction (Fig. 1) on a Mono Q cationic resin (Fig. 2) using the FPLC system (Pharmacia, Uppsala, Sweden);

ii) preparation of neurosecretory granules from the cortex by previously reported techniques (12) and banding of the vesicles on either Percoll or sucrose gradients (12,13). After osmotic shock, the activity was spun down with the membranes of the granules and was only released as a soluble activity by further treatment of the granule ghosts by mild ionic strength solutions (Gomez, S et al., in preparation).

The activity obtained after the ion exchange step was essentially free of degrading activity producing the Asn-Tyr*(NH_2) fragment. It released Peptide II from Peptide I (scheme 1) as assessed by:

i) N-terminal analysis of the product; a single Ala residue was measured;
ii) comparison with reference synthetic Peptide II.

A Km approximating 20 μM and a Vmax of 2.1 pmol$\cdot g^{-1}$ per hr were measured with Peptide I as substrate. The activity was insensitive to classical serine-protease inhibitors but was completely abolished by thiol-protease blocking agents like iodoacetamide. Optimal activity was observed over a broad range of pH (above 6-8), but below pH 5 the reaction was drastically slowed down (11).

The selectivity of the proteolytic cleavage was tested on synthetic S-28 as substrate. Under neutral pH conditions, S-28 was converted into a product indistinguishable from S-14 by HPLC (Fig. 3). N-terminal analysis of the generated product, showed unequivocally that a peptide bond had been cleaved at the Lys-Ala level, releasing an S-14 with an alanine N-terminal residue.

In contrast, under similar conditions, the 15 K precursor was not affected by the protease and was recovered unmodified after incubation (11). If trivial reasons for this failure are excluded, this implies that the Arg-Lys doublet belonging to S-28 is not readily available to the protease system in the precursor.

Anglerfish S-28 - A New Product of Prosomatostatin II Processing in Anglerfish Brockmann Organs

cDNA cloning predicts two somatostatin genes in anglerfish pancreas

In mammalian, analysis of gene expression as well as of the protein products together indicate that both S-28 and S-14 are

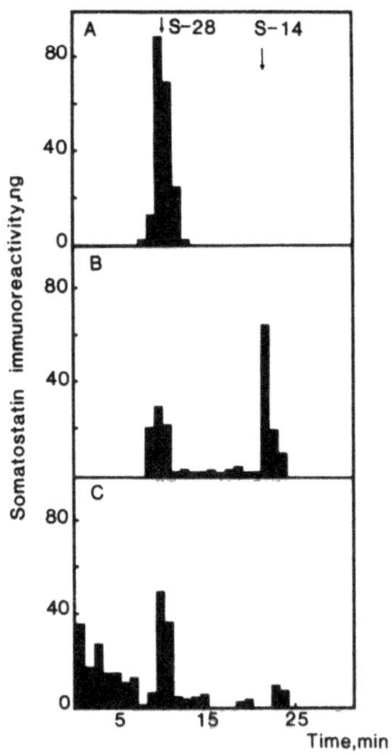

Fig. 3. HPLC analysis of the product of S-28 processing by the Arg-Lys esteropeptidase activity purified from experiment shown in Fig. 2. (A) Control; (B) S-28 exposed to the purified enzyme fraction; (C) S-28 exposed to contaminating degrading activities (from ref. 11).

encoded by a single common precursor (9). In the anglerfish (Lophius piscatorius) pancreatic islets, cloning of two cDNA, corresponding to distinct populations of mRNA, predicts the existence of two genes coding for two prosomatostatins called I and II (2). While prosomatostatin I determines the synthesis of a tetradecapeptide identical to S-14, the predicted sequence of prosomatostatin II indicates that this second precursor should yield a tetradecapeptide modified at positions 7 and 10 ([Tyr^7,Gly^{10}]S-14 or S-14 II).

Characterization of a new octacosapeptide: anglerfish S-28

Analysis of anglerfish Brockmann organs (collected on live fishes thanks to the cooperation of Captain Riou and his crew, Le Conquet, Finistère, France) was performed, after gel permeation of extracts, by radioimmunoassay using polyclonal antibodies directed towards both the central and C-terminal sequences of S-14. The pattern observed, (Fig. 4) consisted of a major peak and two minor components corresponding respectively to S-14, S-28 and a larger molecular weight (Mr ≃ 15,000) species. HPLC analysis of the molecules collected as S-14 species indicated the presence of a single product indistinguishable from hypothalamic S-14 as reference (14). No trace of a tetradecapeptide eluting as synthetic [Tyr^7 ,Gly^{10}]S-14 (kindly donated by Dr. Jean Rivier, the Salk Institute for Biological Studies, La Jolla, California) was detected, a fact also observed by others (15). In contrast, when the S-28 species was analyzed in the same way under reverse phase HPLC resolving S-28 from S-14, two species of S-28 were observed (numbered I and II, repectively, on Fig. 5). Repetitive fractionation on the same column resolved the two peaks (Fig. 5). Determination of the N- terminal amino acids by the manual double coupling of Chang (DABITC/PITC) (16) revealed that the compound of peak II has a N-terminal sequence identical to the S-28 II predicted from prosomatostatin II primary structure (2). Therefore the comparative ability of peptides from peaks I and II to react with ^{125}I were evaluated. While no incorporation of ^{125}I was

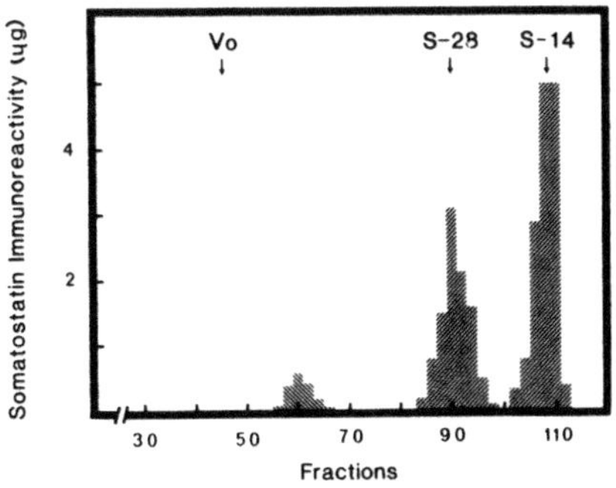

Fig. 4. Fractionation on Sephadex G-50 of anglerfish Brockmann organ extracts.

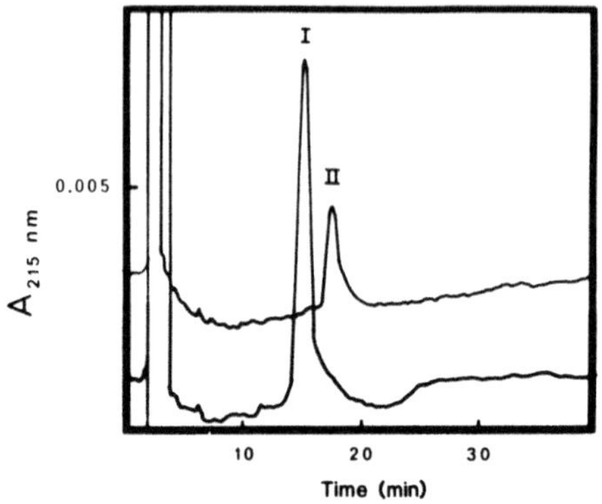

Fig. 5. HPLC separation of the two S-28 species recovered from Fig. 4 experiment (from ref. 14).

observed with the species of peak I, the peptide of peak II was quantitatively labeled suggesting the presence of a tyrosine residue absent in peptide I. Finally the brain cortex converting activity described above, transformed quantitatively the peptide from peak II into a S-14 species indistinguishable from synthetic [Tyr^7,Gly^{10}]S-14 (Fig. 6).

Definitive demonstration of the structure of the S-28 II was achieved by the following experiments (in collaboration with Dr. J.Y. Chang, Ciba-Geigy Limited, Basle, Switzerland (17)).

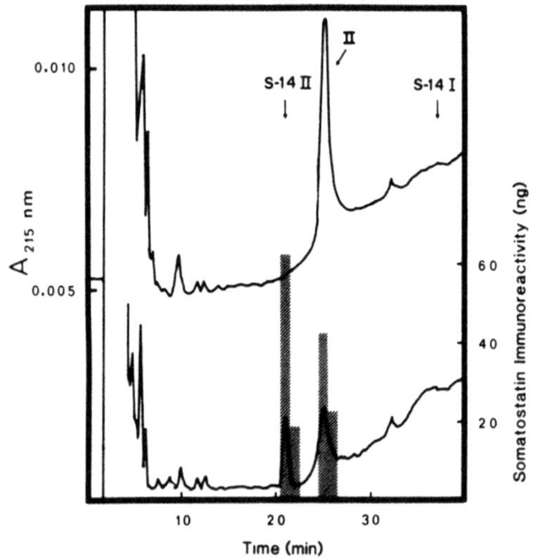

Fig. 6. Conversion of anglerfish S-28 II to [Tyr^7,Gly^{10}] S-14 (S-14 II) by the Arg-Lys esteropeptidase purified from brain cortex extracts. S-14 I refers to hypothalamic S-14 (ref. 14).

i) Firstly, the amino acid composition determined after DABSCl derivatization of the hydrolysate of a sample of peptide from peak II confirmed the presence of a tyrosine and of an extra glycine and the loss of a phenylalanine and a threonine residue (compared with S-28 I).

ii) Partial determination of the sequence was accomplished after endolysine digestion of the new S-28 form. The fragments were analyzed for their N-terminal sequence by the manual double coupling technique (DABITC/PITC) (16).

iii) Finally the complete sequence of the compound was obtained by automated Edman degradation (17).

The determined sequence of S-28 II, i.e.,

```
                        5                   10
Ser Val Asp Ser Thr Asn Asn Leu Pro Pro Arg Glu Arg Lys
 15                  20                  25
Ala Gly Cys Lys Asn Phe Tyr Trp Lys Gly Phe Thr Ser Cys
```

corresponds to an octacosapeptide containing in its C-terminal half the Tyr^{7}, Gly^{10} derivative of S-14 (17). It is in complete agreement with the primary sequence predicted from the cDNA nucleotide sequence of Hobart et al. (2).

A Model

These observations demonstrate that, _in vivo_, the post-translational processing of prosomatostatin II is interrupted at the S-28 II level while S-14 I is produced from the corresponding precursor (prosomatostatin I) in anglerfish pancreatic islets (Fig. 7). The fact that _in vitro_ further enzymatic conversion of S-28 II into S-14

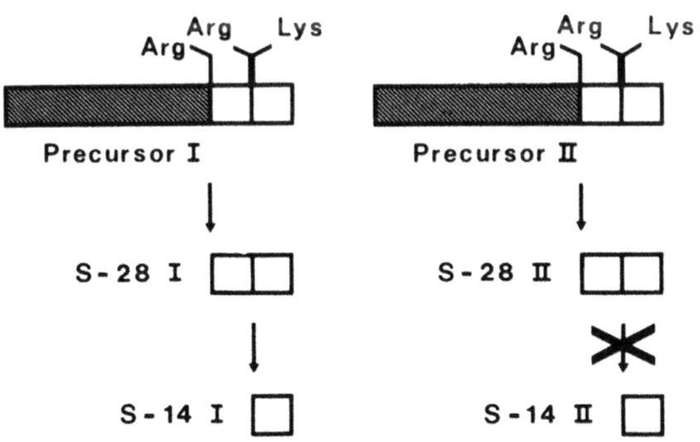

Fig. 7. Differential processing of prosomatostatins I and II in the anglerfish pancreatic islets. A model (from ref. 14).

II could be achieved indicates that this interrupted processing *in vivo* results from a topological segregation of the precursors either in different cells or else in different granules possessing a different processing enzyme equipment. Moreover, these observations provide the first indirect evidence for a proper biological function of a S-28 form. Therefore, its biological potency was tested in an heterologous system using inhibition of GH release from rat anterior pituitary cells (14). Under the experimental conditions used for this test, S-28 II was found to exhibit a strong biological potency (about 95% of the activity of S-14). The relevant biological function of this octacosapeptide, in the gastrointestinal tract, remains to be discovered, although evidence by others suggests differential effects on either insulin or glucagon secretion by the islet cells.

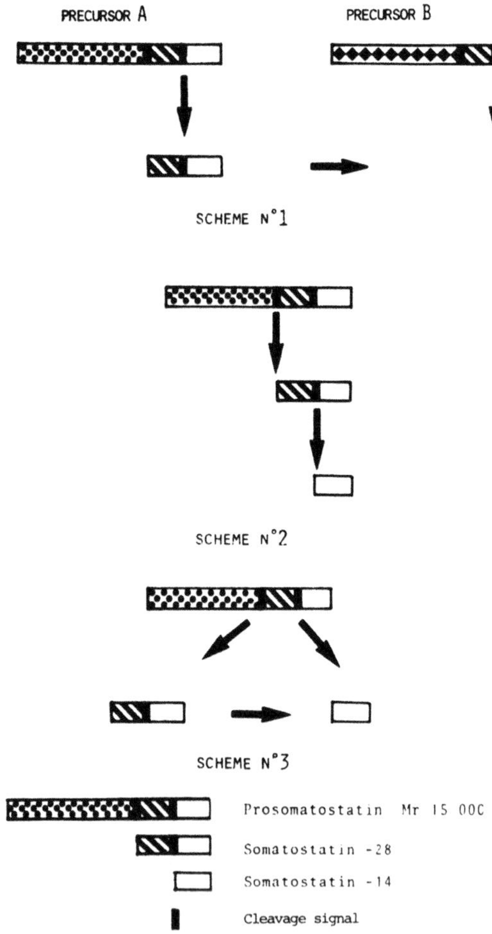

Fig. 8. Hypothetical scheme of biosynthetic conversion of prosomatostatin into S-28 and S-14 in neural tissues.

DISCUSSION

One of the main problems related to S-14 and S-28 expression concerns the routes by which these peptides are generated. Fig. 8 summarizes a few possibilities for the processing pathways. It is clear that, in mammalian systems, scheme 1 should be excluded since no evidence for two distinct precursors is available at this time. In contrast, the Teleostean fish model suggests multigene control for prosomatostatin biosynthesis. Taken together, our findings argue in favor of a biosynthetic pathway in which S-28 is first released from the precursor, before S-14 is detached from the latter (scheme no. 2; Fig. 8). However, the alternative possibility that part of the S-14 produced in somatostatinergic neurones derives directly from the large precursor should be considered. In this context the finding by Benoit et al. (18) of an 8 K fragment lacking the S-14 extremity and reacting with antibodies directed towards the 1-12 N-terminal portion of S-28 is an interesting one. Although it remains to be seen how biologically relevant the cleavages generating this fragment are, one should notice that the formation of an 8 K fragment necessarily implies the removal of an extra-piece of precursor at its C-terminal end. This could be taken as further adding support to the conclusion that the 15 K precursor conformation must be first remodeled by cleavage before the S-14 sequence can be detached from its structure.

In any event, if as believed, the S-28 form results from cleavage by a protease different from the maturase involved in S-28 cleavage, this system remains to be characterized. The interplay between a double enzymatic system could contribute to the regulation of S-28 and S-14 production in various somatostatinergic cells, at the post-translational level. No doubt, the <u>in situ</u> characterization of the enzymes both in the organelles and neural cell types will help considerably in clarifying these issues.

ACKNOWLEDGMENT

This work was supported in part by funds from the Université Pierre et Marie Curie, the Centre National de la Recherche Scientifique (Unité Associée no. 554 et Programme Interdisciplinaire de Recherches sur les Bases Scientifiques des Médicaments), the Ministère de l'Industrie et de la Recherche (contract no. 81-E-0396), the Institut National de la Santé et de la Recherche Médicale (CRL no. 814003 and CRE no. 834006), the Fondation pour la Recherche Médicale Française and the Département de Biologie du Centre d'Etudes Nucléaires de Saclay for the supply of radiochemicals. S.G. is a recipient of a predoctoral fellowship from the Ministère de l'Industrie et de la Recherche and P.G. received fellowships from the Programme Interdisciplinaire de Recherches sur les Bases Scientifiques des Médicaments and from the Association pour le Dévelopement de la Recherche sur le Cancer.

REFERENCES

1. Turner AJ 1984 Neuropeptide processing enzymes. Trends in Neurosciences 7:258.
2. Hobart P, Crawford R, Shen L-P, Pictet R, Rutter WJ 1980 Cloning and sequence analysis of cDNAS encoding two distinct somatostatin precursors found in the endocrine pancreas of anglerfish. Nature 288:137.
3. Shen L-P, Pictet R, Rutter WJ 1982 Human somatostatin-I. Sequence of the cDNA. Proc Natl Acad Sci (USA) 76:6004.
4. Lauber M, Camier M, Cohen P 1979 Higher molecular weight forms of immunoreactive somatostatin in mouse hypothalamic extracts. Evidence of processing in vitro. Proc Natl Acad Sci (USA) 76:6004.
5. Ivell R, Richter D 1982 In vitro messenger ribonucleic acid directed synthesis and processing of an immunologically identified precursor to tetradecapeptide somatostatin from bovine hypothalamus. Biochemistry 21:1204.
6. Pradayrol L, Jørnvall H, Mutt V, Ribet A 1980 N-terminally extended somatostatin: the primary structure of somatostatin-28. FEBS Lett 109:55.
7. Esch F, Böhlen P, Ling N, Benoit R, Brazeau P, Guillemin R 1980 Primary structure of ovine hypothalamic somatostatin-28 and somatostatin-25. Proc Natl Acad Sci USA 77:6827.
8. Spiess J, Villareal J, Vale W 1981 Isolation and sequence analysis of a somatostatin-like polypeptide from ovine hypothalamus. Biochemistry 20:1982.
9. Morel A, Nicolas P, Cohen P 1983 Evidence for a predominant form of Mr = 15000 prosomatostatin in the mouse hypothalamus. J Biol Chem 258:8273.
10. Morel A, Lauber M, Cohen P 1981 Selective processing of the 15000 Mr prosomatostatin by mouse hypothalamic extracts releases the tetradecapeptide. FEBS Lett 136:316.
11. Gluschankof P, Morel A, Gomez S, Nicolas P, Fahy C, Cohen P 1984 Enzymes processing somatostatin precursors. An Arg-Lys esteropeptidase from the rat brain cortex converting somatostatin-28 into somatostatin-14. Proc Natl Acad Sci (USA) 81:6682.
12. Bonne D, Nicolas P, Lauber M, Camier M, Tixier-Vidal A, Cohen P 1977 Evidence for an adenylate cyclase activity in neurosecretory granule membranes from bovine neurohypophysis. Eur J Biochem 78:337.
13. Masse MJO, Desbois-Perichon P, Cohen P 1982 Identification of neurophysin-related proteins in bovine neurosecretory granules. Eur J Biochem 127:609.
14. Morel A, Gluschankof P, Gomez S, Fafeur V, Cohen P 1984 Characterization of a somatostatin-28 containing the (Tyr-7, Gly-10) derivative of somatostatin-14. A terminal active product of prosomatostatin II processing in anglerfish pancreatic islets. Proc Natl Acad Sci (USA) 81:7003.

15. Noe BD 1981 Synthesis of one form of pancreatic islet somatostatin predominates. J Biol Chem 256:9397.
16. Chang JY, Brauer D, Wittmann-Liebold B 1978 Micro-sequence analysis of peptides and proteins using 4-MN-dimethylaminobenze 4'-isothiocyanate/phenylisothiocyanate double coupling method. FEBS Lett 93:205.
17. Morel A, Chang JY, Cohen P 1984 The complete aminoacid sequence of anglerfish somatostatin-28 II: A new octacosapeptide containing the (Tyr-7, Gly-10) derivative of somatostatin-14 I. FEBS Lett 175:21.
18. Benoit R, Ling N, Alford B, Guillemin R 1982 Seven peptides from pro-somatostatin in rat brain. Biochem Biophys Res Commun 107:944.

8

POST-TRANSLATIONAL PROCESSING OF ANGLERFISH ISLET SOMATOSTATIN PRECURSORS

BRYAN D. NOE AND JOACHIM SPIESS

Department of Anatomy
Emory University School of Medicine
Atlanta, GA 30322
Peptide Biology Laboratory
The Salk Institute
La Jolla, CA 92037

ABSTRACT

Two distinct somatostatin precursors are synthesized in anglerfish (AF) islets. In addition to a precursor which has somatostatin 14 (SS-14) as a C-terminal cleavage product, a precursor which contains at its C-terminus [Tyr^7,Gly^{10}] SS-14 as a potential cleavage product is also synthesized. However, even though an Arg-Lys pair is located immediately N-terminal to Ala^1 of the C-terminal tetradecapeptide, [Tyr^7,Gly^{10}]SS-14 was not found in significant amounts in extracts of AF islets. Instead, a 28 residue peptide having [Tyr^7,Gly^{10}]SS-14 (AF SS-28) at its C-terminus was found to be a primary cleavage product of this form of pro-SS. A question which arises from these observations is whether the differential cleavage of pro-SS-14 (PSS-I) and pro-SS-28 (PSS-II) is the result of differences in primary and/or secondary structure of the two precursors which in turn modulate the activity of the same converting enzyme, or whether separate cleavage enzymes exist for each precursor. Experiments were designed to address this question.

Microsomes (M) and secretory granules (SG) were isolated from AF pancreatic islets. Fraction purity was monitored by RIA for islet hormones, and by assays for plasma membrane and lysosomal enzymes. The ability of lysed M and SG preparations to mediate conversion of radiolabeled islet prohormones to products was monitored by gel filtration and HPLC analysis of the products. The pH optimum for converting activity in M and SG was found to be near 5.0. Incubations in the presence of selective proteinase inhibitors and prohormones containing Arg and Lys analogs demonstrated that a cysteine proteinase(s) which cleaves at basic amino acid residues is involved in granule-mediated conversion. A significant proportion of the converting activity in granules was found to co-precipitate with SG membranes. Washing these membranes with 1M KCl resulted in dissociation of most of the converting activity from the membranes suggesting that the proteinase(s) involved is membrane-associated. The processing activities for proinsulin and pro-SS-28 which were observed in SG were also found to be active, and membrane-associated, in M. However, converting activity for pro-SS-14 was found only in SG. Much of the PSS-I to SS-14 processing activity was membrane-associated in SG. By contrast, pro-SS-28 converting activity in SG was entirely soluble. These results suggest that two or more separate enzymes are involved in processing pro-SS-14 and pro-SS-28 and that these enzymes have differential activity in M and SG. No significant differences in the converting activity of Golgi- and RER-enriched subfractions of microsomes were observed. This finding is consistent with the hypothesis that converting enzymes are synthesized at the RER and translocated across the ER membrane along with the precursors.

INTRODUCTION

The pancreatic islet tissue of the anglerfish (Lophius americanus) is anatomically separate from the exocrine pancreas. One can routinely obtain 100-350 mg of uncontaminated islet tissue from a single animal. Moreover, the somatostatin producing D cell content of this tissue comprises up to 30% of the tissue mass (1). For these reasons, the anglerfish islet presents an excellent model system in which to examine processing of somatostatin precursors at the subcellular levels. Results from cell free translation of mRNAs from anglerfish have demonstrated the existence of multiple preprosomatostatin mRNAs in this tissue (2). However, at the present time, expression of only two of these messages has been demonstrated in intact anglerfish islets. These are the two (pre)prosomatostatins discussed in the abstract, one (PSS-1) which yields SS-14 as a primary cleavage product, and the other (PSS-II) which yields AF SS-28, a 28 residue peptide having $[Tyr^7,Gly^{10}]$SS-14 as its COOH-terminus (3-7). Schematic representations of the structures of these two peptides which show the positions of their primary cleavage sites are shown in Fig. 1.

Neither the 28 residue peptide which forms the COOH-terminus of PSS-I nor the 14 residue peptide which forms the COOH-terminus of PSS-II ($[Tyr^7,Gly^{10}]$SS-14) can be found as cleavage products in intact tissue (3-7). It therefore seems clear that SS-14 is the predominant cleavage product of PSS-I and that the 28 residue COOH-terminal sequence of PSS-II (AF SS-28) is the predominant product of this second form of somatostatin precursor. Despite marked

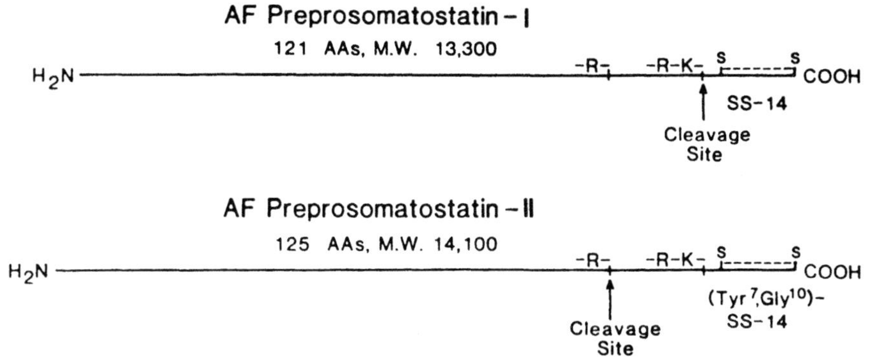

Fig. 1. Diagram showing the relative sizes of anglerfish preprosomatostatins I and II. The vertical arrows indicate the primary post-translational cleavage sites in both precursors. In PSS-I this cleavage occurs at the COOH-terminus of an Arg-Lys pair, whereas in PSS-II the primary cleavage occurs at the COOH-terminus of a single Arg residue.

similarities in the COOH-terminal amino acid sequence in the two precursors, especially in the terminal hexadecapeptides, the processing pattern differs significantly. A question which arises from this observation is whether cleavage of these two precursors is mediated by the same or different enzyme(s). The data to be discussed in this chapter were derived from experiments designed to address this question. Before discussing these results, however, we will review the information which is currently available regarding prohormone converting enzymes in general, and what is known about the characteristics of anglerfish islet converting enzymes in particular.

General Characteristics of Converting Enzymes

Soon after the discovery of proinsulin, Steiner and his co-workers demonstrated that insulin could be cleaved from proinsulin by employing carefully monitored digestion with trypsin and carboxypeptidase B (8). This led to the proposal that processing of prohormones *in vivo* may be mediated through sequential cleavage by a trypsin-like endopeptidase followed by the action of a carboxypeptidase B-like (CPB-like) exopeptidase. The trypsin-like enzyme could cleave at the COOH-terminus of a single basic amino acid or pair of basic amino acids, and the CPB-like enzyme would be necessary to remove the basic amino acids from the COOH-terminal end of the hormone or the remaining non-hormonal fragment(s) of the precursor. The evidence which has been generated to support this proposal is compelling. Kemmler et al. (9) first demonstrated that proinsulin to insulin conversion could be inhibited by the cysteine proteinase inhibitor, p-chloromercuribenzoate (PCMB), but not by serine proteinase inhibitors. Subsequently, Zühlke et al. (10, 11), using synthetic substrates, demonstrated trypsin-like and CPB-like activities in a crude secretory granule preparation from rat islets. Results from studies performed in other laboratories have identified numerous other candidate converting enzymes.

Trypsin-Like Enzymes

Over the years, a number of enzymes having trypsin-like cleavage specificity, i.e. enzymes which cleave at COOH-termini of basic amino acids, have been proposed as the initial converting enzymes in the processing of a variety of prohormones. Most of these enzymes have been demonstrated to be distinctly different from trypsin with regard to characteristics other than cleavage specificity. Many have pH optima in the 5.0-6.5 range and inhibitor spectra which differentiate them from serine proteinases, the class to which trypsin belongs (see Noe, ref. 12 and Loh et al., ref. 13 for recent reviews). A significant number of the "trypsin-like" enzymes characterized in secretory granules from different tissues of various species have been found to be thiol (cysteine) proteinases which are distinct from cathepsin B (determined by inhibitor susceptibility). This is the case for enzymes assayed in rat and bovine pituitary neural lobe, rat intermediate pituitary lobe and rat anterior pituitary lobe by Loh and co-workers (13-17). Very similar enzymatic activity(ies) has been characterized in secretory granules from anglerfish islets by Fletcher et al. (18, 19). In addition, results from several laboratories have demonstrated the presence of cysteine proteinases with proenkephalin converting activity in bovine adrenal medulla chromaffin granules. These enzymes have pH optima of 5-6 (20-22).

Other enzymes which have been implicted in prohormone processing have characteristics which not only differentiate them from trypsin, but also indicate that they are different from the acid cysteine proteinases discussed above. One of these is porcine pituitary granule enzyme having a pH optimum of 8.8 (23). Another is an enzyme from bovine parathyroid glands having a pH optimum between 7 and 9 and sensitivity to benzamidine, choloroquine and Ca^{++}, but not trypsin inhibitor. This enzyme was identified and characterized by MacGregor et al. (24) and Habener et al. (25). A third is a serine proteinase having a pH optimum of 7.5-8.0 which has been implicated in proenkepalin processing in the adrenal medulla (26). Establishing the precise role of these enzymes in prohormone processing and their relationship, if any, to the more widely distributed acid cysteine proteinases will require further investigation.

It should be apparent from the preceding discussion that the "trypsin-like" enzymes which apparently initiate prohormone processing are similar to trypsin only to the extent that they cleave at the COOH-terminus of basic amino acid residues. Therefore, it would be more accurate to refer to them as prohormone converting enzymes rather than trypsin-like enzymes.

Carboxypeptidase B-Like Enzymes

As indicated in the introduction to this section, the early work of Steiner and collaborators (8, 9) and Zühlke et al. (10, 11) suggested that the action of a carboxypeptidase B-like (CPB-like) enzyme might be necessary to complete the conversion of prohormones to products. The CPB-like enzyme would remove residual COOH-terminal basic amino acid residues after the initial cleavage is performed. Recently, significant progress has been made in elucidating the characteristics of CPB-like enzymes which may complete prohormone to hormone processing *in vivo*. Fricker and co-workers (27-29) have isolated and characterized a CPB-like enzyme from bovine adrenal chromaffin granules, whole brain and whole pituitary. The enzyme can act upon enkephalin precursors consisting of [Met]- or [Leu]-enkephalins extended from the COOH-terminus by one or two basic residues to convert them to enkephalin. The enzyme has a pH optimum in the 5.5-6.0 range, is activated by Co^{++} and is inhibited by iodoacetamide, $HgCl_2$, EDTA, guanidinopropylsuccinic acid and guanidinoethylmercaptosuccinic acid. The enzyme from all three sources is a glycoprotein and has an apparent molecular weight of 50,000 daltons.

An enzymatic activity with similar characteristics has been identified in purified secretory granules from rat pituitary neural intermediate and anterior lobes (13, 30). This enzymatic activity has been demonstrated to process ACTH[1-17] which has a C-terminal Lys-Lys-Arg sequence to ACTH[1-14] by stepwise removal of the basic residues. A lysate of neural lobe granules also processed arginine vasopressin (AVP)-Gly-Lys-Arg to AVP-Gly by sequential removal of the Arg and Lys. The pH optimum and inhibitor spectrum of the enzyme(s) from the pituitary source were very similar to those observed for the enzyme from bovine adrenal medulla, brain and pituitary by Fricker and co-workers. The pH optima and inhibition by cysteine proteinase inhibitors differentiate these "CPB-like" enzymes from pancreatic CPB. They also differ from lysosomal CPB which is not stimulated by Co^{++}. The evidence accumulated to date suggests that this unique subset of CPB-like enzymes may be involved in prohormone processing in the tissues from which they have been derived. The determination of whether other prohormone producing tissues will be found to contain similar enzymes awaits further investigation.

Characteristics of Converting Enzymes in Anglerfish Islets

Secretory granules. Because a significant proportion of prohormone conversion occurs in secretory granules, we chose to perform our initial studies on islet prohormone converting enzymes using purified secretory granules from anglerfish islets. The large amounts of islet tissue which can be obtained free of exocrine tissue from these animals allows the preparation of secretory granules which are minimally contaminated with lysosomes (18, 19, 31). Control experiments demonstrated the absence of non-specific degradation of islet peptides when labeled islet prohormones were incubated with lysed secretory granule preparations (19). The characteristics of enzymes which are involved in processing prosomatostatins, proglucagon and proinsulin in this tissue were determined. The converting enzymes for each of these prohormones were sensitive to inhibition by antipain, leupeptin, and the cysteine proteinase inhibitors PCMB or dithiodipyridine (DDP). The inhibition of PCMB and DDP was reversed by DTT. Chloroquine, DFP, EDTA, p-nitrophenyl guanidinobenzoate, soybean trypsin inhibitor and TLCK were ineffective as inhibitors of prohormone processing. A significant proportion of the converting activity was secretory granule membrane-associated and the pH optimum for the conversion of all the prohormones was near 5.2 (18, 19). By incorporating canavanine and thialysine, (analogs of arginine and lysine) into the precursors, prohormone conversion was inhibited (32). This demonstrated the absolute requirement for the presence of Arg or Lys at cleavage sites for processing to occur. In addition, it was shown that porcine proinsulin was less effective as a competitive inhibitor of prohormone conversion than equivalent concentrations of unlabeled natural substrate (18, 19, 33). Since the porcine proinsulin provided at least as many pairs of basic amino acids as potential cleavage sites, these results suggested that the converting enzyme(s) requires the presence of a prohormone sequence located NH_2- and/or COOH-terminal to the cleavage sites at basic pairs for substrate recognition and binding. The characteristics of the pro-hormone converting enzyme(s) are similar, but not identical, to those of lysosomal cathepsin B. Cathepsin B differs in that it would be likely to mediate non-specific degradation of the precursors.

It is proposed that the membrane-associated acid cysteine proteinases having a cleavage specificity for Arg and/or Lys residues are the enzymes responsible for performing the initial cleavages of the anglerfish islet prohormones. If prohormone processing in this system involves a two step mechanism, one would expect to find CPB-like activity in anglerfish islet secretory granules as well. Studies designed to identify and characterize CPB-like enzymes in these secretory granules are currently in progress. Preliminary results obtained using the substrate, [^{3}H]benzoyl-Phe-Ala-Arg-OH indicate the presence of significant amounts of CPB-like activity in the islet granules. (R. Mackin and B. Noe, unpublished results). Additional studies with various inhibitors of enzyme activity should further clarify the nature of this enzyme(s).

Microsomes

An assessment of the nature of islet prohormone converting enzyme activity in microsome fractions (RER and Golgi components) from anglerfish islet demonstrated that the pH optimum for this activity is near pH 5.2 and that processing of all prohormones was inhibited by the cysteine proteinase inhibitor, PCMB (34). A subsequent determination of cleavage accuracy showed that the islet prohormones which were processed by microsomal lysate enzymes yielded accurately cleaved products (see below). It was therefore assumed that the microsomal converting enzymes were the same as those found in secretory granules. Microsomes from anglerfish islets have also been found to contain CPB-like activity. Work designed to characterize this activity more fully is currently in progress.

pH Optimum for Converting Activity

It is of interest that the converting enzymes which are thiol proteinases and are often observed experimentally, as well as the CPB-like enzymes found in secretory granules, have pH optima in the 5-6 range. This is consistent with the acidic intragranular pH (between 5.0-6.2) of virtually all secretory granules which have been examined. Those examined include: chromaffin granules from adrenal medulla (35, 36), platelet secretory vesicles (37), neurosecretory vesicles from neurohypophysis (38, 39), anterior pituitary "dense granules" (40), and islet secretory granules (41). It is possible that maintenance of the internal pH of secretory granules near the pH optimum of converting enzymes facilitates prohormone conversion. Moreover, alteration of intragranular pH may provide a mechanism whereby the rate of processing could be modulated. It has not yet been determined whether a significant amount of prohormone processing occurs in the RER and Golgi. If prohormone converting enzymes are present, processing activity may be regulated by intracisternal pH in these compartments as well. If the intracisternal pH is near 7, it would be improbable that significant converting activity would occur because of the rather narrow pH range in which converting enzymes are active (12, 13, 42, 43). Most of the available evidence suggests that processing of prohormones does not begin until after transport to the Golgi apparatus (12, 13, 42, 43), which is consistent with estimates of intracisternal pH of the RER being in the neutral range.

Comparison of Prohormone Processing Activities in Anglerfish Islet Microsomes and Secretory Granules

In an attempt to identify potential differences in either distribution or activity of converting enzymes for the various anglerfish islet prohormones, we initiated a study to examine the processing activity(ies) which exists either in membrane-associated or soluble form in either microsomes or secretory granules. The initial results of this investigation have been recently reported (34). The data and conclusion will be summarized here.

Experiments were performed by preparing microsome and secretory granule fractions from islet tissue as previously described (18, 19, 31). These subcellular fractions were lysed by repeated freezing and thawing and then the membranous and soluble components were separated by centrifugation. These sub-fractions were incubated in vitro with anglerfish islet prohormones labeled with either [^{3}H] tryptophan and [^{14}C] isoleucine or with [^{3}H] tryptophan and [^{35}S] cysteine as described previously (18, 19, 32). Incubations were terminated by bringing the concentration of acetic acid in the media to 2.0 M. Extracts were screened initially by gel filtration (18, 19, 32) and product peptides recovered from appropriate portions of the gel filtration eluates were analyzed by reverse phase HPLC (6, 19, 34). Accuracy of cleavage was monitored by comparing the retention time (RT) of products generated during in vitro processing (mediated by subfraction components) with the RT of products produced in intact tissue. Even though the processing of proglucagon(s) and proinsulin was monitored simultaneously with the conversion of prosomatostatins, the results regarding the generation of the cleavage products of PSS-I (SS-14) and PSS-II (AS SS-28) will be emphasized here.

Processing of PSS-I and PSS-II by Membranous and Soluble Fractions of Secretory Granules

Complete granule lysate, granule lysate supernatant and granule membranes all generated a Mr = 1,000-2,000 peptide having an RT on HPLC identical with synthetic SS-14. These results indicate that both the soluble and membranous components of islet secretory granules contain an enzyme(s) capable of accurately cleaving PSS-I to yield SS-14. In contrast, only the granule supernatant fraction generated appreciable AF SS-28 from PSS-II, (both supernatant and membranous components showed proglucagon and proinsulin converting activity). The converting enzyme(s) for PSS-II to AF SS-28 conversion is apparently primarily soluble in secretory granules. When granule membrane preparations were washed with 1M KCl (a treatment known to promote dissociation of membrane-associated proteins) prior to incubation, a significant reduction of granule membrane-mediated conversion of proglucagon(s), PSS-I and proinsulin resulted. This suggests that a significant proportion of the enzyme(s) involved in processing these prohormones (at least those responsible for initial cleavages at basic residues) is a membrane-associated protein in secretory granules.

Processing of PSS-I and PSS-II by Membranous and Soluble Fractions of Microsomes

When incubated with labeled prohormones, lysates of microsome fractions depleted the prohormone content in the incubates and generated products with labeling patterns, molecular sizes and RT on HPLC identical to many of the products found in extracts of intact tissue and to products generated by granule subfractions. However, some distinct differences between products produced by granule and microsome subfractions were observed. Microsomal lysates were found to be incapable of cleaving SS-14 from PSS-I. This suggests that the PSS-I processing enzyme(s) is either not present or, if present, is inactive in microsomes. For reasons to be discussed later, the latter alternative is more likely to be the correct interpretation. The enzymatic activity(ies) involved in processing proglucagon(s), PSS-II and proinsulin was found in both the membranous and soluble fractions of the microsomes.

It should be emphasized here that these results do not imply that the microsomal components (RER and Golgi) have a significant role in prohormone processing in the intact cell. All of the conversion assays were performed at pH 5.2, the optimum pH for converting activity. As mentioned earlier, if the intracisternal pH of RER and Golgi are near neutral in the intact cell, then most of the microsomal processing activity which is monitored *in vitro* at pH 5.2 would be inhibited.

To determine whether there was a difference in the relative contribution of Golgi components and RER to the composite converting activity of microsomes, Golgi enriched and RER enriched subfractions of microsomes were prepared by discontinuous density gradient centrifugation and tested for their ability to convert islet prohormones (34). It was found that both Golgi enriched and RER enriched microsomal subfractions, when lysed and incubated with labeled precursors, could mediate accurate conversion of proglucagon(s), proinsulin and PSS-II to release their respective products. This observation indicates that both the RER and Golgi subfractions contain the enzymes necessary to mediate processing of these precursors. The demonstration that the RER fractions have these enzymes is consistent with the hypothesis that converting enzymes are synthesized along with the (pre)prohormones at the RER, internalized into RER cisternae and transported through the Golgi and to secretory granules in parallel with the hormone precursors. If this is true, then it is probable that the converting enzyme for PSS-I to SS-14 processing is present, but inactive, in microsome fractions. This would be consistent with our finding that PSS-I processing activity was not observed in microsomes, but was present in secretory granules. Perhaps the PSS-I converting enzyme is activated in secretory granules as a result of a conformational change or an alteration of the intragranular ionic microenvironment.

Conclusions Regarding the Differential Processing of PSS-I and PSS-II in Secretory Granules and Microsomes

The diagram in Fig. 2 summarizes the results with regard to the differential conversion of PSS-I and PSS-II by subfractions of anglerfish islet microsomes and secretory granules.

The PSS-I to SS-14 processing enzyme was found to be active only in secretory granules and showed granule membrane-association. The enzymatic activity for PSS-II to AF SS-28 conversion was observed in microsomes (RER and Golgi) and secretory granules. This activity was membrane-associated in microsomes only. The implications of these findings is that (at least) two separate enzymes which have differential distribution or activity are involved in processing PSS-I and PSS-II. Another observation which is consistent with the suggestion that two different enzymes may be involved in converting these two precursors is that the cleavage sites in these prohormones are distinctly different. The PSS-I cleavage site is on the COOH side of an Arg-Lys sequence at positions -1 and -2 in PSS-I (44, 45) whereas the PSS-II cleavage

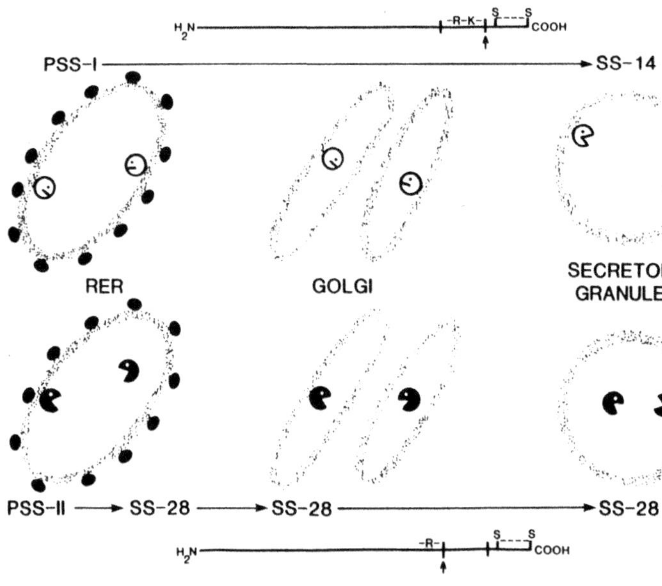

Fig. 2. Distribution and activity of enzymes involved in processing islet prosomatostatins. The enzymes for PSS-I (upper) and PSS-II (lower) processing are represented in three different subcellular compartments by the light and dark Pac-Man symbols, respectively. A symbol close to the membrane indicates membrane-association of the enzyme in that subcellular compartment. An open mouth indicates an active enzyme and a closed mouth indicates an inactive enzyme.

site is on the COOH side of a single Arg at position -15 in PSS-II (7, 44). If separate enzymes are involved in processing PSS-I and PSS-II, it might be postulated that the most efficient way in which this could be accomplished would be for the two precursors to be produced in separate cells. In support of this idea, we have recently obtained preliminary immunohistochemical evidence that SS-14 and [Tyr^7,Gly^{10}]SS-14 can be localized in different cells in anglerfish islets (unpublished results).

Although not emphasized in the presentation of the results, the distribution of the converting enzymes for the proglucagons and proinsulin differed from the distribution of the enzymes for PSS-I and PSS-II. Proglucagon and proinsulin processing was mediated by enzymes in both the membranous and soluble fractions of both microsomes and secretory granules. This observation indicates that enzymes different from those that process PSS-I and PSS-II are involved in conversion of proinsulin and the proglucagons. Taken together, the results from assessing islet prohormone processing in microsome and granule subfractions indicate that a relatively extensive family of related, but not identical, converting endopeptidases exist. It is probable that several different forms of "convertase" are present in the same cell and within different cells of the same tissue. It is possible that there is a specific endopeptidase for each initial prohormone cleavage, or that the same enzyme may mediate cleavage of precursors only at sites where basic pair sequence or some other feature of primary or secondary structure are very similar or identical. One would then predict that converting enzymes should show species specificity. This is, in fact, the case. It has been found that lysed secretory granules from rat neurointermediate lobe do not convert anglerfish islet prohormones and that lysed secretory granules from anglerfish islet cannot process toad pro-opiomelanocortin (Y.P. Loh and B.D. Noe, unpublished results). This reinforces the proposal that converting enzymes from various sources are not identical.

Membrane-Association of Converting Enzymes and Prohormones

Some consideration must be given to the observation that many of the acid cysteine converting enzymes which have been identified appear to be granule membrane-associated. This has been demonstrated in secretory granules from anglerfish islet (18, 19, 34), rat anterior pituitary (17), rat neurointermediate lobe (14) and in rat hypothalamic synaptosomes (46). Although the reasons for association of converting enzymes with granule membranes are not completely understood, there is some evidence that the intragranular segregation may facilitate prohormone transport or conversion.

Using protein-A gold immunolocalization of glicentin and glucagon in the pancreatic A-cells of several different species, Ravazzola and Orci (47) and Garaud et al. (48) demonstrated a preferential distribution of glicentin immunoreactive components at the periphery of A-cell secretory granules and glucagon immunoreactivity at the granule core. The glicentin antisera which were employed did not cross-react with glucagon. Since glicentin forms a portion of pancreatic proglucagons (49, 50), the results were interpreted to indicate that proglucagon is relegated to the granule periphery. Cleavage product (glucagon) would then accumulate at the center of the granule after proglucagon processing.

This information, combined with the knowledge that some converting enzymes are membrane-associated, provided the stimulus for us to investigate the possibility that newly synthesized prohormones may be membrane-associated in microsome and secretory granules from anglerfish islets. We have recently completed studies which demonstrate that 78% to 88% of the newly synthesized proinsulin, proglucagon(s) and prosomatostatin(s) found both in lysed microsomes and secretory granules was membrane-associated. Incubation of these membranes in a high salt solution (1M KCl) prior to centrifugation reduced prohormone association to non-specific binding levels. When labeled prohormones were incubated at 4 C with KCl-washed secretory granule membranes from unlabeled tissue, association of prohormones with membranes increased with incubation time to plateau at 15 to 30 min of incubation. The association was inhibited completely by addition of 10^{-4} M unlabeled prohormones and to a limited extent by anglerfish insulin, but not by BSA, RNase, bacitracin or bovine insulin (51).

These results provide preliminary evidence that there may be prohormone-specific receptors in RER, Golgi and secretory granule membranes. Others have made parallel observations. Orci and Ravazzola (52) have recently reported results from an immunocytochemical study which demonstrate that insulin immunoreactive determinants are associated with the cisternal membrane of the Golgi apparatus in rat pancreatic B-cells. This suggests that (pro)hormones may be associated with Golgi membranes in mammalian islets as well. The association of prohormones with the RER, Golgi and secretory granule membranes may be functionally advantageous to the cell in one or more of the following ways. Association of prohormones with intracellular membranes might: a) facilitate prohormone transport from RER to Golgi and secretory granules, b) target prohormones to secretory granules rather than lysosomes, c) maintain the prohormone substrates in juxtaposition with membrane-associated converting enzymes. Confirmation or refutation of these hypotheses will require further investigation.

SUMMARY

Over the past 4-5 years, a significant amount of new information regarding the characteristics of prohormone converting enzymes has been generated. The evidence available supports the proposal that cleavage at single, pairs or triplets of basic amino acids occurs by a two-step mechanism. The initial cleavage is performed at the COOH-terminus of the last basic amino acid by an endopeptidase having greater specificity than that required for the second cleavage step. The endopeptidase which performs the initial cleavage in many tissues has been characterized as a unique membrane-associated cysteine proteinase with a pH optimum of 5-6, an inhibitor spectrum which differentiates it from cathepsin B, and significant substrate specificity. In some tissues, the second step in the cleavage mechanism is performed by a cobalt activated carboxypeptidase B-like exopeptidase having a pH optimum (5.5-6.0) and an inhibitor spectrum different from that of either lysosomal or pancreatic carboxypeptidase B. This enzyme shows less substrate specificity than the endopeptidase and cleaves residual carboxyl terminal basic residues from hormone products and the non-hormonal "pro-peptides" (e.g. C-peptide of proinsulin). CPB-like enzymes which are thought to be involved in prohormone processing in adrenal, brain and pituitary have been isolated and purified to homogeneity (29). It remains to be determined whether CPB-like enzymes will be found in secretory granules of other cell types which synthesize hormone precursors. None of the endopeptidases involved in precursor processing have yet been isolated. Purification and characterization of these prohormone converting enzymes are essential for providing a more complete understanding of the mechanisms and regulation of post-translational proteolytic processing of prohormones.

The differential distribution and activity of the processing enzymes for PSS-I and PSS-II (34) provide the first direct evidence for the existence of two distinct converting enzymes for islet prosomatostatins. The results of this study may be useful in the interpretation of the differential processing of prosomatostatin which occurs in mammals as well. Results from several studies have demonstrated variable distribution of both SS-28 and SS-14 in different tissues (53-56) and release of both peptides into the circulation (56-59). The amount of either peptide which is produced in various tissues undoubtedly depends on differential cleavage of prosomatostatin. The determination of whether the cleavage mechanism in mammals involves two separate enzymes, as is the case in fish islets, will require further investigation in mammalian islets.

Finally, the observation that newly synthesized prohormones are associated with microsomal and secretory granule membranes (51) may have a number of potentially important implications with regard to prohormone transport, targeting to secretory granules and/or facilitation of prohormone processing. These intriguing possibilities should provide the stimulus for future investigations.

ACKNOWLEDGMENT

Our appreciation to G. Debo, F. Greiner, J. Heil and R. Lee for expert technical assistance. We also wish to thank J. Mackin and G. Morton for assistance in the preparation of the manuscript. Work performed in the authors' laboratories was supported by the following grants from NIH: AM 16921, AM 19890 and AM 26378. From 1977 through 1981, Dr. Noe was also supported by a Research Career Development Award from NIH, AM 00142.

REFERENCES

1. Johnson DE, Torrence JL, Elde RP, Bauer GE, Noe BD, Fletcher DJ 1976 Immunohistochemical localization of somatostatin, insulin and glucagon in the principal islets of the anglerfish (Lophius americanus) and the channel catfish (Ictalurus punctatus). Amer J Anat 147:119.
2. Warren TG, Shields D 1982 Cell-free bioisynthesis of somatostatin precursors: Evidence for multiple forms of preprosomatostatin. Proc Natl Acad Sci (USA) 79:3729.
3. Noe BD, Fletcher DJ, Bauer GE, Weir GC, Patel Y 1978 Somatostatin biosynthesis occurs in pancreatic islets. Endocrinology 102:1675.
4. Noe BD, Fletcher DJ, Spiess J 1979 Evidence for the existence of a biosynthetic precursor for somatostatin. Diabetes 28:724.
5. Noe BD 1981 Synthesis of one form of pancreatic islet somatostatin predominates. J Biol Chem 256:9397.
6. Noe BD, Spiess J 1983 Evidence for biosynthesis and differential posttranslational proteolytic processing of different (pre)prosomatostatins in pancreatic islets. J Biol Chem 258:1121.
7. Noe BD, Spiess J Identification and characterization of a primary cleavage product of (pre)prosomatostatin-II in pancreatic islets. Program of the 65th Annual Meeting of the Endocrine Society, San Antonio, June 1983, p 85 (Abstract).
8. Kemmler W, Peterson JD, Steiner DF 1971 Studies of the conversion of proinsulin to insulin I. Conversion in vitro with trypsin and carboxypeptidase B. J Biol Chem 246:6786.
9. Kemmler W, Steiner DF, Borg J 1973 Studies on the conversion of proinsulin to insulin III. Studies in vitro with a crude secretion granule fraction isolated from islets of Langerhans. J Biol Chem 248:4544.

10. Zühlke H, Steiner DF, Lernmark A, Lipsey C 1976 Carboxypeptidase B-like and trypsin-like activities in isolated rat pancreatic islets, CIBA Symposium No. 41. In: Porter R, Fitzsimons DW (eds) Polypeptide Hormones. Elsevier, New York, p 183.
11. Zühlke H, Kohnert K-D, Jahr H, Schmidt S, Kirschke H, Steiner DF 1977 Proteolytic and transhydrogenolytic activities in isolated pancreatic islets of rats, Acta Biol Med Germ 36:1695.
12. Noe BD 1984 Converting enzymes. In: Polak JM, Bloom SR (eds) Current Trends in Tumour Pathology, vol. 1; Endocrine Tumours. Churchill Livingstone, Edinburgh, (in press).
13. Loh YP, Brownstein MJ, Gainer H 1984 Proteolysis in neuropeptide processing and other neural functions. Ann Rev Neurosci 7:189.
14. Loh YP, Gainer H 1982 Characterization of pro-opiocortin-converting activity in purified secretory granules from rat pituitary neurointermediate lobe. Proc Natl Acad Sci (USA) 79:108.
15. Loh YP, Chang T-L 1982 Pro-opiocortin converting activity in rat intermediate and neural lobe secretory granules. FEBS Letters 137:57.
16. Chang T-L, Gainer H, Russell JT, Loh YP 1982 Proopiocortin-converting enzyme activity in bovine neurosecretory granules. Endocrinology 111:1607.
17. Chang T-L, Loh YP 1983 Characterization of proopiocortin converting activity in rat anterior pituitary secretory granules. Endocrinology 112:1832.
18. Fletcher DJ, Noe BD, Bauer GE, Quigley JP 1980 Characterization of the conversion of a somatostatin precursor to somatostatin by islet secretory granules. Diabetes 29:593.
19. Fletcher DJ, Quigley JP, Bauer GE, Noe BD 1981 Characterization of proinsulin and proglucagon converting activities in isolated islet secretory granules. J Cell Biol 90:312.
20. Evangelista R, Ray P, Lewis RV 1982 A "Trypsin-like" enzyme in adrenal chromaffin granules: A proenkephalin processing enzyme. Biochem Biophys Res Commun 106:895.
21. Troy CM, Musacchio JM 1982 Processing of enkephalin precursors by chromaffin granule enzymes. Life Sciences 31:1717.
22. Mizuno K, Miyata A, Kangawa K, Matsuo H 1982 A unique proenkephalin-converting enzyme purified from adrenal chromaffin granules. Biochem Biophys Res Commun 108:1235.
23. Smyth DG, Austen BM, Bradbury AF, Geisow MJ, Snell CR 1977 Biogenesis and metabolism of opiate active peptides. In: Hughes JR (ed) Centrally Acting Peptides. Macmillan Press, New York, p 231.
24. MacGregor RR, Chu LLH, Cohn DV 1976 Conversion of proparathyroid hormone to parathyroid hormone by a particulate enzyme of the parathyroid gland. J Biol Chem 251:6711.
25. Habener JR, Chang HT, Potts JT Jr 1977 Enzymic processing of proparathyroid hormone by cell-free extracts of parathyroid glands. Biochemistry 16:3910.

26. Lindberg I, Yang H-Y, Costa E 1982 An enkephalin-generating enzyme in bovine adrenal medulla. Biochem Biophys Res Commun 106:186.
27. Fricker LD, Snyder SH 1982 Enkephalin convertase: Purification and characterization of a specific enkephalin-synthesizing carboxypeptidase localized to adrenal chromaffin granules. Proc Natl Acad Sci (USA) 79:3886.
28. Fricker LD, Supattapone S, Snyder SH 1982 Enkephalin convertase: A specific enkephalin synthesizing carboxypeptidase in adrenal chromaffin granules, brain, and pituitary gland. Life Sci 31:1841.
29. Fricker LD, Snyder SH 1983 Purification and characterization of enkephalin convertase, an enkephalin-synthesizing carboxypeptidase. J Biol Chem 258:10950.
30. Hook VYH, Eiden LE, Brownstein MJ 1982 A carboxypeptidase processing enzyme for enkephalin precursors. Nature 295:341.
31. Noe BD, Baste CA, Bauer GE 1977 Studies on proinsulin and proglucagon biosynthesis and conversion at the subcellular level. I. Fractionation procedure and characterization of the subcellular fractions. J Cell Biol 74:578.
32. Noe, BD 1981 Inhibition of islet prohormone to hormone conversion by incorporation of arginine and lysine analogs. J Biol Chem 256:4940.
33. Noe BD, Fletcher DJ, Bauer GE 1981 Biosynthesis of glucagon and somatostatin. In: Cooperstein SJ, Watkins DT (eds), The Islets of Langerhans, Biochemistry, Physiology and Pathology. Academic Press, New York, p 189.
34. Noe BD, Debo G, Spiess J 1984 Comparison of prohormone processing activities in islet microsomes and secretory granules: Evidence for distinct converting enzymes for separate islet prosomatostatins. J Cell Biol 99:578.
35. Pollard HB, Zinder O, Hoffman PG, Nikodejevic O 1976 Regulation of the transmembrane potential of isolated chromaffin granules by ATP, ATP analogs, and external pH. J Biol Chem 251:4544.
36. Johnson RG, Scarpa A 1976 Internal pH of isolated chromaffin vesicles. J Biol Chem 251:2189.
37. Johnson RG, Scarpa A 1978 The internal pH of isolated serotonin containing granules of pig platelets. J Biol Chem 253:7061.
38. Russell JT, Holz RW 1981 Measurement of pH and membrane potential in isolated neurosecretory vesicles from bovine neurohypophyses. J Biol Chem 256:5950.
39. Scherman D, Nordmann JJ 1982 Internal pH of isolated newly formed and aged neurohypophysial granules. Proc Natl Acad Sci (USA) 79:476.
40. Carty SE, Johnson RG, Scarpa A 1982 Electrochemical proton gradient in dense granules isolated from anterior pituitary. J Biol Chem 257:7269.
41. Hutton JC 1982 The internal pH and membrane potential of the insulin-secretory granule. Biochem J 204:171.

42. Docherty K, Steiner DF 1982 Post-translational proteolysis in polypeptide hormone biosynthesis. Ann Rev Physiol 44:625.
43. Lazure C, Seidak NG, Pelaprat D, Chretien M 1983 Proteases and posttranslational processing of prohormones: A review. Can J Biochem Cell Biol 61:501.
44. Hobart P, Crawford R, Shen L-P, Pictet R, Rutter WJ 1980 Cloning and sequence analysis of cDNAs encoding two distinct somatostatin precursors found in the endocrine pancreas of anglerfish. Nature 288:137.
45. Goodman RH, Jacobs JW, Dee PC, Habener JF 1982 Somatostatin-28 encoded in a cloned cDNA obtained from a rat medullary thyroid carcinoma. J Biol Chem 257:1156.
46. Zingg HH, Patel YC 1983 Processing of somatostatin-28 to somatostatin-14 by rat hypothalamic synaptosomal membranes. Life Sciences 33:1241.
47. Ravazzola M, Orci L 1980 Glucagon and glicentin immunoreactivity are topologically segregated in the α granule of the human pancreatic A cell. Nature 284:66.
48. Garaud JC, Eloy R, Moody AJ, Stock C, Greiner JF 1980 Glucagon- and glicentin-immunoreactive cells in the human digestive tract. Cell & Tissue Res 213:121.
49. Moody AJ, Holst JJ, Thim L, Jensen SL 1981 Relationship of glicentin to proglucagon and glucagon in the porcine pancreas. Nature 289:514.
50. Holst JJ 1983 Gut glucagon, enteroglucagon, gut glucagonlike immunorectivity, glicentin: current status. Gastroenterology 84:1602.
51. Noe BD, Moran MN 1984 Association of newly synthesized islet prohormones with intracellular membranes. J Cell Biol 99:418.
52. Orci L, Ravazzola M, Perrelet A 1983 Insulin antigenic sites are associated with the cisternal membrane of the Golgi apparatus in pancreatic B-cells. C R Acad Sci Paris 297:467.
53. Fitz-Patrick D, Patel YC 1981 Evidence for somatostatin precursors in human stomach, placenta, and amniotic fluid. J Clin Endocrinol Metab 53:372.
54. Newgard CB, Holst JJ 1981 Heterogeneity of somatostatin like immunoreactivity (SLI) in extracts of porcine, canine and human pancreas. Acta Endocrinol 98:564.
55. Benoit R, Ling N, Alford B, Guillemin R 1982 Seven peptides derived from pro-somatostatin in rat brain. Biochem Biophys Res Commun 107:944.
56. Patel YC, Wheatley T, Ning C 1981 Multiple forms of immunoreactive somatostatin: Comparison of distribution in neural and non-neural tissues and portal plasma of the rat. Endocrinology 109:1943.
57. Schusdziarra V, Zyznar E, Rouiller D, Harris V, Unger RH 1980 Free somatostatin in the circulation: Amounts and molecular sizes of somatostatin-like immunoreactivity in portal, aortic, and vena caval plasma of fasting and meal-stimulated dogs. Endocrinology 107:1572.

58. Shoelson S, Polonsky K, Dockerty H, Jaspan J, Rubenstein A, 1982 Evidence for the presence of somatostatin 28 in plasma. Diabetes 31:474.
59. Peterfreund RA, Vale W 1982 High molecular weight somatostatin secretion by cultured rat brain cells. Brain Res 239:463.

9

ANGLERFISH PANCREATIC ISLETS PRODUCE TWO FORMS OF SOMATOSTATIN-28

JOACHIM SPIESS AND BRYAN D. NOE

Peptide Biology Laboratory
The Salk Institute
10010 North Torrey Pines Road
La Jolla, CA 92037
Department of Anatomy
Emory University School of Medicine
Atlanta, GA 30322

ABSTRACT

It has been predicted on the basis of cDNA sequence analysis that anglerfish pancreatic islets contain at least two different preprosomatostatins (I and II). The C-terminal amino acid sequences of preprosomatostatin I and II were predicted to be identical to mammalian hypothalamic somatostatin-14 (SS-14) and its analog [Tyr^7,Gly^{10}]SS-14, respectively. That SS-14 is expressed in anglerfish pancreatic islets, has been shown earlier in pulse-chase experiments and by chemical characterization. However, it was observed that [Tyr^7,Gly^{10}]SS-14 was not expressed as such, but as part of larger polypeptides.

Pulse-chase experiments combined with reverse-phase high pressure liquid chromatography, amino acid analysis with two different chromatographic systems, and complete Edman degradation indicated that preprosomatostatin II is processed in anglerfish islets to two different forms of somatostatin-28 (SS-28). The primary structure of the major form containing hydroxylysine (Hyl) was determined to be:

H-Ser-Val-Asp-Ser-Thr-Asn-Asn-Leu-Pro-Pro-Arg-Glu-Arg-Lys-
Ala-Gly-Cys-Lys-Asn-Phe-Tyr-Trp-Hyl-Gly-Phe-Thr-Ser-Cys-OH

The amino acid sequence of the minor form differs only at residue 23 by substitution of lysine for hydroxylysine. This is the first time that hydroxylysine, an amino acid which characteristically occurs in collagen or collagen-like structures has been identified in a potential regulatory peptide. It can be speculated that this amino acid is formed by post-translational hydroxylation of a lysine C-terminally linked to a glycine residue and thus modified at a site which has been recognized as hydroxylation site in collagen or collagen-like structures. The biological consequences of this unusual modification are being investigated.

INTRODUCTION

Somatostatin (SS) was discovered on the basis of its inhibitory effect on the secretion of growth hormone from the anterior pituitary (1). It has been recognized with immunologic assays that somatostatin is widely distributed in various tissues such as hypothalamus, extra-hypothalamic brain, spinal cord, gastrointestinal tract, endocrine pancreas (see 2 for review), thyroid (3) and retina (4), and occurs in multiple forms differing in size and amino acid sequence. The most abundant form, somatostatin-14 (SS-14), a tetradecapeptide, was first isolated from ovine (5, 6) and later porcine (7) hypothalamus and completely characterized chemically by sequence analysis. Subsequently, a peptide identical to ovine SS-14 was found by sequence analysis to be also present in extracts of pigeon pancreas (8), anglerfish pancreatic islets (9) and channel catfish pancreas (10). Thus, the primary structure of SS-14 was observed to be completely conserved in different species and tissues.

From mammalian tissues such as porcine intestine (11) and porcine (12) and ovine (13, 14) hypothalamus, a 28-residue somatostatin (SS-28) has been isolated and shown by sequence analysis to contain at its C-terminus, the amino acid sequence of SS-14 linked to the residual peptide by a pair of basic residues. The assumption that SS-14 (15) and mammalian SS-28 (16) represent primary cleavage products and that mammalian SS-28 probably does not serve as a precursor to SS-14 (16) has been supported by pulse-chase experiments. On the basis of nucleotide sequence analysis of cDNAs obtained from human and rat tumors (17, 18, 32), it has been predicted that the corresponding preprosomatostatins contained at their C-termini the amino acid sequence of mammalian SS-28. Thus, it can be speculated that mammalian SS-28 as well as SS-14 may be derived in mammalian cells from identical genes by differential post-translational processing.

It has been observed that the endocrine pancreas of anglerfish (19, 20) or catfish (21, 33, 34) (in contrast to mammalian tissues) contains at least two different somatostatin genes. From cDNA analysis (19-21, 34), it was concluded that one of these genes in either fish species encoded the amino acid sequence of SS-14, whereas the additional genes encoded amino acid sequences similar, but not identical, to SS-14.

Thus, anglerfish preprosomatostatin II, predicted on the basis of cDNA analysis (19) was found to contain the structure of [Tyr^{7},Gly^{10}]SS-14 at its C-terminus. By sequence analysis of tryptic fragments and pulse-chase experiments (22), we demonstrated previously that this analog of SS-14 is not expressed as such, but as part of larger polypeptides. We herein provide evidence that preprosomatostatin II is processed to two different forms of SS-28 containing [Tyr^{7},Gly^{10}]SS-14 or its hydroxylated analog.

Search for a Somatostatin Containing [Tyr^{7},Gly^{10}]SS-14

Since we assumed that [Tyr^{7},Gly^{10}]SS-14 was expressed as part of larger polypeptides, we performed experiments to identify islet polypeptides which would possibly contain the structure of this SS analog at their C-terminus. Accordingly, islets were incubated for five hours at 20 C in the presence of pairs of amino acids labeled with [^{3}H] and either [^{14}C] or [^{35}S] (15). Especially those amino acids were selected which were predicted (19) to be present in the C-terminal structure of anglerfish pancreatic preprosomatostatin II.

After incubation, islet tissue was homogenized with a Potter-Elvehjem homogenizer in 2 M acetic acid and centrifuged at low speed. The radiolabeled polypeptides of the supernatant were separated from salts and free amino acids by gel filtration through a Bio-Gel P-2 column. The islet extracts thus prepared were subsequently screened by gel filtration through a Bio-Gel P-30 column and reverse-phase high-pressure liquid chromatography (HPLC) on Vydac C_{18} columns. With this approach, we observed that the smallest species, which could qualify as an extended form of [Tyr^{7},Gly^{10}]SS-14, was eluted in the pool of the 2500-8000 dalton polypeptides together with glucagon-like peptides. This species could apparently be radiolabeled with tyrosine, glycine, tryptophan, cysteine, asparagine, threonine, valine, arginine, lysine, and leucine and thus was suspected to represent a polypeptide containing the C-terminal 28 residues of anglerfish preprosomatostatin II.

Under high resolving conditions of reverse-phase HPLC (Fig. 1), it was determined that the SS-like species S-carboxymethylated, as described (14), consisted of at least two components which were later identified as anglerfish SS-28 (aSS-28) and [Lys^{23}]aSS-28.

On the basis of the distribution of radioactivity in the eluates of gel filtration and reverse-phase HPLC, it was estimated that 88-90% of the radioactivity of SS-like polypeptides of molecular weights of less than 8000 was incorporated into SS-14. The residual 10-12% of the radioactivity appeared with the 28 residue SS-like polypeptides. Approximately 95% of the total radioactivity of the two 28 residue peptides was associated with aSS-28 which thus was identified as the predominant form of SS-28 in anglerfish pancreatic islets.

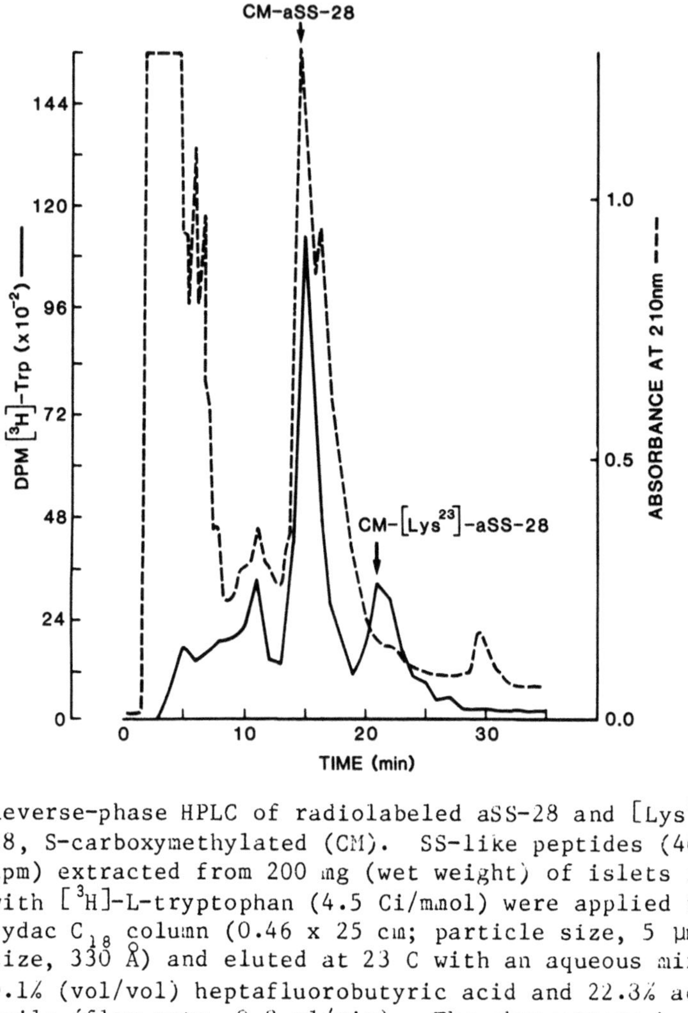

Fig. 1. Reverse-phase HPLC of radiolabeled aSS-28 and [Lys^{23}]aSS-28, S-carboxymethylated (CM). SS-like peptides (46,000 dpm) extracted from 200 mg (wet weight) of islets incubated with [^{3}H]-L-tryptophan (4.5 Ci/mmol) were applied to a Vydac C_{18} column (0.46 x 25 cm; particle size, 5 μm; pore size, 330 Å) and eluted at 23 C with an aqueous mixture of 0.1% (vol/vol) heptafluorobutyric acid and 22.3% acetonitrile (flow rate, 0.8 ml/min). The chromatography was carried out with a Perkin-Elmer Series 3B liquid chromatograph equipped with an LC-75 spectrophotometer.

Purification of Two Forms of Somatostatin-28

The approach used for the chromatographic characterization of the radiolabeled SS-like species as described above was applied to the purification of a sufficient amount of peptide for sequence analysis. From 110 mg (wet weight) of islet tissue (corresponding to one Brockmann body), approximately 16 μg of SS-28, as determined by amino acid analysis (14), was obtained after homogenization with a Potter-Elvehjem homogenizer, gel filtration through Bio-Gel P-2 and P-30 columns and reverse-phase HPLC of the S-carboxymethylated peptides.

Chemical Characterization of Somatostatin-28

The primary structure of the main form of aSS-28 was established by amino acid analysis of the acid and alkaline peptide hydrolysates, complete Edman degradation and peptide mapping on reverse-phase HPLC (Fig. 2). The most interesting result of this analysis which is described in detail elsewhere (23), was the finding of the presence of hydroxylysine in aSS-28.

This amino acid has been considered to be a typical component of collagen or collagen-like structures (see 24 for review) in which it serves as a cross-linker (after oxidative desamination of its amino group) or carbohydrate acceptor (24).

From the observation that hydrolysis of aSS-28 with 2 M NaOH or 6 M HCl did not significantly affect the recovery of hydroxylysine,

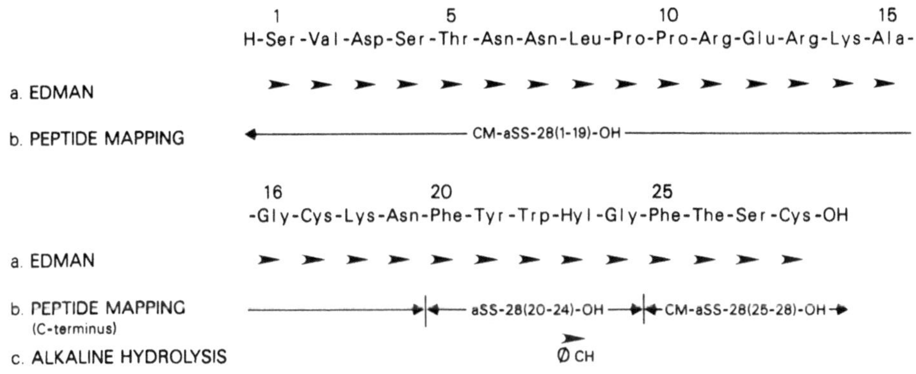

Fig. 2. Strategy of sequence analysis of the main form of anglerfish pancreatic SS-28 (aSS-28).

a. Approximately 2.0 nmol of CM-aSS-28 was subjected to automated Edman degradation in a spinning cup sequencer. Identified residues are marked by arrow. PTH-amino acid yields ranged from 1.6 nmol (valine-2) to 0.06 nmol (CM-cysteine-28).

b. Three main fragments were cleaved from CM-aSS-28 thermolysin and resolved by reverse-phase HPLC. On the basis of chromatographic evidence, it was demonstrated that the C-terminal residue carried a free carboxylic group.

c. It was observed by amino acid analysis of the acid and alkaline hydrolysates of CM-aSS-28 that hydroxylysine-23 was not glycosylated (see text).

it was concluded that hydroxylysine-23 was not glycosylated. In control experiments with glycosylated collagen, we recovered more hydroxylysine from the acid than from the alkaline hydrolysate. This latter difference in recovery of hydroxylysine probably reflected the high stability of acetalic bonds (linking the carbohydrate to hydroxylysine) under alkaline conditions.

The strategy of sequence analysis of the minor form of anglerfish SS-28 ([Lys^{23}]aSS-28) S-carboxymethylated (CM) was similar to the strategy followed in the analysis of aSS-28 (Fig. 2). Amino acid analysis of CM-[Lys^{23}]aSS-28 indicated a significant contamination of this peptide with CM-aSS-28 (Table 1). Based on the amino acid ratios of lysine and hydroxylysine (Table 1), it was estimated that as much as 30-40% of the peptide in this fraction was represented by CM-aSS-28.

Table 1. Amino Acid Composition of the Minor Form of Anglerfish SS-28

Amino acid	acid hydrolysis[a]	Edman[c]
CM-Cys	2.0 (2)[b]	2
Asx	4.0 (4)	4
Thr	1.9 (2)	2
Ser	2.8 (3)	3
Glx	1.2 (1)	1
Pro	2.1 (2)	2
Gly	2.3 (2)	2
Ala	1.0 (1)	1
Val	0.9 (1)	1
Leu	1.3 (1)	1
Tyr	0.9 (1)	1
Phe	1.7 (2)	2
Hyl	0.3 (0)	0
Lys	2.5 (3)	3
Trp	0.8 (1)	1
Arg	2.2 (2)	2

[a]Approximately 0.8 μg of peptide was hydrolyzed at 110 C for 24 hr with 4 M methanesulfonic acid and 0.2% tryptamine in the presence of norleucine as internal standard. The hydrolysate was analyzed with a Beckman 121 MB analyzer using sodium citrate buffers for elution and ninhydrin for detection. Details of the procedure are described elsewhere (14).

[b]Amino acid ratios are presented; the nearest integers are given in parentheses.

[c]The amino acid composition was derived from Edman degradation.

In view of the small deviation of the amino acid ratios from integers (Table 1), a major contamination of CM-[Lys^{23}]aSS-28 with peptides other than CM-aSS-28 was improbable.

Based on the data of complete Edman degradation of CM-[Lys^{23}] aSS-28 (Fig. 3), only one major component was found in the fraction applied to the sequencer. In some Edman cycles, minor amounts of phenylthiohydantoin (PTH) amino acids, which could not be assigned to the main peptide, were detected. However, the yields of these PTH-amino acids never exceeded 10% of the yields of the major PTH-amino acids of the same cycle. In cycle 23, mainly the PTH derivative of lysine was found. However, in view of the detection of a small amount of the PTH derivative of hydroxylysine, it was suggested in agreement with the interpretation of the amino acid analysis (Table 1) that the analyzed fraction was contaminated with CM-aSS-28.

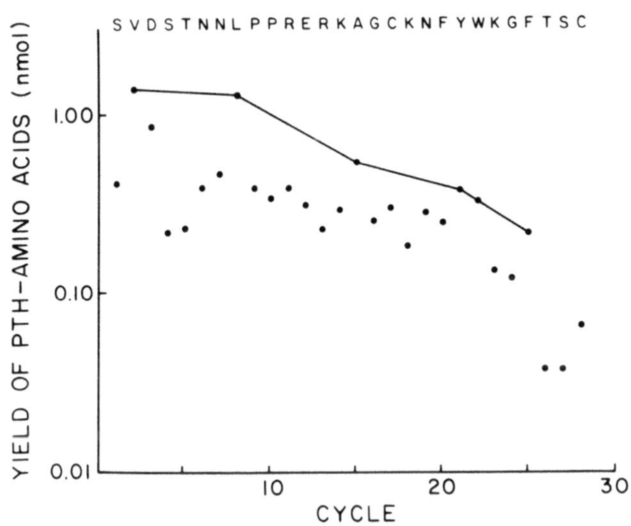

Fig. 3. Edman degradation of CM-[Lys^{23}]aSS-28. Approximately 1.7 nmol of peptide as determined by amino acid analysis was applied to an automated Beckman 890C spinning cup sequencer modified and programmed as described earlier (25, 26, 27). The phenylthiohydantoin (PTH) amino acids were identified and quantified with reverse-phase HPLC (coefficient of variation, 1-6%; minimal detectable amount, <10 pmol) (26). The repetitive yields calculated for stable PTH-amino acids were approximately 98%. Total PTH-amino acid yields per cycle are presented. The solid line interconnecting yields of stable PTH-amino acids indicates the decreasing amount of peptide in the cup during Edman degradation.

The Edman degradation data were confirmed and supplemented with results of reverse-phase HPLC of fragments cleaved from CM-[Lys^{23}] aSS-28 with thermolysin which has been shown (28) to catalyze the cleavage of peptides at the N-terminal side of hydrophobic amino acids. The absorbance profile (Fig. 4) was similar to the profile of the reverse-phase HPLC of CM-aSS-28 digested with thermolysin (23). Three main fragments, containing residues 1-19, 20-24 and 25-28 of CM-[Lys^{23}]aSS-28, were identified by amino acid analysis. The retention time of the C-terminal fragment, H-Phe-Thr-Ser-(CM)Cys-OH, did not deviate significantly from the retention time of CM-SS-14(11-14)-OH derived enzymatically from carboxymethylated synthetic SS-14. However, the C-terminal fragment cleaved from CM-[Lys^{23}]aSS-28 was eluted significantly later than CM-SS-14(11-14)-NH_2 derived from synthetic C-terminally amidated SS-14 (Fig. 4). It was therefore concluded that [Lys^{23}]aSS-28 carried a free C-terminal carboxylic group.

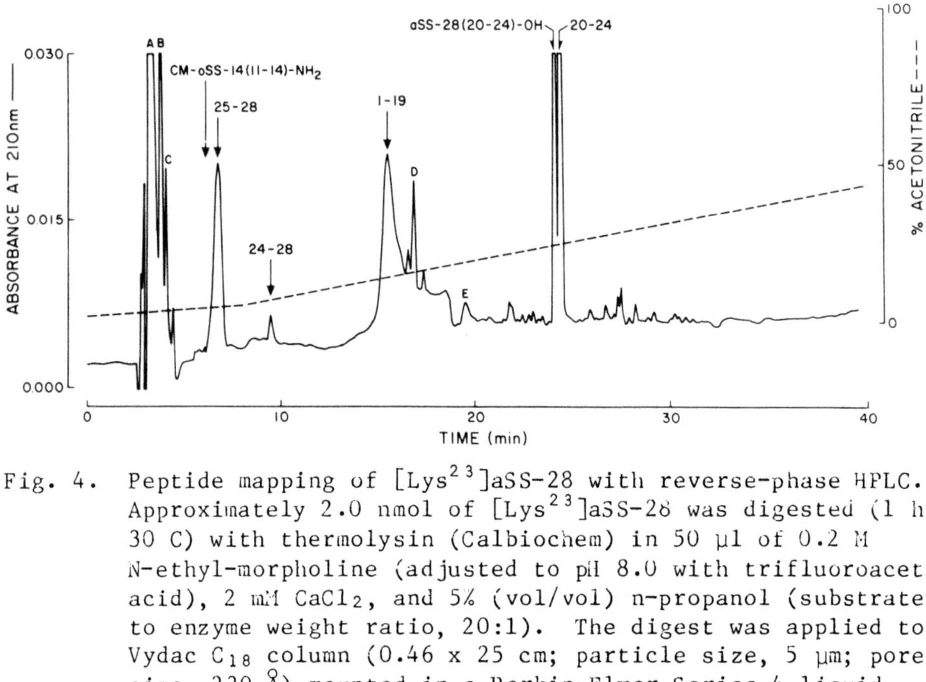

Fig. 4. Peptide mapping of [Lys^{23}]aSS-28 with reverse-phase HPLC. Approximately 2.0 nmol of [Lys^{23}]aSS-28 was digested (1 hr, 30 C) with thermolysin (Calbiochem) in 50 µl of 0.2 M N-ethyl-morpholine (adjusted to pH 8.0 with trifluoroacetic acid), 2 mM $CaCl_2$, and 5% (vol/vol) n-propanol (substrate to enzyme weight ratio, 20:1). The digest was applied to a Vydac C_{18} column (0.46 x 25 cm; particle size, 5 µm; pore size, 330 Å) mounted in a Perkin-Elmer Series 4 liquid chromatography and eluted with an aqueous mixture of 0.05% trifluoroacetic acid and actonitrile (flow rate, 1.0 ml/min; 23 C). All products were subjected to amino acid analysis as described in Table 1. Residue numbers refer to the sequence of [Lys^{23}]aSS-28 (Fig. 3). Products A-D could not be unambiguously identified. The amounts of peptide in the eluate were <0.3 µg (A-D), 0.6 µg (CM-[Lys^{23}]aSS-28(25-28)-OH), 0.07 µg (CM-[Lys^{23}]aSS-28(24-28)-OH), 1.4 µg (CM-[Lys^{23}]-aSS-28(1-19)-OH, 0.31 µg (aSS-28(20-24)-OH), 0.54 µg ([Lys^{23}]aSS-28(20-24)-OH.

Digestion of the CM-[Lys^{23}]aSS-28 preparation with thermolysin produced not only [Lys^{23}]aSS-28(20-24)-OH, H-Phe-Tyr-Trp-Lys-Gly-OH, as expected on the basis of the data of Edman degradation (Fig. 3), but also H-Phe-Tyr-Trp-Hyl-Gly-OH corresponding to aSS-28(20-24)-OH. The amount of the latter peptide represented approximately 36% of the total amount of [Lys^{23}]aSS-28(20-24)-OH and aSS-28(20-24)-OH in the eluate. Hence, it was concluded that this relative amount indicated the extent of the contamination of CM-[Lys^{23}]aSS-28 with CM-aSS-28.

On the basis of the Edman degradation data, peptide mapping and amino acid analysis, the primary structure of the minor form of anglerfish pancreatic somatostatin-28 was established (Fig. 5). This primary structure was found to be identical to the amino acid sequence of the C-terminal 28 residues of preprosomatostatin II as predicted from cDNA analysis (19). The sequence of [Lys^{23}]aSS-28 differed from the one of aSS-28 by the substitution of lysine-23 by hydroxylysine-23 (Fig. 5).

The biologic activities of aSS-28 and [Lys^{23}]aSS-28 have not yet been tested. Since the central part of SS-14, residues 6-9 and residue 11, has been determined to be essential for the potent inhibition of the secretion of growth hormone from cultured rat anterior pituitary cells (29), it is expected that neither aSS-28 nor its non-hydroxylated analog, both of which differ in the corresponding sequence part from SS-14 (Fig. 5), are potent inhibitors of the hypophyseal growth hormone secretion. It appears possible that this peptide may exhibit (pancreatic) biologic activities which differ significantly from the activities of SS-14, especially in view of the unusual presence of hydroxylysine in the main form of anglerfish SS-28.

Processing of Somatostatin Precursors

The experimental data presented here demonstrate that aSS-28 and [Lys^{23}]aSS-28 are the smallest SS-like polypeptides (extracted from pancreatic islets) which contain at their C-termini the structure of [Tyr^{7},Gly^{10}]SS-14 or its hydroxylated analog. That the predominant form of the 28 residue SS-like polypeptides, aSS-28, represents a primary cleavage product derived from preprosomatostatin II has been indicated by the results of pulse-chase experiments (unpublished data).

Based on these experiments and our knowledge of the biosynthesis of collagen (24), it appears probable that the hydroxylation of lysine-23 of aSS-28 occurs before the cleavage of aSS-28.

It has been demonstrated (24) that 5-hydroxylysine is introduced into collagen by enzymatic hydroxylation of lysine residues during translation. Evidence has been provided (30) that the

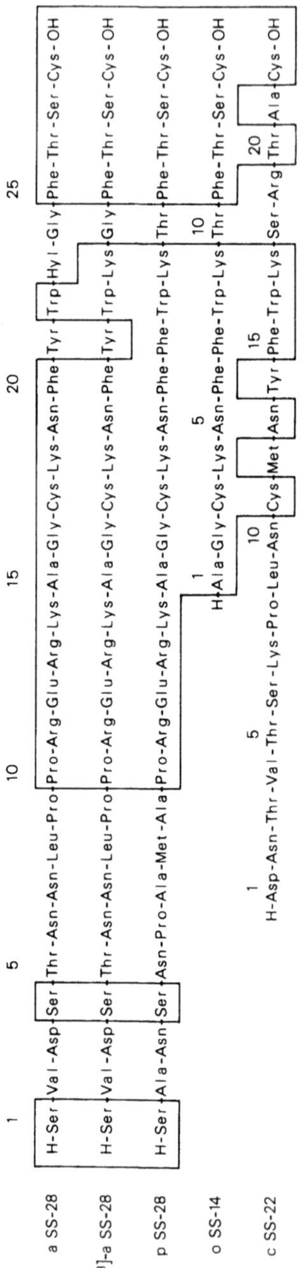

Fig. 5. Sequence homologies of the members of the somatostatin family. A high degree of homology within this peptide family is indicated by areas within solid lines.

catalyzing enzyme, lysyl hydroxylase, hydroxylates only lysine residues which are located N-terminally to glycine residues as neighbors. We assume that a similar mechanism may be followed in the hydroxylation of aSS-28. However, in view of the location of the hydroxylation site at lysine-23 in the C-terminal structure of aSS-28 and the intracellular distances involved, it appears improbable that hydroxylation of aSS-28 could be a cotranslational event. In this instance, we would expect that this modification of lysine may occur post-translationally.

Thus, we propose that preprosomatostatin II may be modified by signal peptidase (removing the signal sequence) and (in part) lysyl hydroxylase before cleavage at the C-terminal side of a single arginine residue to release aSS-28 or [Lys^{23}]aSS-28 (Fig. 6).

It is interesting that the pair of basic residues in the structure of aSS-28 or [Lys^{23}]aSS-28 does not represent a cleavage site, whereas the identical site marks the cleavage of SS-14 from prosomatostatin I (Fig. 6). One can speculate that this difference in processing of the somatostatin precursors I and II reflects high substrate specificity of the proteases involved (31) or the expression of the two precursors in different cells, or both.

ACKNOWLEDGMENT

We thank Dr. J. Rivier for providing synthetic peptides, David Karr, Wilson Woo, Gail Debo and Patricia Moxley for excellent technical assistance, and Susan Logan for manuscript preparation. This

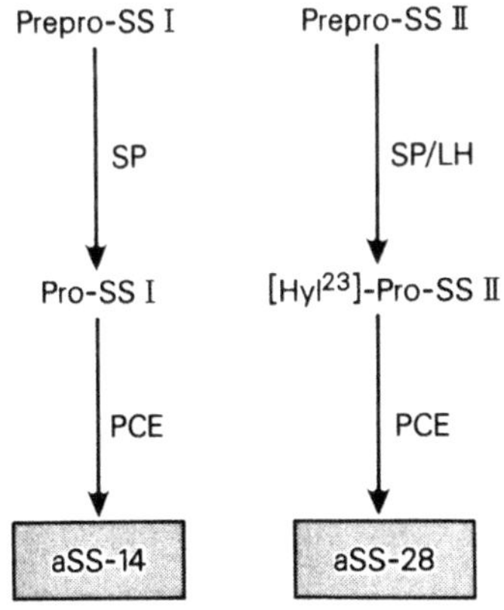

Fig. 6. Processing of preprosomatostatin I and II to the two main forms of somatostatin-28 in anglerfish pancreatic islets. SP, signal peptidase; LH, lysyl hydroxylase; PCE, prohormone converting enzyme.

research was supported by NIH grants AM-26378 and AM-16921, and the Clayton Foundation for Research - California Division. J. Spiess is a Clayton Foundation Investigator.

REFERENCES

1. Krulich L, Dhariwal APS, McCann SM 1968 Stimulatory and inhibitory effects of purified hypothalamic extracts on growth hormone release from rat pituitary in vitro. Endocrinology 83:783.
2. Vale W, Rivier C, Brown M 1977 Regulatory peptides of the hypothalamus. Ann Rev Physiol 39:473,
3. Yamada Y, Ito S, Matsubara Y, Kobayashi S 1977 Immunohistochemical demonstration of somatostatin containing cells in the human, dog and rat thyroid. Tohoku J Exper Med 122:87.
4. Rorstad OP, Brownstein MKJ, Martin JB 1979 Immunoreactive and biologically active somatostatin-like material in rat retina. Proc Natl Acad Sci (USA) 76:3019.
5. Brazeau P, Vale W, Burgus R, Butcher M, Rivier J, Guillemin R 1973 Hypothalamic polypeptide that inhibits the secretion of immunoreactive pituitary growth hormone. Science 179:77.
6. Burgus R, Ling N, Butcher M, Guillemin R 1973 Primary structure of somatostatin, a hypothalamic peptide that inhibits the secretion of pituitary growth hormone. Proc Natl Acad Sci (USA) 69:684.
7. Schally AV, DuPont A, Arimura A, Redding TW, Nishi N, Linthicum GL, Schlesinger DH 1976 Isolation and structure of somatostatin from porcine hypothalami. Biochemistry 15:509.
8. Spiess J, Rivier J, Rodkey JA, Bennett CD, Vale W 1979 Isolation and characterization of somatostatin from pigeon pancreas. Proc Natl Acad Sci (USA) 76:2974.
9. Noe BD, Spiess J, Rivier J, Vale W 1979 Isolation and characterization of somatostatin from anglerfish pancreatic islet. Endocrinology 105:1410.
10. Andrews PC and Dixon J 1981 Isolation and structure of a peptide hormone predicted from a mRNA sequence. J Biol Chem 256:8267.
11. Pradayrol L, Jørnvall H, Mutt V, Ribet A 1980 N-terminally extended somatostatin: the primary structure of somatostatin 28. FEBS Lett 109:55.
12. Schally AV, Huang WY, Chang LC, Arimura A, Reeding TW, Millar RP, Millar MW, Hunkapiller W, Hood LE 1980 Isolation and structure of pro-somatostatin: a putative somatostatin precursor from pig hypothalamus. Proc Natl Acad Sci (USA) 77:4489.
13. Esch F, Böhlen P, Ling N, Benoit R, Brazeau P, Guillemin R 1980 Primary structure of ovine hypothalamic somatostatin-28 and somatostatin-25. Proc Natl Acad Sci (USA) 77:6827.

14. Spiess J, Villarreal J, Vale W 1981 Isolation and sequence analysis of a somatostatin-like polypeptide from ovine hypothalamus. Biochemistry 20:1982.
15. Noe BD, Fletcher DJ, Spiess J 1979 Evidence for the existence of a biosynthetic precursor for somatostatin. Diabetes 28:724.
16. Patel YC, Zingg HH, Srikant CB 1985 Somatostatin-14 like immunoreactive forms in the rat: characterization, distribution, and biosynthesis. In: Patel YC, Tannenbaum GS (eds) Somatostatin. Plenum Publishing Corporation, New York.
17. Goodman RH, Jacobs JW, Dee PC, Habener JF 1982 Somatostatin-28 encoded in a cloned cDNA obtained from a rat medullary thyroid carcinoma. J Biol Chem 257:1156.
18. Shen L-P, Pictet RL, Rutter WJ 1982 Human somatostatin I: sequence of the cDNA. Proc Natl Acad Sci (USA) 79:4575.
19. Hobart P, Crawford R, Shen L-P, Pictet R, Rutter WJ 1980 Cloning and sequence analysis of cDNAs encoding two distinct somatostatin precursors found in the endocrine pancreas of anglerfish. Nature 288:137.
20. Goodman RH, Jacobs JW, Chin WW, Lund PK, Dee PC, Habener JF 1980 Nucleotide sequence of a cloned structural gene coding for a precursor of pancreatic somatostatin. Proc Natl Acad Sci (USA) 77:5869
21. Magazin M, Minth CD, Funckes C, Deschenes R, Tavianini M, Dixon J 1982 Sequence of a cDNA encoding pancreatic preprosomatostatin-22. Proc Natl Acad Sci (USA) 79:5152.
22. Noe BD, Spiess J 1983 Evidence for biosynthesis and differential posttranslational proteolytic processing of different (pre)prosomatostatins in pancreatic islets. J Biol Chem 258:1121.
23. Spiess J, Noe B 1985 Processing of an anglerfish somatostatin precursor to a hydroxylysine containing somatostatin-28. Proc Natl Acad Sci (USA) in press.
24. Prockop DJ, Kivirikko KI, Tuderman L, Guzman NA 1979 The biosynthesis of collagen and its disorders. New Engl J Med 301:13.
25. Wittmann-Liebold B 1982 An evaluation of the current status of protein sequencing. In: Elzinga M (ed) Methods in Protein Sequence Analysis. Humana Press, Clifton, NJ, p 27-63.
26. Spiess J, Rivier J, Rivier C, Vale W 1982 Micro-sequence analysis of ovine hypothalamic corticotropin-releasing factor, In: Elzinga M (ed) Methods in Protein Sequence Analysis. Humana Press, Clifton, NJ, p 131-138.
27. Spiess J, Rivier J, Vale W 1983 Sequence analysis of rat hypothalamic corticotropin-releasing factor with the o-phthalaldehyde strategy. Biochemistry 22:4341.
28. Heinrikson RL 1977 Applications of thermolysin in protein structural analysis. Methods Enzymol 47:175.
29. Vale W, Rivier J, Ling N, Brown M 1978 Biologic and immunologic activities and applications of somatostatin analogs. Metabolism 27:1391.

30. Kivirikko KI, Myllyla R 1980 The hydroxylation of prolyl and lysyl residues. In: Freedman RB, Hawkins HC (eds) Enzymology of Post-translational Modifications of Proteins. Academic Press, London, vol. 1, p 53-104.
31. Noe BD, Debo G, Spiess J 1984 Comparison of prohormone processing activities in islet microsomes and secretory granules: evidence for distinct converting enzymes for separate islet prosomatostatins. J Cell Biol 99:578.
32. Funckes CL, Minth CD, Deschenes R, Magazin M, Tavianini MA, Sheets M, Collier K, Weith HL, Aron DC, Roos BA, Dixon JE 1983 Cloning and characterization of a mRNA encoding rat preprosomatostatin. J Biol Chem 258:8781.
33. Oyama H, Bradshaw RA, Bates OJ, Permutt A 1980 Amino acid sequence of catfish pancreatic somatostatin I. J Biol Chem 255:2251.
34. Taylor WL, Collier KJ, Deschenes RJ, Weith HL, Dixon J 1981 Sequence analysis of a cDNA coding for a pancreatic precursor to somatostatin. Proc Natl Acad Sci (USA) 78:6694.

BIOSYNTHESIS AND PROCESSING OF SOMATOSTATIN

PANEL DISCUSSION

MODERATOR: P. BRAZEAU

DR. P. BRAZEAU (La Jolla): It seems that from studying the genes and studying the clipping of the precursors, one dimension had, most of the time, been completely forgotten. What about the physiological effect of the produced materials? Would that be a wiser approach or at least it might shed a lot more light in terms of what the terminal issue is. That is which tissue produced more S-28 than S-14, are there other biologically active forms of somatostatin, etc? And are there different clipping enzymes from one tissue to another giving rise to different molecular forms of somatostatin in different tissues? For instance, Dr. Patel had raised a very interesting question from the beginning, namely that we find more somatostatin-28 in the gut, compared to the hypothalamus where we find more somatostatin-14. Would there be different clipping enzymes in the two tissues? The other question raised by Dr. Benoit was that, we have the possibility of generating a variety of peptides. But, is it really the case in nature, is it really the case from different species, is it really the case from different tissues of a certain species? So, it is more or less open to discussion to all five of you and I hope somebody can take over here because in terms of precursors and processing I know very little. Who would feel confident to discuss first the enzyme clipping process in different tissues?

DR. J. HABENER (Boston): There are a number of interesting questions that have come out of this. It seems that the new information presented here is the rather interesting post-translational modification of amino acids involving hydroxylation and glycosylation. Let me just make a comment, and ask Dr. Noe a question. If I am not mistaken it seems like this marked diversification of molecules resulting from amino acid derivatization is limited to the fish. For example, it is the catfish somatostatin-22 that is glycosylated and the anglerfish S-28 peptide that is hydroxylated. So it brings up some interesting questions about what it might be doing in the mammal. The question for Dr. Noe was that I think some time in the past you had some evidence for tissue-specific or cell-specific expression of the two fish somatostatin genes, so that would bring up the question whether the enzymes are specialized for certain cell types.

DR. B. NOE (Atlanta): Yes, we are still not finished with the immunohistochemistry analysis. We have some antisera that are generated against the Tyr^7-Gly^{10} form, and of course antisera that are generated against the S-14 form. And unfortunately, the antisera that we have so far generated for the Tyr^7-Gly^{10} form, have some cross reactivity with S-14 although they do show some very nicely dense-stained cells that are different from the somatostatin-14 containing cells. And so, even though we can't come out and say clearly that it is the case, it seems very suggestive at this point that preprosomatostatin-I and preprosomatostatin-II in the anglerfish at least, are produced in separate cell types. This would mean that the enzymes that are processing the two are probably segregated into different subsets of secretory granules. And in fact, as I pointed out during my presentation we do not see any [Tyr^7-Gly^{10}]S-14, produced in the intact tissue. I did not show it during my presentation but *in vitro* when we take the tissue and homogenize it and put all the secretory granules together - which would be a combination of the secretory granules from all of the cell types of the islet - lyse them and incubate in the presence of the precursor, a minor form in the lysates from granules is the Tyr^7-Gly^{10} form, but that is produced only *in vitro*. So that again, possibly supports that in the intact tissue the two enzymes are in separate cells but when you bring them together *in vitro* you can get conversion.

DR. J. GERICH (Rochester): I may have misunderstood, but I got the impression that Dr. Patel and Dr. Cohen arrived at different conclusions from their experiments regarding the formation of somatostatin-14. Is that correct? One suggested that it came directly from the precursor, the large molecular weight somatostatin, and the other suggested that it came through S-28. Is that correct?

DR. P. COHEN (Paris): Not exactly, what I was saying is that the enzyme activity we have characterized using the model peptide *in vitro* was not able to convert the large molecular weight form into S-14. In contrast S-28 was converted to S-14 by cleavage of the lysine-alanine bond. Whether this cleavage is a result of one step or multi-step enzyme system is not clear at this time. It could well be that we have an esteropeptidase cleaving between Arg-Lys and an amino-peptidase removing the lysine. What I want to say is that from this indirect evidence, I believe that S-28 must be an intermediary form, a prerequisite to the formation of S-14 as an indirect proof; and indirect evidence is not a metabolic demonstration. So, my feeling is that we have to release S-28 from the larger molecular weight prosomatostatin form, before S-14 can be released, unless, failure to release S-14 from the precursor could be due to trivial reasons, but this is unlikely.

DR. Y.C. PATEL (Montreal): Yes, we do seem to disagree on that point. I think the question is not whether there are two separate cleavages occurring but, what we feel the order of the cleavages are, as well as their relative importance. I think the kinetic studies show that in both the rat hypothalamus and islets, there is direct dislocation of S-14 from prosomatostatin, that it occurs fairly rapidly and appears to be an important cleavage mechanism for the generation of S-14. This is backed up by the finding in these tissues of high concentrations of the residual cleavage product equivalent to prosomatostatin without the S-14 sequence. As to whether Dr. Cohen is right and whether there is conversion of S-28 to S-14, our kinetic data don't seem to support it, but, perhaps this is because the conversion is very rapid. We are using 20-30 min pulse-chase incubations, but already it may have got converted. Thus, while we cannot completely exclude very rapid cleavage of S-28 to S-14, our inability so far to see any kind of precursor-product relationship between the two forms leads us to believe that S-14 production via S-28 is probably relatively unimportant in our systems.

DR. P. BRAZEAU: Could there be a tissue specificity here in that we are not dealing with the same tissue, nor with the same specific enzyme, and therefore we don't see the same thing? It is just a naive question.

DR. M.D. RUGGERE (Montreal): This is very interesting. It would seem that S-14 can be made either from the precursor directly, or probably through S-28. I have several questions. One is, do you think the same enzyme would cleave off S-14 from either S-28 or the precursor. If Dr. Cohen was right, however, the longer sequence of the precursor molecule might inhibit the action of his particular cleavage enzyme. The second question I have is - how sure are we that these enzymes are so very specific? In the case of other peptides such as vasopressin, the vasopressin cleaving enzymes which are also surface bound and not receptor mediated, similar sorts of enzymes cleave other neuropeptides. And my third question is to Dr. Cohen: Did his synthetic product with the Arg-Lys in it, lose the dibasic amino acids following cleavage?

DR. P. COHEN: So what do you want me to answer? All the questions? Let's start with the last one. I would be happy to show dipeptidyl peptidase which should cleave the Arg-Lys bond as such and would give the S-28(1-12) fragment which would be very nice for everybody. But I am a bit reluctant to follow this because we have no experimental evidence. I refer to a very nice work published in Nature a few days ago from a Japanese group who have been looking for the prohormone cleavage of the mating factor in yeast, by technology very similar to the one we have used. To identify this esteropeptidase which recognizes an Arg-Lys-doublet, they have bought from a commercial source metenkephalin and leuenkephalin analogs containing arginine-lysine and an extension of the C-terminal end. They have found that they could never generate pure metenkephalin or leuenkephalin but they could generate only met- or leuenkephalin with an arginine extension. That means the cleavage was occurring between arginine and lysine. Therefore unless we find that the purified enzyme we have is not the result of the combined activity of two enzymes topologically related, we have to leave open the door to the possibility of a two-step mechanism. We know that our enzyme is closely related to the granule. We have agreement with Dr. Noe about this localization. We can prepare it from neurosecretory granules from various organs and we have found that it can be released easily from membrane by ionic shock. If the cleavage process involves more than one step it would have to be very complicated because to release S-14 we would need the esteropeptidase to cleave between Arg and Lys plus a basic aminopeptidase to remove the lysine and a carboxypeptidase B to remove the arginine and release the S-28(1-12) fragment.

DR. M.D. RUGGERE: Question #2. It seems that S-14 can be made either from S-28 or from the precursor, although perhaps not in your system. It would seem to me that similar enzymes would attack similar sequences unless inhibited. Would it seem that it would be the same enzyme that would make S-14 from either S-28 or from the precursor and the real controller of S-28 in tissues would be whatever cleaved S-28 out of the precursor and whether you went through that step or not. It does not seem that S-14 from S-28 has been a major pathway.

DR. P. COHEN: From a simple glimpse at the sequence and the structure and some attempts we have made to evaluate the secondary structure of both sides of the putative cleavage point, I would not expect that it is the same enzyme doing the two jobs although this has to be proven. We have shown that the 15000 molecular weight prosomatostatin species exposed to this activity is recovered unchanged under various conditions. We cannot exclude that it is a trivial reason that is responsible for the failure to generate S-14. But I would expect that release of the S-28 must occur before S-14 is cleaved from S-28. We can easily imagine that conformationally, the Arg-Lys bond of the S-14 cleavage site in S-28 is masked in the precursor and that would go in the direction of what we are postulating.

DR. M.D. RUGGERE: So you would postulate that tertiary structure would be very important for the activity of this enzyme on the Arg-Lys bond and that there would possibly be two enzymes, instead of one acting on the same site.

DR. P. COHEN: But we have good reason to believe that the enzyme we have does not cut arginine alone at either the S-14 or S-28 cleavage points but it does cut lysine alone, so I don't think that this is the case. I think we are dealing with two different enzymes. We are trying to chase the second enzyme using the synthetic peptide reproducing the sequence between the prosequence and the N-terminal end of the S-28. Maybe we can fish out a different enzyme but this will be more difficult to detect.

DR. W. RUTTER (San Francisco): First I want to compliment these people for providing a lovely story in which certainly the whole scientific work complements the work on the gene so we can try to begin to understand how these molecules exist and in what forms. It seems the work of Drs. Noe and Paul Cohen to a great extent simplifies our understanding of how cleavage can occur and it seems like the simplest hypothesis is that there are multiple enzymes. That explains why in different organs you have different proportions. It also explains why the kinds of kinetic experiments that Dr. Patel has carried out are difficult to interpret, because by varying the ratios of the various enzymes that are present you could get one result or another. So I would first like to present the simplifying hypothesis: that the enzymes are similar or identical. The two or three cleavage enzymes must operate in different cells which then explains I think, the result which we found rather early in the gene - that the somatostatin-II gene was certainly not present in the human somatostatinoma from which we isolated somatostatin-I. If it turns out that the two genes are in fact expressed in different cells, and if the tumor cells were clonal as we expect, then we expect a single somatostatin and that is exactly what we got. So I still then raise the issue about a second cell type which makes somatostatin-II in humans. The second point is that the cDNA levels of anglerfish somatostatin-I and somatostatin-II, were approximately of the order of 10:1 which is about the ratio that Joachim Spiess is finding for the level of the two peptides. Now that does not mean that one activity is inconsequential; it simply means that that is the state of the affairs. That sort of emphasizes the importance of looking at the fragments that each of you are getting. And the first question to Dr. Benoit would be whether each of the sequences that you have, correspond precisely to the sequences which are determined from the cDNAs. Because at one level the easiest way to now ask whether there are going to be multiple somatostatins would be to get some protein sequence information because it is not necessarily going to be easy for us to find a genetic inroad into their absent methods of hybridization from probes that we have.

DR. R. BENOIT (Montreal): Until now the work we have done has been virtually all in rats and until now the sequence information from rat brain corresponds completely with the work done by direct recombinant DNA on the gene itself. I do not have extensive information yet in humans but there is no reason yet according to data combining immunohistochemistry and also radioimmunoassay to believe that there would be a difference there. So up till now so far as I know from my own data in the rat and other animal species, everything seems to correspond rather well with data supporting just one gene.

DR. W. RUTTER: One of the nicest approaches would be to assume that there would be some amino acid crossreaction with the somatostatin-II species, to make antibodies against a putative somatostatin-II proregion and then to use those to see if you could detect a pro-somatostatin-II like molecule in other animal species higher-up stream evolutionarily.

DR. J. DIXON (West Lafayette): I would like to make a comment and then ask a question. We have also looked at the anglerfish somatostatin-II product. We did this actually in search of the corresponding 22 peptide that we had found in catfish, and like the results that Dr. Spiess has presented, we also find that there is hydroxylated lysine. We have analyzed this both directly by mass spectrometry as well as by analyzing the entire peptide by FAB mass spectrometry and we find it to be consistent with his observations. I might also add that we have not been able to find the glycosylated form which is again consistent with his observations. The question that I think is really most interesting is regarding the discussion on the processing enzyme that several of the speakers alluded to. We have heard a lot about the nature of the products that are produced as a result of the processing events; and yet, in fact, the substantial purifications that have been obtained on these enzymes would also suggest that there is probably something known about the enzymology of the processing enzymes, and so the direct question is: Have experiments been carried out on the purified processing enzymes to characterize them in terms of enzymology. This is really to Dr. Noe and to Dr. Cohen.

DR. B. NOE: We are of course heading in that direction but we do not have sufficient amounts of any of the processing enzymes with which to do those kinds of studies yet.

DR. P. COHEN: Maybe I could ask a question to one of the speakers and to Dr. Noe also. At this point in time we only have limited information on the purified enzyme I have shown. It looks to be sensitive to SH reagents. The activity is 100% abolished by PCMB or by iodoacetamide and is absolutely indifferent to trypsin- like serine protease inhibitors. Secondly, in contrast to what Dr. Noe has said, the pH range we have found is between 5 and 8, a relatively broad range, and our enzyme is completely inactivated under pH 5. But Dr. Noe was talking about the microsomal compartment and we are talking about the granule compartment and I think there is agreement that going from the saccule to the granule you have an increase of the optimal pH of the processing enzyme.

DR. B. NOE: We actually find that the pH optimum in the granules is also around 5 and it is fairly sharp. That's the case for the processing enzymes for prosomatostatin, proglucagon, and proinsulin, and it is also consistent with results that have been generated from other laboratories. Peng Loh for instance has results very similar to ours.

DR. P. COHEN: But as Dr. Dixon has said, determining a pH optimum must be with a purified fraction otherwise you cannot get a sharp curve. I do not know to which extent the enzyme has been purified to be able to say what is the pH range optimum for your enzyme. I am very skeptical about extrapolating a pH optimum from *in vitro* experiments to the optimal pH which is occurring inside the granule which is measured most of the time by diffusion of the dye. The dielectric constants, and the condition of the neurosecretory compound inside the granule is completely different. I think this optimal pH concept is to be cautiously taken.

DR. J. SPIESS (La Jolla): I would like to make one comment which came up, especially on the specificity of the release of somatostatin-14. We have very early on, done some model experiments with trypsin which very nicely released somatostastin-14 from prosomatostatin without affecting any of the bonds within the somatostatin unit. This implies that a double basic residue may not be the very best model to investigate some of these questions. It may well be that somatostatin-14 could be released by enzymes which are not involved in the physiology of the processing and therefore the investigation of the larger somatostatin-28 processing may be more revealing in that respect and that could explain for example also some of the experiments Dr. Cohen has presented.

DR. J. ENSINCK (Seattle): If I may preface my questions to Drs. Benoit and Patel by a comment based upon some data that we have been achieving in man. We have recently demonstrated that the 5K-LI measured with the 1-12 immunoassay rises precipitously in the plasma of man after eating. In the rat also it would seem that this material in a single 5K peak is found in intestinal extracts reputedly in the epithelial cells with no demonstration of a 1-14 form. My question therefore is: Is it possible that there is another gene that is coded to synthesize a macromolecular S-28 precursor, if you will, without a terminal S-14 which is related to the known mammalian precursor only by sharing the S-28 (1-12) sequence.

DR. Y.C. PATEL: The idea of two somatostatin genes and precursors in mammals is a nice one since their existence would help to tie in the fish data with the mammalian data and I see that Dr. Rutter is sort of hinting towards something along those lines. So far, the evidence is for a single mammalian gene. He has implied that the possibility of multiple genes cannot be excluded. The presence of 2 separate precursors, one for S-28 and the other for S-14 would certainly simplify our understanding of tissue-specific processing that seems to be so characteristic of mammalian tissues and at the same time bridge the gap between the fish and the mammalian somatostatin systems. I guess that we will have to wait and see. I have a couple of questions for Bryan Noe - can you give us any information as yet on the biological activity of the second product, the 28 form in the anglerfish, and have your localization studies reached a level whereby you can comment on the relationship between the cells that contain each of the two products (S-14 and S-28) and the other islet cells in the anglerfish.

DR. B. NOE: The answer to both of those questions is basically no. We have not yet obtained synthetic anglerfish S-28 that is hydroxylated. The obvious next step is to try to obtain that peptide and check it for biological activity because after all that is the normal cleavage product of the second precursor. Tests of the activity of [Tyr^7-Gly^{10}] S-14 that have been carried out so far probably do not mean that much because that is not the cleavage product of this particular precursor. With regard to your second question, because of the problem with a little bit of crossreactivity in the antisera for the [Tyr^7-Gly^{10}] S-14, we have not really done the morphometric studies that would require answering that question.

DR. J. SPIESS: To the question of the biological activities of these new peptides I would say that based on the structure-activity relationships worked out by Rivier and Wylie Vale, whatever one would do to this molecule at the N-terminus or C-terminus, it would not be expected to be active on the pituitary. Consequently, that does not seem to be the route to go for, but one certainly cannot exclude, that there might be novel pancreatic activities and other types of activities. Certainly, we have only been discussing the endocrine area, but maybe that is a mistake - especially for the larger pro forms. I have gone to quite a few of Bill Rutter's seminars and presentations and have written down all the data about the insulin selective actions of [Tyr^7-Gly^{10}] somatostatin-28 and every time I see it I ask again the people in our laboratory who have performed similar tests and they don't find any activity. However, these two sets of data may not necessarily be contradictory because Bill Rutter uses the perfused pancreas whereas our assays use *in vivo* systems.

DR. P. LOH (Bethesda): I just want to support Dr. Noe in that in the POMC system of proopiomelanocortin, where the enzyme has been purified now, the pH is acidic so the question raised earlier by Dr. Cohen as to whether crude homogenates or purified enzymes have been used for studying pH optima no longer applies. The question I have is for Dr. Noe: Are you absolutely sure that the cleavage site is really on the carboxyl site of the paired basic residue? Can you entertain possibilities of a cleavage in between as in the yeast α factor cleavage?

DR. B. NOE: You mean in the prosomatostatin-I where it is cleaving S-14? We have not looked at the C-terminus of what would be the 1-14 N-terminal segment of S-28, so I cannot answer that question.

DR. J. SPIESS: But isn't it thought in your group that it is reversed; that the lysine is before the arginine in your cleavage group which your enzyme works on?

DR. P. LOH: It is in between, yes, and we also have now an aminopeptidase B-like enzyme that is very specific for taking off the arginine.

DR. B. NOE: Yes, you would have to postulate the removal of the extra basic from the amino end if it cleaved in the middle.

DR. P. LOH: Yes, and there is an enzyme to do that.

DR. FRANCIS (Seattle): This question is directed to Dr. Benoit. In doing gel permeation chromatography and trying to determine molecular weights, I find it difficult to put credence on finding molecular weight of a peptide that might have a linear structure as opposed to a globular structure in these particular gels and to maintain that that is the particular molecular weight. I would like you to comment on what you think the molecular weights really would be if Stokes radius is involved in determining the true molecular weights of these substances.

DR. R. BENOIT: The only answer I can give you on this is that for the three peptides, I discussed here, the molecular weight in general as evaluated by gel filtration was slightly smaller than what the exact molecular weight in reality is. There is about 500 dalton difference. For sure, molecular weights by gel filtration are always an approximation.

DR. W. VALE (La Jolla): The trouble we are having in finding the second gene for anglerfish somatostatin or the equivalent of it in mammalians may be, as pointed out, due to the fact that there is too much difference between them so I think one strategy would be to look back in an intermediate species such as amphibia and see if maybe there you can find something more closely related to the anglerfish.

III

BRAIN SOMATOSTATIN

10

IMMUNOCYTOCHEMICAL STUDIES OF SOMATOSTATIN NEURONS IN BRAIN

ROBERT ELDE, OLLE JOHANSSON AND TOMAS HOKFELT

Department of Anatomy
University of Minnesota
Minneapolis, MN (RE), and

Department of Histology
Karolinska Institute
Stockholm, Sweden (OJ & TH)

ABSTRACT

Immunohistochemical studies with antisera to somatostatin have, in many instances, led the way to our present understanding of the peptidergic nervous system. Somatostatin was among the first of the hypophysiotropic hormones shown to be contained in diverse neuronal circuits outside of the hypothalamus. For example, somatostatin is found within neurons ranging in location from the cerebral cortex to primary sensory neurons to enteric neurons within the gut wall. Somatostatin was also the first neuropeptide demonstrated to coexist within vertebrate neurons that also produce a classical neurotransmitter. Since this initial demonstration in sympathetic ganglionic neurons, somatostatin and numerous other neuropeptides have been demonstrated to coexist with a variety of classical neurotransmitters. The "rules" for coexistence are not clear, since somatostatin coexists in some instances with norepinephrine, in other cases with GABA, and probably with other classical transmitters as well. In some neurons, somatostatin also coexists with certain other neuropeptides. Finally, the specificity of immunohistochemical localizations of somatostatin has now been confirmed by virtue of the co-staining of somatostatin neurons with antisera to other portions of the biosynthetic precursor to somatostatin.

INTRODUCTION

The distribution of immunoreactive somatostatin (IRS) within the brain has been studied in many vertebrate species by numerous investigators and has thus been the topic of several previous reviews (1-7). Comprehensive studies on the distribution of somatostatin immunoreactivity in rodents have been reported by Hökfelt and colleagues (8), Finley and colleagues (9) and in great detail in the recent mapping study of Johansson et al. (10).

Somatostatin as a Hypophysiotropic Hormone

The initial characterization of a 14 amino acid peptide isolated from hypothalamic extracts as a somatotropin release inhibiting hormone (11) strongly suggested that such a peptide must exist within hypothalamic neurons. As antisera were generated to somatostatin, radioimmunoassay studies confirmed the presence of IRS within the hypothalamus (12). More details of the distribution of somatostatin within the hypothalamus were obtained by radioimmunoassay of somatostatin in extracts of hypothalamic nuclei individually isolated by the micropunch method of Palkovits (13). Concomitant with such studies, immunohistochemical analyses using several antisera to somatostatin revealed a dense network of IRS containing fibers in the external layer of the median eminence (14-16). These findings were crucial in establishing that IRS was present in a neuronal system with terminals in a position to release IRS into the hypothalamo-hypophyseal portal system and thereby gain access to somatotrophs in the anterior pituitary. Physiological confirmation of the release of IRS into the portal system and action upon somatotrophs soon followed (17).

The initial immunohistochemical reports of IRS in the hypothalamus failed to detect the neuronal cell bodies that give rise to the immunostained terminals in the external layer of the median eminence. However, with more potent antisera it soon became possible to localize neuronal cell bodies in the periventricular nucleus of the hypothalamus (8, 18, 19). Lesions of the periventricular nucleus established that these cell bodies were, in fact, the origin of the IRS axons in the median eminence (1, 5, 20-25). It should also be noted that at least some IRS neurons within the periventricular zone of the paraventricular nucleus project to the brainstem and spinal cord (26). The organum vasculosum lamina terminalis also contains a high density of IRS terminals and fibers in a neurohemal arrangement (13, 27, 28), although the function of this structure is not as clearly defined as in the case of the median eminence.

More recently, intracerebroventricular administration of colchicine has been used to block the axonal transport of substances from neuronal cell bodies and thereby build up the amount of neuropeptides in cell bodies (29). This maneuver has enabled a greater appreciation of the extent of IRS cell bodies in the periventricular and other nuclei (see below).

Additional organizational features of the IRS neuroendocrine system have been reported for rats (9, 30-37), guinea pigs (38), primates (39, 40), dogs (41) and non-mammalian vertebrates (42-47). It is noteworthy that in each case a hypothalamic nucleus that may be homologous to the periventricular nucleus of the rat contains IRS cell bodies. In addition, the external layer of the median eminence in all species studied contains a high density of IRS fibers and terminals.

Somatostatin as a Putative Neurotransmitter

The occurrence of most hypophysiotropic hormones in widely-distributed neuronal circuits is now an accepted fact. However, studies of somatostatin were among the first to suggest that hypophysiotropic peptides might exist in neurons in diverse brain regions (8, 12, 22, 48), in the peripheral nervous system (49-51) and possibly function as neurotransmitters at these sites. The following is a very limited summary of the distribution of major groups of IRS neuronal cell bodies in the rat central nervous system. Highly schematic representations of the major cell groups are depicted in Figs. 1 and 2. More comprehensive accounts of the cellular distribution of IRS can be found in original papers, including the recent very detailed study by Johansson et al. (10). It should also be noted that the following summary, for the most part, does not discuss the distribution of IRS nerve fibers and terminals, which occur in most areas rich in neuronal cell bodies, as well as in many other brain regions.

Spinal cord

Initial immunohistochemical studies of extrahypothalamic sites reported IRS in small diameter primary afferent neurons whose axons terminate in the superficial zones of the grey matter of the dorsal horn of the spinal cord of rats (52). This finding has been confirmed in other mammalian species (53). The presence of IRS, plus the occurrence of substance P immunoreactivity in a separate but essentially parallel population of primary afferent neurons (52), generated considerable excitement because no viable candidates for neurotransmitters had been determined in these neurons which represent the first link in somatosensory pathways that mediate modalities such as pain.

In addition, IRS is found within neuronal cell bodies intrinsic to the spinal cord (10, 54), including lamina II, near the central canal (lamina X (10, 55)), and within the sacral parasympathetic nucleus and dorsal grey commissure (55-57). Many ventral horn cells transiently express IRS during late fetal and neonatal development

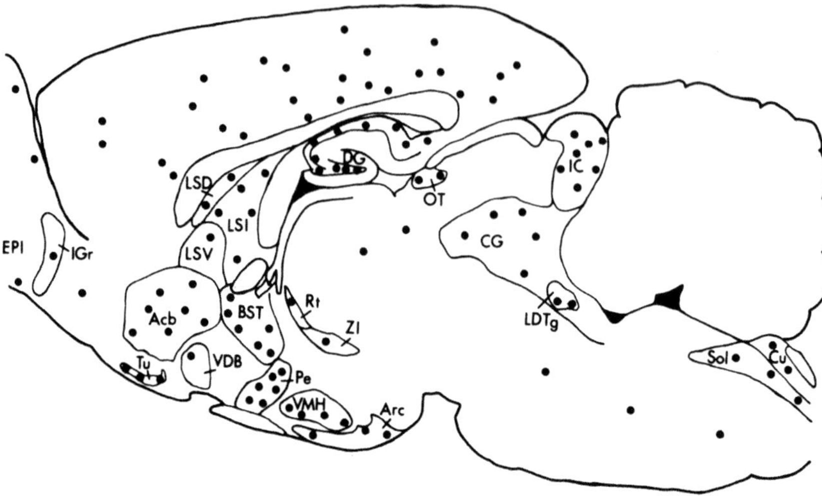

Fig. 1. Highly schematic depiction of major concentrations of IRS containing neuronal cell bodies in rat brain from the mid-saggital plane to a parasaggital plane approximately 1.5 mm lateral to the midline. Landmarks based upon the rat brain atlas of Paxinos and Watson (105).
Abbreviations: Acb, accumbens n.; Arc, arcuate n. (hypothalamus); BST, bed n. stria terminalis; CG, central grey; Cu, cuneate n.; DG, dentate gyrus; EPl, external plexiform layer olfactory bulb; IC, inferior colliculus; IGr, internal layer olfactory bulb; LDTg, laterodorsal tegmental n.; LSD, lateral septal n., dorsalis; LSI, lateral septal n., intermediate; LSV, lateral septal n., ventralis; OT, n. optic tract; Pe, periventricular n. (hypothalamus); Rt, reticular n. (thalamus); Sol, n. solitary tract; Tu, olfactory tubercle; VDB, n. vertical limb diagonal band (Broca); VHM, ventromedial n.; ZI, zona incerta (hypothalamus).

(58). The occurrence of IRS nerve fibers and terminals within the spinal cord has been further studied in rodents (59, 60), and found to be a feature of all vertebrate spinal cords examined, including oppossum (53, 61), bird (62), amphibian (63) and fish (64).

<u>Rhombencephalon</u>

Some sensory cranial nerve nuclei, including the spinal nucleus of the trigeminal nerve (10, 54, 65) and the nucleus of the solitary tract (10, 65, 66, 67) contain low to moderate numbers of IRS neuronal cell bodies. Large numbers of IRS cells are found in the dorsal cochlear nucleus (10, 68) and in the dorsal column nuclei. Certain of the nuclei in the medullary and pontine reticular

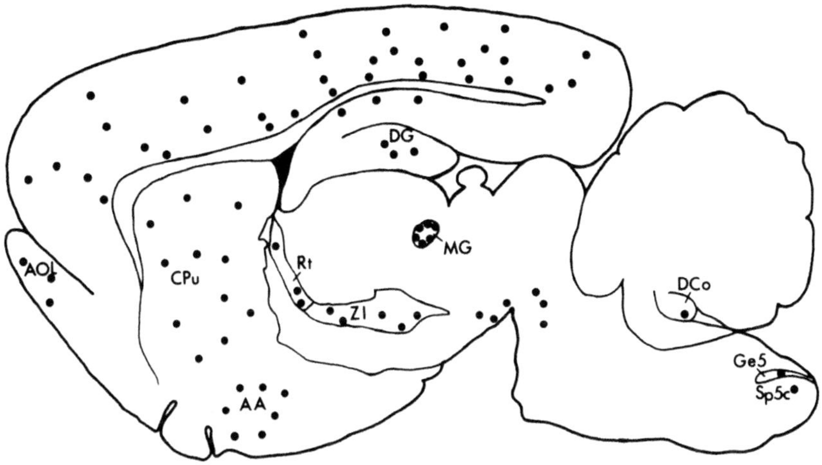

Fig. 2. Highly schematic depiction of major concentrations of IRS containing neuronal cell bodies in rat brain between parasaggital planes approximately 1.5 to 3.0 mm lateral to the midline. Abbreviations: AA, amygdaloid area; AOL, anterior olfactory n., lateralis; CPu, caudate putamen; CDo, dorsal cochlear n.; Ge5, substantia gelatinosa of the caudal sub-nucleus of the spinal trigeminal n.; MG, medial geniculate; Rt, reticular n. (thalamus); Sp5C, n. spinal tract of trigeminal nerve, caudal subnucleus; ZI, zona incerta.

formation also contain moderate numbers of IRS neurons. Near the rostral part of the fourth ventricle IRS cells exist in moderate numbers in the dorsal parabrachial nucleus, the locus coeruleus, the dorsal tegmental nucleus of Gudden and in the periventricular central grey matter.

Mesencephalon

Many IRS cells are found in the inferior colliculus whereas fewer cells are found in the nucleus of the optic tract. The periaqueductal central grey, ventrolateral to the aqueduct, contains numerous IRS cells (10, 69). Fewer IRS-positive cells occur in the mesencephalic reticular formation lateral to the red nucleus. A small number of IRS-positive cells is found in nucleus cuneiformis. An additional collection of IRS cells is found immediately lateral to the substantia nigra (10).

Diencephalon

The hypothalamus contains several nuclei with very high numbers of IRS containing cell bodies. As discussed above, the periventricular area above the caudal portion of the optic chiasm includes one of the most prominent collections of IRS perikarya in the brain. These cell bodies are thought to give rise to axons which terminate in the median eminence and thereby comprise the neuroendocrine system (discussed above; see also 70-72). Other hypothalamic nuclei with high or moderate proportions of IRS cells include the paraventricular nucleus (26), arcuate nucleus (73), ventromedial nucleus and the dorsolateral aspect of the medial forebrain bundle. Smaller proportions of cells are found in the suprachiasmatic nucleus, the retrochiasmatic area and the supramammillary region.

In general, few IRS cells are found in the thalamus, except in the central nucleus of the medial geniculate body (10) and in the reticular nucleus of the thalamus (10, 79). The latter cells merge with a large group of IRS neurons in the zona incerta of the subthalamus.

Telencephalon

The mammalian telencephalon is large in relation to other brain regions and includes numerous groups of neurons with IRS. Numerous subcortical nuclei and regions contain moderate to high numbers of neurons with IRS. These areas include the lateral septal nucleus, the diagonal band of Broca, the interstitial nucleus of the stria terminalis (75, 76), several of the amygdaloid nuclei (75, 76), nucleus accumbens, the caudate-putamen (77-83), the olfactory tubercle, the anterior olfactory nucleus, and the granule cell layer of olfactory bulb (84).

Numerous non-pyramidal neurons in neocortical layers II, III, V and VI contains IRS (83, 85-91). More primitively-organized regions of cerebral cortex also contain high to moderate numbers of IRS neurons. The hippocampal formation contains numerous IRS neurons, especially in the outer part of stratum oriens and in the hilus of the dentate gyrus (92-94).

In summary, IRS-positive neurons are widely distributed throughout many regions of the central nervous system. However, it is of interest to note the occurrence of IRS in neurons at initial sites of synaptic processing in somatic sensory systems (dorsal horn and lamina X of spinal cord, dorsal column nuclei). In addition, IRS neurons are present at several levels in some special sensory systems, including the olfactory system (olfactory bulb, olfactory nuclei and tubercle), the visual system (retina (95-98)), and the auditory system (dorsal cochlear nucleus, inferior colliculus, medial geniculate body). In addition, IRS neurons are present in most areas of the cerebral cortex. Thus, it is reasonable to presume that IRS neurons may participate in regulation of a wide variety of sensory phenomena. The limbic system and basal ganglia also contain many collections of IRS neurons and thus, it is likely that somatostatin is an important modulator of neuronal activity in functions mediated by these vast systems.

Coexistence of Somatostatin with Other Transmitter Candidates

The coexistence of neuropeptides with classical neurotransmitters has now been widely established (99). The first example of such coexistence in vertebrates was the study by Hökfelt and colleagues in which IRS was shown to coexist within a majority of the noradrenergic projection neurons of the inferior mesenteric ganglion of the guinea pig (100). Similarly, IRS coexists with GABA in a majority of the neurons of the thalamic reticular nucleus of the cat (101). It should be noted that many GABAergic neurons in nearby brain regions do not contain IRS, and conversely, many other IRS neurons fail to exhibit GABAergic markers. However, more recent studies have shown IRS in numerous GABAergic neurons of rat neocortex (89). Thus, the rules for the coexistence of IRS with classical neurotransmitters are not clear. The coexistence of IRS and GABA is notable in that such neurons possess two substances whose actions are principally inhibitory.

The coexistence of neuropeptides is not restricted to classical neurotransmitters (99). Many forebrain neurons contain both IRS and a substance stained with antisera against pancreatic polypeptide (81-83, 91). It is likely that the peptide that coexists with IRS in these neurons is more closely related to neuropeptide Y than to pancreatic polypeptide (see 82).

Coexistence of Somatostatin with Other Portions of Prosomatostatin

Several studies (10, 102-104, R. Franco-Bourland & R. Elde, unpublished) have now shown a close correspondence in the staining of neurons with antisera to somatostatin-14 and antisera to various other portions of the prosomatostatin sequence. Such findings are of great interest in that they verify the specificity of immunostaining obtained over the past decade by numerous investigators using a variety of antisera to the tetradecapeptide somatostatin.

REFERENCES

1. Elde R, Hökfelt T 1978 Distribution of hypothalamic hormones and other peptides in the brain. In: Ganong WF, Martini L (eds) Frontiers in Neuroendocrinology. Raven Press, New York, vol. 5:1.
2. Elde R, Hökfelt T, Johansson O, Schultzberg M, Efendic S, Luft R 1978 Cellular localization of somatostatin. Metabolism 27:1151.

3. Elde R, Hökfelt T 1979 Localization of hypophysiotropic peptides and other biologically active peptides within the brain. Ann Rev Physiol 41:587.
4. Hökfelt T, Elde R, Fuxe K, Johansson O, Ljungdahl Å, Goldstein M, Luft R, Efendic S, Nilsson G, Terenius L, Ganten D, Jeffcoate SL, Rehfeld J, Said S, Perez de la Mora M, Possani L, Tapia R, Teran L, Palacios R 1978 Aminergic and peptidergic pathways in the nervous system with special reference to the hypothalamus. In: Reichlin S, Baldessarini RJ, Martin JB (eds) The Hypothalamus. Raven Press, New York, p 69.
5. Johansson O, Hökfelt T 1980 Immunohistochemical distribution of thyrotropin-releasing hormone, somatostatin and enkephalin with special reference to the hypothalamus. In: Wuttke W, Weindl A, Voigt KH, Dries RR (eds) Brain and Pituitary Peptides. S. Karger, Basel, p 202.
6. Parsons JA, Erlandsen SL, Hegre OD, McEvoy RC, Elde RP 1976 Central and peripheral localization of somatostatin. Immunoenzyme immunocytochemical studies. J Histochem Cytochem 24:872.
7. Pelletier G 1980 Immunohistochemical localization of somatostatin. Prog Histochem Cytochem 12:1.
8. Hökfelt T, Efendic S, Hellerström C, Johansson O, Luft R, Arimura A 1975 Cellular localization of somatostatin in endocrine-like cells and neurons of the rat with special references to the A_1-cells of the pancreatic islets and to the hypothalamus. Acta Endocrinol 80:1.
9. Finley JC, Maderdrut JL, Roger LJ, Petrusz P 1981 The immunocytochemical localization of somatostatin-containing neurons in the rat central nervous system. Neuroscience 6:2173.
10. Johansson O, Hökfelt T, Elde RP 1984 Immunohistochemical distribution of somatostatin-like immunoreactivity in the central nervous system of the adult rat. Neuroscience, in press.
11. Brazeau P, Vale W, Burgus R, Ling N, Butcher M, Rivier J, Guillemin R 1973 Hypothalamic polypeptide that inhibits the secretion of immunoreactive pituitary growth hormone. Science 179:77.
12. Brownstein M, Arimura A, Sato H, Schally AV, Kizer JS 1975 The regional distribution of somatostatin in the rat brain. Endocrinology 96:1456.
13. Palkovits M, Brownstein MJ, Arimura A, Sato H, Schally AV, Kizer JS 1976 Somatostatin content of the hypothalamic ventromedial and arcuate nuclei and the circumventricular organs in the rat. Brain Res 109:430.
14. Hökfelt T, Efendic S, Johansson O, Luft R, Arimura A 1974 Immunohistochemical localization of somatostatin (growth hormone release-inhibiting factor) in the guinea pig brain. Brain Res 80:165.
15. Dubois MP, Barry J, Leonardelli J 1974 Mise en evidence par immunofluorescence et repartition de la somatostatin (SRIF) dans l'eminence mediane des Vertebres (Mammiferes, Oiseaux, Amphibiens, Poissons). CR Acad Sc Paris 279:1899.

16. Pelletier G, Labrie F, Arimura A, Schally AV 1974 Electron microscopic immunohistochemical localization of growth hormone-release inhibiting hormone (somatostatin) in the rat median eminence. Am J Anat 140:445.
17. Arimura A, Smith WD, Schally AV 1976 Blockade of the stress-induced decrease in blood GH by anti-somatostatin serum in rats. Endocrinology 98:540.
18. Elde RP, Parsons JA 1975 Immunocytochemical localization of somatostatin in cell bodies of the rat hypothalamus. Am J Anat 144:541.
19. Alpert LC, Brawer JR, Patel YC, Reichlin S 1976 Somatostatinergic neurons in anterior hypothalamus: immunohistochemical localization. Endocrinology 98:255.
20. Brownstein MJ, Arimura A, Fernandez-Durango R, Schally AV, Palkovits M, Kizer JS 1977 The effect of hypothalamic deafferentation on somatostatin-like activity in the rat brain. Endocrinology 100:246.
21. Kawano H, Daikoku S, Saito S 1982 Immunohistochemical studies of intrahypothalamic somatostatin-containing neurons in rat. Brain Res 242:227.
22. Epelbaum J, Willoughby JO, Brazeau P, Martin JB 1977 Effects of brain lesions and hypothalamic deafferentation on somatostatin distribution in the rat brain. Endocrinology 101:1495.
23. Epelbaum J, Arancibia LT, Herman JP, Kordon C, Palkovits M 1981 Topography of median eminence somatostatinergic innervation. Brain Res 230:412.
24. Crowly WR, Terry LC 1980 Biochemical mapping of somatostatinergic systems in rat brain: effects of periventricular hypothalamic and medial basal amygdaloid lesions on somatostatin-like immunoreactivity in discrete brain nuclei. Brain Res 200:283.
25. Patel YC, Hoyte K, Martin JB 1979 Effect of anterior hypothalamic lesions on neurohypophysial and peripheral tissue concentrations of somatostatin n the rat. Endocrinology 105:712.
26. Sawchenko PE, Swanson LW 1982 Immunohistochemical identification of neurons in the paraventricular nucleus of the hypothalamus that project to the medulla or to the spinal cord in the rat. J Comp Neurol 205:260.
27. Dube D, Leclerc R, Pelletier G, Arimura A, Schally AV 1975 Immunohistochemical detection of growth hormone-release inhibiting hormone (somatostatin) in the guinea-pig brain. Cell Tissue Res 161:385.
28. Krause R 1979 Comparative distribution of LH-RH and somatostatin in the supraoptic crest (OVLT) of the rat. Neurosci Lett 11:177.
29. Hökfelt T, Elde R, Johansson O, Terenius L, Stein L 1977 The distribution of enkephalin-immunoreactive cell bodies in the rat central nervous system. Neurosci Lett 5:25.
30. Baker BL, Yu Y 1976 Distribution of growth hormone-release-inhbiting hormone (somatostatin) in the rat brain as observed with immunocytochemistry. Anat Rec 186:343.

31. Daikoku S, Hisano S, Kawano H, Okamura Y, Tsuruo Y 1983 Ontogenetic studies on the topographical heterogeneity of somatostatin-containing neurons in rat hypothalamus. Cell Tissue Res 233:347.
32. Dierickx K, Vandesande F 1979 Immunocytochemical localization of somatostatin-containing neurons in the rat hypothalamus. Cell Tissue Res 201:349.
33. Ibata Y, Fukui K, Obata HL, Tanaka M, Hisa Y, Sano Y, Ishigami T, Imagawa K, Sin S 1982 Postnatal ontogeny of catecholamine and somatostatin neuron systems in the median eminence of the rat as revealed by a colocalization technique. Brain Res Bull 9:407.
34. King JC, Gerall AA, Fishback JB, Elkind KE, Arimura A 1975 Growth hormone-release inhibiting hormone (GH-RIH) pathway of the rat hypothalamus revealed by the unlabeled antibody peroxidase-antiperoxidase method. Cell Tiss Res 160:423.
35. Krisch B 1980 Immunocytochemistry of neuroendocrine systems: vasopressin, somatostatin, luliberin. Prog Histochem Cytochem 13:1.
36. Krisch B 1979 Immunohistochemical results on the distribution of somatostatin in the hypothalamus and in limbic structures of the rat. J Histochem Cytochem 27:1389.
37. Makara GB, Pakovits M, Antoni FA, Kiss JZ 1983 Topography of the somatostatin-immunoreactive fibers to the stalk-median eminence of the rat. Neuroendocrinology 37:1.
38. Tramu G, Beauvillain JC, Croix D, Leonardelli J 1981 Comparative immunocytochemical localization of enkephalin and somatostatin in the median eminence, hypothalamus and adjacent areas of the guinea-pig brain. Brain Res 215:235.
39. Desy L, Pelletier G 1977 Immunohistochemical localization of somatostatin in the human hypothalamus. Cell Tissue Res 184:491.
40. Filby AB, Gross DS 1983 Distribution of immunoreactive somatostatin in the primate hypothalamus. Cell Tissue Res 233:69.
41. Hoffman GE, Hayes TA 1979 Somatostatin neurons and their projections in dog diencephalon. J Comp Neurol 186:371.
42. Blahser S, Fellmann D, Bugnon C 1978 Immunocytochemical demonstration of somatostatin-containing neurons in the hypothalamus of the domestic mallard. Cell Tissue Res 195:183.
43. Dierickx K, Goossens N, Vandesande F 1981 The origin of somatostatin fibers in the median eminence and neural lobe of Rana temporaria. Cell Tissue Res 215:41.
44. Doerr-Schott J, Dubois MP 1977 Immunohistochemical demonstration of an SRIF-like system in the brain of the reptile: Lacerta muralis Laur. Experientia 33:947.
45. Fasolo A, Gaudino G 1982 Immunohistochemical localization of somatostatin-like immunoreactivity in the hypothalamus of the lizard, Lacerta sicula. Gen Comp Endocrinol 48:205.

46. Vandesande F, Dierickx K 1980 Immunocytochemical localization of somatostatin-containing neurons in the brain of Rana temporaria. Cell Tissue Res 205:43.
47. Goossens N, Dierickx K, Vandesande F 1980 Immunocytochemical localization of somatostatin in the brain of the lizard, Ctenosauria pectinata. Cell Tissue Res 208:499.
48. Patel YC, Reichlin S 1978 Somatostatin in hypothalamus, extra-hypothalamic brain, and peripheral tissues of the rat. Endocrinology 102:523.
49. Schultzberg M, Dreyfus CF, Gershon MD, Hökfelt T, Elde RP, Nilsson G, Said S, Goldstein M 1978 VIP-, enkephalin-, substance P-, and somatostatin-like immunoreactivity in neurons intrinsic to the intestine: immunohistochemical evidence from organotypic tissue cultures. Brain Res 155:239.
50. Schultzberg M, Hökfelt T, Nilsson G, Terenius L, Rehfeld JF, Brown M, Elde R, Goldstein M, Said S 1980 Distribution of peptide- and catecholamine-containing neurons in the gastro-intestinal tract of rat and guinea-pig: immunohistochemical studies with antisera to substance P, vasoactive intestinal polypeptide, enkephalins, somatostatin, gastrin/cholecystokinin, neurotensin and dopamine B-hydroxylase. Neuroscience 5:689.
51. Costa M, Furness JB, Smith IJ, Davies B, Oliver J 1980 An immunohistochemical study of the projections of somatostatin-containing neurons in the guinea-pig intestine. Neuroscience 5:841.
52. Hökfelt T, Elde R, Johansson O, Luft R, Nilsson G, Arimura A 1976 Immunohistochemical evidence for separate populations of somatostatin-containing and substance P-containing primary afferent neurons in the rat. Neuroscience 1:131.
53. DiTirro FJ, Ho RH, Martin GF 1981 Immunohistochemical localization of substance-P, somatostatin, and methionine-enkephalin in the spinal cord and dorsal root ganglia of the North American opossum, Didelphis virginiana. J Comp Neurol 198:351.
54. Forssmann WG, Burnweit C, Shehab T, Triepel J 1979 Somatostatin-immunoreactive nerve cell bodies and fibers in the medulla oblongata et spinalis. J Histochem Cytochem 27:1391.
55. Dalsgaard CJ, Hökfelt T 1981 Somatostatin immunorective cell bodies in the dorsal horn and the parasympathetic intermedio-lateral nucleus in the rat spinal cord. Neurosci Lett 27:335.
56. Schroder HD 1984 Somatostatin in the caudal spinal cord: an immunohistochemical study of the spinal centers involved in the innervation of pelvic organs. J Comp Neurol 223:400.
57. Sasek CA, Seybold VS, Elde RP 1984 The immunohistochemical localization of nine peptides in the sacral parasympathetic nucleus and the dorsal gray commissure in the rat spinal cord. Neuroscience 12:855.
58. Ho RH 1983 Widespread distribution of substance P- and somatostatin-immunoreactive elements in the spinal cord of the neonatal rat. Cell Tissue Res 232:471.

59. Hunt SP, Kelly JS, Emson PC, Kimmel JR, Miller RJ, Wu JY 1981 An immunohistochemical study of neuronal populations containing neuropeptides or gamma-aminobutyrate within the superficial layers of the rat dorsal horn. Neuroscience 6:1883.
60. Seybold V, Elde R 1980 Immunohistochemical studies of peptidergic neurons in the dorsal horn of the spinal cord. J Histochem Cytochem 28:367.
61. DiTirro FJ, Martin GF, Ho RH 1983 A developmental study of substance-P, somatostatin, enkephalin, and serotonin immunoreactive elements in the spinal cord of the North American opossum. J Comp Neurol 213:241.
62. Lavalley AL, Ho RH 1983 Substance P, somatostatin, and methionine enkephalin immunoreactive elements in the spinal cord of the domestic fowl, Gallus domesticus. J Comp Neurol 213:406.
63. Lorez HP, Kemali M 1981 Substance P-, met-enkephalin- and somatostatin-like immunoreactivity distribution in frog spinal cord. Neurosci Lett 26:119.
64. Ritchie TC, Leonard RB 1983 Immunohistochemical studies on the distribution and origin of candidate peptidergic primary afferent neurotransmitters in the spinal cord of an elasmobranch fish, the Atlantic stingray (Dasyatis sabi). J Comp Neurol 213:414.
65. Douglas FL, Palkovits M 1982 Distribution and quantitative measurements of somatostatin-like immunoreactivity in the lower brainstem of the rat. Brain Res 242:369.
66. Maley B, Elde R 1982 Immunohistochemical localization of putative neurotransmitters within the feline nucleus tractus solitarii. Neuroscience 7:2469.
67. Kalia M, Fuxe K, Agnati LF, Hökfelt T, Harfstrand A 1984 Somatostatin produces apnea and is localized in medullary respiratory nuclei: a possible role in apneic syndromes. Brain Res 296:339.
68. Takatsuki K, Shiosaka S, Sakanaka M, Inagaki S, Senba E, Takagi H, Tohyama M 1981 Somatostatin in the auditory system of the rat. Brain Res 213:211.
69. Beitz AJ, Shepard RD, Wells WE 1983 The periaqueductal gray-raphe magnus projection contains somatostatin, neurotensin and serotonin but not cholecystokinin. Brain Res 261:132.
70. Bennett-Clarke C, Romagnano MA, Joseph SA 1980 Distribution of somatostatin in the rat brain: Telencephalon and diencephalon. Brain Res 188:473.
71. Romagnano MA, Pilcher WH, Bennett CC, Chafel TL, Joseph SA 1982 Distribution of somatostatin in the mouse brain: effects of neonatal MSG treatment. Brain Res 234:387.
72. Shiosaka S, Takatsuki K, Sakanaka M, Inagaki S, Takage H, Senba E, Kawai Y, Minagawa H, Tohyama M 1981 New somatostatin-containing sites in the diencephalon of the neonatal rat. Neurosci Lett 25:69.

73. Ohtsuka M, Hisano S, Daikoku S 1983 Electron microscopic study of somatostatin-containing neurons in rat arcuate nucleus with special reference to neuronal regulation. Brain Res 263:191.
74. Graybiel AM, Elde RP 1983 Somatostatin-like immunoreactivity characterizes neurons of the nucleus reticularis thalami in the cat and monkey. J Neurosci 3:1308.
75. Roberts GW, Woodhams PL, Polak JM, Crow TJ 1982 Distribution of neuropeptides in the limbic system of the rat: The amygdaloid complex. Neuroscience 7:99.
76. Sakanaka M, Shiosaka S, Takatsuki K, Inagaki S, Takagi H, Senba E, Kawai Y, Matsuzaki T, Tohyama M 1981 Experimental immunohistochemical studies on the amygdalofugal peptidergic (substance P and somatostatin) fibers in the stria terminalis of the rat. Brain Res 221:231.
77. DiFiglia M, Aronin N 1982 Ultrastructural features of immunoreactive somatostatin neurons in the rat caudate nucleus. J Neurosci 2:1267.
78. Graybiel AM, Ragsdale CW Jr, Yoneoka ES, Elde RP 1981 An immunohistochemical study of enkephalins and other neuropeptides in the striatum of the cat with evidence that the opiate peptides are arranged to form mosaic patterns in register with the striosomal compartments visible by acetylcholinesterase staining. Neuroscience 6:377.
79. Krisch B, Leonhardt H 1980 An intermittent somatostatin-immunoreactivity in the cortex and basal ganglia of the rat. Cell Tissue Res 205:327.
80. Takagi H, Somogyi P, Somogyi J, Smith AD 1983 Fine structural studies on a type of somatostatin-immunoreactive neuron and its synaptic connections in the rat neostriatum: a correlated light and electron microscopic study. J Comp Neurol 214:1.
81. Vincent SR, Johansson O 1983 Striatal neurons containing both somatostatin- and avian pancreatic polypeptide (APP)-like immunoreactivities and NADPH-diaphorase activity: A light and electron microscopic study. J Comp Neurol 217:264.
82. Vincent SR, Johansson O, Hokfelt T, Skirboll L, Elde RP, Terenius L, Kimmel J, Goldstein M 1983 NADPH-diaphorase: A selective histochemical marker for striatal neurons containing both somatostatin- and avian pancreatic polypeptide (APP)-like immunoreactivities. J Comp Neurol 217:252.
83. Vincent SR, Skirboll L, Hökfelt T, Johansson O, Lundberg JM, Elde RP, Terenius L, Kimmel J 1982 Coexistence of somatostatin- and avian pancreatic polypeptide (APP)-like immunoreactivity in some forebrain neurons. Neuroscience 7:439.
84. Davis BJ, Burd GD, Macrides F 1982 Localization of methionine-enkephalin, substance P, and somatostatin immunoreactivities in the main olfactory bulb of the hamster. J Comp Neurol 204:377.
85. Johansson O 1978 Localization of somatostatin-like immunoreactivity in the Golgi apparatus of central and peripheral neurons. Histochemistry 58:167.

86. Laemle LK, Feldman SC, Lichtenstein E 1982 Somatostatin-like immunoreactivity in the central visual pathway of the prenatal rat. Brain Res 251:365.

87. McDonald JK, Parnavelas JG, Karamanlidis AN, Brecha N, Koenig JI 1982 The morphology and distribution of peptide-containing neurons in the adult and developing visual cortex of the rat. I. Somatostatin. J Neurocytol 11:809.

88. Morrison JH, Benoit R, Magistretti PJ, Bloom FE 1983 Immunohistochemical distributin of pro-somatostatin-related peptides in cerebral cortex. Brain Res 262:344.

89. Schmechel DE, Vickrey BG, Fitzpatrick D, Elde RP 1984 Gabaergic neurons of mammalian cerebral cortex: widespread subclass defined by somatostatin content. Neurosci Lett 47:227.

90. Sorensen KV 1982 Somatostatin: localization and distribution in the cortex and the subcortical white matter of human brain. Neuroscience 7:1227.

91. Vincent SR, Johansson O, Hökfelt T, Meyerson B, Sachs C, Elde RP, Terenius L, Kimmel J 1982 Neuropeptide coexistence in human cortical neurones. Nature 298:65.

92. Feldman SC, Dreyfus CF, Lichtenstein ES 1982 Somatostatin neurons in the rodent hippocampus: an in vitro and in vivo immunocytochemical study. Neurosci Lett 33:29.

93. Kohler C, Chan Palay V 1982 Somatostatin-like immunoreactive neurons in the hippocampus: an immunocytochemical study in the rat. Neurosci Lett 34:259.

94. Morrison JH, Benoit R, Magistretti PJ, Ling N, Bloom FE 1982 Immunohistochemical distribution of pro-somatostatin-related peptides in hippocampus. Neurosci Lett 34:137.

95. Brecha N, Karten HJ, Schenker C 1981 Neurotensin-like and somatostatin-like immunoreactivity within amacrine cells of the retina. Neuroscience 6:1329.

96. Ishimoto I, Fukuda M, Kuwayama Y, Shimizu Y, Shiosaka S, Takagi H, Senbe E, Sakanaka M, Inagaki S, Takatsuki K, Minagawa H, Tohyama M 1982 Phylogenetical development of somatostatin-containing cells in the retina from teleosts to mammals: immunohistochemical analysis. J Hirnforsch 23:127.

97. Lin CT, Li HZ, Wu JY 1983 Immunocytochemical localization of L-glutamate decarboxylase, gamma-aminobutyric acid transaminase, cysteine sulfinic acid decarboxylase, aspartate aminotransferase and somatostatin in rat retina. Brain Res 270:273.

98. Rorstad OP, Brownstein MJ, Martin JB 1979 Immunoreactive and biologically active somatostatin-like material in rat retina. Proc Natl Acad Sci (USA) 76:3019.

99. Hökfelt T, Johansson O, Ljungdahl A, Lundberg JM, Schultzberg M 1980 Peptidergic neurones. Nature 284:515.

100. Hökfelt T, Elfvin LG, Elde R, Schultzberg M, Goldstein M, Luft R 1977 Occurrence of somatostatin-like immunoreactivity in some peripheral sympathetic noradrenergic neurons. Proc Natl Acad Sci (USA) 74:3587.

101. Oertel WH, Graybiel AM, Mugnaini E, Elde RP, Schmechel DE, Kopin IJ 1983 Coexistence of glutamic acid decarboxylase- and somatostatin-like immunoreactivity in neurons of the feline nucleus reticularis thalami. J Neurosci 3:1322.
102. Bakhit C, Koda L, Benoit R, Morrison JH, Bloom FE 1984 Evidence for selective release of somatostatin-14 and somatostatin-28(1-12) from rat hypothalamus. J Neurosci 4:411.
103. Ho RH, Berelowitz M 1984 Somatostatin 28(1-14) immunoreactivity in primary afferent neurons of the rat spinal cord. Neurosci Lett 46:161.
104. Lechan RM, Goodman RH, Rosenblatt M, Reichlin S, Habener JF 1983 Prosomatostatin-specific antigen in rat brain: localization by immunocytochemical staining with an antiserum to a synthetic sequence of preprosomatostatin. Proc Natl Acad Sci (USA) 80:2780.
105. Paxinos G, Watson C 1982 The Rat Brain in Stereotaxic Coordinates. Academic Press, Sydney.

11

SOMATOSTATIN SECRETION FROM THE HYPOTHALAMUS

ROBERT A. PETERFREUND AND WYLIE W. VALE

Peptide Biology Laboratory
The Salk Institute for Biological Studies
San Diego, California 92037

Comprehensive understanding of the physiologic role of somatostatin (SS) encompasses the question of the control of SS itself. Thus the biosynthesis, storage, secretion and degradation of the peptide became topics for investigation. This chapter will focus on secretion of SS from the hypothalamus, including a discussion of experimental systems and a review of data concerning the characterization and regulation of SS secretion.

I. A variety of model systems have been employed to investigate the regulation of SS secretion from the hypothalamus, including *in vivo* and *in vitro* preparations. Experimental endpoints in intact animal studies have consisted of assessments of SS concentrations in tissues (1-8), measurements of the circulating concentrations of target peptides such as GH (9-13), or direct quantitation of SS levels in pituitary portal blood (14-19) or median eminence (20). Such preparations have theoretical and practical disadvantages which limit their utility in addressing the question of the control of SS secretion.

Tissue depletion of SS, used as a measure of secretion following an experimental manipulation in the intact animal, may actually reflect modulation of synthesis, storage or degradation of the peptide. Multiple levels of modulation are also possible so that an observed tissue concentration may result from two or more opposing or complementary processes such as enhanced peptide synthesis plus enhanced secretion. Circulating concentrations of target hormones may be the product of multiple influences. Plasma GH levels, for example, reflect the level of stimulation by GRF and the degree of inhibition by SS, as well as the influence of other regulatory agents such as thyroid hormones or glucocorticoids (21). Thus, the indirect assessment of SS secretion in the intact animal by quantitation of SS in tissues or GH in the circulation is potentially confounded by the complexity of modulation.

An alternative approach, portal vessel cannulation, affords a means to directly measure secreted SS in the intact animal. This painstaking and technically difficult procedure requires the use of anesthesia, which may itself influence hypothalamic secretion of peptides (22). Direct measurement of SS secretion into the median eminence through the use of sampling with push-pull cannulae involves the destruction of some tissue, although possibly eliminating the need for anesthesia during experimentation. Thus, direct assay protocols also have limitations.

In general, interpretation of the results of an in vivo manipulation may be hampered by the route of administration of the experimental challenge. For example, a test substance administered into the cerebral ventricle of the intact animal could exert its influence at the level of the SS cell in the hypothalamus, or it could act elsewhere in the brain to indirectly influence hypothalamic SS cells, or it could even leak into the periphery and potentially exert a direct effect on the pituitary or some other tissue. It would thus appear that the complexity of the brain, in terms of anatomy and physiology, imposes barriers to the ready assessment of SS secretion from the hypothalamus in vivo.

To circumvent the problems of intact animal models, a variety of in vitro preparations have been devised as experimental systems with which to study the control of hypothalamic SS. These include synaptosomal (23, 24), brain slice or fragment (25-38) and dispersed cell (39-43) preparations. Advantages of these in vitro preparations include more direct access to secreted peptide for measurement, relative isolation of systems from influences which may operate in the intact animal, and improved targeting of experimental manipulations. However, these preparations have inherent disadvantages which also must be considered. Anatomic relationships present in the intact animal, of potential significance in the regulation of SS secretion, may be disrupted by the dissection of tissues. In slice or fragment preparations, tissue perfusion and oxygenation may be uneven resulting in questionable health and responsiveness of the individual cells. Access by test substances to all of the cells within a fragment or slice may be nonuniform which complicates analysis of data. Degradation of secreted peptide within a tissue block before release into the incubation medium provides another confounding variable.

Some of the problems inherent in model systems based on chunks or slices of tissue are potentially circumvented with dispersed cell preparations. Such preparations, using monolayer or suspension techniques, have the advantage of complete cell exposure to perfusing medium, oxygen and experimental challenges such as the administration of transmitters or drugs. Secreted peptide has direct access to the incubation medium and is thus more readily available for measurement. The long-term survival and responsiveness of dispersed cells, particularly in monolayer culture, has been documented (41). Dish-to-dish uniformity of responsiveness within and between preparations is readily achieved.

Dispersed cell preparations, however, have potential disadvantages which must always be considered. Anatomic relationships are maximally disrupted. In short-term preparations of acutely dispersed tissue, cells may lack sufficient time to regain physiologic responsiveness following the preparatory steps. The morphological evolution of dispersed neuron-like cells over days to weeks in culture (41) is noteworthy in this regard. Moreover, long-term preparations of dispersed cells have only been consistently successful with immature brain as a source of tissue. Finally, the artificial incubation and nutrient conditions of dispersed cell preparations may fail to reproduce essential components of the cell's environment _in situ_, so that responsiveness may be altered. In fact, one of the interesting problems for _in vitro_ investigations is that of the minimum essential requirements for culture conditions to permit physiologic response characteristics. Thus, the applicability of the _in vitro_ findings to the intact, mature animal is subject to question.

In excellent summaries of the available data obtained in a variety of model systems, Reichlin (44) and Arimura (45) have tabulated a number of substances capable of modifying SS secretion by hypothalamus, extrahypothalamic brain or peripheral tissues. Identified regulatory factors include drugs, transmitters, peptides, hormones and ions. Some of these data are incomplete, and some are difficult to compare because of the differences in experimental design or conditions. Thus, the question of SS secretion from the hypothalamus has been only partially answered in reliable experimental systems.

II. The remainder of this chapter will focus on secretion of SS as studied in the model system of dispersed fetal rat hypothalamic cells maintained in long-term primary monolayer culture. While disadvantages of this model, such as those cited above, were well recognized, the advantages of viability, uniformity and direct access to cells and secretory products proved very attractive. Two general categories of questions were addressed concerning the secretion of SS from the hypothalamus:

1. What is the nature of the secreted form(s) of SS?
2. What factors control secretion of SS?

Primary cultures were prepared from collagenase dispersed fetal rat hypothalamic tissue as previously described in detail (46). Motivated by the detection and characterization of several SS-like peptides or SS-containing peptides in extracts of mammalian hypothalamus (47-50), experiments were directed toward characterizing the nature of the SS-like immunoactivity (SSLI) which was secreted after stimulation with a variety of agents.

Stimulation of cells with depolarizing concentrations of potassium released substantial quantities of SSLI in a calcium dependent fashion (Fig. 1). Fractionation of high potassium incubation medium by either gel filtration chromatography (41) or reverse phase high performance liquid chromatography (RP-HPLC) (51), followed by radioimmunoassay, revealed the presence of at least two identifiable forms of SS-like peptides, one resembling SS-14 and one resembling SS-28 (Fig. 2). These observations exploited the availability of an

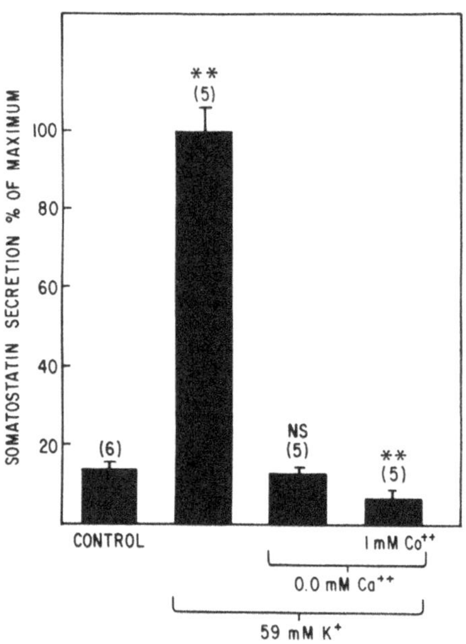

Fig. 1. Secretion of SSLI in response to depolarization with high medium potassium. Cells were incubated in basal medium, isotonic medium containing 59 mM K^+, or medium lacking added calcium but which contains cobalt ion, a blocker of Ca^{++} channels. Each bar represents mean secretion ± SE of 5-6 separate dishes of cells in a treatment group. NS or **, respectively, indicate not significantly ($p > 0.05$) or significantly ($p < 0.01$) different from control. Absolute basal level of secretion was about 70 fmol/dish. See ref. 41 for details.

antiserum directed toward the center of the SS-14 molecule and thus cross-reacting with SS-28, and an antiserum directed toward the amino terminus of SS-14 and incapable of detecting SS-28. Quantitative analysis using RP-HPLC suggested that treatment with three separate stimuli, high potassium, phorbol 12-myristate 13-acetate (52) or picrotoxinin (53), was associated with the augmented release of both SS-28-like and SS-14-like peptides (51). Representative data appear in Fig. 3. Taken together, these findings are consistent with the possibility that an SS-28-like molecule, as well as an SS-14-like molecule, may play an extracellular modulatory role in the intact animal.

The second general question addressed was that of the regulation of SS secretion by the hypothalamus. Reproducibility and uniformity of responsiveness obtained with the dispersed cell preparation was exploited in the construction of dose response curves, analysis of potential interactions between different regulatory agents, and the specification of ion dependence for secretion. Representative data for the cholinergic agonist carbachol appear in Fig. 4, demonstrating a stimulatory action for this analog of acetylcholine (53). Stimulation of SSLI secretion is also seen in response to norepinephrine (Table 1) (Peterfreund and Vale, unpublished observations) and the phorbol ester tumor promoter PMA (52). Inhibition of secretion could be demonstrated with serotonin and

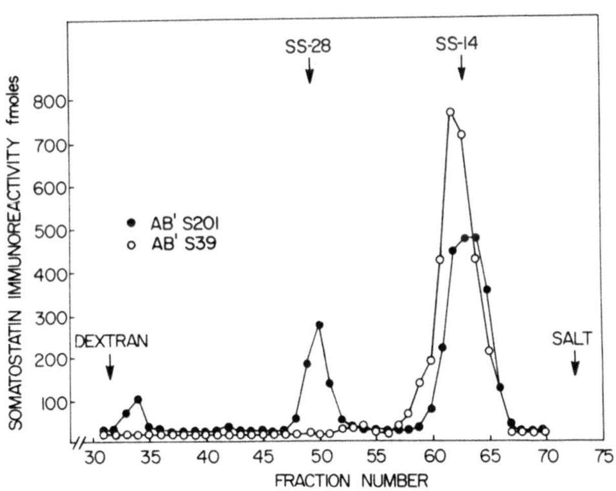

Fig. 2. Gel filtration chromatography profile of SS secretory products. Medium from cells stimulated with high potassium was concentrated and applied to a Sephadex column eluted with acetic acid. Elution profile was determined with two anti-SS sera directed to read different portions of the SS-14 molecule. Arrows indicate migration positions of standards. See text and ref. 41 for details.

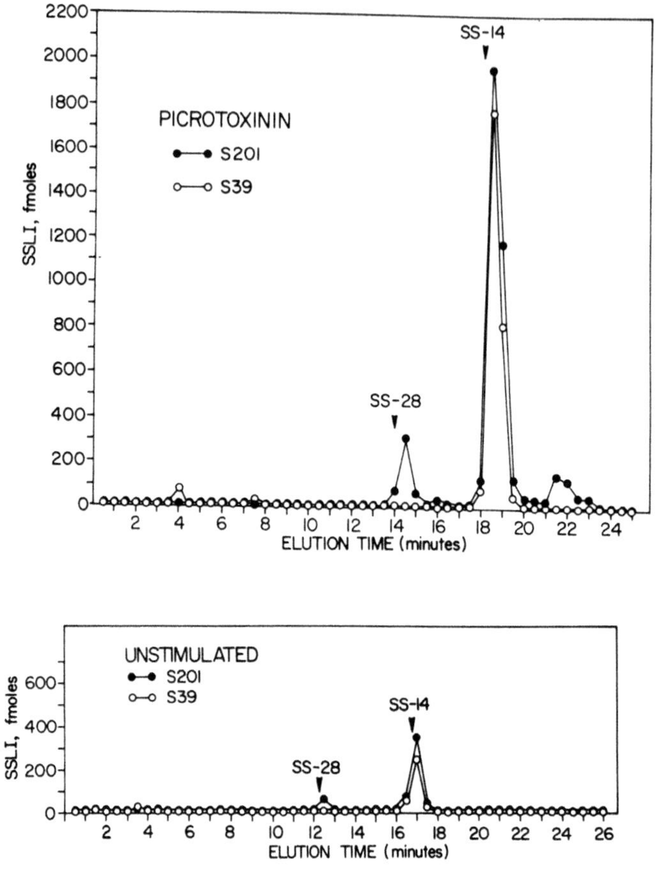

Fig. 3. HPLC profile of SS secretory products. Top: stimulation conditions with picrotoxinin (PTX). Bottom: basal conditions. Incubation medium was concentrated and applied to a C-18 reverse phase column eluted with a gradient of acetonitrile. Elution profile was determined with two separate antisera as described in legend to Fig. 1. Arrows indicate migration positions for synthetic standards. See text and ref. 51 for details.

analogs as well as GABA and analogs (53). Fig. 5 depicts the inhibition of the significant response to PMA by treatment with either GABA or muscimol and illustrates the ability of the dispersed cell model system to directly demonstrate interactions between modulators. Noteworthy was the inhibitory activity of barbiturates such as sodium pentobarbital in this model system (Fig. 6) (52), an observation which suggests potential interactions between brain peptide sytems and a variety of CNS-active drugs often used in experimental or therapeutic settings.

Table 1. SSLI Secretion by Hypothalamic Cells: Response to Norepinephrine

Treatment	SSLI fmoles/dish ± SE	Difference from control
Control	30.9 ± 2	--
Norepinephrine 0.1 nM	31.4 ± 1	NS
Norepinephrine 1.0 nM	36.2 ± 1	**
Norepinephrine 10.0 nM	49.0 ± 2	**
Norepinephrine 100 nM	50.8 ± 2	**
Norepinephrine 1000 nM	42.7 ± 1	**

Buffer contained sodium ascorbate, 10^{-4} M as an antioxidant. N = 4 or 5 per treatment. NS = not significantly different from control ($p > .05$). ** = different from control ($p < .01$).

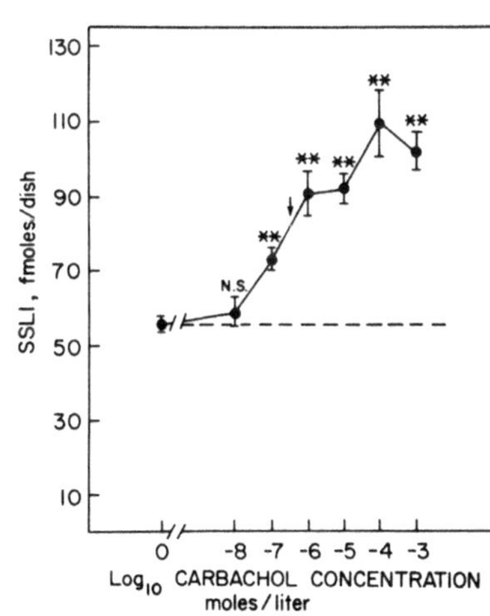

Fig. 4. Secretion of SSLI in response to doses of carbachol. Cells were incubated in the presence of one of several doses of carbachol. Each point represents mean secretion ± SE of 4-5 separate dishes of cells in a treatment group. Arrow indicates dose of carbachol for one-half maximal response. See ref. 53 for details.

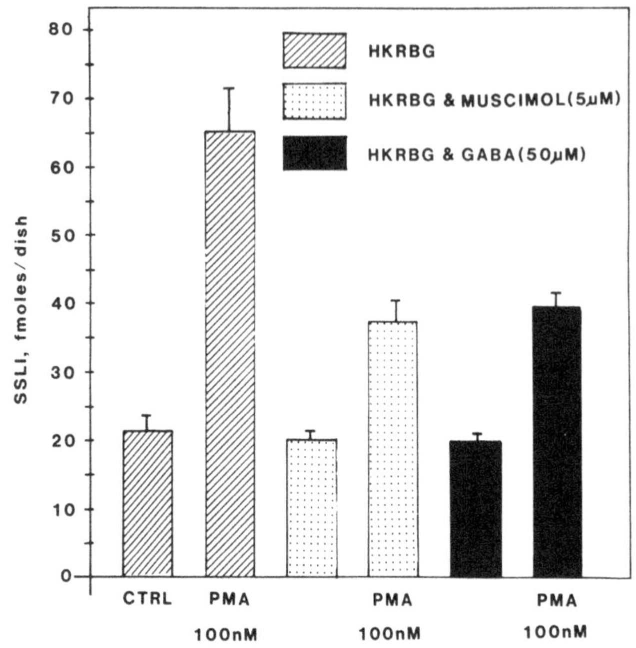

Fig. 5. Effect of GABA or muscimol pretreatment in response to PMA. Cells were incubated in regular medium, medium containing GABA or medium containing the GABA agonist muscimol, with or without PMA. Symbols are defined in legend to Fig. 1. GABA or muscimol treated dishes of cells also receiving PMA had a significantly depressed response when compared to cells receiving PMA alone. See ref. 52 for details.

Of particular interest has been the action of SS to affect brain functions, independent of the pituitary gland. One aspect of this question is the effect of SS on its own secretion, a possibility suggested by in vivo experiments (54) and also by work on the endocrine pancreas (55, 56). The availability of biologically active and immunologically inactive synthetic analogs of SS, which fail to cross-react with particular SS radioimmunoassays, made possible an assessment of the effect of biologically active SS-like peptides on secretion of native SSLI (57). Representative data appear in Fig. 7, demonstrating inhibition of carbachol stimulated SSLI secretion at doses of analog on the order of 1 nM. These data are consistent with the possibility that SS participates in the regulation of its own secretion, possibly by "ultra-shortloop" mechanisms as has been suggested for other neuromodulator systems (58, 59). The data definitely indicate a brain action of SS within the hypothalamus.

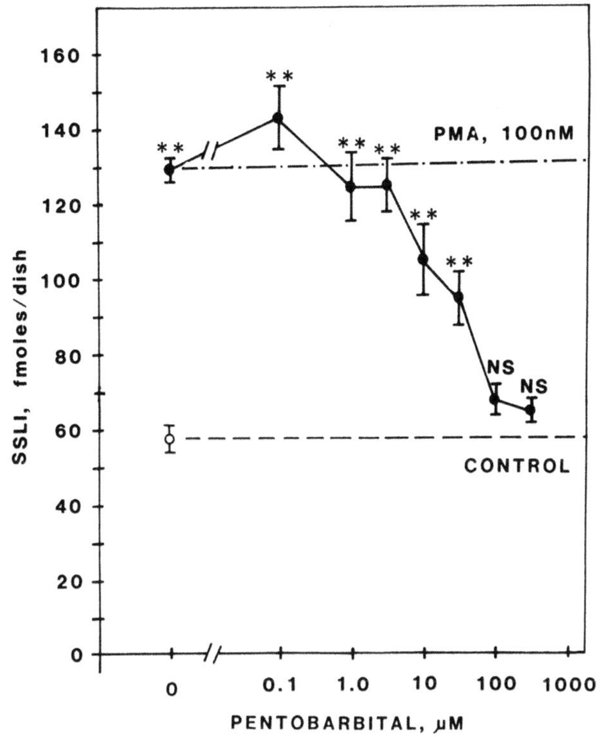

Fig. 6. Secretion of SSLI in response to PMA; effect of doses of sodium pentobarbital. Cells were incubated in basal conditions (open circle) or with PMA (100 nM) after pre-treatment with one of several doses of sodium pentobarbital (closed circles). Symbols are defined in legend to Fig. 1. See ref. 52 for details.

A tabulation of the regulatory findings made with the collagenase dispersed fetal rat hypothalamic cell preparation appears in Table 2A. Some of the findings confirm and extend the observations of Gamse et al. (40) who detected inhibition of SS secretion by GABA and augmentation by GABA antagonists. The fundamental soundness of the approach to the study of hypothalamic SS secretion is supported by the concordance of observations. However, other data are at variance with those made elsewhere, notably the observation in an acute slice system that cholinergic agonists increase SS secretion (30). The basis for this discordance remains unclear, but may be explained by differences in the model systems studied.

The data provided by the dispersed cell system suggest the possibility that SS cells exhibit a tonic, basal level of secretion. SS cells may thus have an intrinsic level of excitation *in vivo*

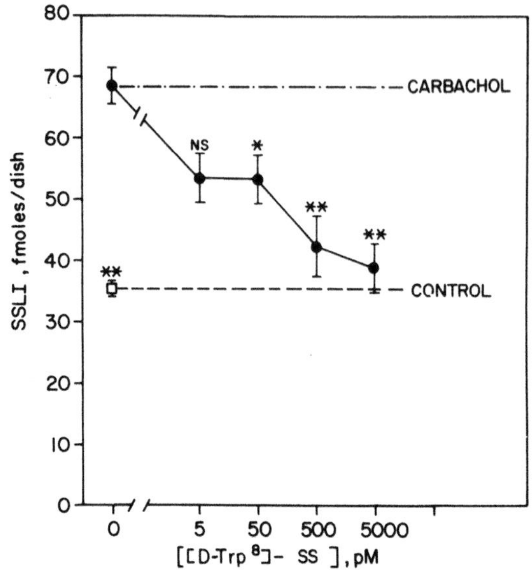

Fig. 7. Secretion of SSLI stimulated by carbachol; effect of agonist analog of SS. Cells were incubated in basal conditions (box), or with carbachol after pretreatment with one of several doses of [D-Trp^{8}]-SS (closed circles). NS indicates not significantly different from carbachol-only treated cells. * and ** indicate different from carbachol-only treated cells, $p < 0.05$ or $p < 0.01$, respectively. See ref. 57 for details.

which is modified positively or negatively to achieve quantitative control over secretions. Alternatively, SS cells within the culture may be driven to secrete by the influence of cells which coculture in the dishes. This raises the interesting possibility that functional communication between brain cells may be established in vitro. The observation that GABA blockers such as bicuculline or picrotoxinin stimulate SS secretion in vitro supports the hypothesis that GABAergic cells coculturing in the dishes tonically exert an inhibitory influence on the SS cells. By extension of the concept of functional communication between coculturing cells, an experimental treatment applied to the population in a dish could act on a cell type which in turn influences SS cells. Unless a direct influence on the SS cell can be demonstrated for a particular manipulation, there is a theoretical limit of resolution to an analysis of the data in the dispersed cell model system. Thus, the only possible definitive conclusion wold be that a particular treatment exerts its influence at the level of the hypothalamus.

Table 2. Modulation of SS Secretion from Cultured Brain Cells: Summary

A. Hypothalamus

Agent	Effects on SS Secretion: Basal	Effects on SS Secretion: Stimulated
High medium potassium	↑	NT
Muscarinic cholinergic agonists	↑	NT
Muscarinic cholinergic antagonists	→	↓
CRF and active analogs	↑	NT
Phorbol diesters	↑	NT
GABA agonists	↓ →	↓
GABA blockers	↑	↑
5HT agonists	↓ →	↓
Tetrodotoxin	↓	↓
Low sodium conditions	↓	↓
Cobalt ions	↓	↓
Verapamil	↓	↓
Somatostatin analogs (active)	NT	↓
Barbiturates	↓ →	↓
Thyroid hormones (chronic)	→	→
Glucocorticoids (chronic)	→	→
Norepinephrine	↑	NT

(continued)

The present data from the dispersed cell system also do not permit any firm statements to be made about the control of anterior pituitary GH or TSH secretion, as mediated by hypothalamic secretion of SS, because SS from the hypothalamus may subserve other roles, in addition to the role of regulating the anterior pituitary. Thus, observations about hypothalamic secretion of SS may pertain more to the brain biology of this peptide than to its neuroendocrine functions. However, in some instances a concordance of in vivo and in vitro observations had been made. For example, CRF, a peptide originally isolated as a hypothalamic regulator of pituitary ACTH secretion, has been demonstrated to stimulate the secretion of SS

Table 2 (continued)

B. Cerebral Cortex

Agent	Effects on SS Secretion	
	Basal	Stimulated
High medium potassium	↑	NT
Muscarinic cholinergic agonists	↑	NT
Muscarinic cholinergic antagonists	→	↓
CRF and active analogs	↑	NT
Phorbol diesters	↑	NT
GABA agonists	↓ →	↓
GABA blockers	↑	↑
Tetrodotoxin	↓	↓
Low sodium conditions	↓	↓
Cobalt ions	↓	↓
5HT	→	→
Thyroid hormones (chronic)	↓	↓
Glucocorticoids (chronic)	→	→
Sex steroids (chronic)	→	→

↑ = increase
↓ = decrease
→ = no effect
NT = not evaluated

from hypothalamic cells *in vitro* (60). Recent experiments *in vivo* (61) have demonstrated a brain action of CRF to suppress GH secretion, which is consistent with the *in vitro* finding of augmented SS secretion. This set of observations also extends the activity spectrum of CRF to the brain, in addition to its corticotrophic function.

For comparison with the results from studies on collagenase dispersed hypothalamic cells, a summary is presented for the data from cerebral cortical cells prepared and studied in a similar fashion (Table 2B). Similarities in responsiveness are striking, including augmented secretion in response to CRF, several monoamines and phorbol ester compounds. There remain, however, some apparent differences between hypothalamic cells and cerebral cortical cells which can only be firmly established with future work.

The present in vitro data therefore identify a number of regulatory candidates which may modulate SS secretion from the hypothalamus in the intact animal. Some of these individual agents may interact to produce a net influence on secretion. However, the data from in vitro work do not suggest which influences may predominate in vivo, nor which functions of SS in the brain or in the pituitary are modulated by particular agents.

III. In summary, an overview of the types of systems employed to study somatostatin secretion from the hypothalamus has been presented, along with a discussion of some of the merits and disadvantages of the various preparations.

Results from the model system consisting of collagenase dispersed fetal rat brain cells maintained in long-term primary culture were reviewed. Emphasis was placed on the secretion of a high molecular weight, amino-terminally extended form of SS resembling SS-28. In addition, results from a number of experiments examining the regulation of SS secretion suggested that monoamines, peptides, a variety of drugs and other biologically active compounds could modulate SS secretion in a highly reproducible fashion. Interaction between different agents, such as GABA and PMA, or SS analogs and carbachol, was demonstrated. Taken together, the data identified specific agents which could influence SS secretion in the intact animal by acting at the level of the hypothalamus, and demonstrated the advantages of the dispersed cell model system.

ACKNOWLEDGMENT

This work was supported by NIH grants AM26741 and AA03504, and a grant from The March of Dimes-Birth Defects Foundation. Research conducted in part by the Clayton Foundation for Research-California Division. WWV is a Clayton Foundation Investigator. RAP is the recipient of a Medical Scientist Training Program Award PHS GM 07198.

The authors would like to thank Carolyn Douglas and Pamela Resch for technical assistance and Susan Logan and Susan McCall for expert manuscript preparation.

REFERENCES

1. Itoh M 1979 Immunoreactive somatostatin in the hypothalamus and other regions of the rat brain: effects of insulin, glucose, alpha- or beta blocker and L-dopa. Endocrinol Jpn 26:41.
2. Berelowitz M, Maeda K, Harris S, Frohman LA 1980 The effect of alterations in the pituitary-thyroid axis on hypothalamic content and in vitro release of somatostatin-like immunoreactivity. Endocrinology 107:24.
3. Berelowitz M, Firestone SL, Frohman LA 1981 Effects of growth hormone excess and deficiency on hypothalamic somatostatin content and release and on tissue somatostatin distribution. Endocrinology 109:714.
4. Terry L, Crowley W 1980 The effect of exercise stress on somatostatin concentrations in discrete brain nuclei. Brain Res 197:543.
5. Walker P, Dussault JH 1980 Hypothalamic somatostatin and pituitary and serum growth hormone concentrations during postnatal development in rats exposed chronically to propylthiouracil or a low iodine diet. J Develop Physiol 2:111.
6. Hoffman D, Baker B 1977 Effect of treatment with growth hormone on somatostatin in the median eminence of hypophysectomized rats. Proc Soc Exp Biol Med 156:265.
7. Kanatsuka A, Makino H, Matsushima Y, Osegawa M, Yamamoto H, Kumagai A 1979 Effect of hypophysectomy and growth hormone administration on somatostatin content in the rat hypothalamus. Neuroendocrinology 29:186.
8. Takahara J, Yunoki S, Hasogi H, Yahushiji W, Kageyama J, Ofuji T 1980 Concomitant increases in serum growth hormone and hypothalamic somatostatin in rats after injection of γ-aminobutyric acid, aminooxyacetic acid or γ-hydroxybutyric acid. Endocrinology 106:343.
9. Eden S, Ericson E, Martin JB, Modigh K 1981 Evidence for a growth hormone releasing factor mediating alpha adrenergic influence on growth hormone secretion in the rat. Neuroendocrinology 33:24.
10. Willoughby JO, Kablar S, Jervas PM, Menodue MF, Oliver JR 1983 Evidence that the regulation of growth hormone secretion is mediated predominantly by a growth hormone releasing factor. Neuroendocrinology 36:358.
11. Willoughby JO, Martin JB 1978 Pulsatile growth hormone secretion: inhibitory role of medial preoptic area. Brain Res 148:240.
12. Willoughby J, Terry L, Brazeau P, Martin JB 1977 Pulsatile growth hormone, prolactin and thyrotropin secretion in rats with hypothalamic deafferentation. Brain Res 127:137.
13. Critchlow V, Abe S, Urman S, Vale W 1981 Effects of lesions of the periventricular nucleus of the preoptic-anterior hypothalamus on growth hormone and thyrotropin secretion and brain somatostatin. Brain Res 222:267.

14. Abe H, Kato Y, Chiba T, Taminoto T, Fujita T 1973 Plasma immunoreactive somatostatin levels in rat hypophyseal portal blood: effect of glucagon administration. Life Sci 23:1647.
15. Chihara K, Arimura A, Kubli Gorfias C, Schally A 1979 Enhancement of immunoreactive somatostatin release into hypophyseal portal blood by electrical stimulation of the preoptic area in the rat. Endocrinology 105:1416.
16. Chihara K, Arimura A, Schally AV 1979 Effect of intraventricular injection of dopamine, norepinephrine, acetylcholine, and 5-hydroxytryptamine on immunoreactive somatostatin release into rat hypophyseal portal blood. Endocrinology 104:1656.
17. Chihara K, Minamitani N, Kaji H, Arimura A, Fujita T 1981 Intraventricularly injected growth hormone stimulates somatostatin release into rat hypophyseal portal blood. Endocrinology 109:2279.
18. Gilling P, Giraud P, Conte-Devalx B, Jaquet P, Codaccioni JL, Oliver C 1979 Immunoreactive somatostatin in rat hypophyseal portal blood. Endocrinology 104:1407.
19. Millar RP, Sherwood WJ, Wegener I, Fink G 1983 Somatostatin-28 is a hormonally active peptide secreted into hypophysal portal blood. Brain Res 260:334.
20. Kasting NW, Martin JB, Arnold MA 1981 Pulsatile somatostatin release from the median eminence of the unanesthetized rat and its relationship to plasma growth hormone levels. Endocrinology 109:1739.
21. Vale W, Vaughan J, Yamamoto G, Spiess J, Rivier J 1983 Effects of synthetic human pancreatic (tumor) GH releasing factor and somatostatin, triiodothyronine and dexamethasone on GH secretion in vitro. Endocrinology 112:1553.
22. Saito H, Ogawa T, Ishimaru K, Oshima I, Saito S 1979 Effect of pentobarbital and urethane on the release of hypothalamic somatostatin and pituitary growth hormone. Horm Metab Res 11:550.
23. Bennet G, Edwardson J, Marcano de Cotte D, Berelowitz M, Pimstone B, Kronheim S 1979 Release of somatostatin from rat brain synaptosomes. J Neurochem 32:1127.
24. Epelbaum J, Brazeau P, Tsang D, Brawer J, Martin JB 1977 Subcellular distribution of radioimmunoassayable somatostatin in brain. Brain Res 126:309.
25. Berelowitz M, Dudlak D, Frohman LA 1982 Release of somatostatin-like immunoreactivity from incubated rat hypothalamus and cerebral cortex. J Clin Invest 69:1293.
26. Berelowitz M, Szabo M, Frohman LA, Firestone L, Chu R, Hintz RL 1981 Somatomedin-C mediates growth hormone negative feedback by effects on both hypothalamus and pituitary. Science 212:1279.
27. Negro-Vilar A, Ojeda SR, Arimura A, McCann SM 1978 Dopamine and norepinephrine stimulate somatostatin release by median eminence fragments in vitro. Life Sci 23:1493.
28. Ojeda S, Negro-Vilar A, Arimura A, McCann S 1980 On the hypothalamic mechanism by which prostaglandin E_2 stimulates growth hormone release. Neuroendocrinology 31:1.

29. Maeda L, Frohman LA 1980 Release of somatostatin and thyrotropin releasing hormone from rat hypothalamic fragments in vitro. Endocrinology 106:1837.
30. Richardson SB, Hollander CS, D'Eletto R, Greenleaf PW, Thaw C 1980 Acetylcholine inhibits the release of somatostatin from rat hypothalamus in vitro. Endocrinology 107:122.
31. Richardson SB, Hollander C, Prasad J, Hirooka Y 1981 Somatostatin release from rat hypothalamus in vitro - Effects of melatonin and serotonin. Endocrinology 109:602.
32. Sheppard MC, Kronheim S, Pimstone BL 1978 Stimulation by growth hormone of somatostatin release from the rat hypothalamus in vitro. Clin Endocrinol 9:583.
33. Sheppard MC, Kronheim S, Pimstone BL 1978 Effect of substance P, neurotensin and the enkephalins on somatostatin release from the rat hypothalamus in vitro. J Neurochem 32:647.
34. Shimatsu A, Kato Y, Matsushito M, Katakami H, Yanaihara N, Stimulation by glucagon and neurotensin of somatostatin release from perfused rat hypothalamus. Program of the 63rd Annual Meeting of the Endocrine Society, 1981 (Abstract 198).
35. Shimatsu A, Kato Y, Matsushita N, Katakami H, Yanaihara N, Imura H 1982 Effects of glucagon, neurotensin and vasoactive intestinal polypeptide on somatostatin release from perfused rat hypothalamus. Endocrinology 11:2113.
36. Zingg H, Patel Y 1979 Somatostatin precursors: evidence for presence in and release from rat median eminence and neurohypophysis. Biochem Biophys Res Commun 90:466.
37. Ensinck JW, Laschansky EC, Kanter R, Fujimoto W, Koerker D, Goodner C 1978 Somatostatin biosynthesis and release in the hypothalamus and pancreas of the rat. Metabolism 27:1207.
38. Iversen LL, Iversen SD, Bloom F, Douglas C, Brown M, Vale W 1978 Calcium dependent release of somatostatin and neurotensin from rat brain in vitro. Nature 273:161.
39. Denizeau F, Dube D, Antakly T, Lemay A, Parent A, Pelletier G, Labrie F 1981 Attempts to demonstrate peptide localization and secretion in primary cultures of fetal rat hypothalamus. Neuroendocrinology 32:96.
40. Gamse R, Vaccaro D, Gamse G, Dipace M, Fox TO, Leeman SE 1980 Release of immunoreactive somatostatin from hypothalamic cells in culture, inhibition by gamma aminobutyric acid. Proc Natl Acad Sci (USA) 77:5552.
41. Peterfreund RA, Vale WW 1982 High molecular weight somatostatin secretion from cultured rat brain cells. Brain Res 239:463.
42. Richardson SB, Greenleaf P, Hollander CS 1983 Somatostatin release from dispersed hypothalamic cells - effects of membrane depolarization, calcium and glucose deprivation. Brain Res 266:75.
43. Richardson SB, Nguyen T, Hollander CS 1983 Dopamine stimulates somatostatin release from perfused hypothalamic cells. Amer J Physiol 244:E560.

44. Reichlin S 1983 Somatostatin. In: Krieger DT, Brownstein M, Martin JB (eds) Brain Peptides. John Wiley and Sons, New York, p 711.
45. Arimura A, Fishback JB 1981 Somatostatin: regulation of secretion. Neuroendocrinology 33:246.
46. Shoemaker W, Peterfreund R, Vale W 1983 Methodological considerations in culturing peptidergic neurons. In: Conn PM (ed) Methods of Enzymology, Academic Press, New York, vol. 103:347.
47. Esch F, Bohlen P, Ling N, Benoit R, Brazeau P, Guillemin R 1980 Primary structure of ovine hypothalamic SS-28 and SS-25. Proc Natl Acad Sci (USA) 77:6827.
48. Spiess J, Vale W 1980 Multiple forms of somatostatin-like activity in rat hypothalamus. Biochemistry 19:2861.
49. Spiess J, Villarreal J, Vale W 1980 Immunological, enzymological and chemical characterization of a large somatostatin-like peptide. In: Koch G, Richter D (eds) Biosynthesis, Modification and Processing of Cellular and Viral Proteins. Academic Press, New York, p 79.
50. Spiess J, Villarreal J, Vale W 1981 Isolation and sequence analysis of somatostatin-like peptide from ovine hypothalamus. Biochemistry 20:1982.
51. Peterfreund R, Vale W 1984 Picrotoxinin and phorbol-12-myristate-13-acetate stimulate the secretion of multiple forms of somatostatin from cultured rat brain cells. J Neurochem 43:126.
52. Peterfreund RA, Vale WW 1983 Phorbol diesters stimulate somatostatin secretion from cultured brain cells. Endocrinology 113:200.
53. Peterfreund RA, Vale WW 1983 Muscarinic cholinergic stimulation of somatostatin secretion from long-term dispersed cell cultures of fetal rat hypothalamus: inhibition by γ aminobutyric acid and serotonin. Endocrinology 112:526.
54. Lumpkin MD, Negro-Vilar A, McCann SM 1981 Paradoxical elevation of growth hormone by intraventricular somatostatin: possible ultrashort-loop feedback. Science 211:1072.
55. Ipp E, Rivier J, Dobbs RE, Brown M, Vale W, Unger RH 1979 Somatostatin analogs inhibit somatostatin release. Endocrinolology 104:1270.
56. Patel YC, Amherdt M, Orci L 1982 Quantitative electron microscopic autoradiography of insulin, glucagon and somatostatin binding sites on islets. Science 217:1155.
57. Peterfreund R, Vale W 1984 Somatostatin analogs inhibit somatostatin secretion from cultured hypothalamus cells. Neuroendocrinology, in press.
58. Langer SZ 1977 Presynaptic receptors and their role in the regulation of transmitter release. Br J Pharmacol 60:481.
59. Starke K 1977 Regulation of noradrenaline release by presynaptic receptor systems. Rev Physiol, Biochem & Pharmacol 77:1.

60. Peterfreund RA, VAle WW 1983 Ovine corticotropin-releasing factor stimulates somatostatin secretion from cultured brain cells. Endocrinology 112:1275.
61. Rivier C, Vale W 1984 Corticotropin-releasing factor (CRF) acts centrally to inhibit growth hormone secretion in the rat. Endocrinology 114:2409.

12

SOMATOSTATIN AND THE CEREBRAL CORTEX

RICHARD ROBBINS

Neuroendocrine Section, Endocrinology Division
University of Colorado Health Sciences Center
Denver, Colorado 80262

ABSTRACT

A unique subset of interneurons which are rich in immunoreactive somatostatin (IRS) exists in the cerebral cortex. The regulation of IRS secretion by these cells is reviewed. Acetylcholine, glutamic acid and several neuropeptides including VIP, CCK, and met-enkephalin have been identified as IRS secretagogues. The types of molecules which stimulate IRS release, the electrophysiologic effects of somatostatin, and the recognition of abnormal IRS levels in human CNS diseases were all used to formulate a working model of the role of the somatostatinergic cell in ongoing cerebral cortical function.

INTRODUCTION

The extrahypothalamic brain is rich in immunoreactive somatostatin (IRS). Immunohistochemical studies have demonstrated complex systems of IRS positive neurons in the cerebral cortex (1, 2), hippocampus (3), thalamus (4), caudate (5), brainstem nuclei (6), and in the spinal cord (7). Neuronal elements outside the central nervous system have also been localized in autonomic ganglia (8), and in neuronal plexi in the gastrointestinal tract (9).

Extensive studies exploring the release of IRS from the hypothalamus, the gut, and from pancreatic islets have been reported and recently reviewed (10, 11). This chapter will summarize the data on regulation of IRS release from cerebral cortical neurons and will compare results obtained from these studies with those exploring IRS release from other tissues.

IRS Release from Cerebral Cortex

Brownstein et al. (12) were the first to report the presence of IRS in the cerebral cortex. These observations were soon confirmed by several other investigators (13-15). Petrusz et al. (16) and Finley et al. (17) were the first to demonstrate cortical nerve terminals, and cell bodies, respectively, which were positive for IRS, confirming the earlier observations of Brownstein et al. (18) that IRS in many extrahypothalamic areas was not dependent on hypothalamic connections. The observations of Delfs et al. (19) that isolated cerebral cortical cell cultures accumulated IRS confirmed the anatomical suspicions that the cortical IRS system was autonomous. More recent detailed anatomical and developmental analyses have demonstrated that the IRS positive cells in the cerebral cortex are non-pyramidal interneurons with dendritic and axonal fields entirely within this structure (1, 20, 21). Sheppard et al. (22) have demonstrated that the IRS released from cortical synaptosomes is virtually identical in immunogenicity, chromatographic character, and bioactivity with synthetic somatostatin-14 (S-14).

That somatostatin may play a role in ongoing cortical activity is further supported by studies which have demonstrated direct electrophysiologic effects of the peptide on *in situ* or *in vitro* cerebral cortical cells (23-26). A physiologic role for somatostatin is further supported by the demonstration of specific somatostatin receptors in cortical membrane preparations (27, 28). Recent reports in fact demonstrate that the cerebral cortex has the highest specific somatostatin binding of any major brain region (27, 29).

Studies on the release of IRS from cerebral cortical cells *in vitro* have been carried out (Table 1). Cultured fetal rat cortical cells have been shown to synthesize prosomatostatin (30) and to process it to somatostatin tetradecapeptide (S-14). My laboratory has extensively explored the factors which regulate the release of IRS from these cortical cell cultures. Previous immunohistochemical studies on these cultures demonstrated that only neuronal elements contained IRS (19). We therefore equate IRS release from these cultures with neuronal secretion.

Ionophores

As in virtually every other tissue, chemical depolarization of cerebral cortical cells leads to enhanced IRS secretion. Physiologic buffers containing high (60 mM) potassium increase IRS release in a calcium dependent manner (31). Enhanced IRS release induced by the sodium ionophore, veratridine, can be blocked by coincubation with calcium flux inhibitors (cobalt and verapamil), or a specific sodium channel blocker, tetrodotoxin (31). Similar results have been reported in hypothalamus (32-34), in the pancreas (35-36), in

Table I. Release of IRS from Cerebral Cortical Cells *in vitro*

	Stimulants	No effect	Inhibitors
Ionophores	KCL (60mM) Veratridine Picrotoxin		Verapamil Tetrodotoxin
Neurotransmitters	Acetylcholine Dopamine	Serotonin Norepinephrine	Histamine
Amino acids	Glutamic acid Aspartic acid	Taurine Glycine Arginine	GABA
Neuropeptides	VIP CCK-8 Neurotensin Met-enkephalin	Insulin TRH	
Others	Cyclic AMP IBMX Glucopenia	Bromocriptine	

the amygdala (37), and in studies employing freshly prepared cortical slices (38) or cortical synaptosomes (39).

Significant increases in IRS release from cultured cortical cells can be induced by 3', 5', dibutyryl cyclic AMP and by the phosphodiesterase inhibitor 1,3 dimethylxanthine (40) implicating cyclic AMP as a second messenger system capable of mediating stimulatory inputs to cortical somatostatinergic neurons.

Neurotransmitters

Dopamine (DA). Although DA caused a slight enhancement of IRS release from cerebral cortical cells, this response was complex. Both 10 and 100 nM DA stimulated IRS release whereas lower or higher concentrations had no effect on IRS release (Fig. 1). DA has no apparent effect on IRS release from pancreatic islets (41). Conversely, DA has been shown to be a reliable IRS secretagogue in the hypothalamus (33, 42-44), and in the stomach (45).

Norepinephrine (NE). NE at concentrations from 100 pM to 10 μM had no effect on IRS release from cortical cells (40). This result is inconsistent with an earlier one suggesting that high levels of

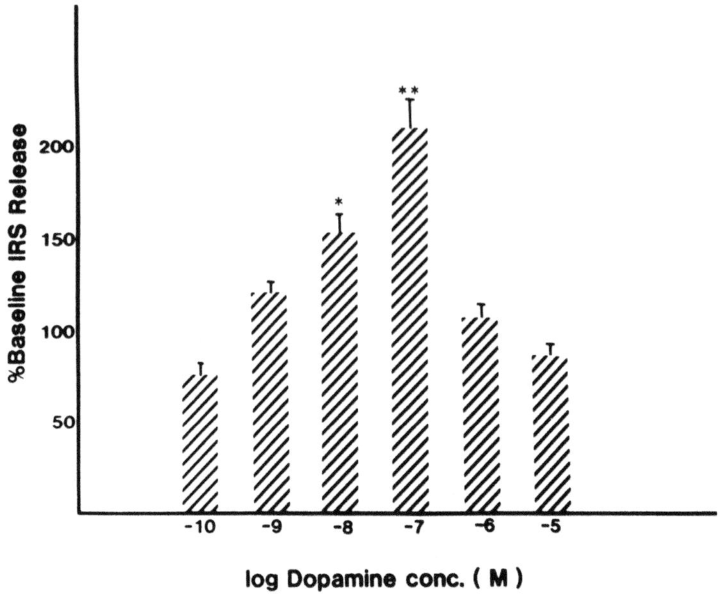

Fig. 1. The effect of dopamine on IRS release from cerebral cortical cell cultures. Dose-response relationship.

NE were stimulatory to IRS release from cortical synaptosomes (39). However, the absence of an effect of NE in our system is similar to the observations of Maeda and Frohman (33) using rat hypothalamic tissue. Enhanced IRS release from hypothalamic preparations, however, has been reported in response to NE (43, 44, 46). IRS release from pancreatic islets is inhibited by noradrenergic (alpha) stimuli (47, 48). These observations are further complicated by the anatomical observations of IRS in sympathetic noradrenergic neurons (8). The lack of an effect of NE in intact cortical cells may reflect the fact that although there are noradrenergic nerve terminals in the rat cerebral cortex (predominantly in layer 1), very few (5%) are forming synaptic complexes (see 49, for review). In addition, the recent observations of Vizi (50) that NE inhibits cortical acetylcholine (ACh) release may be important as we have shown that ACh is an IRS secretogogue (vide infra).

Acetylcholine. ACh at 1 and 10 μM concentrations significantly increased IRS release. Lesser amounts (100 pM - 100 nM) had no apparent effect on IRS secretion. Atropine markedly decreased this effect but hexamethonium, a nicotinic receptor blocker, slightly augmented the ACh-induced IRS rise, indicating that muscarinic receptors mediate this response (40). ACh has been reported to increase (51) and to decrease (47) IRS release from the pancreas and likewise to increase (44), have no effect (33, 52), or decrease (53) IRS release from hypothalamic tissue. Lesions of the nucleus basalis which caused greater than 50% decrease in choline acetyltransferase in the cerebral cortex, however, were not associated with any change in cortical IRS concentration (54).

Others. Serotonin (10 pM - 1 μM) had no influence on the rate of IRS secretion from cultured cortical cells (40). Two separate groups examining IRS release from hypothalamic tissue similarly found no effect of serotonin (33, 44). Histamine had no dramatic effect on cerebral cortical cell IRS release at concentrations up to 1 μM (40).

Peptides

The effects of several neuropeptides on the release of IRS from cerebral cortical cells were examined by exposing the cells to short (10 min) incubations of the freshly prepared peptide in a physiologic buffer. No effects of any peptide were seen below 1 μM concentrations. At 1 μM both neurotensin and vasoactive intestinal polypeptide (VIP) stimulated IRS release. At 10 μM sulfated cholecystokinin octapeptide (CCK-8) and met-enkephalin increased IRS release. Further examination of the neurotensin-induced IRS release mechanism revealed that the effect could be blocked by phentolamine, propranolol, and haloperidol. These results demonstrate a new level of potential intracortical communication, that is, between two peptidergic interneurons. Immunohistochemical studies would predict that such interactions are most likely to occur in the molecular layer (layer I) of the neocortex.

Neurotensin has been shown to be a reliable stimulant of IRS release in both hypothalamic (33, 55, 56) and pancreatic islet preparations (57). VIP, like neurotensin, stimulates IRS release from several other tissues including pancreatic islets (58, 59) and hypothalamic and cerebrocortical cells *in vitro* (60). Of note, however, is a previous report that VIP was inhibitory to IRS release from adult hypothalamic tissue *in vitro* (61). The excitatory effect of VIP may be due in part to the ability of this peptide to increase cyclic AMP levels in brain cells (62). CCK has been shown to stimulate IRS release from islet preparations (63, 64) but its effects on other IRS secreting tissues have not been examined. Met-enkephalin and other opiates have been found to have no effect on IRS release (52, 55) from the hypothalamus but are inhibitory to IRS release from the gut (65, 66). This pattern of tissue specificity of certain peptides on IRS release is reminiscent of that seen for neurotransmitters reinforcing the concept that IRS release has been evolutionarily modified by each tissue for its unique requirements.

Amino acids

Unlike the hypothalamus, which uses modified amino acids as the major neurotransmitters (e.g. catecholamines, serotonin, histamine) the cerebral cortex relies on native amino acids such as glutamate, glycine, gamma aminobutyric acid (GABA), and aspartate as a major source of chemical information transduction. The effects of these amino acids were therefore carefully examined in regard to IRS release from cerebral cortical cells (67).

Glutamate and aspartate were potent stimulants of IRS release. The dose response curve for glutamate demonstrated activity at concentrations as low as 10 μM and had half maximal activity at 100 μM. Analogs of these amino acids were also active in the following hierarchy: N-methyl d-aspartic acid > kainic acid > quisqualic acid. Glycine and taurine were very weak stimulants of IRS release. Arginine, an amino acid with marked activity in the gut and pancreas (51, 57) had no effect on cerebrocortical IRS release, further supporting the concept of tissue specificity.

Glucose

Supraphysiologic glucose concentrations enhance IRS release from islet preparations (48, 68) although complex interislet cross-talk makes a direct effect on D cells difficult to document. Berelowitz et al. (56) have demonstrated that IRS release from both hypothalamic and cerebral cortical tissue is sensitive to changes in medium glucose concentration, the most dramatic effect being an inverse relationship between hypothalamic IRS release and glucose concentration. Our studies (69) have demonstrated a sharp increase in cortical IRS secretion associated with a sudden drop in glucose concentration, but no change with a sudden increase. The possibility that IRS could participate in the marked change in cortical electrical activity seen with sudden drops in blood sugar in humans deserves further investigation.

Effects of Somatostatin on Cerebral Cortical Cells

Although the initial report of the effect of S-14 on electrical activity of cerebral cortical neurons found it inhibitory to 47% of the cells (23) subsequent reports have revealed a more complex relationship. Using iontophoretic techniques, Ioffe et al. (70), Olpe et al. (25), and Phillis and Kirkpatrick (71) found that more than half of the cerebral cortical neurons tested were excited by S-14. The effects of S-14 in other CNS regions has also been reported to be either predominantly inhibitory (72-74) or excitatory (75-76).

The most detailed analysis of the influence of S-14 on cortical cells has recently been reported by Delfs and Dichter (26). These investigators using monolayer cultures of rat cerebral cortical cells found that S-14 directly depolarized 34% of the cells and increased incoming activity in 58% of cells. In addition, S-14 decreased the ongoing inhibitory inputs by increasing membrane resistance in six of nine such cells tested. Although some cells were directly inhibited, they demonstrated that the overall excitatory nature of S-14 was present only at "physiologic" concentrations, and that tachyphylaxis to S-14 did exist. These results are extremely important in that they establish cerebral cortical neurons as one of the rare cell types which are not inhibited by this generally inhibitory peptide. Dichter and Delfs (77) have further provided evidence that the effect of S-14 may be due to enhanced delivery or action of glutamate, an excitatory amino acid, which suggets that S-14 effects are not entirely due to post-synaptic actions on the neuron being monitored.

Actions of S-14 on biochemical events in the telencephalon have also been observed. An increase in cortical DA turnover but no effect on serotonin turnover has been reported (78). Chesselet and Reisine (79) reported that S-14 enhanced H-DA release from neostriatum. Tanaka and Tsujimoto (80) noted that S-14 enhanced serotonin release from cortex, and Tsujimoto and Shokichi (81) found increased NE release from cortex in response to S-14. No change in NE release from cortex slices was noted by Gothert (82), although S-14 did decrease NE release from hypothalamic slices. Somatostatin-14 has also been reported to decrease basal and VIP-induced cyclic AMP levels in cultured brain cells (62).

Abnormal IRS Levels in Human CNS Disease

Cerebrospinal fluid (CSF) levels of IRS have been reported to be decreased in depression (83), multiple sclerosis (84), Huntington's chorea (85), senile dementia (86, 87), and Parkinson's disease (88, 89). Tissue levels of IRS in the cerebral cortex are depleted in Alzheimer's disease and the senile dementia of the Alzheimer's type (90, 91). The co-localization of IRS and acetylcholinesterase in cultured cerebral cortical neurons (92) make the somatostatinergic interneuron a subject of prime interest in the pathophysiology of Alzheimer's type dementia, as deficits in Ach are the only other reliable biochemical marker of this disease (93).

A Hypothetical Model of the Cortical Somatostatinergic Cell

The modular concept of cerebral cortical structure (94), predicts that there are functional neocortical units (modules), made up of 2000-3000 cells each, which communicte with other cortical modules, both ipsilateral and contralateral. These units are vertically organized and therefore contain neurons from all six layers of the cerebral cortex. Incoming information from brainstem, thalamic, or cortical sources is encoded into chemical signals by a network of interneurons which modulate the output of the major efferents, the pyramidal neurons (95).

The somatostatinergic cell, like other peptide (e.g. VIP, CCK-8, CRF)-containing cortical cells is morphologically neuronal with processes contained entirely within the cortex, resulting in its designation as an interneuron (1). Our studies on the regulation of IRS release from these cells predict a minor role for catecholamines, but potentially important roles for glutamate and certain neuropeptides.

The inhibitory nature of somatostatin in other tissues suggests that its excitatory influence on cortical neurons may represent a disinhibition. The major inhibitory interneuronal secretion in the mammalian cerebral cortex is GABA (96). Our proposed model consists of a somatostatinergic neuron which is depolarized by excitatory amino acids, and which communicates with other neuropeptidergic neurons, presumably in the dendritic meshwork of layer 1. Enhanced electrical activity induces increased IRS release which hyperpolarizes GABA-containing interneurons thereby releasing the tonic GABAergic inhibition of certain pyramidal neurons. A very close anatomical relationship between IRS positive and GABAergic neurons in a thalamic nucleus which modulates thalamocortical connections has been reported (4).

This hypothesis was initially tested in monolayer cultures of cerebral cortical cells which had been pre-loaded with [^{3}H] GABA. Somatostatin-14 (10 μM) caused a significant reduction in [^{3}H] GABA release while an equimolar concentration of CCK-8 resulted in enhanced release. This initial result suggests that our hypothesis may be a valid working model.

CONCLUSION

The clinical and basic research of the past five years firmly establishes somatostatin as an important element in cerebral cortical function. The studies on the secretion of IRS from cerebrocortical cells in vitro demonstrates similarities with its secretion from hypothalamic and pancreatic islet cells, and unique features such as resistance to catecholamines and sensitivity to native amino acids such as glutamate. Further understanding of human dementias may be advanced significantly by elucidation of the exact role of the somatostatinergic cell. Clinical studies, especially in patients with Alzheimer's disease, involving somatostatin therapy, are still premature considering our rudimentary understanding of its role. Further studies of this unique cell, however, may provide the basis upon which to design such clinical studies.

ACKNOWLEDGMENT

I would like to thank Roxanne Landon, and Richard Sutton for invaluable technical assistance and Drs. Seymour Reichlin and Bill

Leidy for helpful comments. The secretarial abilities of Ms. Wendy Hall are gratefully acknowledged. Studies summarized in this review were supported by NIH grants AM 30451 and BRSG 05357.

REFERENCES

1. McDonald J, Parnavelas J, Karamanlidis A, Brecha N, Koenig J 1982 The morphology and distribution of peptide-containing neurons in the adult and developing visual cortex of the rat. I. Somatostatin. J Neurocytology 11:809.
2. Shiosaka S, Takatsuki K, Saknaka M, Inagaki S, Takagi H, Senba E, Kawai Y, Iida H, Minagawa H, Hara Y, Takashi M, Tohyama M 1982 Ontogeny of somatostatin-containing neuron system of the rat; immunohistochemical analysis II. Forebrain and diencephalon. J Comp Neurol 204:211.
3. Roberts G, Woodhams P, Polak J, Crow T 1984 Distribution of neuropeptides in the limbic system of the rat: the hippocampus. Neurosci 11:35.
4. Oertel W, Graybiel A, Mugnaini E, Elde R, Schmechel D 1983 Coexistence of glutamic acid decarboxylase and somatostatin immunoreactivity in neurons of the feline nucleus reticularis thalami. J Neurosci 3:1322.
5. Takagi H, Somogyi P, Somogyi J, Smith A 1983 Fine structural studies on a type of somatostatin-immunoreactive neuron and its synaptic connections in the rat neostriatum. J Comp Neurol 214:1.
6. Forssman WG, Burnweit C, Shehab T, Triepol J 1979 Somatostatin immunoreactive cell bodies and fibers in the medulla oblongata and spinalis. J Histochem Cytochem 27:1391.
7. Hokfelt T, Elde R, Johansson O, Luft R, Nilsson G, Arimura A 1976 Immunohistochemical evidence for separate populations of somatostatin containing and substance-P containing primary afferent neurons in the rat. Neuroscience 1:131.
8. Hokfelt T, Elfin L, Elde R, Schultzberg M, Goldstein M, Luft R 1977 Occurrence of somatostatin-like immunoreactivity in some peripheral sympathetic noradrenergic neurons. Proc Natl Acad Sci (USA) 74:3587.
9. Costa M, Patel Y, Furness JB, Arimura A 1977 Evidence that some intrinsic neurons of the intestine contain somatostatin. Neurosci Lett 6:215.
10. Reichlin S 1981 Systems for the study of regulation of neuropeptide secretion. In: Martin JB, Reichlin S, Bick K (eds) Neurosecretion and Brain Peptides. Raven Press, New York, p 573.
11. Arimura A, Fishback J 1981 Somatostatin: regulation of secretion. Neuroendocrinology 33:246.
12. Brownstein M, Arimura A, Sato H, Schally AV, Kizer JS 1975 The regional distribution of somatostatin in the rat brain. Endocrinology 96:1456.

13. Kobayashi RM, Brown M, Vale W 1977 Regional distribution of neurotensin and somatostatin in rat brain. Brain Res 126:584.
14. Epelbaum J, Willoughby J, Brazeau P, Martin J 1977 Effects of brain lesions and hypothalamic deafferentation on somatostatin distribution in the rat brain. Endocrinology 101:1495.
15. Patel Y, Reichlin S 1978 Somatostatin in hypothalamus, extra-hypothalamic brain and peripheral tissues of the rat. Endocrinology 102:523.
16. Petrusz P, Sar M, Grossman G, Kizer JS 1977 Synaptic terminals with somatostatin-like immunoreactivity in the rat brain. Brain Res 137:181.
17. Finley J, Grossman G, Dimeo P, Petrusz P 1978 Somatostatin containing neurons in the rat brain. Amer J Anat 153:483.
18. Brownstein MJ, Arimura A, Fernandez-Durango R, Schally AV, Kizer JS 1977 The effect of hypothalamic deafferentation on somatostatin-like activity in the rat brain. Endocrinology 100:246.
19. Delfs J, Robbins R, Connolly JL, Dichter M, Reichlin S 1980 Somatostatin production by rat cerebral neurons in dissociated cell cultures. Nature 283:676.
20. Bennett-Clarke C, Romagnano M, Joseph S 1980 Distribution of somatostatin in the rat brain telencephalon and diencephalon. Brain Res 188:473.
21. Sorensen K 1982 Somatostatin: localization and distribution in the cortex and the subcortical white matter of human brain. Neuroscience 7:1227.
22. Sheppard M, Hendricks S, Hudson A, Kronheim S 1982 Characterization of immunoreactive somatostatin release from rat nervous system in vitro. Biochem J 201:321.
23. Renaud L, Martin J, Brazeau P 1975 Depressant action of TRH, LH-RH, and somatostatin on the activity of central neurons. Nature 255:233.
24. Ioffe S, Havlicek V, Friesen H, Chernick V 1977 SRIF excitatory to cortical neurons in awake rabbits. Fed Proc 36:364.
25. Olpe H, Balcar V, Bittiger H, Rink H, Seiber P 1980 Central actions of somatostatin. Eur J Pharmacol 63:127.
26. Delfs J, Dichter M 1983 Effects of somatostatin on mammalian cortical neurons in culture: physiological actions and unusual dose-response characteristics. J Neurosci 3:1176.
27. Srikant CB, Patel YC 1981 Somatostatin receptors: Identification and characterization in rat brain membranes. Proc Natl Acad Sci (USA) 78:3930.
28. Reubi JC, Rivier J, Perrin M, Brown M, Vale W 1982 Specific high affinity binding sites for somatostatin-28 on pancreatic β-cells: differences with brain somatostatin receptors. Endocrinology 110:1049.
29. Czernik A, Petrack B 1983 Somatostatin receptor binding in rat cerebral cortex. J Biol Chem 258:5525.

30. Robbins R, Reichlin S 1983 Somatostatin biosynthesis by cerebral cortical cells in monolayer culture. Endocrinology 113:574.
31. Robbins RJ, Sutton RE, Reichlin S 1982 Sodium and calcium dependent somatostatin release from dissociated cerebral cortical cells in culture. Endocrinology 110:496.
32. Berelowitz M, Kronheim S, Pimstone B, Sheppard M 1978 Potassium stimulated calcium dependent release of immunoreactive somatostatin from incubated rat hypothalamus. J Neurochem 31:1537.
33. Maeda K, Frohman LA 1980 Release of somatostatin and thyrotropin-releasing hormone from rat hypothalamic fragments in vitro. Endocrinology 106:1837.
34. Patel YC, Zingg HH, Dreifuss JJ 1978 Somatostatin secretion from the rat neurohypophysis and stalk median eminence in vitro: calcium-dependent release by high potassium and electrical stimulation. Metabolism 27:1243.
35. Hermansen K 1980 The role of sodium in somatostatin secretion: Evidence for the involvement of Na^+ channels in the release mechanism. Endocrinology 106:1843.
36. Frankel B, Heldt A, Grodsky G 1982 Effects of K^+ and arginine on insulin, glucagon, and somatostatin release from the in vitro rat pancreas. Endocrinology 110:428.
37. Iversen LL, Iversen DS, Bloom F, Douglas C, Brown M, Vale W 1978 Calcium dependent release of somatostatin and neurotensin from rat brain in vitro. Nature 273:161.
38. Lee S, Havlicek V, Panerai A, Friesen HG 1978 High K^+-induced release of somatostatin from the cortical preparation of rat brain. Experientia 35:351.
39. Bennett G, Edwardson J, Marcano de Cotte D, Berelowitz M, Pimstone B, Kronheim S 1979 Release of somatostatin from rat brain synaptosomes. J Neurochem 32:1127.
40. Robbins RJ, Sutton RE, Reichlin S 1982 Effects of neurotransmitters and cyclic AMP on somatostatin release from cultured cerebral cortical cells. Brain Res 234:377.
41. Barden N, Cote JP, Lavoie M, Dupont A 1978 Secretion of somatostatin by rat islets of Langerhans and gastric mucosa and a role for pancreatic somatostatin in the regulation of glucagon release. Metabolism 27:1215.
42. Wakabayashi I, Miyazawawa H, Kanda M, Miki N, Demura R, Demura R, Shizume K 1977 Stimulation of immunoreactive somatostatin release from hypothalamic synaptosomes by high K and dopamine. Endocrinol Japon 24:601.
43. Negro-Vilar A, Ojeda SR, Arimura A, McCann SM 1978 Dopamine and norepinephrine stimulate somatostatin release by median eminence fragments in vitro. Life Sci 23:1493.
44. Chihara K, Arimura A, Schally AV 1979 Effect of intraventricular injections of dopamine, norepinephrine, acetylcholine, and 5-hydroxy-tryptamine on immunoreactive somatostatin release into rat hypophysial portal blood. Endocrinology 104:1656.

45. Unvas-Wallensten K, Efendic S, Luft R 1978 Release of somatostatin into the antral lumen of cats. Metabolism 27:1233.
46. Epelbaum J, Tapia-Arancibia L, Kordon C 1981 Noradrenaline stimulates somatostatin release from incubated slices of the amygdala and the hypothalamic preoptic area. Brain Res 215:393.
47. Samols E, Weir GC, Ramseur R, Day JA, Patel YC 1978 Modulation of pancreatic somatostatin by adrenergic and cholinergic agonism and by hyper- and hypoglycemic sulfonamides. Metabolism 27:1219.
48. Sorenson R, Elde R, Seybold V 1979 Effect of norepinephrine on insulin, glucagon and somatostatin secretion in isolated perfused rat islets. Diabetes 28:899.
49. Moore RY, Bloom FE 1979 Central catecholamine neuron systems: anatomy and physiology of the norepinephrine and epinephrine systems. In: Ann Rev Neurosci, Annual Reviews Inc, Palo Alto, p 113.
50. Vizi S 1980 Modulation of cortical release of acetylcholine by noradrenaline released from nerves arising from the rat locus coeruleus. Neuroscience 5:2139.
51. Hermansen K, Christensen SE, Orskov H 1979 Characterization of somatostatin release from the pancreas. Diabetologia 16:261.
52. Terry LC, Rorstad OP, Martin JB 1980 The release of biologically and immunologically reactive somatostatin from perifused hypothalamic fragments. Endocrinology 107:794.
53. Richardson SB, Hollander CS, D'Eletto R, Greenleaf PW, Thaw C 1980 Acetylcholine inhibits the release of somatostatin from rat hypothalamus in vitro. Endocrinology 107:122.
54. McKinney M, Davies P, Coyle J 1982 Somatostatin is not co-localized in cholinergic neurons innervating the rat cerebral cortex-hippocampal formation. Brain Res 243:169.
55. Sheppard MC, Kronheim S, Pimstone BL 1979 Effect of substance P, neurotensin and the enkephalins on somatostatin release from the rat hypothalamus in vitro. J Neurochem 32:647.
56. Berelowitz M, Dudlak D, Frohman L 1982 Release of somatostatin-like immunoreactivity from incubated rat hypothalamus and cerebral cortex. J Clin Invest 69:1293.
57. Dolais-Kitabgi J, Kitabgi P, Brazeau P, Freychet P 1979 Effect of neurotensin on insulin, glucagon, and somatostatin release from isolated perfused pancreatic islets. Endocrinology 105:256.
58. Ipp E, Dobbs R, Unger RH 1978 Vasoactive intestinal peptide stimulates pancreatic somatostatin release. FEBS Lett 90:76.
59. Hermansen K 1980 Effects of Substance P, and other peptides on the release of somatostatin, insulin, and glucagon in vitro. Endocrinology 107:256.
60. Tapia-Arancibia L, Reichlin S, VIP and PHI stimulate somatostatin secretion from fetal cerebral cortical and diencephalic cells in dispersed culture. Program of the 7th International Congress of Endocrinology, Quebec City, July 1984, #2509 (Abstract).

61. Epelbaum J, Tapia-Arancibia L, Besson J, Rotsztejn W, Kordon C 1979 Vasoactive intestinal peptide inhibits release of somatostatin from hypothalamus in vitro. Eur J Pharm 58:493.
62. van Calker D, Muller M, Hamprecht B 1980 Regulation by secretin, VIP, and somatostatin of cAMP accumulation in cultured brain cells. Proc Natl Acad Sci (USA) 77:6907.
63. Hermansen K 1984 Effects of CCK-4, non-sulfated CCK-8 and sulfated CCK-8 on pancreatic somatostatin, insulin and glucagon secretion in the dog. Endocrinology 114:1770.
64. Ipp E, Dobbs RE, Harris V, Arimura A, Vale W, Unger RH 1977 The effects of gastrin, gastric inhibitory polypeptide, secretin, and the octapeptide of cholecystokinin upon immunoreactive somatostatin release by the perfused canine pancreas. J Clin Invest 60:1216.
65. Chiba T, Taminato T, Kadowaka Y, Inove Y, Mori K, Seino H, Abe H, Chira S, Matsukura S, Fujita T, Goto Y 1980 Effects of various gastrointestinal peptides on gastric somatostatin release. Endocrinology 106:145.
66. Ipp E, Unger R 1979 Bombesin stimulates the release of insulin and glucagon but not somatostatin from the isolated perfused dog pancreas. Endo Res Commun 6:37.
67. Robbins R, Landon RM 1983 Somatostatin release from cerebral cortical cells: influence of amino acid neurotransmitters. Brain Res 273:374.
68. Schauder P, McIntosh C, Arends J, Arnold R, Frerichs H, Cruetzfeldt W 1976 Somatostatin and insulin release from isolated rat pancreatic islets stimulated by glucose. FEBS Lett 68:225.
69. Robbins R 1983 Influence of glucose on somatostatin synthesis and secretion in isolated cerebral cortical cells. J Neurochem 40:1430.
70. Ioffe S, Havlicek V, Friesen H, Chernick V 1978 The post-synaptic changes and effect of L-glutamate, GABA, and naloxone on SRIF sensitive cells in cerebral cortex of awake, non-paralyzed rabbits. Fed Proc 37:523.
71. Phillis J, Kirkpatrick J 1980 The actions of motilin, LH-RH, CCK-8, somatostatin, vasoactive intestinal peptide and other peptides on rat cerebral cortical neurons. Can J Physiol Pharm 58:612.
72. Randic M, Miletic V 1978 Depressant actions of methionine-enkephalin and somatostatin in cat dorsal horn neurones activated by noxious stimuli. Brain Res 152:196.
73. Pittman QJ, Siggins GR 1981 Somatostatin hyperpolarizes hippocampal pyramidal cells in vitro. Brain Res 221:402.
74. Chan-Palay V, Ito M, Tongroach P, Sakurai M, Palay S 1982 Inhibitory effects of motilin, somatostatin, leu-enkephalin, met-enkephalin and taurine on neurons in the lateral vestibular nucleus. Proc Natl Acad Sci (USA) 79:3355.
75. Dodd J, Kelly J 1978 Is somatostatin an excitatory transmitter in the hippocampus? Nature 273:674.

76. Macdonald RL, Nowak LM 1981 Substance P and somatostatin actions on spinal cord neurons in primary dissociated cell culture. In: Martin JB, Reichlin S, Bick KL (eds) Neurosecretion and Brain Peptides. Raven Press, New York, p 159.
77. Dichter MA, Delfs JR 1981 Somatostatin and cortical neurons in cell culture. In: Martin JB, Reichlin S, Bick K (eds) Neurosecretion and Brain Peptides. Raven Press, New York, p 145.
78. Garcia-Sevilla J, Magnusson T, Carlsson A 1978 Effect of intracerebroventricularly administered somatostatin on brain monoamine turnover. Brain Res 155:159.
79. Chesselet M, Reisine T 1983 Somatostatin regulates dopamine release in rat striatal slices and cat caudate nuclei. J Neurosci 3:232.
80. Tanaka S, Tsujimoto A 1981 Somatostatin facilitates serotonin release from cerebral cortex, hippocampus and hypothalamic slices. Brain Res 208:219.
81. Tsujimoto A, Shokichi T 1981 Stimulatory effects of somatostatin on norepinephrine release from rat brain cortex slices. Life Sci 28:903.
82. Gothert M 1980 Somatostatin selectively inhibits norepinephrine release from hypothalamic neurons. Nature 288:86.
83. Rubinow D, Gold P, Post R, Ballinger J, Cowdry R, Bollinger J, Reichlin S 1983 CSF somatostatin in affective illness. Arch Gen Psych 40:409.
84. Sorensen K, Christensen S, Dupont E 1980 Low somatostatin content in cerebrospinal fluid in multiple sclerosis. Acta Neurol Scand 61:186.
85. Schrober E 1981 Huntington's chorea - measurements of somatostatin, substance P and cyclic nucleotides in the cerebrospinal fluid. J Neurol 225:183.
86. Oram J, Edwardson J, Millard P 1981 Investigation of cerebrospinal fluid neuropeptides in idiopathic senile dementia. Gerontology 27:216.
87. Wood P, Lal E, Cajal S, Gauthier S, Nair N 1982 Reduced lumbar CSF somatostatin levels in Alzheimer's disease. Life Sci 31:2073.
88. Dupont E, Christensen S, Hanson A, Olivarius A, Orskov H 1982 Low cerebrospinal fluid somatostatin in Parkinson's disease: An irreversible abnormality. Neurology 32:312.
89. Epelbaum J, Ruberg M, Moyse E, Javog-Agid F, Dubois B, Agid Y 1983 Somatostatin and dementia in Parkinson's disease. Brain Res 278:376.
90. Davies P, Katzman R, Terry RD 1980 Reduced somatostatin-like immunoreactivity in cerebral cortex from cases of Alzheimer's disease and Alzheimer senile dementia. Nature 288:279.
91. Rossor MN, Emson P, Mountjoy C, Roth M, Iversen LL 1980 Reduced amounts of immunoreactive somatostatin in the temporal cortex in senile dementia of Alzheimer type. Neurosci Lett 20:373.

92. Delfs J, Znu C, Dichter M 1984 Coexistence of acetylcholinesterase and somatostatin-immunoreactivity in neurons cultured from rat cerebrum. Science 223:61.
93. Davies P 1979 Neurotransmitter related enzymes in senile dementia of the Alzheimer's type. Brain Res 171:319.
94. Szentagothai J 1978 The neuron network of the cerebral cortex: a functional interpretation. Proc Roy Soc Biol 201:219.
95. Eccles J 1981 The modular operation of the cerebral neocortex considered as the material basis of mental events. Neuroscience 6:1839.
96. Tapia R 1983 GABA: metabolism and biochemistry of synaptic transmission. In: Lajtha A (ed) Handbook of Neurochemistry. Plenum Press, New York, vol 3:423.

13

CENTRAL NERVOUS SYSTEM ACTIONS OF SOMATOSTATIN-RELATED PEPTIDES

MARVIN R. BROWN AND LAUREL A. FISHER

Peptide Biology Laboratory
The Salk Institute
10010 North Torrey Pines Road
La Jolla, California 92037

ABSTRACT

Somatostatin-related peptides act within the central nervous system to influence adrenomedullary epinephrine secretion and thermoregulation. Cysteamine-induced depletion of brain somatostatin-related peptides or central administration of a somatostatin receptor antagonist alters adrenomedullary epinephrine secretion and thermoregulation in a predictable manner. The actions of cysteamine and the somatostatin receptor antagonist are reversed by administration of somatostatins into the central nervous system, supporting the hypothesis that endogenous brain somatostatin-related peptides are involved in the regulation of adrenomedullary epinephrine secretion and thermoregulation.

INTRODUCTION

Somatostatins comprise a family of peptides, some of which may be derived from the same high-molecular-weight protein precursor and others from different precursors and different genes (1, 2). Radioimmunological (3) and immunocytochemical (4) detection of somatostatin-like peptides throughout the central nervous system (CNS) suggests that somatostatins may participate in mediating other brain functions in addition to controlling pituitary hormone secretion. Indeed, somatostatin-related peptides modify neuronal excitability and neurotransmitter release and act within the CNS to influence motor activity, sleep and feeding behavior (5). The following discussion focuses on the CNS actions of somatostatin-14 (SS-14), somatostatin-28 (SS-28) and related peptides on adrenomedullary epinephrine secretion and thermoregulation.

Effects of Somatostatins on Plasma Glucose and Epinephrine Concentrations

Initial investigations into the neuropharmacology of somatostatins utilized an eight-amino acid rigid-ring analog of SS-14, desAA^{1,2,4,5,12,13} [D-Trp^8]-somatostatin (ODT8-SS) (6). This analog, but not SS-14 itself, was found to act within the brain to prevent hyperglycemia induced by stress and other neurally active stimuli, such as drugs (6). The subsequent discovery of SS-28 led to the demonstration that this endogenous peptide, like ODT8-SS, was extremely potent in preventing stress-induced hyperglycemia (7). Somatostatin-related peptides prevent stress-induced hyperglycemia by inhibiting adrenomedullary epinephrine secretion (7, 8). Intracerebroventricular (icv) administration of ODT3-SS or SS-28 prevents epinephrine secretion normally observed after stress, insulin-induced hypoglycemia, and a variety of pharmacologic manipulations (Fig.1). Recent studies indicate that SS-28 acts within the dorsal hypothalamic area of animals to produce this inhibitory action on adrenomedullary epinephrine secretion (9).

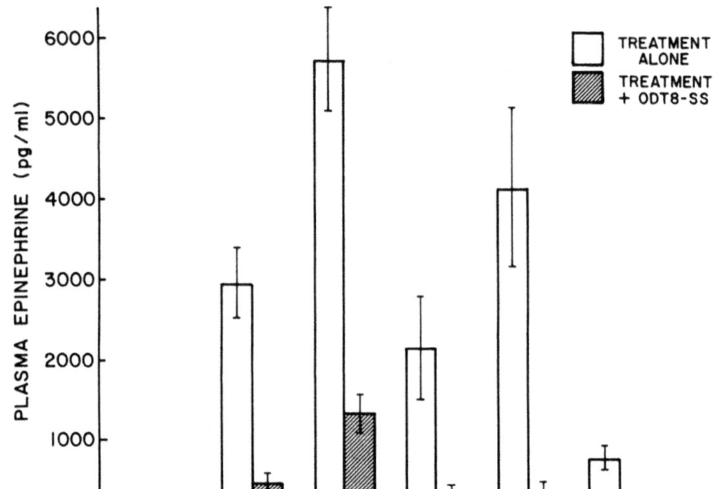

Fig. 1. Effects of desAA^{1,2,4,5,12,13} [D-Trp^8]-somatostatin (1nmol, ODT8-SS) on basal and bombesin (570 pmol)-, carbachol (54 nmol)-, 2-deoxy-glucose (18 μmol)-, insulin (1 U)- and stress-induced elevations of plasma epinephrine concentrations. ODT8-SS, bombesin, carbachol and 2-deoxy-glucose were given icv and insulin was given intravenously. Stress consisted of noise. All experiments were carried out in awake, unrestrained rats. The values shown represent those obtained 60 min after initial treatments.

Effects of Somatostatins on Thermoregulation

Somatostatin-14 was initially demonstrated by Cohn (10) to reduce body temperature while other investigators reported that SS-14 had little effect on body temperature (11, 12). ODT8-SS administered icv was found to produce significant elevations of body temperature (13) (Fig. 2). These potent hyperthermic actions of the oligosomatostatins suggested the possibility that other somatostatin-like ligands, e.g., SS-28, might exist within the CNS and that the hyperthermic actions of this endogenous somatostatin were being mimicked by the oligosomatostatins. Indeed, SS-28 given icv elevates body temperature (Fig. 2) and moreover, both SS-28 and ODT8-SS act within the CNS to prevent hypothermia induced by a variety of pharmacologic methods. Fig. 3 shows the dose-dependent inhibition of bombesin-induced hypothermia by SS-28 and ODT8-SS. The antagonistic actions of bombesin and somatostatin-related peptides are not limited to their opposite effects on adrenomedullary epinephrine secretion and thermoregulation. Recent studies demonstrate that ODT8-SS acts within the CNS to reverse bombesin-induced bradycardia into tachycardia (Fig. 4).

Evidence for a possible physiological role of somatostatin-related peptides in regulating body temperature has been obtained from studies performed in the ob/ob mouse (14). Homozygous ob/ob mice exposed to cold develop lethal hypothermia if not removed from

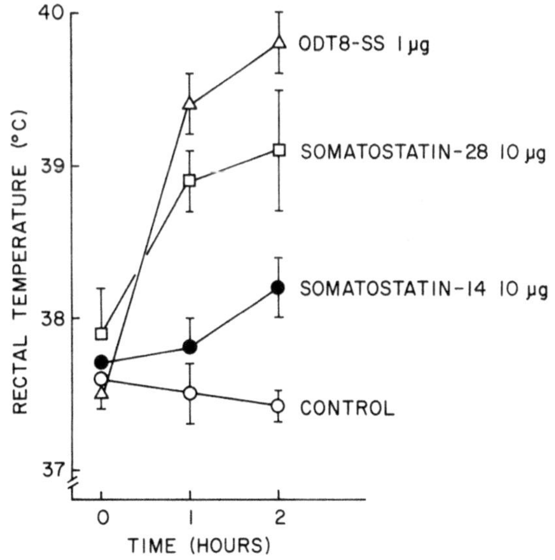

Fig. 2 Effects of desAA^{1,2,4,5,12,13} [D-Trp^8]-somatostatin (ODT8-SS), somatostatin-14 and somatostatin-28 given icv on body temperature of rats at ambient temperature of 23 C.

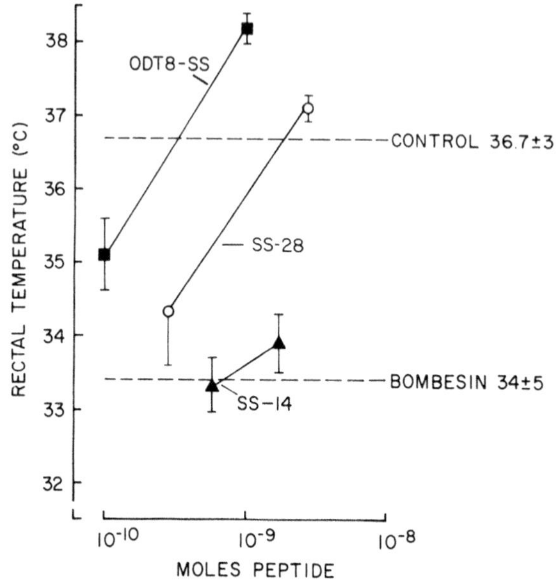

Fig. 3. Reversal of bombesin (57 pmol)-induced hypothermia by the desAA^{1,2,4,5,12,13} [D-Trp^{8}]-somatostatin (ODT8-SS), somatostatin-14 (SS-14) and somatostatin-28. All peptides were given icv and the rats were placed at 4 C. Body temperatures were measured at 60 min following peptide injection.

the cold and rewarmed. Intracerebroventricular administration of ODT-8 to these animals completely prevents cold-induced hypothermia. Since these animals have decreased brain levels of somatostatin-like activity (Brown and Vale, unpublished data), the possibility exists that their failure to thermoregulate results from a defect in a CNS somatostatinergic pathway involved in thermoregulation.

Depletion of Tissue Somatostatin Levels by Cysteamine

Until recently, a major drawback in assessing the neurobiological significance of somatostatin-related peptides has been the inability to deplete endogenous stores or to block the receptors through which these peptides exert their actions. In the past two years, both of these methods have become available.

Cysteamine (β-mercaptoethylamine) administration has been demonstrated to decrease the concentrations of somatostatin-like peptides in pancreas, gut and brain (15-19). Current data support the concept that cysteamine specifically lowers brain concentrations of SS-14 and SS-28 since it does not alter the concentrations of vasopressin, substance P, luteinizing hormone-releasing factor, enkephalin, vasoactive intestinal peptide and cholecystokinin (15, 17, 18).

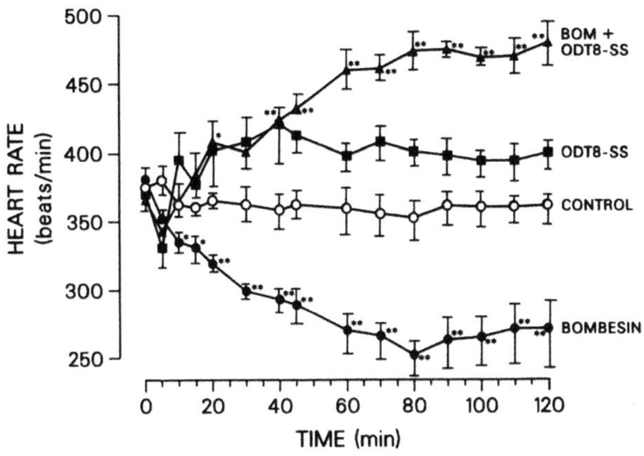

Fig. 4. Effects of ODT8-SS (1 nmol, icv) and bombesin (570 pmol, icv) on heart rate in conscious, unrestrained rats. ODT8-SS produced a slight elevation of heart rate and totally reversed bombesin-induced bradycardia into tachycardia. *, $p < 0.05$; **, $p < 0.01$ compared to zero time point.

Cysteamine administration (90 and 300 mg/kg, sc) decreases brain concentrations of somatostatin-like immunoactivity (SLI), but does not modify the concentration of two other sulphur containing peptides, calcitonin gene-related peptide and vasopressin. Recent studies demonstrate that cysteamine placed into specific hypothalamic regions depletes concentrations of SLI at the injection site without affecting SLI levels in adjacent brain regions (Brown and Vale, unpublished observations). Cysteamine does not interact in any of several radioimmunoassay systems nor does it interfere with the biological action of SS-14 to inhibit growth hormone secretion from anterior pituitary cells in culture (17).

We have shown previously that cysteamine abolishes somatostatin, but not vasopressin, immunocytochemical staining in rat brains (17). These results and those of others (15, 18) strongly suggest that cysteamine specifically depletes brain somatostatin levels over the time course tested. For this reason, cysteamine has been used recently as a pharmacologic tool to investigate the neurobiological role of brain somatostatins in the regulation of adrenomedullary epinephrine secretion and body temperature (17).

Effects of Cysteamine on Adrenomedullary Epinephrine Secretion

As noted above, CNS administration of SS-28 or ODT8-SS inhibits adrenomedullary secretion of epinephrine induced by a variety of neurally active stimuli (7, 8). In contrast, administration of cysteamine and, thus, depletion of brain somatostatin levels results in a prolonged elevation of plasma glucose and epinephrine concentrations without influencing plasma norepinephrine levels (17) (Fig. 5). Administration of ODT8-SS into the CNS lowers plasma concentrations of epinephrine following treatment with cysteamine (17). The rise of plasma glucose levels following cysteamine treatment is probably dependent on adrenomedullary epinephrine secretion since the cysteamine-induced hyperglycemia is prevented by icv administration of ODT8-SS. These results demonstrate that depletion of brain somatostatin using cysteamine increases adrenomedullary epinephrine secretion and are consistent with the hypothesis that brain somatostatins are involved in the physiologic regulation of adrenomedullary release of epinephrine.

Effects of Cysteamine on Thermoregulation

SS-28 and ODT8-SS placed into the CNS prevent hypothermia induced by a variety of pharmacologic methods and these somatostatins by themselves produce a prostaglandin-independent hyperthermia (13, 14). Consistent with the hypothesis that somatostatins may play a role in thermoregulation, cysteamine administration produces a dose-

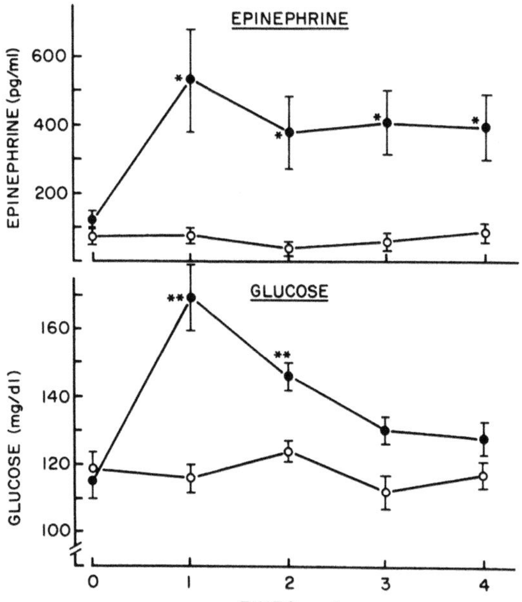

Fig. 5. Effects of cysteamine administration on plasma epinephrine and glucose levels. Cysteamine (300 mg/kg, sc) was injected immediately after the time zero sample. Experiments were carried out in awake rats and blood was collected through indwelling jugular catheters. *, $p < 0.05$; **, $p < 0.01$ compared to time zero values.

dependent lowering of body temperature in cold-exposed rats (17) (Fig. 6). This lowering of body temperature in cold- exposed rats results in part from an inability to increase heat production as evidenced by the effects of cysteamine on preventing cold-induced increases in oxygen consumption (17). Cysteamine- induced hypothermia is reversed by icv administration of SS-28 or ODT8-SS (17).

Cysteamine-treated animals kept at 22 C exhibit a slight reduction of body temperature and cysteamine treatment does not prevent ODT8-SS-induced hyperthermia (Fig. 7). In contrast, cysteamine does suppress the hyperthermia induced by prostaglandin E_2 (PGE_2) (Fig. 7). These results suggest the possibility that PGE_2-induced hyperthermia may be in part mediated by, or dependent on, endogenous somatostatinergic pathways. Furthermore, these results demonstrate that cysteamine does not impair an animal's ability to increase body temperature through generalized disruption of thermoregulatory mechanisms.

Effects of a Somatostatin Antagonist on Adrenomedullary Epinephrine Secretion

Fries et al. (20) recently reported the structure of a somatostatin analog that antagonizes the effects of SS-14 on growth hormone, insulin and glucagon secretion. Fig. 8 shows the effects of this somatostatin antagonist, cyclo [7-amino-heptanoyl-Phe-D-Trp-Lys-Thr (Bzl)], given icv on plasma concentrations of epinephrine. The somatostatin antagonist alone elevates plasma concentrations of

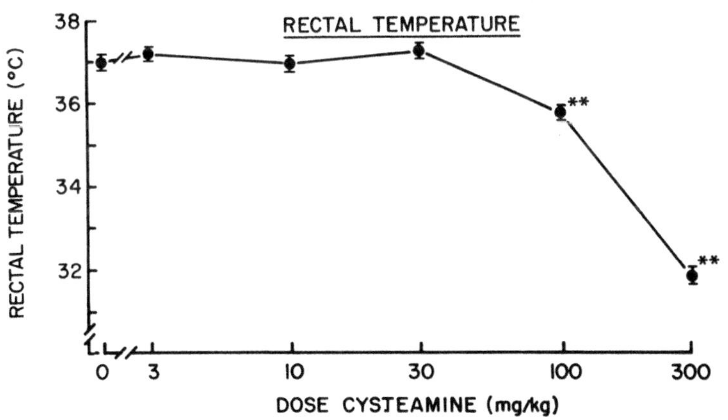

Fig. 6. Effects of various doses of cysteamine injected subcutaneously on rectal temperature of rats. Cysteamine was administered 3 hr prior to 4 C cold exposure. One hour after cold exposure, rectal temperatures were measured. *, $p < 0.05$; **, $p < 0.01$ compared to control (0 mg/kg) value.

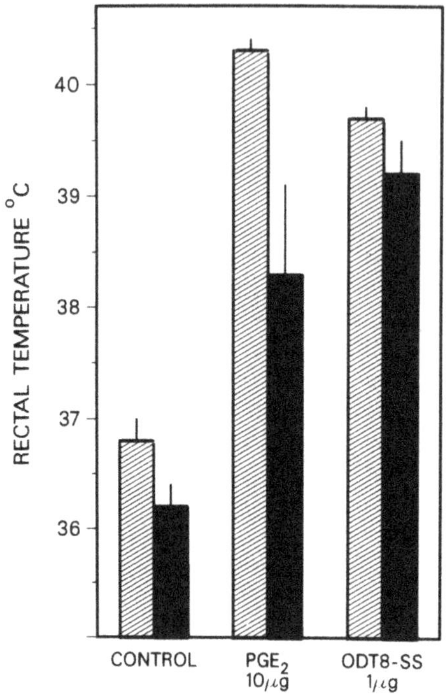

Fig. 7. Effects of ODT8-SS and prostaglandin E_2 (PGE_2) given icv on rectal temperatures of rats treated with cysteamine. Cysteamine (300 mg/kg) was given subcutaneously 3 hr prior to icv injection of ODT8-SS (1 nmol) or PGE_2 (28 nmol). Rectal temperatures were measured 60 min after the icv injections. Experiments were performed at room temperature (22 C). Hatched = saline pretreatment; shaded = cysteamine pretreatment.

epinephrine and this effect is counteracted by icv administration of ODT8-SS. The somatostatin antagonist does not modify plasma concentrations of norepinephrine.

The observed effects of this somatostatin receptor antagonist are similar to those produced by cysteamine and support the hypothesis that brain somatostatins are involved in the regulation of adrenomedullary epinephrine secretion.

Effects of a Somatostatin Antagonist on Thermoregulation

The somatostatin receptor antagonist given icv to rats housed at 22 C prevents ODT8-SS-induced hyperthermia and produces a slight but insignificant decrease in body temperature by itself (Fig. 9). In experiments carried out at 4 C, icv administration of the

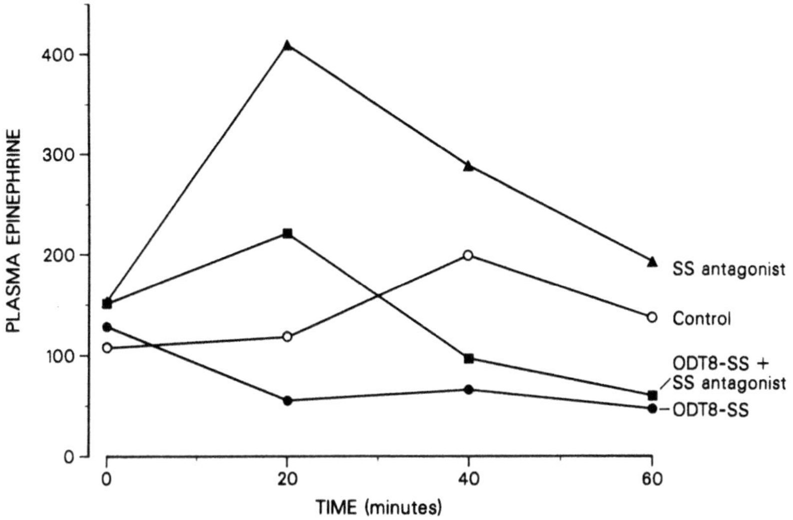

Fig. 8. Effects of a somatostatin receptor antagonist (10 μg) and ODT8-SS (1 nmol) on plasma concentrations of epinephrine in the rat. Peptides were injected icv in awake rats immediately after the time zero sample.

somatostatin receptor antagonist significantly lowers body temperature, suggesting that CNS somatostatinergic pathways may participate in mediating the thermoregulatory response to cold exposure.

CONCLUSIONS

Several lines of evidence now exist to support the hypothesis that peptides related to somatostatin are involved in the regulation of adrenomedullary epinephrine secretion and thermoregulation. First, somatostatin-like immunoactivity is present in brain regions that participate in the regulation of these systems (3, 4). Second, somatostatin-like peptides (in particular the endogenous somatostatin SS-28) act within discrete brain regions, e.g., dorsal hypothalamic area, to inhibit adrenomedullary epinephrine secretion (9), and, in as yet unidentified brain areas, to increase body temperature and prevent hypothermia induced by a variety of methods (13, 14). Third, the genetically obese ob/ob mouse has decreased brain concentrations of somatostatin, impaired ability to thermoregulate and high plasma concentrations of epinephrine (14). Fourth, depletion of brain somatostatins using cysteamine or blockade of brain somatostatin receptors using a somatostatin receptor antagonist results in impaired ability to thermoregulate and elevation of plasma concentrations of epinephrine (17). Recent studies indicate that cysteamine inhibits the synthesis of somatostatin and thus this

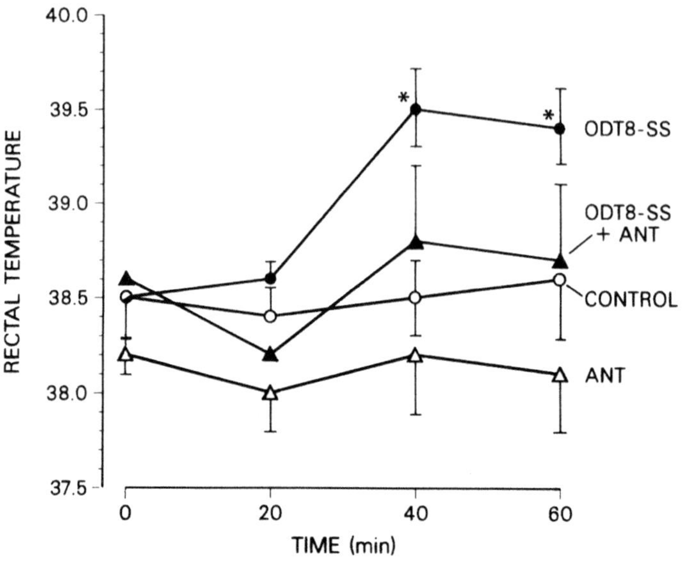

Fig. 9. Effects of a somatostatin receptor antagonist (10 μg) and ODT8-SS (1 nmol) on rectal temperature of rats at 22 C. Peptides were injected icv in awake rats immediately after the time zero value. *, $p < 0.05$ compared to the time zero values.

substance may prove to be a useful tool to study dynamic changes of endogenous somatostatins in animals under different physiologic circumstances. The ability to deplete somatostatins within discrete brain regions by microinjections of cysteamine will provide a powerful method to further investigate the neurobiological role(s) of endogenous somatostatins.

ACKNOWLEDGMENT

Research supported in part by NIH Grant NS-14263. Research conducted in part by the Clayton Foundation for Research-California Division. M. Brown is a Clayton Foundation Investigator. The authors thank R. Allen, V. Webb, R. Kaiser and R. Galyean for technical assistance, and S. Logan for manuscript preparation.

REFERENCES

1. Goodman RH, Lund PK, Jacobs JW 1980 Pre-prosomatostatins. J Biol Chem 255:6549.
2. Hobart P, Crawford R, Shen L, Pictet R, Rutter WJ 1980 Cloning and sequence analysis of cDNAs encoding two distinct somatostatin precursors found in the endocrine pancreas of anglerfish. Nature 228:137.

3. Kobayashi RM, Brown M, Vale W 1977 Regional distribution of neurotensin and somatostatin in rat brain. Brain Res 126:584.
4. Sawchenko PE, Swanson LW 1982 Immunohistochemical identification of neurons in the paraventricular nucleus of the hypothalamus that project to the medulla or to the spinal cord in the rat. J Comp Neurol 205:260.
5. Reichlin S 1983 Somatostatin. In: Krieger DT, Brownstein MJ, Martin JB (eds) Brain Peptides. John Wiley & Sons, Inc, New York, p 711.
6. Brown MR , Rivier J, Vale W 1979 Somatostatin: central nervous system actions on glucoregulation. Endocrinology 104:1709.
7. Brown M, Rivier J, Vale W 1981 Somatostatin-28: selective action on the pancreatic β-cell and brain. Endocrinology 108:2391.
8. Fisher DA, Brown M 1980 Somatostatin analog: Plasma catecholamine suppression mediated by the central nervous system. Endocrinology 107:714.
9. Brown MR 1983 Central nervous system sites of action of bombesin and somatostatin to influence plasma epinephrine levels. Brain Res 276:253.
10. Cohn ML 1975 Cyclic AMP, thyrotropin releasing factor, and somatostatin: key factors in the regulation of the duration of narcosis. In: Fink BR (ed) Molecular Mechanisms of Anesthesia: Progress in Anesthesiology. Raven Press, New York, vol. 1:485.
11. Brown M, Vale W 1980 Peptides and thermoregulation. In: Cox B, Lomax P, Milton AS, Schonbaum E (eds) Thermoregulatory Mechanisms and Their Therapeutic Implications. S. Karger, Basel, p 186.
12. Nemeroff CB, Osbahr AJ, Manberg PJ, Ervin GN, Prange AJ 1976 Alterations in nociception and body temperature after intracisternally administered neurotensin, β-endorphin, other endogenous peptides, and morphine. Proc Natl Acad Sci (USA) 76:5368.
13. Brown M, Tâché Y, Rivier J, Pittman Q 1981 Peptides and regulation of body temperature. In: Martin JB, Reichlin S, Bick KL, (eds) Neurosecretion and Brain Peptides: Implications for Brain Functions and Neurological Diseases. Raven Press, New York, p 397.
14. Brown M, Ling N, Rivier J 1981 Somatostatin-28, somatostatin-14 and somatostatin analogs: effects on thermoregulation. Brain Res 214:127.
15. Arimura A, Szabo S 1982 Selective depletion of somatostatin in rat brain by cysteamine. Brain Res 240:178.
16. Bakhit C, Benoit R, Bloom FE 1983 Effects of cysteamine on prosomatostatin related peptides. Regul Pept 6:169.
17. Brown MR, Fisher LA, Sawchenko PE, Swanson LW, Vale W 1983 Biological effects of cysteamine: relationship to somatostatin depletion. Regul Pept 5:163.

18. Sagar SM, Landry D, Millard WJ, Badger TM, Arnold MA, Martin JB 1982 Depletion of somatostatin-like immunoactivity in the rat central nervous system by cysteamine. J Neurosci 2:225.
19. Szabo S, Reichlin S 1981 Somatostatin in rat tissues is depleted by cysteamine administration. Endocrinology 109:2255.
20. Fries JL, Murphy WA, Sheiras-Diaz J, Coy DH 1982 Somatostatin antagonist analog increases GH, insulin, and glucagon release in the rat. Peptides 3:811.

14

PHYSIOLOGICAL ROLE OF SOMATOSTATIN IN REGULATION OF PULSATILE GROWTH HORMONE SECRETION

GLORIA SHAFFER TANNENBAUM

Departments of Pediatrics, and Neurology and Neurosurgery
McGill University and Montreal Children's Hospital
Montreal, Quebec H3H 1P3, Canada

INTRODUCTION

Regulation of the secretion of anterior pituitary hormones, in general, and growth hormone (GH), in particular, is achieved by the remarkably complex interaction of neural and feedback regulatory components. It is now generally recognized that central nervous system (CNS) control of GH secretion occurs by way of the intricate interplay of at least two hypothalamic hypophysiotrophic hormones - one stimulatory, a GH-releasing factor, GRF, and one inhibitory, a GH-release inhibiting factor, somatostatin. The objective of this chapter is to review our current understanding of the regulatory mechanisms for the control of GH secretion, with particular emphasis on the physiological role of somatostatin in GH regulation.

Spontaneous GH Secretion

A major principle of pituitary hormone secretion that has emerged in recent years is that the release of all hormones from the anterior pituitary gland does not occur in a steady state fashion, as the concept of homeostasis implied, but rather in an episodic or rhythmic manner. In the case of GH, early studies in man suggested that GH was secreted in distinct episodes, although much emphasis was placed on a correlation between the peak secretion of GH and the onset of sleep (1-3). Subsequent studies in a wide variety of species documented spontaneous marked elevations of basal plasma GH for which no reasonable explanation was available (4-6). To clearly define the temporal pattern of spontaneous GH secretion and study the physiological control mechanisms governing this mode of GH release, an experimental model was developed which permits frequent serial sampling of blood, with minimal effects on blood volume, from undisturbed freely-behaving rats over long periods of time (7).

Growth hormone secretion in the rat was found to be entirely pulsatile in nature (Fig. 1). The profile of GH secretion is characterized by high-amplitude GH secretory bursts which have a rapid onset with peak plasma GH values often exceeding 500 ng/ml. The GH secretory episodes are multiphasic in nature and generally show a double or triple peak, and the bursts terminate abruptly with a time-course consistent with the known half-life of GH in the rat. In the intervening trough periods, basal plasma GH levels are undetectable (<1 ng/ml, by standard RIA techniques). The frequency of the GH surges is precisely regulated with a 3.3 hour interval between secretory episodes, and this striking pattern persists unchanged across all phases of the light-dark cycle. Subsequent experiments demonstrated a uniformity in timing of the pulses in relation to clock-time indicating that the GH secretory bursts are entrained to the light-dark cycle. We concluded from these early studies that 1) GH secretion in the rat is regulated primarily by an endogenous ultradian rhythm with a periodicity of 3.3 hours, 2) the alternation of light and darkness probably serves as a Zeitgeber which sets the biological clock for GH secretion but is not necessary for maintenance of the basic ultradian rhythm, and 3) the GH rhythm is not dependent on changes in plasma glucose or insulin levels and continues to function independent of feeding (7, 8).

The secretion of GH has been shown to be pulsatile in nature in every species examined thus far. Recently, we studied spontaneous daytime GH secretory patterns in human male and female subjects at various stages of pubertal development (9). Non-sleep related bursts of GH secretion were evident in children of all ages and stages of puberty. Generally, 2 episodes of GH secretion were

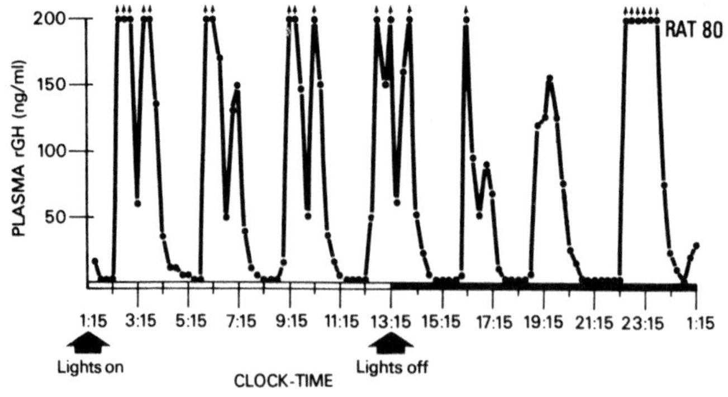

Fig. 1. Rhythmic GH secretory profile of a male rat sampled over a 24-h period.

observed during a 6-h sampling period, very similar indeed to the rat profiles described above. Thus, pulsatile secretion appears to be a generalized physiologic phenomenon of GH release in a wide variety of species ranging from rat to man.

Work in my laboratory has subsequently focused on the mechanisms involved in generating the ultradian rhythm of GH secretion.

Hypothalamic Regulation of GH Secretion

The rhythmic nature of the GH secretory profile and its persistence in constant conditions suggest that neural mechanisms play a crucial role in GH regulation. Evidence for hypothalamic control of GH secretion has been obtained in several species. The major nuclear centres of the hypothalamus that are implicated are schematized on Fig. 2. The ventromedial-arcuate (VMN-ARC) region of the hypothalamus has been implicated as a stimulatory locus in GH control since lesions of this area cause growth retardation (10) and depressed plasma GH levels (11, 12), whereas electrical stimulation results in a rise in plasma GH (13, 14). Evidence for an inhibitory role of the preoptic-anterior hypothalamic area has been obtained using similar techniques with resultant opposite effects; i.e. selective lesion of the preoptic-anterior hypothalamus (15, 16), or disconnection of this area from the medial basal hypothalamus (17,

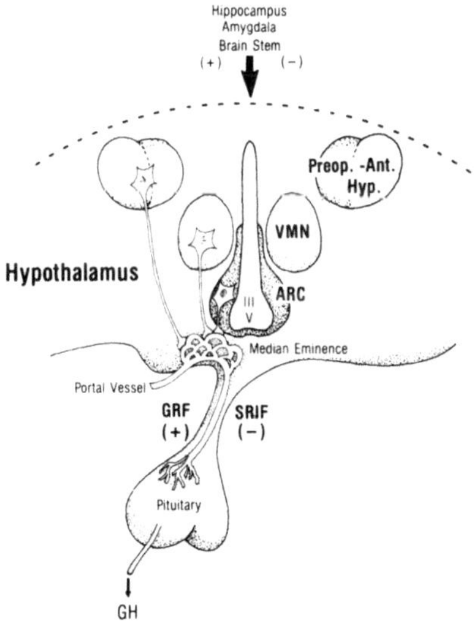

Fig. 2. Major nuclear centres of the hypothalamus implicated in GH regulation. Abbreviations: VMN, ventromedial nucleus; ARC, arcuate nucleus; GRF, GH-releasing factor; SRIF, somatostatin.

18), markedly augments plasma GH levels, whereas electrical stimulation causes inhibition of GH release (19). In addition, extrahypothalamic brain sites with known afferent inputs to the mediobasal hypothalamus, including the hippocampus and the amygdala, have been identified to be effective in either stimulation or inhibition of GH release (20).

We have recently completed a large series of experiments examining the effects of lesions of the VMN-ARC region of the hypothalamus (VMH) on the dynamics of the GH rhythm (21). In these studies, one group of animals received bilateral electrolytic lesions of the VMH, whereas a second group served as controls and received a sham lesion. As shown on Fig. 3, sham-lesioned animals exhibited the typical ultradian rhythm of GH secretion with most peak GH values >400 ng/ml. In striking contrast, VMH-lesioned animals exhibited a dramatic suppression in both amplitude and duration of GH secretory episodes; in these rats, peak GH levels rarely exceeded 90 ng/ml and a large proportion of plasma GH values were undetectable. Similar findings have been reported in rats neonatally administered monosodium glutamate (MSG), an agent which selectively destroys neuronal perikarya in the ARC nucleus of the hypothalamus (22, 23). Taken together, the results of these studies provide support for the view that the VMN-ARC region of the hypothalamus contains the neural substrates for generation and maintenance of the ultradian surges of GH release.

It is currently believed that CNS control of GH secretion is achieved (at least in part) by an interaction of the 2 hypothalamic hormones, GRF and somatostatin, which are released from axon terminals in the median eminence into the hypophyseal portal circulation and transported to the pituitary where they have their effects on GH secretion (see Fig. 2). Consistent with the physiological findings on hypothalamic regulation of GH secretion, immunohistochemical studies have revealed that the principal cell source of somatostatinergic fibers projecting to the median eminence is located in the anterior periventricular region of the hypothalamus (24, Chapter 10, this volume) whereas, to date, the primary neural locus for GRF-immunoreactive neurons appears to be the ARC nucleus (25, 26).

Physiological Role of Somatostatin in Spontaneous GH Secretion

The GH-release inhibiting factor, tetradecapeptide somatostatin (somatostatin-14, SRIF), was originally isolated from sheep hypothalami on the basis of its ability to inhibit GH release from dispersed rat pituitary cells in monolayer cultures (27). This peptide has subsequently been shown to be a potent inhibitor of GH release to virtually all known physiological and pharmacological stimuli, both *in vivo* and *in vitro*, and in a wide variety of species including man (see ref. 28 for review). Despite its multiplicity of effects on hormone secretion and its widespread distribution

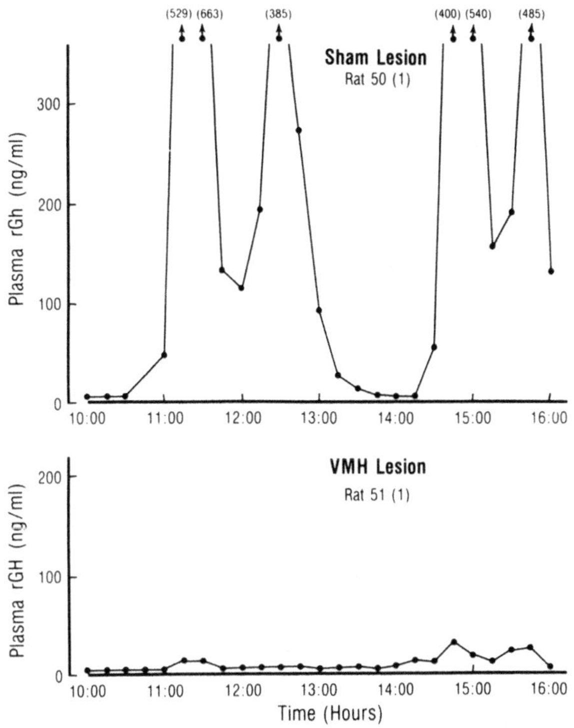

Fig. 3. Effect of lesions of the VMH (VMN-ARC region of the hypothalamus) on pulsatile GH secretion. Sham-lesioned animals exhibited the typical pulsatile pattern of GH release; VMH lesions caused a severe suppression in amplitude and duration of spontaneous GH secretory episodes.

throughout the body, the role of endogenous somatostatin in physiological regulation of GH secretion remains to be fully elucidated.

The availability of a specific antiserum to somatostatin provides a useful tool for assessing the possible involvement of endogenous somatostatin in hormone regulation. While working in the laboratory of Dr. Joseph Martin, an antiserum to somatostatin-14 was generated in sheep (29). This antiserum binds 33% of [^{125}I-Tyr^{1}] somatostatin-14 at a final dilution of 1:25,000 and can detect 10 pg/assay tube of synthetic somatostatin-14. The antiserum is directed toward the central portion of the molecule, corresponding to the sequence of amino acids 4-10 (30). If circulating somatostatin plays a role in maintaining the GH rhythm we hypothesized that its effects might be neutralized or blocked by the administration of a specific antiserum to somatostatin and thus its role in generating the rhythmic pattern of GH secretion might be unmasked.

Two groups of normal, freely-behaving rats were used in these experiments. One group was administered 1 ml of the somatostatin antiserum iv, whereas a second group served as controls and received 1 ml normal sheep serum. As shown on Fig. 4A, normal sheep serum did not alter the typical pulsatile pattern of GH secretion with most peak GH values >500 ng/ml and trough levels below the detectable limit of our present GH RIA (6.2 ng/ml). In contrast, administration of somatostatin antiserum during a trough period caused a rapid surge of GH secretion and significant elevation of subsequent GH trough levels; GH trough values did not reach undetectable levels throughout the 6-h sampling period in somatostatin antiserum-treated animals (Fig. 4B). However, it is of interest to note that the episodic surges of GH release were not abolished by immunoneutralization with anti-somatostatin serum.

A similar elevation of baseline or trough GH levels following anti-somatostatin treatment has been reported in several species (31-35). These data suggest that endogenous circulating somatostatin is a physiologic regulator of GH trough periods and is likely released episodically into the hypophyseal portal circulation to inhibit GH release. Furthermore, since the GH secretory bursts persisted despite somatostatin neutralization, the findings in all of these studies provide support for the view that the secretion of GH must be regulated by the interaction of at least 2 hypothalamic hypophysiotrophic hormones, one inhibitory, somatostatin, and the other excitatory, GRF.

Recently the picture has become even more complex. The existence of larger forms of somatostatin of molecular weight greater than that of somatostatin-14 had been widely documented in several laboratories (36-41), and it was suggested that these substances represented possible precursors of somatostatin-14. The successful isolation and characterization of somatostatin-28, an N-terminally extended form of somatostatin-14 containing 28 amino acids, has now been described by several groups (42-44).

Considerable interest has been aroused concerning the biologic activity of this peptide. Brazeau et al. (45) reported that somatostatin-28 was far more potent than somatostatin-14 in inhibition of GH secretion both _in vitro_ and _in vivo_, whereas Myers and co-workers (46) reported equipotency between the two peptides. These results were somewhat surprising, since precursors have classically been considered to be less biologically active than their products. Thus, we undertook a study to further assess the biological actions of somatostatin-28, in comparison to those of somatostatin-14, on spontaneous GH secretion, using unanesthetized freely-moving rats (47). As illustrated on Fig. 5, the sc administration of somatostatin-14 resulted in a rapid suppression of spontaneous GH secretory bursts; plasma GH levels remained depressed for only 30 min, consistent with

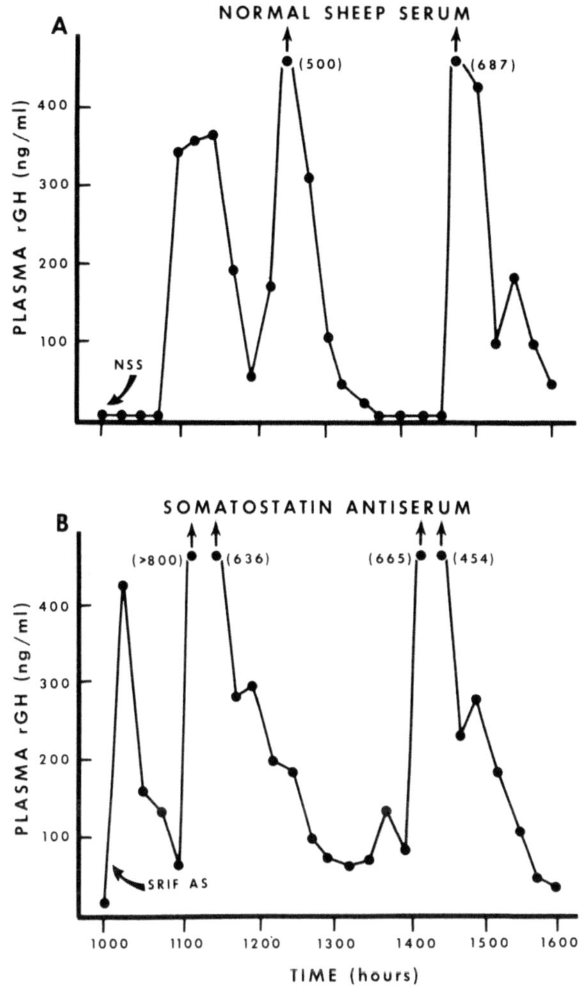

Fig. 4. Effect of passive immunization with somatostatin antiserum (SRIF AS) on spontaneous GH secretory profile. Administration of SRIF AS caused a rapid surge of GH release and significant elevation of GH trough levels compared to normal sheep serum (NSS)-treated controls.

the known short duration of biological activity of somatostatin-14. In contrast, somatostatin-28 caused a marked inhibition of GH release which persisted for a significantly longer period of time (90 min).

These results demonstrated that somatostatin-28 is indeed a potent inhibitor of spontaneous GH secretion and that the duration

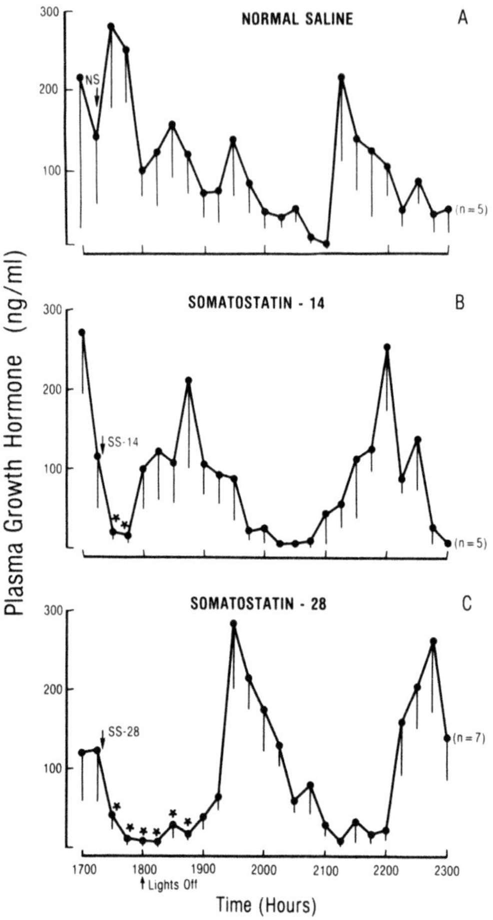

Fig. 5. Comparison of the time course of effects of normal saline (NS), somatostatin-14 (SS-14), and somatostatin-28 (SS-28) on mean 6-h plasma GH levels. The duration of significant GH inhibition by SS-28 was markedly longer than that by SS-14 (90 vs. 30 min). Vertical lines represent the SE. The number of animals in each group is shown in parentheses. *, Significant differences of $p < 0.05$ or less vs. NS-treated controls. (From ref. 47, with permission).

of inhibitory action of somatostatin-28 on physiologic GH release is significantly longer than that of somatostatin-14. The natural occurrence of somatostatin-28 in the hypothalamus (43, 44), and the demonstration of high biological activity on spontaneous GH release, suggests that somatostatin-28 may not merely be a prohormone but may act as a hormone on its own, released into the hypophyseal portal circulation to play an important physiological role in GH regulation.

Support for this view is obtained from recent studies demonstrating that somatostatin-28: 1) is secreted from stalk median eminence synaptosomes under simulated physiological conditions (48), 2) is released into the hypophyseal portal blood (49), and 3) binds to pituitary somatostatin-14 receptors with a greater affinity than that of somatostatin-14 (50). Preliminary passive immunization studies employing an antiserum specific for somatostatin-28 provide some evidence for a physiological role for somatostatin-28, in addition to that of somatostatin-14, in the regulation of basal GH levels (51).

Physiological Role of Somatostatin in Disordered States of GH Secretion

Considerable evidence has accumulated to indicate that the secretion of GH is sensitive to changes in nutritional status. We have demonstrated that the spontaneous pulses of GH release are markedly suppressed in response to food deprivation (52), insulinopenic diabetes (53, 54) and intracellular glucopenia (55). In order to elucidate the mechanism(s) mediating these GH suppression responses we assessed the role of endogenous somatostatin using the technique of passive immunization (29, 53). As summarized on Fig. 6, immunoneutralization with anti-somatostatin serum reversed the GH-inhibitory reactions to both starvation and streptozotocin-induced diabetes suggesting that circulating somatostatin plays a physiological role in these conditions. Alterations in pancreatic, gastrointestinal and blood concentrations of somatostatin-like immunoreactivity have been well documented in starvation (52, 56) and various forms of diabetes (57-61). These findings are compatible with the view that somatostatin may be an important hormonal regulator of nutrient homeostasis (62, Chapter 23, this volume) and suggest that blood-borne somatostatin is capable of exerting an endocrine-like action on distant target organs, such as the pituitary gland, to effect changes in GH secretion.

Circulating somatostatin has also been implicated as a physiologic regulator of stress-induced GH suppression since pretreatment with anti-somatostatin sera partially restores normal GH secretory pulses under stressful conditions (63, 64).

We have examined the mechanism responsible for the impaired GH secretion observed in animals bearing lesions of the VMH (21). It is likely that the decrease in magnitude of the GH surges observed in this model of disordered growth is due to disruption of either excitatory, GRF, or inhibitory, somatostatinergic, neuronal pathways involved in the control of GH secretion. In contrast to our previous studies, administration of somatostatin antiserum to these rats failed to restore the amplitude of the GH pulses or to significantly alter mean 6-h plasma GH levels (Fig. 7). A similar lack of effect of somatostatin antiserum on GH pulse amplitude has

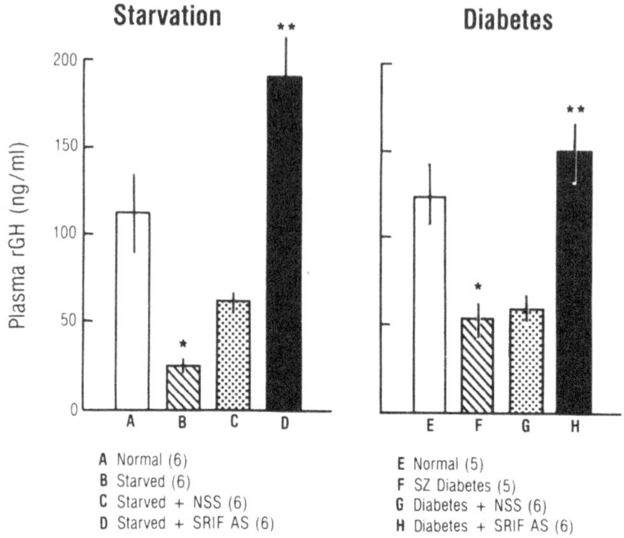

Fig. 6. Summary of effects of immunoneutralization with anti-somatostatin serum (SRIF AS) on the GH suppression response observed in starvation and streptozotocin (SZ) diabetes. Administration of SRIF AS successfully restored high-amplitude GH pulses in both conditions, compared to normal sheep serum (NSS)-treated controls. Each bar represents the mean 6-h plasma GH level ± SE, and the number of animals in each group is shown in parentheses. *, $p < 0.01$, compared to normal; **, $p < 0.005$, compared to NSS controls.

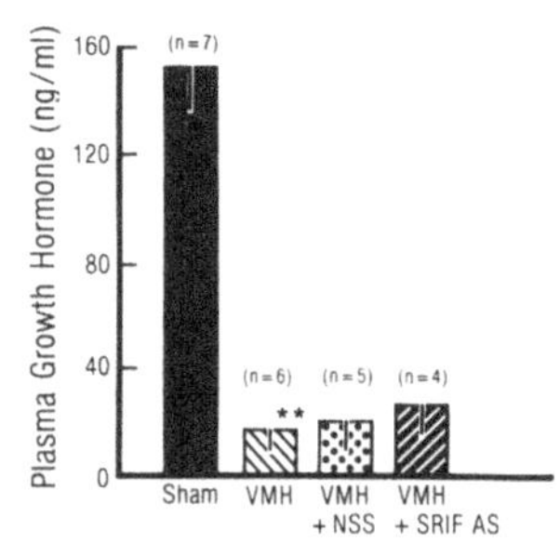

Fig. 7. Effect of somatostatin antiserum (SRIF AS) on mean 6-h plasma GH levels in VMH-lesioned animals. Administration of SRIF AS failed to significantly alter the suppressed GH secretory profile, compared to VMH-normal sheep serum (NSS)-injected controls. Each bar represents the mean ± SE, and the number of animals in each group is shown in parentheses. **, $p < 0.001$ vs. sham lesion.

been reported in MSG-treated rats (23). It is unlikely that inadequate passive immunization can account for the lack of effect since measurement of the somatostatin binding capacity of the plasma of treated animals revealed that significant somatostatin antibody titers were present for the entire sampling period (21). These results provide good evidence that increased somatostatin release is not the mechanism whereby VMN-ARC lesions cause suppression of GH secretion. The findings suggest that the suppression of GH surges observed following damage to this region of the brain is due to interruption of stimulatory pathways involved in GH regulation, namely, GRF neurons.

The Interrelationship of Somatostatin and GRF

Despite an intensive search over the last 20 years for the GH-releasing factor, purification and characterization of this factor had eluded the best efforts of many investigators. Much excitement has been generated during the past 2 years by reports from the laboratories of Guillemin (65) and Vale (66) of the successful isolation, characterization and reproduction by total synthesis of peptides with high intrinsic GH-releasing activity from human pancreatic (hp) islet cell tumors. The synthetic replicates of these peptides (hpGRF-44 and hpGRF-40) were shown to be potent and specific stimulators of pituitary GH release (65-68) and to be identical in both biological activity (69) and structure (70) to the GRF present in human hypothalamus. Recently, Spiess et al. (71) reported the isolation and characterization of a 43-amino acid peptide which they propose to be the long-sought rat hypothalamic (rh) GRF. The availability of such peptides now provides a powerful tool to further delineate the physiological control mechanisms governing the rhythmic secretion of GH.

The first question we raised was whether the GRF peptides could restore high-amplitude GH secretory pulses in GH-deficient animals bearing lesions of the VMH. To address this issue, VMH-lesioned rats were administered 3 iv bolus injections of an hpGRF-40 analog at 90 min intervals. As a control, the same rats received iv injections, at the same time points and same dose (10 μg), of another hypothalamic releasing factor, TRH (72). As shown on Fig. 8, hpGRF caused a dramatic surge of GH within 5 min after injection; plasma GH rose to levels as high as 2900 ng/ml and remained significantly elevated for 15-30 min, compared to TRH-injected controls. These findings clearly demonstrate that hpGRF is a powerful releaser of GH in VMH-lesioned rats, and suggest that the ultradian surges of GH release are likely dependent on the release of GRF from the VMN-ARC region of the hypothalamus. The more recent immunohistochemical detection of hpGRF-like immunoreactivity in both ARC and VMN nuclei of mammalian brain (25, 26) provides strong support for this view.

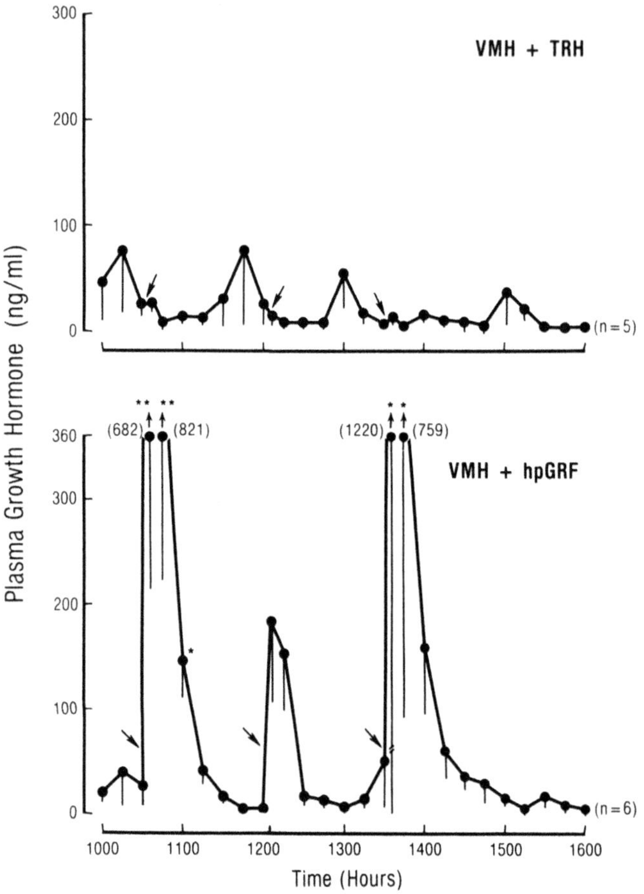

Fig. 8. Mean 6-h plasma GH profiles of VMH-lesioned rats given 3 iv bolus injections of either TRH or hpGRF. Administration of hpGRF caused a dramatic surge of GH release within 5 min. Arrows indicate times of injections. Vertical lines represent the SE. The number of animals in each group is shown in parentheses. *, $p < 0.05$, **, $p < 0.01$, compared to VMH + TRH controls. (From ref. 72, with permission).

The demonstration of powerful GH-releasing activity by hpGRF in animals with hypothalamic damage is promising in that hpGRF and its analogs may provide valuable agents for the diagnosis and treatment of disorders of growth secondary to CNS dysfunction. However, it became evident when examining the individual GH secretory profiles that the magnitude of the GH response to hpGRF varied with the time of administration (see Fig. 8). One possible explanation for the variability of response is that the inhibitory peptide, somatostatin, was interfering with the actions of hpGRF.

To study the interaction between somatostatin and hpGRF *in vivo* we iv administered somatostatin-14 (208 μg) simultaneously with hpGRF (10 μg) to VMH-lesioned animals and compared the GH response to that observed following the administration of hpGRF (10 μg) alone. As shown on Fig. 9, the concomitant administration of somatostatin-14 and hpGRF resulted in a significant inhibition of the hpGRF-induced GH release 5 min after injection, indicating that somatostatin can antagonize the actions of hpGRF, although there was no significant effect 15 min post treatment. This observation fits well with *in vitro* reports demonstrating that somatostatin inhibits hpGRF-induced GH release from dispersed rat pituitary cells in typical non-competitive antagonism (73, 74). Taken together, these findings provide support for the view that GRF and somatostatin have different receptors on the pituitary somatotrophes. Furthermore, the data suggest that the duration of biological activity of GRF may be longer than that of somatostatin-14.

We have continued to utilize the GRF peptides as probes to further elucidate the interrelationship of somatostatin and GRF in generation of the ultradian rhythm of GH secretion. In these studies, normal freely-moving rats were iv administered rhGRF and hpGRF-44 during both peak and trough periods of the GH rhythm (75). As illustrated on Fig. 10A, administration of rhGRF during a time of peak GH secretion (1100 h) resulted in 2- to 3-fold increases in plasma GH. In contrast, injection of rhGRF during a trough period (1300 h) had only a minimal effect on plasma GH levels. Because our previous findings suggested that somatostatin secretion was increased during GH trough periods, we examined the effects of passive immunization with antiserum to somatostatin on GRF-induced GH release.

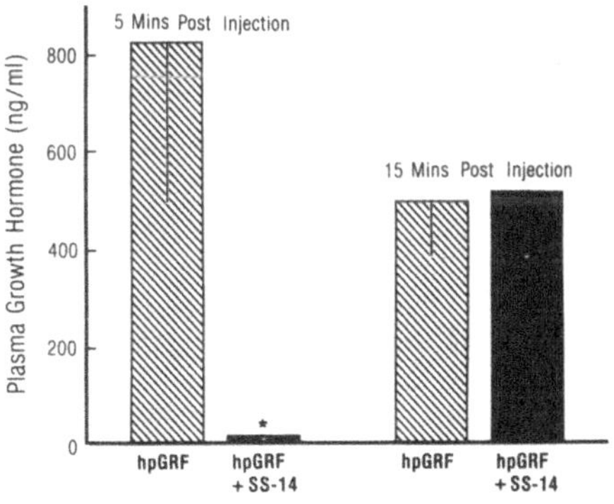

Fig. 9. Effect of the simultaneous iv administration of hpGRF and and somatostatin-14 (SS-14) on plasma GH responsiveness to hpGRF in 4 VMH-lesioned rats. Injection of hpGRF + SS-14 caused a significant inhibition of hpGRF-induced GH release at 5 min, but not at 15 min, post injection. Each bar represents the mean ± SE. *, $p < 0.05$ vs. hpGRF alone.

Immunoneutralization with anti-somatostatin serum eliminated the time-dependent difference and permitted marked rhGRF-induced GH release at 1300 h (Fig. 10B), indicating that the weak GRF-induced GH release observed during trough periods is due to antagonization by endogenous circulating somatostatin. Similar results were obtained with the hpGRF peptide. These findings provide additional support for the view that the release of somatostatin from the hypothalamus into the hypophyseal portal blood is increased episodically during trough periods.

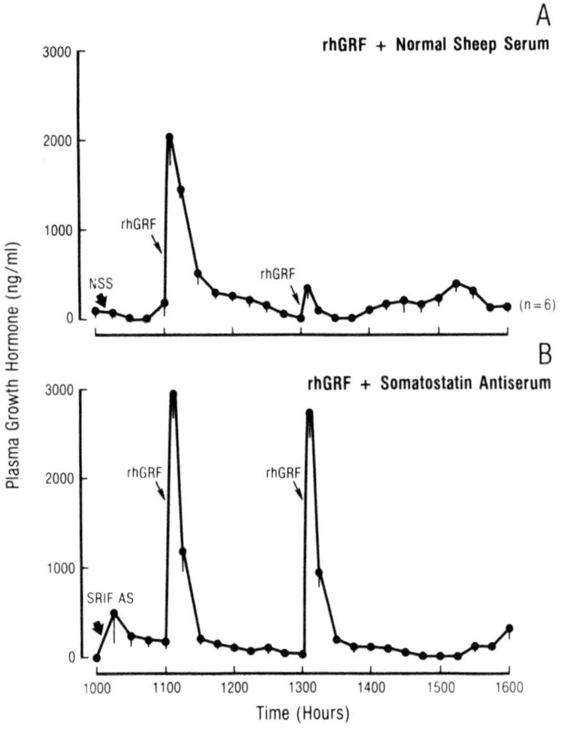

Fig. 10. Mean plasma GH response to rhGRF administered during peak and trough periods of the GH rhythm to rats pretreated with either normal sheep serum (NSS) of somatostatin antiserum (SRIF AS). A, In NSS-treated animals, the plasma GH response to rhGRF was significantly greater during a time of peak GH secretion (1100 h) than during a trough period (1300 h). B, Passive immunization with SRIF AS reversed the weak response at 1300 h and significantly increased the rhGRF-induced GH release at 1100 h. Vertical lines represent the SE. The number of animals is shown in parentheses. (From ref. 75, with permission).

Whereas the GRF peptides have now been shown to possess high GH-releasing activity *in vivo* in several species, including man (76-80), a consistent observation reported by most researchers has been the wide variability of response across subjects. The striking time-dependent difference (peak vs. trough periods) in the magnitude of the GH response to GRF clearly indicates that the intermittent secretion of endogenous somatostatin is an important factor which must be taken into account when assessing the *in vivo* biological activities of the GRF peptides.

It is also of interest to note that immunoneutralization with somatostatin antiserum significantly augmented the GH response to rhGRF during a time of peak GH secretion (Fig. 10B). This finding suggests that the GH-releasing ability of GRF is also somewhat antagonized by endogenous circulating somatostatin during a normal GH secretory episode, and is consistent with previous observations indicating that passive immunization with somatostatin antiserum generally augments the responsiveness of plasma GH to GRF (77, 81). Taken together, the data provide support for the view that somatostatin exerts a tonic inhibitory effect on GH release and that this tonic secretion of somatostatin is increased episodically (every 3-4 h) to achieve the undetectable plasma GH levels observed during trough periods of the GH rhythm.

These results, together with the available evidence to date (see ref. 75 for review), lead to the hypothesis shown schematically on Fig. 11 that both somatostatin and GRF are secreted tonically from the hypothalamus into the hypophyseal portal blood, and that superimposed upon this steady state release is an additional rhythmic surge of each peptide, with a periodicity of 3-4 h, about 180° out of phase, providing for integration of the ultradian rhythm of GH secretion as observed in the peripheral blood. Whether these rhythmic patterns of discharge are intrinsic to the respective peptidergic neurons involved, as has been demonstrated electrophysiologically for other hypothalamic neurosecretory neurons (82), or whether they are dependent on an external oscillator(s) or ultradian clock in another CNS site is a subject for future research.

Feedback Regulation of GH Secretion

"Short-loop" feedback control of GH secretion

Is the secretion of GH determined entirely by hypothalamic events or do feedback mechanisms come into play? Because GH does not stimulate the secretion of a specific endocrine product from any peripheral target organ, it had been postulated that GH itself may act as its own controlling signal via hypothalamic and/or pituitary receptors. Early studies in rats demonstrated that pituitary GH content was altered in response to exogenous administration of GH

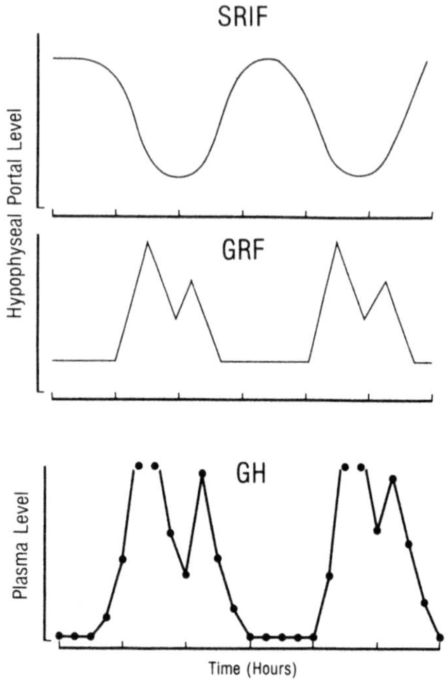

Fig. 11. Postulated rhythmic secretion of somatostatin (SRIF) and GH-releasing factor (GRF) into hypophyseal portal blood, with the net result on GH secretion, as observed in the peripheral plasma. (From ref. 75, with permission).

(83, 84), and was reduced in animals bearing tumors that secreted GH (85). In primates, systemic administration of GH had been shown to inhibit the endogenous GH response to insulin-induced hypoglycemia in both monkey (86) and man (87, 88). While these studies suggested that GH may play a role in inhibiting its own secretion they did not shed light on either the site (pituitary or brain) or mechanism of action for GH negative feedback.

We undertook a study to determine whether GH can regulate its own secretion at the level of the CNS (89). For these experiments, rats were implanted with chronic intracerebroventricular (icv) cannulae in the left lateral ventricle of the brain at the time of venous cannulation. As shown on Fig. 12, icv administration of rat GH caused a marked alteration in the GH secretory profile compared to normal saline icv-injected controls. The most striking effect was a dramatic suppression in amplitude of the GH secretory episodes, with peak GH values not exceeding 76 ng/ml during the latter 3 h of the sampling period. Recent studies employing human GH have confirmed these findings (90, 91). These results provided

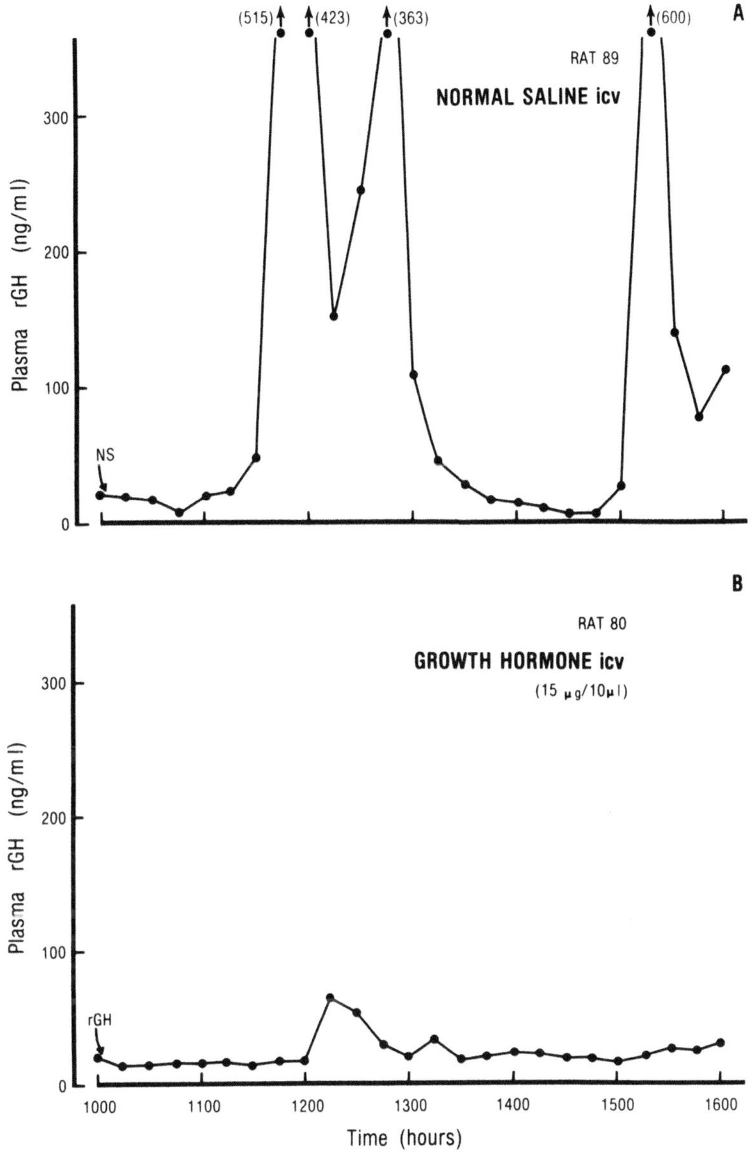

Fig. 12. Effect of intracerebroventricular (icv) administration of rat (r) GH on pulsatile GH secretion. A, Central injection of normal saline did not alter the typical ultradian rhythm of GH secretion. B, The icv injection of rGH resulted in a marked suppression in amplitude of spontaneous GH pulses.

convincing evidence that GH can regulate its own secretion via a "short-loop" negative feedback system. Furthermore, the data indicated that the CNS is an important site for GH autoregulation.

"Long-loop" feedback control of GH secretion

While the regulation of most anterior pituitary hormones by specific peripheral target gland hormones occurs by way of a classic "long-loop" feedback mechanism, such a mechanism has not been apparent for GH. Although GH does not stimulate the secretion of a specific endocrine product from a distinct endocrine target organ, it has been postulated that many of the growth-promoting peripheral actions of GH are mediated by the somatomedins (see ref. 92 for review). Somatomedin is a general term for a family of peptides, under GH control, that exhibits growth-promoting and insulin-like activities on several tissues (93). Several somatomedins have been identified as insulin-like growth factors (IGF's) (94); however, the role of these substances in GH regulation is unclear. Thus, it was relevant to ask whether GH "long-loop" feedback might be mediated by these GH-dependent peptides.

We assessed the involvement, at a CNS level, of ILA's, a preparation enriched in IGF's, in feedback regulation of pulsatile GH secretion (95). Intracerebroventricular administration of ILA's caused a marked decrease in spontaneous GH secretory episodes; this was a specific effect of the somatomedin-enriched preparation and was not seen with either bovine serum albumin, as a protein control, or porcine insulin, another growth factor not directly stimulated by GH. These findings provided *in vivo* evidence that IGF's, or somatomedins, may participate in a GH negative feedback system at the level of the CNS. Similar results have recently been reported using a purified preparation of somatomedin C (91). Others have also made observations consistent with negative feedback of GH secretion. The tapeworm *Spirometra mansonoides* produces a growth-promoting substance, immunologically distinct from GH, which competes in a GH RRA, and stimulates somatomedin production (96); rats infested with this worm show a depletion of pituitary GH content indicating a feedback effect either directly via the tapeworm substance and/or via somatomedin (97). Clinical observations further support the hypothesis that IGF's play a role in GH negative feedback. In Laron dwarfism, where somatomedin generation is lacking, increased concentrations of GH are present (98), whereas in kwashiorkor, low concentrations of somatomedin coexist with high levels of GH (99).

Physiological Role of Somatostatin in Feedback Regulation of GH Secretion

"Short-loop" feedback control

The mechanism whereby GH influences its own secretion is of interest. There is no support, to date, for a direct effect of GH at the level of the pituitary gland, since neither human nor rat GH was able to suppress GH release from rat pituitary cells in culture (100, 101). The results of several recent studies suggest an involvement of the somatostatinergic system in "short-loop" feedback control of GH secretion. Depletion of GH by hypophysectomy causes a significant reduction of median eminence somatostatin (102-106), which is then restored to normal following GH treatment (103, 106). Rats treated systemically with GH exhibit increased hypothalamic somatostatin concentration (106), and *in vitro* administration of rat GH causes a dose-dependent increase in somatostatin release from incubated rat hypothalami (107, 108). Finally, intraventricular administration of rat GH in a dose similar to that used in our study has been reported to stimulate somatostatin release into hypophyseal portal blood (109).

We have recently completed a series of *in vivo* experiments designed to assess the possible involvement of the two hypothalamic peptides, somatostatin and GRF, in mediation of GH autoregulation. In these studies, freely-moving rats were administered rat (r) GH (15 μg/10 μl) via the lateral brain ventricle followed by either a) 1 ml somatostatin antiserum iv, b) 10 μg hpGRF-44 iv or c) somatostatin antiserum + hpGRF-44, iv. As illustrated on Fig. 13, icv injection of rGH caused a severe suppression in GH pulse amplitude compared to normal saline icv-treated controls. Immunoneutralization with anti-somatostatin serum failed to restore the amplitude of GH pulses to normal values (although trough and mean 6-h plasma GH levels were significantly elevated in this group.) Administration of a supramaximal bolus of hpGRF-44 significantly augmented GH pulse amplitude, however peak GH levels in this group still did not reach normal values. Only the combination of hpGRF-44 and passive immunization with somatostatin antiserum permitted restoration of high-amplitude GH secretory bursts in rats administered rGH centrally (Fig. 13). These results provide support for only a partial role for endogenous somatostatin in mediating GH autofeedback. The findings suggest that the mechanism(s) whereby GH inhibits its own secretion likely involves decreased output of hypothalamic GRF concomitant with increased release of somatostatin.

"Long-loop" feedback control

Existing evidence supports the concept that the somatomedin peptides exert "long-loop" negative feedback control of GH secretion by acting at both the pituitary and hypothalamic level. Support for

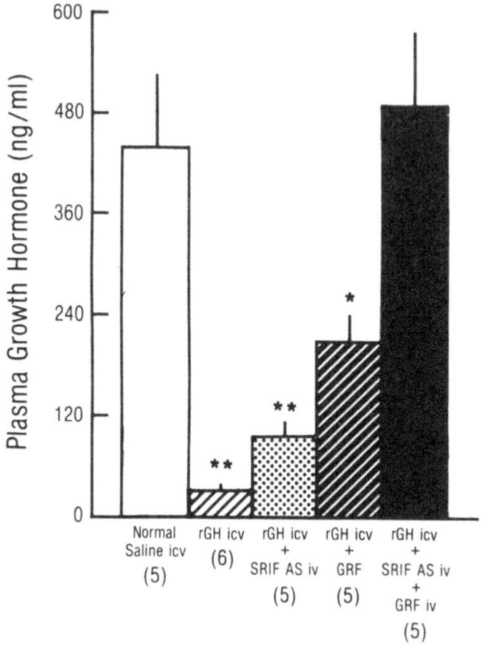

Fig. 13. Assessment of the roles of somatostatin and GRF in mediation of GH autofeedback. Only the combination of GRF + somatostatin antiserum (SRIF AS) permitted restoration of normal GH pulse amplitude in rats administered rGH intracerebroventricularly (icv). Each bar represents the mean peak GH level ± SE, and the number of animals in each group is shown in parentheses. *, $p < 0.05$, **, $p < 0.01$, compared to normal saline icv group.

a pituitary locus comes from in vitro studies which indicate that somatomedin C and the IGF's can inhibit both basal and stimulated (cAMP and GRF) GH release from rat pituitary cells in culture (101, 110, 111), and that specific receptors for IGF's are present on rat anterior pituitary cells (112, 113). At the level of the CNS, the IGF's have been shown to specifically bind to membrane preparations of both rat (112) and human (114) brain and are found in high concentrations in human cerebrospinal fluid (115). Direct evidence for a role for somatostatin in mediating long-loop feedback of GH release comes from studies by Berelowitz et al. which demonstrate that somatomedin C directly stimulates somatostatin release from rat hypothalami in culture (110). These latter findings, together with the in vivo results on spontaneous GH release (91, 95), suggest that the somatomedins/IGF's may be involved in a GH negative feedback loop at a CNS level via the inhibitory mechanism of hypothalamic somatostatin release. However, the possibility that the IGF's have a simultaneous inhibitory effect on hypothalamic GRF release cannot be excluded.

Finally, it is also of interest to note, in relation to feedback control of GH secretion, that both somatostatin (116) and GRF (117) may be capable of inhibiting their own neurosecretion, possibly via an "ultrashort-loop" feedback mechanism. Direct support for this concept comes from recent studies by Peterfreund et al. indicating that somatostatin can inhibit its own release from hypothalamic cells in culture (see Chapter 11, this volume). The presence of recurrent inhibition in the tuberoinfundibular system, whereby axon collateral terminals of peptidergic neurosecretory neurons terminate directly or indirectly on their cells of origin to inhibit their firing, is well documented (118). This could provide the pathway for "ultrashort-loop" feedback, a concept originally postulated for hypothalamic releasing factors by Motta et al. (119). Such a mechanism might function in the mediation of the phasic or rhythmic nature of the GH secretory profile. Disruption of this feedback regulation of either somatostatin or GRF could conceivably play a role in the pathogenesis of pituitary disorders.

CONCLUSION

In summary, Fig. 14 is a rather simplistic schematic representation of an exceptionally complex regulatory system that has evolved for a hormone that is responsible for one of the most important of all endocrine functions, namely growth. It is evident that the remarkable peptide(s), somatostatin, plays an important role, at many levels, in physiological regulation of the secretion of GH. No doubt, future research will unravel additional significant contributions of somatostatin to the intricate pathways of GH modulation.

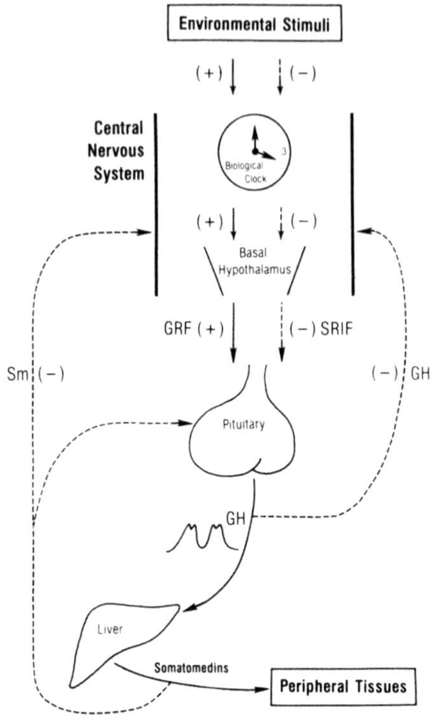

Fig. 14. Schematic representation of the regulatory mechanisms for the control of GH secretion.

ACKNOWLEDGMENTS

I wish to thank Drs. Joseph B. Martin and Paul Brazeau for their encouragement and support in the earlier studies, Dr. Roelof Eikelboom and Ms. Jean-Claude Painson for their valuable contribution in recent experiments, Ms. Wendy Gurd, Laura Wanamaker and Sylvie Trudel Barrett for skillful technical assistance, and Mrs. Mary Youakim for fine secretarial help. I am grateful to the NIADDK for generous supplies of rat GH RIA materials.

The studies conducted in the author's laboratory described herein were supported by grants from the Medical Research Council of Canada, the Quebec Medical Research Council and the National Institutes of Health. G.S.T. is a scholar of the Quebec Medical Research Council.

REFERENCES

1. Quabbe HJ, Schilling E, Helge H 1966 Pattern of growth hormone secretion during a 24-hour fast in normal adults. J Clin Endocrinol Metab 26:1173.
2. Takahashi Y, Kipnis DM, Daughaday WH 1968 Growth hormone secretion during sleep. J Clin Invest 47:2079.
3. Parker DC, Rossman LG 1973 Physiology of human growth hormone release in sleep. In: Scow RO (ed) Endocrinology. Excerpta Medica Foundation, Amsterdam, p 655.
4. Jacoby JH, Sassin JF, Greenstein M, Weitzman ED 1974 Patterns of spontaneous cortisol and growth hormone secretion in rhesus monkeys during the sleep-wake cycle. Neuroendocrinology 14:165.
5. McIntyre HB, Odell WD 1974 Physiological control of growth hormone in the rabbit. Neuroendocrinology 16:8.
6. Chamley WA, Fell LR, Alford FP, Goding JR 1975 Twenty-four hour secretory profiles of ovine prolactin and growth hormone. J Endocrinol 61:165.
7. Tannenbaum GS, Martin JB 1976 Evidence for an endogenous ultradian rhythm governing growth hormone secretion in the rat. Endocrinology 98:562.
8. Tannenbaum GS, Martin JB, Colle E 1976 Ultradian growth hormone rhythm in the rat: effects of feeding, hyperglycemia, and insulin-induced hypoglycemia. Endocrinology 99:720.
9. Miller JD, Tannenbaum GS, Colle E, Guyda HJ 1982 Daytime pulsatile growth hormone secretion during childhood and adolescence. J Clin Endocrinol Metab 55:989.
10. Reichlin S 1960 Growth and the hypothalamus. Endocrinology 67:760.
11. Frohman LA, Bernardis LL 1968 Growth hormone and insulin levels in weanling rats with ventromedial hypothalamic lesions. Endocrinology 82:1125.
12. Martin JB, Renaud LP, Brazeau P 1974 Pulsatile growth hormone secretion: suppression by hypothalamic ventromedial lesions and by long-acting somatostatin. Science 186:538.
13. Frohman LA, Bernardis LL, Kant KJ 1968 Hypothalamic stimulation of growth hormone secretion. Science 162:580.
14. Martin JB 1972 Plasma growth hormone (GH) response to hypothalamic or extrahypothalamic electrical stimulation. Endocrinology 91:107.
15. Rice RW, Critchlow V 1976 Extrahypothalamic control of stress-induced inhibition of growth hormone secretion in the rat. Endocrinology 99:970.
16. Willoughby JO, Martin JB 1978 Pulsatile growth hormone secretion: inhibitory role of medial preoptic area. Brain Res 148:240.

17. Mitchell JA, Hutchins M, Schindler WJ, Critchlow V 1973 Increases in plasma growth hormone concentration and naso-anal length in rats following isolation of the medial basal hypothalamus. Neuroendocrinology 12:161.
18. Willoughby JO, Terry LC, Brazeau P, Martin JB 1977 Pulsatile growth hormone, prolactin, and thyrotropin secretion in rats with hypothalamic deafferentation. Brain Res 127:137.
19. Martin JB, Tannenbaum GS, Willoughby JO, Renaud LP, Brazeau P 1975 Functions of the central nervous system in regulation of pituitary GH secretion. In: Motta M, Crosignani PG, Martini L (eds) Hypothalamic Hormones. Chemistry, Physiology, Pharmacology and Clinical Uses. Academic Press, New York, p 217.
20. Martin JB, Kontor J, Mead P 1973 Plasma GH responses to hypothalamic, hippocampal and amygdaloid electrical stimulation: Effects of variation in stimulus parameters and treatment with α-methyl-p-tyrosine (α-MT). Endocrinology 92:1354.
21. Eikelboom R, Tannenbaum GS 1983 Effects of obesity-inducing ventromedial hypothalamic lesions on pulsatile growth hormone and insulin secretion: evidence for the existence of a growth hormone-releasing factor. Endocrinology 112:212.
22. Terry LC, Epelbaum J, Martin JB 1981 Monosodium glutamate: acute and chronic effects on rhythmic growth hormone and prolactin secretion, and somatostatin in the undisturbed male rat. Brain Res 217:129.
23. Millard WJ, Martin JB Jr, Audet J, Sagar SM, Martin JB 1982 Evidence that reduced growth hormone secretion observed in monosodium glutamate-treated rats is the result of a deficiency in growth hormone releasing factor. Endocrinology 110:540.
24. Alpert LC, Brawer JR, Patel YC, Reichlin S 1976 Somatostatinergic neurons in anterior hypothalamus: Immunohistochemical localization. Endocrinology 98:255.
25. Bloch B, Brazeau P, Ling N, Böhlen P, Esch F, Wehrenberg WB, Benoit R, Bloom F, Guillemin R 1983 Immunohistochemical detection of growth hormone-releasing factor in brain. Nature 301:607.
26. Merchenthaler I, Vigh S, Schally AV, Petrusz P 1984 Immunocytochemical localization of growth hormone-releasing factor in the rat hypothalamus. Endocrinology 114:1082.
27. Brazeau P, Vale W, Burgus R, Ling N, Butcher M, Rivier J, Guillemin R 1973 Hypothalamic peptide that inhibits the secretion of immunoreactive pituitary growth hormone. Science 179:77.
28. Martin JB, Brazeau P, Tannenbaum GS, Willoughby JO, Epelbaum J, Terry LC, Durand D 1978 Neuroendocrine organization of growth hormone regulation. In: Reichlin S, Baldessarini R, Martin JB (eds) The Hypothalamus. Raven Press, New York, p 329.
29. Tannenbaum GS, Epelbaum J, Colle E, Brazeau P, Martin JB 1978 Antiserum to somatostatin reserves starvation-induced inhibition of growth hormone but not insulin secretion. Endocrinology 102:1909.

30. Rorstad OP, Epelbaum J, Brazeau P, Martin JB 1979 Chromatographic and biological properties of immunoreactive somatostatin in hypothalamic and extrahypothalamic brain regions of the rat. Endocrinology 105:1083.
31. Ferland L, Labrie F, Jobin M, Arimura A, Schally AV 1976 Physiological role of somatostatin in the control of growth hormone and thyrotropin secretion. Biochem Biophys Res Commun 68:149.
32. Steiner RA, Stewart JK, Barber J, Koerker D, Goodner CJ, Brown A, Illner P, Gale CC 1978 Somatostatin: a physiological role in the adolescent male baboon. Endocrinology 102:1587.
33. Schusdziarra V, Rouiller D, Arimura A, Unger RH 1978 Antisomatostatin serum increases levels of hormones from the pituitary and gut, but not from the pancreas. Endocrinology 103:1956.
34. Varner MA, Davis SL, Reeves JJ 1980 Temporal serum concentrations of growth hormone, thyrotropin, insulin, and glucagon in sheep immunized against somatostatin. Endocrinology 106:1027.
35. Terry LC, Martin JB 1981 The effects of lateral hypothalamic-medial forebrain stimulation and somatostatin antiserum on pulsatile growth hormone secretion in freely behaving rats: evidence for a dual regulatory mechanism. Endocrinology 109:622.
36. Arimura A, Sato H, Dupont A, Nishi N, Schally AV 1975 Somatostatin: abundance of immunoreactive hormone in rat stomach and pancreas. Science 189:1007.
37. Patel YC, Reichlin S 1978 Somatostatin in hypothalamus, extrahypothalamic brain, and peripheral tissues of the rat. Endocrinology 102:523.
38. Conlon JM, Zyznar E, Vale W, Unger RH 1978 Multiple forms of somatostatin-like immunoreactivity in canine pancreas. FEBS Lett 94:327.
39. Pradayrol L, Chayvialle JA, Carlquist M, Mutt V 1978 Isolation of a porcine intestinal peptide with C-terminal somatostatin. Biochem Biophys Res Commun 85:701.
40. Millar RP 1978 Somatostatin immunoreactive peptides of higher molecular weight in ovine hypothalamic extracts. Endocrinology 77:429.
41. Spiess J, Rivier J, Rodkey J, Bennett C, Vale W 1979 Isolation and characterization of somatostatin from pigeon pancreas. Proc Natl Acad Sci (USA) 76:2974.
42. Pradayrol L, Jörnvall H, Mutt V, Ribert A 1980 N-terminally extended somatostatin: the primary structure of somatostatin-28. FEBS Lett 109:55.
43. Esch F, Böhlen P, Ling N, Benoit R, Brazeau P, Guillemin R 1980 Primary structure of ovine hypothalamic somatostatin-28 and somatostatin-25. Proc Natl Acad Sci (USA) 77:6827.

44. Schally AV, Huang W-Y, Chang RCC, Arimura A, Redding TW, Millar RP, Hunkapiller MW, Hood LE 1980 Isolation and structure of prosomatostatin: a putative somatostatin precursor from pig hypothalamus. Proc Natl Acad Sci (USA) 77:4489.
45. Brazeau P, Ling N, Esch F, Böhlen P, Benoit R, Guillemin R 1981 High biological activity of the synthetic replicates of somatostatin-28 and somatostatin-25. Regul Peptides 1:255.
46. Meyers CA, Murphy WA, Redding TW, Coy DH, Schally AV 1980 Synthesis and biological actions of prosomatostatin. Proc Natl Acad Sci (USA) 77:6171.
47. Tannenbaum GS, Ling N, Brazeau P 1982 Somatostatin-28 is longer acting and more selective than somatostatin-14 on pituitary and pancreatic hormone release. Endocrinology 111:101.
48. Kewley CF, Millar RP, Berman MC, Schally AV 1981 Depolarization- and ionophore-induced release of octacosa somatostatin from stalk median eminence synaptosomes. Science 213:913.
49. Millar RP, Sheward WJ, Wegener I, Fink G 1983 Somatostatin-28 is an hormonally active peptide secreted into hypophysial portal blood. Brain Res 260:334.
50. Srikant CB, Patel YC 1981 Receptor binding of somatostatin-28 is tissue specific. Nature 294:259.
51. Jacovidou N, Patel YC Effects of in vivo immunoneutralization with specific somatostatin-28 antiserum on growth hormone secretory dynamics in the rat. Program of the Satellite Symposium on Somatostatin, Montreal, June 1984, A27 (Abstract).
52. Tannenbaum GS, Rorstad O, Brazeau P 1979 Effects of prolonged food deprivation on the ultradian growth hormone rhythm and immunoreactive somatostatin tissue levels in the rat. Endocrinology 104:1733.
53. Tannenbaum GS 1981 Growth hormone secretory dynamics in streptozotocin diabetes: evidence of a role for endogenous circulating somatostatin. Endocrinology 108:76.
54. Tannenbaum GS, Colle E, Gurd W, Wanamaker L 1981 Dynamic time-course studies of the spontaneously diabetic BB Wistar rat. I. Longitudinal profiles of plasma growth hormone, insulin, and glucose. Endocrinology 109:1872.
55. Painson JC, Ling N, Tannenbaum GS Effects of intracellular glucopenia on pulsatile growth hormone (GH) secretion: mediation by GH-releasing factor (GRF) and somatostatin (SRIF). Program of the 7th International Congress of Endocrinology, Quebec City, July 1984, A1496 (Abstract).
56. Shapiro B, Berelowitz M, Pimstone BL, Kronheim S, Sheppard M 1979 Tissue and serum somatostatin-like immunoreactivity in fed, 15-h fasted, and 72-h-fasted rats. Diabetes 28:182.
57. Petersson B, Elde R, Efendić S, Hökfelt T, Johansson O, Luft R, Cerasi E, Hellerström C 1977 Somatostatin in the pancreas, stomach and hypothalamus of the diabetic Chinese hamster. Diabetologia 13:463.

58. Patel YC, Cameron DP, Bankier A, Malaisse-Lagae F, Ravazzola M, Studer P, Orci L 1978 Changes in somatostatin concentration in pancreas and other tissues of streptozotocin diabetic rats. Endocrinology 103:917.
59. Berelowitz M, Shapiro B, Kronheim S 1979 Growth hormone release inhibitory hormone-like immunoreactivity in pancreas and gut in streptozotocin diabetes in the rat and response to insulin administration. Clin Endocrinol (Oxf) 10:195.
60. Patel YC, Wheatley T, Malaisse-Lagae F, Orci L 1980 Elevated portal and peripheral blood concentration of immunoreactive somatostatin in spontaneously diabetic (BBL) Wistar rats. Diabetes 29:757.
61. Tannenbaum GS, Colle E, Wanamaker L, Gurd W, Goldman H, Seemayer T 1981 Dynamic time-course studies of the spontaneously diabetic BB Wistar rat. II. Insulin-, glucagon-, and somatostatin-reactive cells in the pancreas. Endocrinology 109:1880.
62. Schusdziarra V, Zyznar E, Rouiller D, Boden G, Brown JC, Arimura A, Unger RH 1980 Splanchnic somatostatin: a hormonal regulator of nutrient homeostasis. Science 207:530.
63. Terry LC, Willoughby JO, Brazeau P, Martin JB, Patel Y 1976 Antiserum to somatostatin prevents stress-induced inhibition of growth hormone secretion in the rat. Science 192:565.
64. Arimura A, Smith WD, Schally AV 1976 Blockade of the stress-induced decrease in blood GH by anti-somatostatin serum in rats. Endocrinology 98:540.
65. Guillemin R, Brazeau P, Böhlen P, Esch F, Ling N, Wehrenberg WB 1982 Growth hormone-releasing factor from a human pancreatic tumor that caused acromegaly. Science 218:585.
66. Rivier J, Spiess J, Thorner M, Vale W 1982 Characterization of a growth hormone-releasing factor from a human pancreatic islet tumour. Nature 300:276.
67. Wehrenberg WB, Ling N, Brazeau P, Esch F, Böhlen P, Baird A, Ying S, Guillemin R 1982 Somatocrinin, growth hormone releasing factor, stimulates secretion of growth hormone in anesthetized rats. Biochem Biophys Res Commun 109:382.
68. Thorner MO, Rivier J, Spiess J, Borges JLC, Vance ML, Bloom SR, Rogol AD, Cronin MJ, Kaiser DL, Evans WS, Webster JD, MacLeod RM, Vale W 1983 Human pancreatic growth hormone-releasing factor selectively stimulates growth hormone secretion in man. Lancet 1:24.
69. Böhlen P, Brazeau P, Bloch B, Ling N, Gaillard R, Guillemin R 1983 Human hypothalamic growth hormone releasing factor (GRF): evidence for two forms identical to tumor derived GRF-44-NH_2 and GRF-40. Biochem Biophys Res Commun 114:930.
70. Ling N, Esch F, Böhlen P, Brazeau P, Wehrenberg WB, Guillemin R 1984 Isolation, primary structure, and synthesis of human hypothalamic somatocrinin: Growth hormone-releasing factor. Proc Natl Acad Sci (USA) 81:4302.

71. Spiess J, Rivier J, Vale W 1983 Characterization of rat hypothalamic growth hormone-releasing factor. Nature 303:532.
72. Tannenbaum GS, Eikelboom R, Ling N 1983 Human pancreas GH-releasing factor analog restores high-amplitude GH pulses in CNS lesion-induced GH deficiency. Endocrinology 113:1173.
73. Brazeau P, Ling N, Böhlen P, Esch F, Ying S-Y, Guillemin R 1982 Growth hormone releasing fctor, somatocrinin, releases pituitary growth hormone in vitro. Proc Natl Acad Sci (USA) 79:7909.
74. Vale W, Vaughan J, Yamamoto G, Spiess J, Rivier J 1983 Effects of synthetic human pancreatic (tumor) GH releasing factor and somatostatin, triiodothyronine and dexamethasone on GH secretion in vitro. Endocrinology 112:1553.
75. Tannenbaum GS, Ling N 1984 The interrelationship of growth hormone (GH)-releasing factor and somatostatin in generation of the ultradian rhythm of GH secretion. Endocrinology 115:1952.
76. Leung FC, Taylor JE 1983 In vivo and in vitro stimulation of growth hormone release in chickens by synthetic human pancreatic growth hormone releasing factor (hpGRFs). Endocrinology 113:1913.
77. Chihara K, Minamitani N, Kaji H, Kodama H, Kita T, Fujita T 1983 Human pancreatic growth hormone-releasing factor stimulates release of growth hormone in conscious unrestrained male rabbits. Endocrinology 113:2081.
78. Almeida OFX, Schulte HM, Rittmaster RS, Chrousos GP, Loriaux DL, Merriam GR 1984 Potency and specificity of a growth hormone-releasing factor in a primate and in vitro. J Clin Endocrinol Metab 58:309.
79. Ohmura E, Jansen A, Chernick V, Winter J, Friesen HG, Rivier J, Vale W 1984 Human pancreatic growth hormone releasing factor (hpGRF-1-40) stimulates GH release in the ovine fetus. Endocrinology 114:299.
80. Rosenthal SM, Schriock EA, Kaplan SL, Guillemin R, Grumbach MM 1983 Synthetic human pancreas growth hormone-releasing factor ($hpGRF_{1-44}$-NH_2) stimulates growth hormone secretion in normal men. J Clin Endocrinol Metab 57:677.
81. Wehrenberg WB, Ling N, Böhlen P, Esch F, Brazeau P, Guillemin R 1982 Physiological roles of somatocrinin and somatostatin in the regulation of growth hormone secretion. Biochem Biophys Res Commun 109:562.
82. Yamashita H, Koizumi K, Brooks CM 1979 Rhythmic patterns of discharge in hypothalamic neurosecretory neurons of cats and dogs. Proc Natl Acad Sci (USA) 76:6684.
83. Krulich L, McCann SM 1966 Influences of growth hormone (GH) on content of GH in the pituitaries of normal rats. Proc Soc Exp Biol Med 121:1114.
84. Muller E, Pecile A 1966 Influence of exogenous growth hormone on endogenous growth hormone release. Proc Soc Exp Biol Med 122:1289.

85. MacLeod RM, DeWitt GW, Smith MC 1968 Suppression of pituitary gland hormone content by pituitary tumor hormones. Endocrinology 82:889.
86. Sakuma M, Knobil E 1970 Inhibition of endogenous growth hormone secretion by exogenous growth hormone infusion in the rhesus monkey. Endocrinology 86:890.
87. Abrams RL, Grumbach MM, Kaplan SL 1971 The effect of administration of human growth hormone on the plasma growth hormone, cortisol, glucose, and free fatty acid response to insulin: evidence for growth hormone autoregulation in man. J Clin Invest 50:940.
88. Hagen TC, Lawrence AM, Kirsteins L 1972 Autoregulation of growth hormone secretion in normal subjects. Metabolism 21:603.
89. Tannenbaum GS 1980 Evidence for autoregulation of growth hormone secretion via the central nervous system. Endocrinology 107:2117.
90. Willoughby JO, Menadue M, Zeegers P, Wise PH, Oliver JR 1980 Effects of human growth hormone on the secretion of rat growth hormone. J Endocrinol 86:115.
91. Abe H, Molitch ME, Van Wyk JJ, Underwood LE 1983 Human growth hormone and somatomedin C suppress the spontaneous release of growth hormone in unanesthetized rats. Endocrinology 113:1319.
92. Phillips LS, Vassilopoulou-Sellin R 1980 Somatomedins. New Eng J Med 302:371; ibid: 438.
93. Daughaday WH, Hall K, Raben MS, Salmon WD Jr, Van den Brande JL, Van Wyk JJ 1972 Somatomedin: A proposed designation for the "sulfation factor." Nature 235:107.
94. Zapf J, Rinderknecht E, Humbel RE, Froesch EF 1978 Nonsuppressible insulin-like activity (NSILA) from human serum: recent accomplishments and their physiologic implications. Metabolism 27:1803.
95. Tannenbaum GS, Guyda HJ, Posner BI 1983 Insulin-like growth factors: a role in growth hormone negative feedback and body weight regulation via brain. Science 220:77.
96. Tsushima T, Friesen HG, Chang TW, Raben MS 1974 Studies by radioreceptor assay (RRA) of a factor with growth hormone-like activity in incubation media of spargana of Spirometra mansonoides. Endocrinology 94:A69.
97. Garland JT, Daughaday WH 1972 Feedback inhibition of pituitary growth hormone in rats infected with Spirometra mansonoides. Proc Soc Exp Biol Med 139:497.
98. Laron Z, Pertzelan A, Karp M, Kowadlo-Silbergold A, Daughaday WH 1971 Administration of growth hormone to patients with familial dwarfism with high plasma immunoreactive growth hormone: measurement of sulfation factor, metabolic and linear growth responses. J Clin Endocrinol Metab 33:332.
99. Hintz RL, Suskind R, Amatayakul K, Thanangkul O, Olson R 1978 Plasma somatomedin and growth hormone values in children with protein-calorie malnutrition. J Pediatr 92:153.

100. Richman RA, Weiss JP, Hochberg Z, Florini JR 1981 Regulation of growth hormone release: evidence against negative feedback in rat pituitary cells. Endocrinology 108:2287.
101. Goodyer CG, De Stephano L, Guyda HJ, Posner BI 1984 Effects of insulin-like growth factors on adult male rat pituitary function in tissue culture. Endocrinology 115:1568.
102. Baker BL, Yen Y-Y 1976 The influence of hypophysectomy on the stores of somatostatin in the hypothalamus and pituitary stem. Proc Soc Exp Biol Med 151:599.
103. Hoffman DL, Baker BL 1977 Effect of treatment with growth hormone on somatostatin in the median eminence of hypophysectomized rats. Proc Soc Exp Biol Med 156:265.
104. Wakabayashi I, Demura R, Kanda M, Demura H, Shizume K 1976 Effect of hypophysectomy on hypothalamic somatostatin content in rats. Endocrinol Japon 23:439.
105. Fernandez-Durango R, Arimura A, Fishback J, Schally AV 1978 Hypothalamic somatostatin and LH-RH after hypophysectomy, in hyper- or hypothyroidism, and during anesthesia in rats. Proc Soc Exp Biol Med 157:235.
106. Patel YC 1979 Growth hormone stimulates hypothalamic somatostatin. Life Sci 24:1589.
107. Sheppard MC, Kronheim S, Pimstone BL 1978 Stimulation by growth hormone of somatostatin release from the rat hypothalamus in vitro. Clin Endocrinol 9:583.
108. Berelowitz M, Firestone SL, Frohman LA 1981 Effects of growth hormone excess and deficiency on hypothalamic somatostatin content and release and on tissue somatostatin distribution. Endocrinology 109:714.
109. Chihara K, Minamitani N, Kaji H, Arimura A, Fujita T 1981 Intraventricularly injected growth hormone stimulates somatostatin release into rat hypophysial portal blood. Endocrinology 109:2279.
110. Berelowitz M, Szabo M, Frohman LA, Firestone S, Chu L, Hintz RL 1981 Somatomedin-C mediates growth hormone negative feedback by effects on both the hypothalamus and the pituitary. Science 212:1279.
111. Brazeau P, Guillemin R, Ling N, Van Wyk J, Humbel R 1982 Inhibition par le somatomédines de la sécretion de l'hormone de croissance stimulée par le facteur hypothalamique somatocrinine (GRF) ou le peptide de synthèse hpGRF. C R Seances Acad Sci (Paris) 295:651.
112. Goodyer CG, De Stephano L, Lai WH, Guyda HJ, Posner BI 1984 Characterization of insulin-like growth factor receptors in rat anterior pituitary, hypothalamus, and brain. Endocrinology 114:1187.
113. Rosenfeld RG, Ceda G, Wilson DM, Dollar LA, Hoffman AR 1984 Characterization of high affinity receptors for insulin-like growth factors I and II on rat anterior pituitary cells. Endocrinology 114:1571.

114. Sara VR, Hall K, Von Holtz H, Humbel R, Sjogren B, Wetterberg L 1982 Evidence for the presence of specific receptors for insulin-like growth factors I(IGF-I) and 2(IGF-2) and insulin throughout the adult human brain. Neurosci Lett 34:39.
115. Haselbacher G, Humbel R 1982 Evidence for two species of insulin-like growth factor II (IGF II and "big" IGF II) in human spinal fluid. Endocrinology 110:1822.
116. Lumpkin MD, Negro-Vilar A, McCann SM 1981 Paradoxical elevation of growth hormone by intraventricular somatostatin: possible ultrashort-loop feedback. Science 211:1072.
117. Tannenbaum GS 1984 Growth hormone-releasing factor: direct effects on growth hormone, glucose, and behavior via the brain. Science 226:464.
118. Renaud LP 1978 Neurophysiological organization of the endocrine hypothalamus. In: Reichlin S, Baldessarini RJ, Martin JB (eds) The Hypothalamus. Raven Press, New York, p 329.
119. Motta M, Franschini F, Martini L 1969 "Short" feedback mechanisms in the control of anterior pituitary function. In: Ganong WF, Martini L (eds) Frontiers in Neuroendocrinology. Oxford University Press, New York, p 211.

15

SOMATOSTATIN ALTERATIONS AND BRAIN DISEASES

J. EPELBAUM, Y. AGID*, A. ENJALBERT, M. HAMON**, F. JAVOY-AGID*, C. KORDON, Y. LAMOUR AND E. MOYSE

Unités 159, **114, 161 INSERM and
*Laboratoire de Médecine Expérimentale de la Pitié
Paris, France

INTRODUCTION

Soon after its discovery as a hypothalamic growth hormone inhibiting factor, somatostatin-14 (S-14, SRIF) was localized by radioimmunoassay (1, 2) and immunocytochemistry (3-5) in extra-hypothalamic structures. Present in neurons, S-14 is synthesized as part of a prohormone and transported to nerve terminals from which it is released in response to depolarizing stimuli. The peptide is then degraded *in situ* by enzymes after binding to its specific receptors (6, 7). In the pituitary, S-14 seems to act by inhibiting adenylate cyclase (8-10); but in the brain, its mechanism of action is still poorly understood.

These findings suggest that S-14 serves as a neurotransmitter or neuromodulator in the central nervous system, although its functions in the various brain areas where it is present have not been determined as yet. For instance, electrophysiological effects of the peptide are still a matter of controversy, since it was reported to either stimulate (11) or inhibit (12) spontaneous electrical activity in hippocampal slices *in vitro*. Also, S-14 has been reported to inhibit or stimulate the release of various neurotransmitters and neurohormones (see 13, for review). Many behavioural changes have been observed after intracerebral administration of S-14 or analogs (see 14, for review), but no definite pharmacological characterization of such effects has yet been performed.

Somatostatin Modifications in Brain Diseases

Cerebrospinal fluid measurement

Almost immediately after a specific RIA for S-14 like immunoreactivity (SLI) became available, Patel et al. (15) were able to measure SLI levels in the cerebrospinal fluid (CSF). Since then, a number of studies (Table I) reported changes in CSF SLI levels in various neurological and neuropsychiatric diseases. As shown in Table I, changes in SLI levels are variable and not clearly characteristic of any single disease (15-21). On the other hand, other transmitters measured under the same conditions (18), do not exhibit changes parallel to those of SLI. Furthermore, as SLI is also concentrated in spinal cord neurons, it is very difficult to determine whether modifications observed in CSF levels of SLI are of spinal or of cerebral origin.

In summary, as already stated (19) "the potential interactions are too complex to elucidate further with random CSF levels from individual patients".

Table I. Alterations in CSF and Post-mortem Tissue Levels of SLI in Various Pathological Conditions

	SOMATOSTATIN IN HUMAN CSF		SOMATOSTATIN IN HUMAN TISSUE	
ALZHEIMER	$\downarrow$	BEAL et al, 1984 WOOD et al, 1982	$\downarrow$ Cx	DAVIES et al, 1980 ROSSOR et al, 1980 NEMEROFF et al, 1983 FERRIER et al, 1983
MIXED DEMENTIA	$\downarrow$			
SCHIZOPHRENIA	0		$\downarrow$ limbic lobe or no change	(FERRIER et al, 1983 NEMEROFF et al, 1983)
MULTIPLE SCLEROSIS (on relapse)	$\downarrow$	(SORENSEN et al, 1980)		
PARKINSON	$\downarrow$	(DUPONT et al, 1982)	$\downarrow$ Cx	(EPELBAUM et al, 1983)
HUNTINGTON	$\downarrow$ 0	(CRAMER et al, 1981 BEAL et al, 1984)	$\uparrow$ neostriatum	(ARONIN et al, 1983 NEMEROFF et al, 1983)
DEPRESSION	$\downarrow$	(RUBINOW et al, 1983)		
CORTICAL AND SPINAL CHORD DISEASES	$\uparrow$	(PATEL et al, 1977)		

$\downarrow$ decrease in SLI levels; $\uparrow$ increase in SLI levels;
0 no change in SLI levels.

Tissue concentrations

Transmitter concentrations measured in carefully dissected post-mortem samples provide a better indicator of discrete regional changes. Such studies have revealed a dopaminergic deficiency in Parkinson's disease, and more recently, a cholinergic depletion in Alzheimer's disease. Abnormal concentrations of SLI have been observed in Huntington's chorea (22, 23), schizophrenia (23, 24), Alzheimer'd disease (23, 25-27) and Parkinson's disease in relation to dementia.

Huntington's chorea (HC). HC is genetically inherited as an autosomal dominant trait (the gene has recently been localized (28)) which results in major motor deficits and mental disturbances. Levels of SLI in neostriatum are elevated as compared to controls. However, other peptides, like TRH and neurotensin, and neurotransmitters are also modified in a parallel way (23). On the contrary, in the nucleus accumbens, the rise in SLI levels is not correlated with a rise in TRH and neurotensin concentrations. Histological studies have demonstrated a concomitant loss of volume in the caudate nucleus of HC patients; increased neuropeptide concentrations in this region could thus mainly be due to a selective preservation of the neuronal elements containing these substances. However, there is a marked increase in the density of SLI containing fibers (29) in the neostriatum while SLI containing cell bodies diminish in proportion with tissue volume loss. Such findings could imply a disease-specific process leading to an elevation in the metabolism of SLI in caudate regions. The pathophysiological significance of such modifications remains to be demonstrated.

Schizophrenia. This major psychiatric disorder may be associated with neuropathological alterations of the limbic forebrain; however no definite modification of SLI content was evident from two different studies (23,24).

Senile dementias. Alzheimer's disease (AD) is a dementing organic brain disorder occurring in both the presenile and senile age ranges. It is characterized histopathologically by senile plaque formation and neurofibrillary degeneration (tangles) that are more numerous in the diseased state than in age-matched controls. An intense interest arose from the discovery that a cholinergic defect was observed in the cortex of patients dying with AD while cholinomimetic drugs were able to enhance learning of new information in normal subjects (30). Cholinergic neuronal pathways have recently been characterized by the use of cholineacetyltransferase (CAT) immunocytochemistry (31-33). It was shown that most of the cholinergic innervation in the cortex comes from the basal forebrain (i.e. the nucleus of the diagonal band of Broca and the substantial innominata in rat and the nucleus basalis of Meynert in man). Therefore, AD which is often referred to as a "cortical dementia" is in fact characterized biochemically by subcortical changes in cholinergic parameters. The only intrinsic cortical neurotransmitter-like substance which has consistently been shown to decrease is SLI (34). It has even been possible to inversely correlate SLI concentrations with the plaque counts and the neurofibrillary tangles in temporal cortex (35), while cholecystokinin, vasoactive intestinal peptide, enkephalins, TRH, neurotensin, vasopressin and oxytocin levels were not affected in AD. In one study, it was also possible to correlate SLI levels and CAT activity in selected cases of AD (36).

Alzheimer symptoms are frequently associated with other neurological diseases, in particular Parkinson's disease (PD). We had access to a semi-logically well defined population of brains from PD patients, which were either non-demented, slightly demented, or severely demented. Since neuropathological signs of AD are present (37, 38) and CAT levels are decreased in patients with PD (39, 40), in relation to their state of dementia, we investigated whether SLI levels were modified in these post-mortem brain samples and whether this was related to dementia.

The control population consisted of neurologically and psychiatrically normal subjects matched with PD patients for age, agonal status and post-mortem delay in tissue handling. Dementia was diagnosed on the basis of retrospective analysis of case histories. The patients were rated on a scale of 0 to 2 (0, no clinical evidence of intellectual deterioration; 1, slightly impaired memory, occasional episode of confusion; 2, severe intellectual deterioration including memory, concept formation and orientation in time and space). The clinical diagnosis was confirmed by histological examination for neurofibrillary tangles, senile plaques and granulovascular degeneration. Histological alterations were found in the brains of all clinically demented subjects. The tissue was dissected from serial sections without thawing and pulverized to homogeneous powder on dry ice until assay time. Levels of SLI were measured according to Rorstad et al. (41). The results are summarized in Fig. 1 for frontal cortex. Mean SLI levels were significantly lower in both the slightly and severely demented PD groups. Significantly lower SLI concentrations were also found in the hippocampus (-59%) of severely demented as compared to non-demented PD patients, and in the entorhinal cortex (-54%) of severely demented PD subjects as compared to controls. Non-significant decreases were observed in the temporal (-33%) and cingulate cortex (-38%) of severely demented patients. SLI levels were not modified in occipital cortex, caudate nucleus and hypothalamus. This study shows that SLI levels decrease in certain cortical structures and in the hippocampus of PD subjects who are demented. This decrease was parallel to that of CAT in the same subjects (39, 40) although no significant correlations could be established between these two parameters in individual brains, except for the cingulate cortex.

As in AD, SLI and CAT content of the cortex and hippocampus diminished in demented PD subjects. It cannot be determined from such studies whether reduced SLI levels result from decreased synthesis or from degenerative processes affecting SLI containing neurons in the cortex and hippocampus. Such a process, however, seems associated, both in AD and demented PD, with an impairment of the cortical cholinergic innervation originating in the basal forebrain. In contrast, in Pick's disease, where cortical cholinergic innervation is not modified, SLI levels are not changed (42).

Possible Relationships Between Cholinergic and Somatostatinergic Innervations in the Cortex

Cellular localization

Using immunocytochemical techniques (43), SLI containing perikarya have been localized in most areas of the rat cortex. SLI-positive cell bodies are mainly located in layers II, III and VI. This localization is suggestive of interneurons involved in local regulation. On the other hand, SLI-positive neurons have been visualized in all layers of human cortex, with some fibers also present in the subcortical white matter (44). Thus, somatostatin could interact in various brain areas, not only through cortico-cortical connections but also by influencing the neuronal circuits passing through the subcortical white matter.

Somatostastin innervation of the cortex thus appears intrinsic, while cholinergic elements mainly arise from the basal forebrain (30-32). It has been demonstrated that SLI was not colocalized in

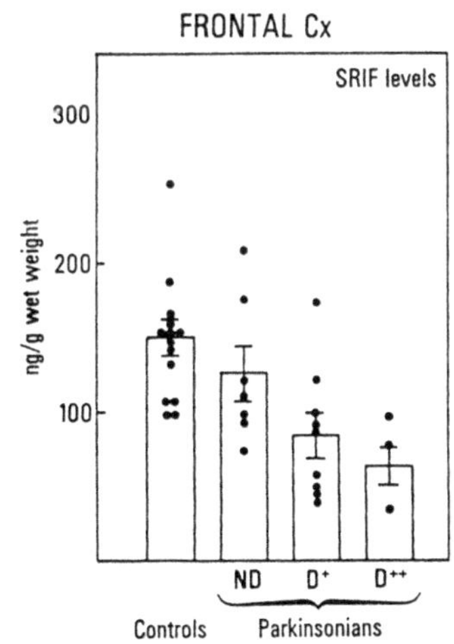

Fig. 1. Concentrations of SLI (shown as SRIF) in frontal cortex of Parkinsonian subjects with(D^+, D^{++}) and without (ND) dementia.

afferent cortical projections, since lesions of the ventral pallidum caused a 64% reduction in cortical CAT levels without modifying SLI concentrations (45). However, the problem is further complicated by the occurrence of a distinct intrinsic CAT-positive network in the cerebral cortex (46, 47) which might account for a non-negligible part of the cholinergic innervation of the cortex. Indeed, coexistence of acetylcholinesterase (ACE) and SLI has been reported in a small percentage (20%) of ACE stained brain neurons in culture (48).

Regional distribution

We measured SLI and CAT concentrations in samples dissected from serial sections of fresh rat brain, according to a previously described method (49). A positive correlation (r = 0.72) was found between the two sets of data (Fig. 2). Using the same approach in the human, a similar pattern of distribution was observed (Fig. 3). These findings lend further support to an anatomical relationship, both in rodents and humans, between SLI and acetylcholine neurons in the cortex, along the rostrocaudal axis.

Laminar distribution

The diffuse laminar distribution of CAT positive fibers, observed by some authors, does not agree with observations made using ACE histochemistry or even CAT immunocytochemistry; the laminar distribution of cholinergic markers in the cerebral cortex is still far from being clearly understood (see 50 for review). It is thus difficult, at the present time, to compare the laminar distribution of cholinergic markers with SLI levels in the whole cortex. However, in rat primary somatosensory cortex, a region which corresponds to the immunocytochemical study of SLI-positive neurons by Morrison et al. (43), the properties of two populations of acetylcholine-sensitive neurons have been described (51, 52). Their laminar distribution is not coincident with SLI containing cell bodies since cholinergic-sensitive neurons are located in layers V to VIA and VIB to underlying white matter, while SLI containing cell bodies are mainly observed in layers II, III and VI. Such a distribution would be compatible with a post- synaptic articulation between SLI and acetylcholine containing neurons only in layer VI of the cortex.

Possible synaptic articulations

A post-synaptic articulation would be consistent with the finding that acetylcholine stimulates SLI release from cultured brain cells in vitro (53). Conversely, S-14 has been reported to stimulate acetylcholine release from cortical synaptosomes (54) and to increase turnover rate of the transmitter in various brain regions, including the cortex (55, 56). SLI fibers could thus regulate cholinergic neurons by direct interactions; S-14 binding sites could be directly located on acetylcholine neurons. In that

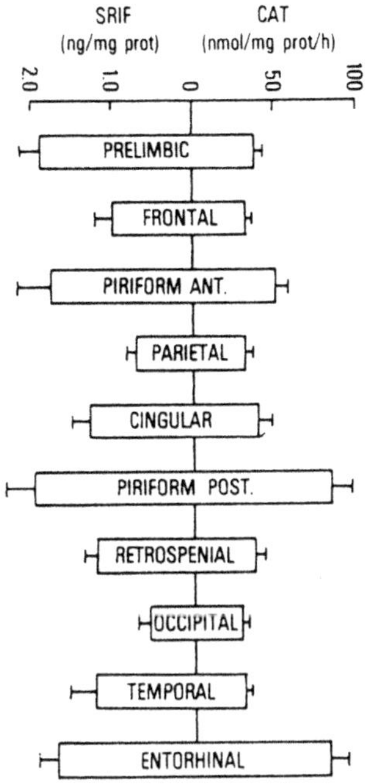

Fig. 2. Intracortical distribution of SLI (shown as SRIF) and CAT activity in rat. Data are expressed as mean ± SE of 6 different animals per group.

case, S-14 binding sites and presynaptic cholinergic markers (CAT) would be similarly localized. In addition, the number of S-14 binding sites should decrease in relation to cholinergic markers in PD demented patients. Using CGP 23996 (des-Ala^1, Gly^2, des amino-Lys^3, Tyr^{11}-dicarba^{3,14} somatostatin), a good ligand for labeling S-14 binding sites in rat brain (57), we tested these propositions.

There was no correlation between [^{125}I]CGP binding and CAT activity in rostrocaudal samples from rat brain (data not shown). As shown in Fig. 4, we characterized the kinetics of [^{125}I]CGP binding to human frontal cortex. According to Scatchard analysis, there is a single class of high affinity binding sites (Kd = 1.5 nM at 37 C and a maximal binding capacity of 215 fmol/mg protein). These values are in the same order of magnitude as those originally reported by Czernik et al. (55) in rat brain, using the same ligand. Samples from the same brains that were already used in previous studies concerning cholinergic parameters (39, 40) and SLI levels (58) in frontal cortex from demented PD subjects were pooled for saturation studies (Table II). There was no modification in either the affinity or maximal binding capacity of[^{125}I]CGP binding in any group tested. However, the variation in maximal binding capacity was very

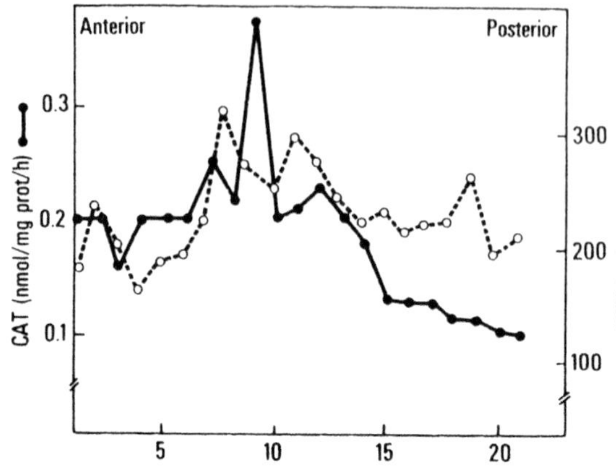

Fig. 3. Intracortical distribution of SLI (shown as SRIF) and CAT activity in man. The measurements were performed on 4 different samples dissected from the same brain. SE omitted for clarity.

important in these experiments. In a preliminary study (59), using [^{125}I-Tyr]-S-14, a tendency to a decrease in S-14 binding sites was noted in demented PD patients. A similar experiment is needed, using [^{125}I]CGP, to really compare the levels of endogenous SLI and S-14 binding sites in various populations of PD patients in relation to dementia.

CONCLUSIONS

Levels of SLI in CSF vary considerably in numerous diseases but there does not seem to be a specific relation between these modifications and a given disease. On the contrary, tissue levels of SLI are specifically increased in neostriatum in Huntington's chorea while they are decreased in cortex of Alzheimer's and Parkinson's

Table II. [^{125}I]CGP 23996 Binding in Frontal Cortex of Parkinsonian Subjects

	Controls	Parkinsonian subjects		
		ND	D+	D++
Kd (nM)	3.4±1.5	2.3±1.0	4.1±2.5	3.0±1.4
Bmax (fmol/mg protein)	310±100	409±114	546±317	331±107

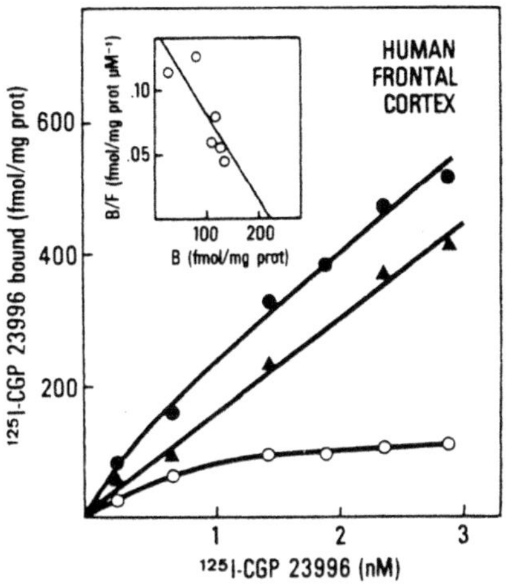

Fig. 4. Binding isotherms of [^{125}I]CGP 23996 to human frontal cortex. ▲ non specific binding; ● total binding; o specific binding; inset: Scatchard representation of the specific binding.

disease in relation to dementia. It is not clear whether these modifications reflect metabolic changes and/or degenerative processes. While a number of biochemical parameters are similarly modified in Huntington's disease, SLI and acetylcholine are mainly affected in Alzheimer's and Parkinson's disease in relation to dementia. This is strongly suggestive of a relationship between the cholinergic and the somatostatinergic modifications observed in demented patients. However, this does not preclude that either degenerative process is really the cause of the other, or whether both might have a common external origin. A number of possible interactions have been postulated (Fig. 5):

1. Ascending cholinergic fibers could innervate somatostatin interneurons.

2. Somatostatin interneurons could make presynaptic contact on cholinergic terminals.

3. Ascending cholinergic fibers could innervate cortical interneurons which have contact with somatostatinergic fibers.

4. Both cholinergic and somatostatinergic fibers synapse on the same neuron.

Since the laminar distribution of CAT and SLI seems different, the first hypothesis is not the most likely. The fact that there is no correlation between CAT and S-14 receptors is not in favor of the second hypothesis. Thus a direct contact between acetylcholine and SLI neurons does not seem to occur and a polysynaptic relationship

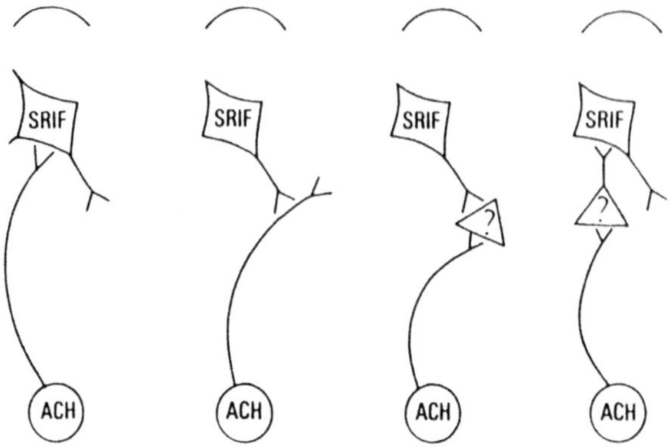

Fig. 5. Possible relationships between SLI positive neurons (shown as SRIF) and acetylcholine innervations in the cortex (see text for explanation).

between the two neurons is more probable. Additional studies are needed to begin to assess the pathophysiological significance of SLI modifications in neurological degenerative diseases.

REFERENCES

1. Brownstein M, Arimura A, Sato H, Kizer JS 1975 The regional distribution of somatostatin in rat brain. Endocrinology 96:1456.
2. Kobayashi RM, Vale M 1977 Regional distribution of neurotensin and somatostatin in rat brain. Brain Res 126:584.
3. Elde R, Hökfelt T 1979 Localization of hypophysiotropic peptides and other biologically active peptides within the brain. Ann Rev Physiol 41:587.
4. Bennett-Clark C, Romagnano MA, Joseph SA 1980 Distribution of somatostatin in the rat brain: telencephalon and diencephalon. Brain Res 188:473.
5. Finley JCW, Maderdrut JL, Rogers LJ, Petrusz P 1981 The immunocytochemical localization of somatostatin-containing neurons in the rat central nervous system. Neuroscience 6:2173.
6. Srikant CB, Patel YC 1981 Somatostatin receptors: identification and characterization in rat brain membranes. Proc Natl Acad Sci 78:3930.
7. Epelbaum J, Tapia Arancibia L, Kordon C, Enjalbert A 1982 Characterization, regional distribution and subcellular distribution of [^{125}I]-Tyr-somatostatin binding sites in rat brain. J Neurochem 38:1515.

8. Rouleau D, Barden N 1981 Inhibition of anterior pituitary prostaglandin stimulated adenylate cyclase activity by somatostatin. Can J Biochem 59:307.
9. Cronin MJ, Rogol AD, Myers GA, Hewlett EL 1983 Pertussis toxin blocks the somatostatin induced inhibition of growth hormone release and adenosine 3'-5' monophosphate accumulation. Endocrinology 113:209.
10. Koch BD, Schonbrunn A 1984 The somatostatin receptor is directly coupled to adenylate cyclase in GH_4C_1 pituitary cell membranes. Endocrinology 114:1784.
11. Dodd J, Kelly JS 1978 Is somatostatin an excitatory transmitter in the hippocampus? Nature 273:674.
12. Pittman QJ, Siggins GR 1981 Somatostatin hyperpolarizes hippocampal pyramidal cells in vitro. Brain Res 221:402.
13. Epelbaum J, Arancibia S, Drouva SV, Kordon C 1982 Mode et régulation de la sécrétion de la somatostatine cérébrale. In: Tixier Vidal A, Richard P (eds) Régulations Cellulaires Multihormonales en Neuroendocrinologie. INSERM, Paris, 110:103.
14. Reichlin S 1983 Somatostatin. N Engl J Med 309:1495 (Part I) and (Part 2) 1556.
15. Patel YC, Rao K, Reichlin S 1977 Somatostatin in human cerebrospinal fluid. N Engl J Med 296:529.
16. Cramer H, Kohler J, Oepen G, Schonberg G, Schroter E 1981 Huntington's chorea-measurements of somatostatin, substance P, and cyclic nucleotides in the cerebrospinal fluid. J Neurol 225:183.
17. Dupont E, Christensen SE, Hansen AP, Olivarias BF, Orskov H 1982 Low cerebrospinal fluid somatostatin in Parkinson's disease: an irreversible abnormality. Neurology 32:312.
18. Wood PL, Etienne P, Lal S, Gauthier S, Cajal S, Nair NPV 1982 Reduced lumbar CSF somatostatin levels in Alzheimer's disease. Life Sci 31:2073.
19. Rubinow DR, Gold PW, Post RM, Ballenger JC, Cowdry R, Bollinger J, Reichlin S 1983 CSF somatostatin in affective illness. Arch Gen Psych 40:409.
20. Sorensen KV, Christensen SE, Dupont E, Hansen AP, Pedersen E, Orskov A 1980 Low somatostatin content in cerebrospinal fluid in multiple sclerosis. Acta Neurol Scandinav 61:186.
21. Beal NF, Martin JB 1984 Somatostatin: normal and abnormal observations in the central nervous system. In: Wurtman RJ, Corkin SH, Growdow JH (eds) Alzheimer's Disease: Advances in Basic Research and Therapies. Center for Brain Sciences and Metabolism, Charitable Trust, p 229.
22. Aronin N, Cooper PE, Lorenz LJ, Bird ED, Sagar SM, Leeman SE, Martin JB 1983 Somatostatin is increased in the basal ganglia in Huntington's disease. Ann Neurol 13:519.
23. Nemeroff CB, Youngblood WW, Manberg, PJ, Prange AJ, Kizer JS 1983 Regional brain concentrations of neuropeptides in Huntington's chorea and schizophrenia. Science 221:972.

24. Ferrier IW, Roberts GW, Crow TJ, Johnstone EC, Owens DGC, Lee YC, O'Shaughnessy DO, Adrian TE, Polak JM, Bloom SR 1983 Reduced cholecystokinin-like and somatostatin-like immunoreactivity in limbic lobe is associated with negative symptoms - in schizophrenia. Life Sci 33:475.
25. Davies P, Katzman R, Terry RD 1980 Reduced somatostatin-like immunoreactivity in cerebral cortex from cases of Alzheimer disease and Alzheimer senile dementia. Nature 288:279.
26. Rossor MN, Emson PC, Mountjoy CQ, Roth M, Iversen LL 1980 Reduced amounts of immunoreactive somatostatin in the temporal cortex in senile dementia of Alzheimer type. Neurosci Lett 20:373.
27. Ferrier IN, Cross AJ, Johnson JA, Robert GW, Crow TJ, Corsellis JAN, Lee YC, O'Shaughnessy D, Adrian TE, McGregor GP, Baracese-Hamilton AJ, Bloom SR 1983 Neuropeptides in Alzheimer type dementia. J Neurol Sci 62:159.
28. Gusella JF, Wexfler N, Conneally PM, Naylor PL, Anderson MA, Tanzi RE, Watkins PC, Ottina K, Wallace MR, Sakaguchi AY, Young AB, Shoulsow I, Bonilla E, Martin JB 1983 A polymorphic DNA marker genetically linked to Huntington's disease. Nature 306:234.
29. Marshall PE, Landis DMD, Williams RS 1983 Fibers containing somatostatin-like immunoreactivity increase in the neostriatum in Huntington's disease. Neurology 33:159.
30. Corkin S, Davies KL, Growdow JH, Usdin E, Wurtman RJ 1984 Aging. Alzheimer's Disease: A Report of Progress in Research. Raven Press, New York, vol. 19.
31. Mesulam MM, Myfson EJ, Levey AI, Wainer BH 1983 Cholinergic innervation of cortex by the basal forebrain; cytochemistry and cortical connections of the septal area, diagonal band nuclei, nucleus basalis (substantia innominata) and hypothalamus in the rhesus monkey. J Comp Neurol 214:170.
32. Armstrong DM, Saper CB, Levei AI, Wainer BH, Terry RD 1983 Distribution of cholinergic neurons in rat brain demonstrated by the immunocytochemical localization of choline acetyltransferase. J Comp Neurol 216:53.
33. McKinney M, Coyle JT, Hedreen JC 1983 Topographic analysis of the innervation of the rat neocortex and hippocampus by the basal forebrain cholinergic system. J Comp Neurol 217:103.
34. Rossor MN, Emson PC, Iversen LL, Mountjoy CD, Roth M, Fahrenkrug J, Rehfeld JF 1982 Neuropeptides and neurotransmitters in cerebral cortex in Alzheimer's disease. In: Corkin S, Davies KL, Growdow JH, Usdin E, Wurtman RJ (eds) Aging. Alzheimer's Disease: a Report of Progress in Research. Raven Press, New York, 19:15.
35. Rossor MN, Emson PC, Iversen LI, Mountjoy CQ, Roth M 1984 Patterns of neuropeptide deficits in Alzheimer's disease. In: Wurtman RJ, Corkin SH, Growdow JH (eds) Alzheimer's Disease: Advances in Basic Research and Therapies. Center for Brain Sciences and Metabolism, Charitable Trust, p 29.

36. Davies P, Katz DA, Crystal HA 1982 Choline acetyl transferase, somatostatin and substance P in selected cases of Alzheimer's disease. In: Corkin S, Davies KL, Growdow JH, Usdin E, Wurtman RJ (eds) Aging. Alzheimer's Disease: A Report of Progress in Research. Raven Press, New York, 15:9.
37. Boller F, Mizutani T, Roesman U, Gambetti P 1980 Parkinson disease, dementia and Alzheimer disease: clinicopathological correlations. Ann Neurol 7:329.
38. Hakim AM, Mathieson G 1979 Dementia in Parkinson's disease: a neuropathologic study. Neurology 29:1209.
39. Dubois B, Ruberg M, Javoy Agid F, Agid Y 1983 A subcortico-cortical cholinergic system is affected in Parkinson's disease. Brain Res 288:213.
40. Ruberg M, Ploska A, Javoy-Agid F, Agid Y 1982 Muscarinic binding and choline acetyltransferase activity in Parkinsonian subjects with reference to dementia. Brain Res 232:129.
41. Rorstad OP, Epelbaum J, Brazeau P, Martin JB 1979 Chromatographic and biological properties of immunoreactive somatostatin in hypothalamic and extrahypothalamic brain regions of the rat. Endocrinology 105:1083.
42. Wood PL, Etienne P, Lal S, Nair NPV, Bird MD 1983 A post mortem comparison of the cortical cholinergic system in Alzheimer's disease and Pick's disease. J Neurol Sci 62:211.
43. Morrison JH, Benoit R, Magistretti PJ, Bloom FE 1983 Immunohistochemical distribution of pro-somatostatin-related peptides in cerebral cortex. Brain Res 262:344.
44. Sorensen KV 1982 Somatostatin: localization and distribution in the cortex and the subcortical white matter of human brain. Neuroscience 7:1227.
45. McKinney M, Davies P, Coyle JT 1982 Somatostatin is not colocalized in cholinergic neurons innervating the rat cerebral cortex-hippocampal formation. Brain Res 243:169.
46. Eckenstein F, Thoenen H 1983 Cholinergic neurons in the rat cerebral cortex demonstrated by immunohistochemical localization of choline acetyltransferase. Neurosci Lett 36:211.
47. Houser CR, Crawford GD, Barber RP, Salvaterra PM, Vaughn JE 1983 Organization and morphological characteristics of cholinergic neurons: an immunocytochemical study with a monoclonal antibody to choline acetyltransferase. Brain Res 266:97.
48. Delfs JR, Zhu CH, Dichter MA 1984 Coexistence of acetylcholineesterase and somatostatin immunoreactivity in neurons cultured from rat cerebrum. Science 223:61.
49. Zigmond RE, Ben Ari Y 1976 A simple method for the serial sectioning of fresh brains and removal of identifiable nuclei from stained sections for biochemical analysis. J Neurochem 26:1279.
50. Fibiger HC 1982 The organization and some projections of cholinergic neurons of the mammalian forebrain. Brain Res Rev 4:327.

51. Lamour Y, Dutar P, Jobert A 1982 Excitating effect of acetylcholine on different types of neurons in the first somatosensory neocortex of the rat laminar distribution and pharmacological characteristics. Neuroscience 7:1483.
52. Lamour Y, Dutar P, Jobert A 1983 A comparative study of two populations of acetylcholine sensitive neurons in rat somatosensory cortex. Brain Res 289:157.
53. Robbins RJ, Sutton RE, Reichlin S 1982 Effects of neurotransmitters and cyclic AMP on somatostatin release from cultured cerebral cortical cells. Brain Res 234:377.
54. Nemeth EF, Cooper JR 1979 Effect of somatostatin on acetylcholine release from rat hippocampal synaptosomes. Brain Res 165:166.
55. Malthe-Sorensen D, Wood PL, Cheney DL, Costa E 1978 Modulation of the turnover rate of acetylcholine in rat brain by intraventricular injections of thyrotropin releasing hormone, somatostatin, neurotensin and angiotensin II. J Neurochem 31:685.
56. Wood PL, Cheney DL, Costa E 1979 Modulation of the turnover rate of hippocampal acetylcholine by neuropeptides; possible site of action of alpha-melanocyte stimulating hormone adrenocorticotrophic hormone and somatostatin. J Pharm Exp Ther 209:97.
57. Czernik AJ, Petrack B 1983 Somatostatin receptor binding in rat cerebral cortex. J Biol Chem 258:5525.
58. Epelbaum J, Ruberg M, Moyse E, Agid FJ, Dubois B, Agid Y 1983 Somatostatin and dementia in Parkinson's disease. Brain Res 278:376.
59. Epelbaum J, Agid Y, Dubois B, Enjalbert A, Javoy F, Moyse E, Ruberg M, Somatostatin levels and binding sites in the cortex of parkinsonian subjects: relationships with dementia. Program of the Meeting on Peptides and Neurological Diseases, Cambridge 1983 (Abstract).

BRAIN SOMATOSTATIN

PANEL DISCUSSION

MODERATOR: W. VALE

DR. W. VALE (La Jolla): I believe we have moved from a descriptive phase in which for the last ten years or so we have been discussing what is somatostatin and its various forms, where is somatostatin formed, and what happens when you give it. This afternoon's discussions are a good example that we are now moving more into an hypothesis-directed system in which we are focusing on particular biological events. Of course, this has always been the case for the hypothalamic-pituitary axis as somatostatin was characterized based on its ability to affect this, and several of the speakers addressed themselves to this issue. There were discussions of sympathetic nervous system, and the possible role of somatostatin there, and there were two talks on possible cortical interactions of somatostatin. Finally, we discussed some possible pathologic correlates of somatostatin. If one looks at Koch's postulates and what we need to satisfy them before we believe that something is a neuromodulator or neurotransmitter, we are doing very well on some, yet, on others, particularly within the central nervous system, I think we have a way to go and this is mainly because of technological limitations. Where we particularly need data is on dynamic measurements of somatostatin in specific sites of the central nervous system under concise situations. Now technologically this is very difficult with the exception of the hypothalamic-pituitary system where people are now measuring portal blood levels of somatostatin and other modulators. We also need specific ways to block somatostatin's action. The antagonists of David Coy are very important in this regard; also passive immunization is very useful, in terms of neutralizing the central nervous system. Well, I think we have come a long way since it was characterized and I would like to now throw the discussion open to the floor, if anyone has questions.

DR. A. ARIMURA (New Orleans): I have a specific question for Dr. Elde. As shown by Dr. Peterfreund and Dr. Robbins, the release of somatostatin from neurons is stimulated by catecholamines and cholinergic stimuli. Did you find any specific synaptic type junction beween the monoaminergic neurons and the somatostatin neurons, especially in the periventricular areas?

DR. R. ELDE (Minneapolis): That has been technically a difficult thing to do at levels of resolution that are satisfying. We noticed some time ago when we were first looking at somatostatin cells in the periventricular nucleus, that they live in a literal nest of dopamine fibres, but at the light microscopic level one says simply that they exist in a dense network of dopamine fibers. However, it is difficult to identify whether they in fact make synaptic and functional contact with somatostatin cells. I think we are only now at the point where we can look at those interactions with microscopic techniques and have some confidence that we can localize two substances simultaneously; the special problem has been looking at the interaction of small diameter structures like nerve fibers with other structures. I think we are only coming to that point now. Other data that would suggest interactions would include receptor autoradiography over regions of somatostatin-rich areas of cell bodies. But again the problem with that is the autoradiographic methods generally have not allowed fixation that is robust enough to preserve somatostatin in the neurons so you can't simultaneously do the immunohistochemistry for somatostatin and, say, phenylclonidine binding for α-2 adrenergic sites. I think some progress is being made but there is not very much data present at this point in time.

DR. A. VINIK (Ann Arbor): May I ask three questions of three different speakers. Dr. Peterfreund, I think that's very exciting data that you have presented in terms of the phorbol esters suggesting that somatostatin release may be under the control of a C kinase system; the question I'd like to ask you is whether this is calcium-dependent the way it is in other tissues. The second question: is there a response to phospholipids, and thirdly: is there a response to inositol tri-phosphates which suggests that this may be a regulatory system for somatostatin and have universal applicability?

DR. R. PETERFREUND (La Jolla): In answer to the question about the phospholipids and the C-kinase: no, we have not looked at that as yet. The effect of phorbol esters is partially blocked in low calcium conditions. We cannot completely inhibit the response but we can knock it down 50-75% and we can mimic that with verapamil, cobalt ions, or low calcium conditions, but we cannot eliminate the effect completely as we can, say, with acetylcholine stimulation.

DR. A. VINIK: Could you get complementary stimulation if you used a phorbol ester together with dibutyryl saying that there are two pathways of activation of somatostatin release?

DR. R. PETERFREUND: We have not done that.

DR. A. VINIK: That would be very exciting. Now, my second question is to Dr. Robbins. The data you presented on the uniqueness of the regulation of somatostatin release looking at the CNS, looking at the gut, etc., I think was super. The one thing, as we will discuss tomorrow, is the uniqueness of regulation of antral somatostatin which responds to calcium depletion in a very unique manner of releasing somatostatin. Did you find evidence for that in your search of 95 papers or so that you referred to, or anywhere else?

DR. R. ROBBINS (Denver): That calcim depletion decreased somatostatin secretion?

DR. A. VINIK: No, that it is a releaser. You only showed zero calcium, not depletion of calcium or the blockade of, let us say, calcium-calmodulin events.

DR. R. ROBBINS: In our system, blockade of calcium channels with cobalt, for instance, decreases basal secretion of somatostatin from the cells. I think there has also been a study on parafollicular cell secretion of somatostatin which shows that it is directly responsive to calcium, but as calcium goes up somatostatin secretion also goes up. Those are the only two I know of.

DR. A. VINIK: Now could I ask my last question. Dr. Brown, your data in terms of the role of centrally regulated epinephrine seemed interesting in terms of the hyperglycemia which was produced and the ability to abolish the hyperglycemia. One of your slides seemed to suggest that if you abolish the epinephrine response it did not affect the rebound from hypoglycemia. Do you think there is an important regulatory mechanism for hyperglycemia in diabetes and not for the counterregulation in response to hypoglycemia?

DR. M. BROWN (La Jolla): If you noticed, the time course of that was one hour. The fact of the matter is that was one unit of insulin over a one-hour period; that's a lot of insulin. What happens is if you look at a longer time point there is a difference between the somatostatin-treated animals and the non-somatostatin-treated animals in terms of the return to euglycemia. So the answer is yes, adrenal epinephrine in the rat, using this as evidence, is playing a role in the return to euglycemia.

DR. S. GUTTMANN (Basle): I have two questions, one for Dr. Peterfreund and the second to Dr. Robbins. Dr. Peterfreund, do you suggest that somatostatin has autoreceptors like neurotransmitters, since you are suggeting the short-loop feedback?

DR. R. PETERFREUND: Well, the data are consistent with that possibility but it is also possible that there are neural communication loops set up within the cultures such that somatostatin could act on a cell which in turn acts on the somatostatin neuron that secretes.

Some of the data that would support that type of circuitry in the culture dishes would be the effect of GABA blockers; with the GABA blocker you get an augmentation of secretion, and that would be consistent with GABA cells within the cultures tonically inhibiting the somatostatinergic cells. So it is possible that when we give a somatostatin analog we are interfering, in some way, with one of these loops that are developing within the culture dishes and it is also possible that there are autoreceptors. I don't think the data at this point allows us to make that distinction. It is the most parsimonious explanation but it may not be correct at this point.

DR. S. GUTTMANN: Dr. Robbins, you have proposed that the GABA uptake is not influenced by 1 μM somatostatin or somatostatin analog, but the release is inhibited by 10 μM. Why did you change the doses and still with 10 μM the increase was very small?

DR. R. ROBBINS: In response to that, I only showed one slide. We've done dose-response curves with somatostatin all the way from 10 nM up to 10 μM for both uptake and release and we find that as far as uptake or reuptake of tritiated GABA is concerned, across the whole spectrum, somatostatin has no effect. Our dose-response curve on the effect of somatostatin on releasing tritiated GABA from these cells starts to appear only at 1 μM, with a maximum effect at 10 μM we have not gone any higher. The effect is apparent for the first - 10-30 min of incubation, but with more prolonged incubations one tends to lose the effect. We have shown that these cells metabolize somatostatin-14 quite rapidly with a half-time in the order of 15 min, so that when we go longer we may be losing somatostatin because of processing or degradation. The other point is that 10 μM is a very high concentration. Does the brain ever, or do these cells ever, see 10 μM somatostatin? That is a hard question to answer. The final point is that these are neonatal cells which we took from 16 day embryos and they had been in culture for 10 days, so they may not have developed. We know that GABA transaminase, the enzyme that degrades GABA, for instance, is virtually absent in these age cultures. On the other hand, glutamic acid decarboxylase that synthesizes GABA is present in these cells at a level about half of what it is in the adult. So there are various things going on in the cells at this age, but I will accept the possibility that 10 μM somatostatin is certainly not physiologic and we need to do more studies to look at that.

DR. S. SZABO (Boston): My questions are not related to cysteamine, or at least not directly. Dr. Brown, you have presented nice data on the correlation of hyperglycemia and somatostatin in the brain, and stress in general. Just to play the devil's advocate, have you looked into the possibility, or have you considered, that part of this is not only mediated through the medulla but also through the cortex? Glucocorticoids would be a good mediator especially since they go to the hypothalamus. Very specifically, have you looked at adrenal medullectomized animals where the medulla would be removed and the cortex would still be operating? Moreover, just to enlarge your hypothesis concerning stress and hyperglycemia; did you look at somatostatin levels in the adrenal since some people claim there is a measurable amount of somatostatin right in the adrenal gland?

DR. M. BROWN: The answer to the first question - the role of glucocorticoids in that response - I cannot unequivocally rule that out. Are you talking about stress inducing the release of glucocorticoids?

DR. S. SZABO: Have you done medullectomy for example?

DR. M. BROWN: No, we've done hypophysectomy.

DR. S. SZABO: And total adrenalectomy also?

DR. M. BROWN: No; well, we've done a hypophysectomy which prevented the rise of corticoids to stress. We still see a rise of glucose, and in that circumstance somatostatin still inhibits the rise of glucose. Does that answer your question?

DR. S. SZABO: Yes, partially, but did you remove the adrenal medulla?

DR. M. BROWN: We have not. I ordered some rats that allegedly were adrenalmedullectomized. I could not measure any epinephrine, but they had horrible adrenocortical problems. They had astronomically high levels of ACTH and I chose not to do the experiment, so that is what happened. The second question about the role of somatostatin in the adrenal medulla itself; somatostatin may indeed have an action or be released from the adrenal medulla. Regarding what effect the administration of exogenous somatostatin may have on adrenomedullary function, I can only say that when somatostatin is given peripherally, and presumably it would have access to the adrenal medulla, it has no effect on inhibition of epinephrine secretion; it is only when it is put in the brain.

DR. S. SZABO: Another short question for Dr. Robbins. You have shown very nicely that there is a biphasic dose response of dopamine to somatostatin. We have special interest in dopamine because of its possible relation to duodenal ulcer disease. Have you ever actually found an inhibition of somatostatin secretion by dopamine and have you tried dopamine antagonists on somatostatin secretion?

DR. R. ROBBINS: We have not tried any dopamine antagonists. On our dose response curve you can see that it was at the nM range that we had stimulatory effects but even when we went up to μM, when the effect went away, it stayed basal, it did not suppress.

DR. S. SZABO: It never went down?

DR. R. ROBBINS: It never went down. I think, also in gut and in the islet, dopamine tends to be stimulatory to somatostatin secretion; but I do not know of any situations in which a dopaminergic ligand would have inhibited somatostatin.

DR. R. BENOIT (Montreal): In terms of peptide-peptide interactions in cortex or in hypothalamus, there are four speakers who spoke about the relationship between VIP and somatostatin: Dr. Goodman, Dr. Robbins, Dr. Epelbaum in the past, and maybe Dr. Peterfreund did some work on that. So what is the effect of VIP on the secretion of somatostatin in the hypothalamus and in the cortex? Does everybody agree that it causes an increase in stimulation?

DR. R. ROBBINS: If you take a look at the literature there are several papers on that point. Dr. Tapia-Arancibia has shown recently that in both hypothalamic and cortical cells, VIP stimulates somatostatin. I think that Dr. Goodman has demonstrated that both somatostatin immunoreactivity and somatostatin mRNA go up with VIP. The only paper negative on that side was Dr. Epelbaum's paper of two or three years ago using an entirely different system, which was an explant system, and maybe I will let him speak for himself.

DR. J. EPELBAUM (Paris): It was not the only one; I think there was another one by Dr. Shimatsu showing exactly the same result that we had. The main question relates to the doses. The doses that we used were much lower than the one being used to demonstrate stimulation. I think that Dr. Tapia-Arancibia said that when she used lower doses she saw a decrease in the hypothalamus.

DR. R. ROBBINS: Our dose response curves for VIP start at 0.5 μM; there is a significant increase at 1 μM and it goes up at 3 μM and 10 μM; below 0.5 μM we do not see an effect.

DR. H. KATAKAMI (Cincinnati): One question, one comment. The question is about the discrepancy between the *in vivo* and the *in vitro* results. In view of previous data from Kyoto, we have reported that central GABA stimulates growth hormone secretion and antisomatostatin serum does not block the GH release induced by GABA. In contrast, destruction of GRF-containing neurons by neonatal treatment with monosodium glutamate almost completely suppressed GH release induced by GABA, suggesting the involvement of hypothalamic GRF in GH release induced by GABA. Did you ever look at some discrepancy or some modulation by the experimental conditions, such as the age of rat or the incubation period, if it will modify the effects? I'm asking whether the experimental condition *in vitro* would modify the results, such as fetal age or the medium, etc?

DR. R. PETERFREUND: There are a couple of points. First, I think it is very hard to immediately draw parallels or contrasts between *in vivo* and *in vitro* work at this stage, because in some of the *in vivo* experiments it is hard to say exactly where an applied substance might be working. If it is administered in the periphery, how well does it access into the brain; if it is administered into the brain how well does it get to the different brain regions that we are looking at? In the *in vitro* work, such as Dr. Robbins does and that I have been working on, I think we can say that things work at the level of the hypothalamus or at the level of the region of the cerebral cortex. So the findings, when you take those considerations into account, are not necessarily contradictory. I am a little unclear on one portion of what you said; that is, if you administer antisomatostatin serum you do not abolish the effect of GABA. Well, it would seem to me that the idea with the GABA would be that you would already be inhibiting somatostatin secretion so that I am not sure what antisomatostatin serum would do in addition to that inhibition. The qualitative effects of those manipulations should be the same.

DR. H. KATAKAMI: Before the injection of GABA, antisomatostatin serum did elevate the basal plasma GH level. Sixty minutes after the injection of antisomatostatin serum we injected GABA centrally and we got a further increase by GABA. My comment relates to the suppressive effect of hpGRF-44 in the conscious rat reported by Dr. Tannenbaum. In our studies, 1 μg of hpGRF-40 did elevate plasma GH transiently, 20 min after injection, whereas a small dose of hpGRF-40 suppressed spontaneous GH secretion in the non-stressed conscious male rat. Antisomatostatin sera blocked the suppressive effects of the small dose of GRF. So I would like to make a comment on the difference between GRF 1-40 and GRF 1-44.

DR. G.S. TANNENBAUM (Montreal): Recently, we have examined the effects of intracerebroventricular administration of GRF-44 on spontaneous growth hormone secretion. What we found was a striking suppression in amplitude of the growth hormone surges in response to central administration of GRF, which was a rather surprising effect. We did a careful dose-response study and found that this response was dose-dependent. We started with a rather high dose, 10 μg, and went down to 0.5 μg. There was never any evidence of leakage into the systemic circulation. That is always a concern; Marvin Brown raised it and I feel very much the same about those studies in which we administer peptides centrally because there can be significant leakage into the hypophyseal portal circulation. At no time did we see release of growth hormone; there was always a suppression. We then examined the possibility that this suppressive effect of central GRF was mediated by an increased release of somatostatin; that is, that the centrally administered GRF was acting on somatostatinergic neurons to cause somatostatin release. Passive immunization with antisomatostatin serum in these GRF-treated animals had absolutely no effect on restoration of the growth hormone pulses. At this point, my view on these data is that we do have some evidence to suggest that GRF may participate in an ultra-short-loop feedback system similar to that which has been described for somatostatin, originally by McCann in vivo, and today, as well, by Dr. Peterfreund in vitro.

DR. J. TABORSKY (Seattle): I have one comment which relates to Dr. Vale's comment and also to some data by Dr. Peterfreund. Dr. Vale's comment was "we need some tools to take a look at what the physiological role of brain somatostatin is." Dr. Peterfreund showed that certain non-immunoreactive analogs of somatostatin can inhibit the release of brain somatostatin. I have employed one of these non-immunoreactive analogs of somatostatin to inhibit the release of somatostatin from the pancreas and have shown that insulin and glucagon go up. It would seem feasible at this point to try some of these non-immunoreactive analogs of somatostatin in selected brain areas as a probe to inhibit the release of brain somatostatin and possibly observe the effects resulting from that inhibition. It is a tool I think that is worthy of some effort.

DR. W. VALE: That is a very good point; the problem is that many of those analogs are also biologically active in their own regard.

DR. J. TABORSKY: The clear thing that has to be done is a very careful log-dose response.

DR. W. VALE: So you would need one that is selective.

DR. J. TABORSKY: Well, there is no such thing for any analog; if the dose gets high enough it will inhibit. But, if you are careful about the dose-response curve I think you can gain some information. I have a question for Dr. Epelbaum. It concerns CSF somatostatin. You have shown that there is a decrease in the somatostatin concentration in the frontal cortex and in CSF in Alzheimer's disease. Do you mean to imply, by that, that the somatostatin in the CSF is coming from the frontal cortex and if it is not from there, where is it from and why is it decreased?

DR. J. EPELBAUM: It could come from the cortex but it could also come from the spinal cord or any place near the ventricles, and that is why it is difficult to conclude anything from the CSF data. My point was that at the present time, with the tools that we have, it is more accurate to assay the levels in the brain structures.

DR. W. RUTTER (San Francisco): I have a couple of questions out of pure ignorance, not out of any aggressive tendency. They have to do with concentrations. Dr. Tannenbaum, in your nice experiments you had a curve with GRF which suggested to me that the levels of GRF that were responsible for the effects were of the order of nanomolar; you had it in micrograms. First of all, can you tell the audience more or less what concentration ranges are effective, and I wondered whether you had similar titrations for somatostatin to show the levels of somatostatin which are effective in these kinds of experiments?

DR. G.S. TANNENBAUM: We have not done it for somatostatin; we have been trying to do it for GRF. Part of the problem in the literature right now is that there is some confusion in terms of trying to obtain a dose-response effect for GRF. I think part of that problem is the result of what we have discussed here today. That is, depending on the time of administration of the GRF peptide, you can get a very different response - we see tremendous variability in the magnitude of the response to the very same dose of the peptide, and I believe that this is due to interference by endogenous somatostatin *in vivo*. If you administer the same 10 μg dose, during a time when you normally have endogenous secretion of GRF, you will get a much higher response than if you administer it during a trough period of GH secretion.

DR. W. RUTTER: I thought you might have done that in the presence of antibody to somatostatin.

DR. G. TANNENBAUM: We have not done it as yet but it is certainly worth doing right now.

DR. W. RUTTER: The question related to that was, of course, the very high levels that were required in Dr. Robbins' experiments and then really, initially, the responses obtained by Dr. Peterfreund; in those cases the responses seemed modest and the levels of agents required for the response seemed very high. For PMA, if I remember correctly, there were 100 nM concentrations required; for carbachol, very high concentrations, and for barbiturates, almost mM concentrations, or 10^{-1} mM concentrations, and so I wondered what you thought of the biology in this particular situation because of that circumstance?

DR. R. PETERFREUND: The concentrations for the barbiturates, for example, are actually pretty standard for the literature on barbiturate experiments; in fact, a lot of times you will see people using concentrations well up into the mM range, 10 mM and so on, for the effects of various barbiturates. We're actually under that seeing some of our effects; so in that sense we are lower. For PMA, again I think we are well within reason in terms of the concentrations that are employed in a lot of *in vitro* systems. The K_D for binding for PMA and for phorboldibutyrate in our lab is of the order of about 10 nM and we see significant effects. It reaches a maximum at about between 10 and 100 nM so we are working around the range of the K_D, and that is around the range that people work in the various literature reports. For the cholinergic drugs, again I think we may be a little high on those but I think Dr. Robbins' data and mine are fairly congruent in the general dose ranges that we are using.

DR. W. RUTTER: What do you think about the size of the response that you get in a system like that? Quite obviously it is a dispersed cell system so that there can be other kinds of effects, but the thing that was going on in my mind is whether you were having a direct effect of these agents on the cells themselves or an indirect effect on some other cell, and that's one of the reasons that the responses were so modest?

DR. R. PETERFREUND: Firstly, I agree that there is always the possibility that there are multiple things going on. Secondly, these cells really do not store large amounts of peptide; the quantity that is released relative to the quantity that is stored is a fairly substantial proportion. The basal release might be about 10% of the total concentration, something like 5% or 10%, so that in terms of percentage of what's actually within the cells you are releasing a fairly substantial amount, and then interactions such as you suggested may be possible, we can't rule those out.

DR. S. RICHARDSON (New York): Dr. Peterfreund, using a different system of acutely dispersed adult rat hypothalamic cells we have found that both basal and ouabain-stimulated somatostatin release could be inhibited by somatostatin and I was very interested in your data with the carbachol stimulation. Have you tried any other stimulatory agents in an attempt to demonstrate the inhibitory effect of the S-14 analog?

DR. R. PETERFREUND: No, we just used the carbachol because that was a well-characterized stimulus in our hands and it's also more physiologically relevant perhaps than the PMA which we've used in other studies.

DR. S. RICHARDSON: That is very interesting, thank you.

DR. A. SCHONBRUNN (Boston): I have one question relating to the effects of VIP on somatostatin secretion. Becaue it has been shown in other systems that GRF can bind, or at least maybe exert some of its actions through VIP receptors and possibly vice versa, and since the effects that you see of VIP on somatostatin secretion occur at such high concentrations of VIP, I was wondering if you had looked at GRF or other homologous peptides to see whether they might be more potent at stimulating somatostatin secretion?

DR. R. ROBBINS: No, we have not but there are a number of other interesting overlaps there. For instance, Van Calker reported that VIP is a very potent stimulator of cyclic AMP in cultured brain cells. Somatostatin secretion increases when intracellular cyclic AMP is raised. VIP may be very important in glycogenolysis in the cerebral cortex in breaking down glycogen to glucose and, as we showed, glucose is an important element in basal somatostatin secretion but we have not looked at GRF receptors.

DR. A. SCHONBRUNN: Or any of the other, PHI, or secretin, or any of the others?

DR. R. ROBBINS: No, we have not.

DR. J. EPELBAUM: May I have a comment on this topic; because, as Dr. Schonbrunn said, it is very strongly suggestive of something looking like GRF. The release by VIP that has been shown this morning is a tremendous amount - nothing to compare with the acetylcholine release of somatostatin that you have shown. It is quite comparable with the release that you get on GH secretion with GRF; and in both events, the GRF effect is linked to the stimulation of cyclase as is VIP, which is also a very potent stimulator of cyclase.

DR. J. DELFS (Boston): I have two questions, the first is to Dr. Epelbaum. We have observed in cultures of dispersed cells from fetal rats that there is a co-existence of somatostatin and acetylcholinesterase. We are now analyzing data in sections of adult rat brain and there seems to be even a greater coincidence of those two markers. Have you looked at that in your models or in human tissue?

DR. J. EPELBAUM: Well, I did not want to complicate the story because, as you know, there is an interesting cholinergic neuronal system in the cortex - it is very clear from your experiments and from others with choline acetyltransferase immunocytochemistry. This accounts for about 30% of the acetylcholine in the cortex and we are sure that in the Alzheimer and Parkinson demented patient it is not the intrinsic acetylcholine neurons which are touched; those are the ascending projections from the ventral forebrain. But perhaps there is a plasticity of the cortex and maybe the intrinsic cholinergic innervation could account for some recuperation.

DR. R. ROBBINS: If I may make a comment, maybe Dr. Delfs can respond to this. The question about acetylcholinesterase and how specific it is in metabolizing acetylcholine, and maybe some other peptides, comes up. A recent paper which lesioned the nucleus basalis caused over 50% depletion in acetylcholinesterase in the cerebral cortex but did not change the somatostatin content, for instance. I wonder how you might put those two together with your results?

DR. J. DELFS: There certainly is the existence of a cholinergic system which is intrinsic to cortex. It has been a subject of debate for a number of years and I think in the last 18 months a number of groups utilizing panels of monoclonal antibodies against choline acetyltransferase have really, to the satisfaction of most people, demonstrated an intrinsic cholinergic system within cortex. The morphological characteristics of the neurons are really not similar to those of the somatostatinergic neurons. Secondly, there is increasing evidence that suggests that the overlap between choline acetyltransferase and acetylcholinesterase is not good in cortex, if it exists at all. And certainly that goes along with the lesioning studies. I would think that the possible importance of the findings of acetylcholinesterase and somatostatin immunoreactivity coexistent in the same neurons would more likely suggest, perhaps, a postsynaptic role for the somatostatinergic neuron. But I think that's, at best, circumstantial and I think that, as in all histochemical studies, you have to say it's this way. We say it's this way because we observe it and perhaps at some point we will understand its importance. Acetylcholinesterase is certainly a valid marker for a subset of neurons - but I don't think that we know what it means when they are not cholinergic.

DR. J. EPELBAUM: Your study was done in cultured cells; did you see any coexistence of acetylcholinesterase and somatostatin *in situ*?

DR. J. DELFS: Yes. We are in the process of analyzing that. In fact, there is a much more considerable coexistence of acetylcholinesterase and somatostatin immunoreactivity in intact sections of adult rat brain which, perhaps, may be a bit more preponderant in the deeper layers, i.e. layers 5 and 6.

I have a second question and this will be to Dr. Robbins. It is prefaced by noting that in intracellular studies that we have done, examining the effects of somatostatin on cortical neurons in culture, we observed two phenomena which you are familiar with. One is tachyphylaxis; with as little as a couple of seconds of exposure to a very low dose of somatostatin, perhaps in the range of 100 pmol, the excitatory and depolarizing effects of somatostatin on those neurons disappear. The second was a phenomenon in which as the number of applications of somatostatin was increased, and as the dose of somatostatin was increased, there was a tendency to see more inhibitory effects, whereas at smaller doses for briefer periods of time, it tended to be excitatory effects. Have you looked in your systems, at very brief time intervals, to examine the effects of either the changes in secretion or the changes in release of the GABA by somatostatin?

DR. R. ROBBINS: Yes we have looked at 1, 5, 10, 20 and 30 min time periods and we see no effect at any time under 10 min. The concentration also works at 30 min. So that presumably it is not working immediately at a membrane level but it is inducing something that is changing in the cell - that takes up to 30 min to see.

DR. S. HEISLER (Quebec City): My question is addressed to Dr. Peterfreund. You have showed some results with a phorbol methylester which, as you know, is a pharmacological tool although there is some discussion that it may resemble, structurally at least, diazoglycerol. I wanted to know whether the inhibitory effects that you had with GABA and muscimol extended to some of the other secretory agonists, such as carbachol and CRF, or whether we have two sets of post-receptor mechanisms that might be involved in the secretory pathway?

DR. P. PETERFREUND: They do extend. GABA will inhibit the carbachol effect as will muscimol. I showed it mostly in cerebrocortical cultures. The response to CRF is markedly inhibited by the GABA agents, so they seem to work on all the stimuli that we have tried.

IV

MECHANISM OF ACTION / ANALOGS OF SOMATOSTATIN

16

SOMATOSTATIN RECEPTORS

C. B. SRIKANT* AND Y. C. PATEL

Fraser Laboratories, McGill Univ. Depts. of Medicine, and Neurology and Neurosurgery, Royal Victoria Hospital

Montreal Neurological Inst., Montreal Quebec, Canada

ABSTRACT

It is now well established that the biological actions of tetradecapeptide somatostatin (somatostatin-14, S-14) are receptor-mediated. These receptors were first quantified in GH_4C pituitary tumor cells using [^{125}I-Tyr^{1}] S-14 as radioligand which was found to exhibit high non-specific binding to membrane receptor preparations from normal tissues. Our studies have shown that [^{125}I-Tyr^{11}] S-14 in which the radiolabel is situated away from the N-terminus exhibits significantly lower non-specific binding and therefore is more suitable for S-14 receptor studies. In the CNS, highest concentration of S-14 receptors was found in the cerebral cortex, followed by thalamus, hypothalamus, striatum, amygdala and hippocampus while medulla-pons, cerebellum and spinal cord exhibited negligible binding. Outside the CNS membrane receptors for S-14 have been characterized in pituitary, adrenal cortex and pancreatic acini. In all these tissues a single class of high affinity binding sites for S-14 were present, the receptors in pancreatic acinar cells exhibiting significantly greater affinity for binding S-14 than in other tissues.

---

*C.B. Srikant is a Chercheur-Boursier of the Fondation de la Recherche en Santé du Québec and Y.C. Patel is a Senior Scientist of the Medical Research Council of Canada. This work was supported by grants from the Medical Research Council (MT 6832) and USPHS (AM 21373).

Structure-activity relationship studies using a number of structural analogs of S-14 have shown that the cyclic structure of the molecule is essential and that amino acid residues 7-11 (Phe-Trp-Lys-Phe-Phe) constitute the active recognition site for receptor binding. D-Trp^{8} modified analogs, in particular halogenated [D-Trp^{8}] S-14 analogs, exhibited greater receptor binding affinity than S-14. The relative potencies of some of the analogs, e.g. [D-Trp^{8}]S-14, [L-Br$_{5}$-Trp^{8}]S-14,[L-F$_{5}$-Trp^{8}]S-14 and [des AA^{1,2,4,5,12,13}, D-Trp^{8}] S-14 were different between tissues suggesting that the S-14 receptors in these tissues are heterogeneous.

Somatostatin-28 (S-28) bound to S-14 receptors in all the tissues but with significantly different affinities. Its affinity for binding to S-14 receptors was greater than that of S-14 in the pituitary but not in brain and exocrine pancreas whereas in the adrenal cortex both S-28 and S-14 exhibited comparable binding affinities. These data coupled with the observed greater biological potency of S-28 in some tissues suggest that separate receptors for S-28 distinct from those of S-14 may exist. Receptor sites quantitated with a radioligand prepared from a Tyr analog of S-28 - [Leu^{8}, D-Trp^{22}, ^{125}I-Tyr^{25}] S-28 - were found to exhibit binding parameters comparable to those quantitated with [^{125}I-Tyr^{11}]S-14 in each tissue. Furthermore, both S-28 and S-14 inhibited the receptor biding of these two radioligands with the same relative potencies. It appears, therefore, that both [^{125}I-Tyr^{11}] S-14 and [Leu^{8}, D-Trp^{22}, ^{125}I-Tyr^{25}] S-28 interact with the same receptor sites. <u>In vivo</u> radioautographic studies in the rat, however, indicate that [Leu^{8}, D-Trp^{22}, ^{125}I-Tyr^{25}] S-28 preferentially labels binding sites in median eminence which interact poorly with [^{125}I-Tyr^{11}] S-14. Thus the presence of distinct S-14 and S-28 receptors at least in discrete areas of rat brain appears likely. Further studies using more selective analogs of S-28 will be necessary to identify these receptors in direct binding studies.

These receptors are regulated by changes in ligand concentration. Down-regulation of S-14 receptors following exposure to high concentrations of S-14 has been demonstrated in pituitary tumor cells GH_4C_1 and AtT-20. Such homologous regulation of S-14 receptors in normal tissues may occur in pathophysiological conditions associated with elevated tissue and plasma somatostatin levels, but remains to be demonstrated by direct binding studies. Depletion of brain somatostatin by cysteamine was found to result in up-regulation of cerebrocortical S-14 receptors in the rat. Heterologous regulation of S-14 receptors by TRH and glucocorticoids has been reported in GH_4C_1 cells; such a regulation of S-14 in normal tissues has not been observed.

INTRODUCTION

The cyclic tetradecapeptide somatostatin (somatostatin-14, S-14) exerts a number of hormonal and neuroendocrine effects in several tissues. Its actions have now been shown to be receptor-mediated (1-13). The presence of functional receptors for S-14 was first demonstrated by direct binding studies in a rat pituitary tumor cell line (GH_4C_1) (1). Studies in our laboratory led to the identification and characterization of these receptors in normal rat brain (2, 3). Subsequently we and others have characterized the S-14 receptors in rat pituitary (4-7), exocrine pancreas (8-10, 14) and adrenal cortex (11-13). These studies suggest that S-14 receptors in these tissues are heterogeneous and exhibit distinctly different ligand specificities. In this chapter the current state of knowledge in this field is reviewed.

Methodological Aspects

Schonbrunn and Tashjian used an N-terminally labelled Tyr analog of S-14- [^{125}I-Tyr^1] S-14 as the radioligand to demonstrate the presence of high affinity S-14 receptors in GH_4C_1 cells (1). Initial attempts to demonstrate S-14 binding in normal tissues using this ligand however proved unsuccessful; only poor binding to extremely low affinity sites could be discerned in such tissues as bovine pituitary (15), rat pancreas (16) and human blood cells (17). Marks et al. (18) have shown that the N-terminal end of S-14 is extremely susceptible to degradation by aminopeptidase-like enzymes in normal tissues. Thus, the failure to detect high affinity S-14 binding sites in the above studies could have resulted from the binding of radiolabelled fragments [^{125}I-Tyr] or [^{125}I-Tyr-Gly] (resulting from N-terminal degradation of [^{125}I-Tyr^1]S-14) to sites that are not specific for S-14. Studies in our laboratory have shown that during incubation with rat brain synaptosomal membane preparations, >70% loss of radiolabel occurred from two radioligands containing ^{125}I at the N-terminal end ([^{125}I-Tyr]-S-14 and [^{125}I-Tyr^1]S-14). In the presence of added proteolytic inhibitors, degradation of these ligands was reduced but remained unacceptably high ($\simeq$30%) (3). In contrast, [^{125}I-Tyr^{11}] S-14 in which the radiolabel is situated away from the N-terminal end, was found to be relatively more stable, exhibiting less than 5% degradation under identical conditions and enabled the identification of high affinity S-14 receptors in rat brain synaptosomal membranes (3). Using this radioligand we have subsequently characterized S-14 receptors in rat pituitary (4), adrenal cortex (12, 13) and exocrine pancreas (10). Recently a conformationally restricted analog - [des Ala^1, Gly^2, des amino Cys^3, ^{125}I-Tyr^{11}, dicarba^{3,4}] somatostatin - has also been shown to be stable and suitable as a radioligand for S-14 receptor studies (19). Despite the problems of greater instability of N-terminally labelled ligands, several groups have employed radioligands such as [^{125}I-Tyr]-S-14, [^{125}I-Tyr^1] S-14 and [^{125}I-Tyr^1,

D-Trp[8]] S-14 and reported binding constants comparable to those obtained using [^{125}I-Tyr^{11}]S-14 in our laboratory (5, 7, 8, 9, 12, 20, 21) (Table 1). The presence of S-14 binding sites on pancreatic A, B and D cells has been shown by autoradiographic technique using [^{125}I-Tyr^{1}]S-14 (22). Direct binding studies have been carried out using whole rat islets only (26). Because of the inherent heterogeneity of islet cells, quantitation of S-14 receptors on individual islet cells will require binding studies with separated fractions of islet cells. In adition the existence of intra-cellular receptors for S-14 in rat liver (23), pancreas (24, 25), and stomach (26) have been reported but remain to be confirmed. In all the above studies and in our own experience N-terminally labelled S-14 ligands were found to exhibit very high non-specific binding (up to 60% of total binding), presumably due to interaction of radiolabelled fragments such as [^{125}I-Tyr], [^{125}I-Tyr-Gly] or [^{125}I-Tyr-Ala-Gly] with sites that are not specific for S-14. By contrast [^{125}I-Tyr^{11}] S-14 exhibited markedly lower non-specific binding which constituted ~ 25%

Table 1. Comparison of Binding Constants of S-14 Receptors in Normal Rat Tissues Obtained Using Different Radioligands

Tissue	Radioligand	Bmax (fmol/mg)	Kd (nM)	Ref.
Cerebral cortex	[^{125}I-Tyr^{11}] S-14	410 ± 40	1.7 ± 0.12	3
	[^{125}I-Tyr^{11}] S-14	200	1.02	6
	[^{125}I-Tyr^{1}] S-14	53	0.8	19
	[^{125}I-Tyr^{11}]CGP-23996*	450 ± 30	2.4 ± 0.1	21
Pituitary	[^{125}I-Tyr^{11}] S-14	305 ± 25	1.1 ± 0.1	4
	[^{125}I-Tyr^{11}] S-14	101 ± 15	2.43±0.23	6
	[^{125}I-Tyr^{1}] S-14	104 ± 19	0.9 ± 0.22	5
	[^{125}I-Tyr^{1}, D-Trp^{8}] S-14	54 ± 2.6	0.12	7
Pancreatic acinar cells	[^{125}I-Tyr^{11}] S-14	266 ± 22	0.5 ± 0.04	11
	[^{125}I-Tyr^{11}] S-14	178 ± 18**	0.15±0.03	8
	[^{125}I-Tyr^{11}] S-14	72.2±10**	0.28±0.02	10
	[^{125}I-Tyr^{1}] S-14	600 ± 54	0.32±0.03	9
Adrenal cortex	[^{125}I-Tyr^{11}] S-14	350 ± 40	1.1 ± 0.11	13,14
	[^{125}I-Tyr^{1}] S-14	193 ± 3.2	0.66	12

* CGP-23996:[des Ala^{1}, Gly^{2} desamino Cys^{3} Tyr^{11} dicarba^{3,14}]somatostatin.

** Guinea pig.

of total binding thus enabling more reliable mesurements of S-14 receptor binding in normal tissues. Similar conclusions were reached by Esteve et al. in their studies on pancreatic acinar cell S-14 receptors (10).

The binding of [^{125}I-Tyr^{11}] S-14 to synaptosomal membrane receptors was specific and was not influenced by other peptide hormones. The specific binding of this radioligand was inhibited by S-14 in a dose-dependent manner and analysis of the binding data revealed the presence of a single class of high affinity sites present in highest concentration in the cerebral cortex. Medulla-pons, cerebellum and spinal cord exhibited very low binding while thalamus, hypothalamus, striatum, amygdala and hippocampus were found to contain intermediate receptor densities (Fig. 1). Outside the CNS, S-14 receptors have been quantitated using [^{125}I-Tyr^{11}] S-14 in rat pituitary, adrenal cortex and pancreatic acinar cells. As illustrated in Fig. 2 (left panel) the S-14 receptors in each of these tissues consisted of a single class of high affinity sites. The receptors present in pancreatic acinar cell membranes exhibited significantly higher affinity for S-14 than those present in other tissues (Fig. 2, right panel).

Ligand Specificity for Receptor Binding

Using a wide variety of synthetic analogs of S-14 which exhibit greater potency and/or selectivity of action in different tissues (27-29) we and others have investigated the structural requirements of the ligand for optimal receptor binding. Such structure-activity relationship studies in our laboratory (4, 12, 13, 30, 31) and those of others (5, 7, 32, 33) have shown that the cyclic structure of the molecule is essential and that the amino acid residues 7-11 (Phe-Trp-Lys-Thr-Phe) constitute the ligand recognition site for S-14

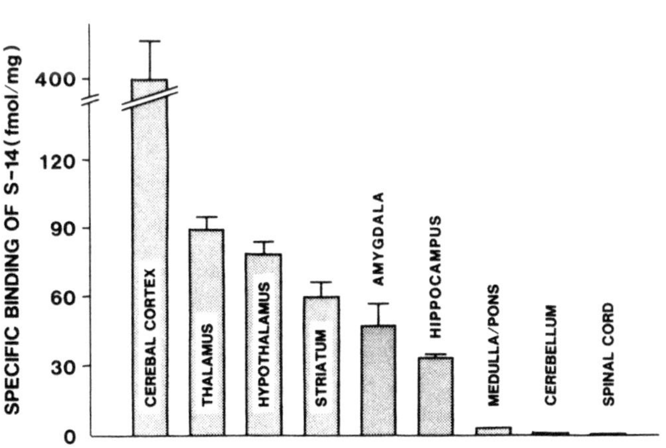

Fig. 1. Regional distribution of S-14 receptors in rat CNS.

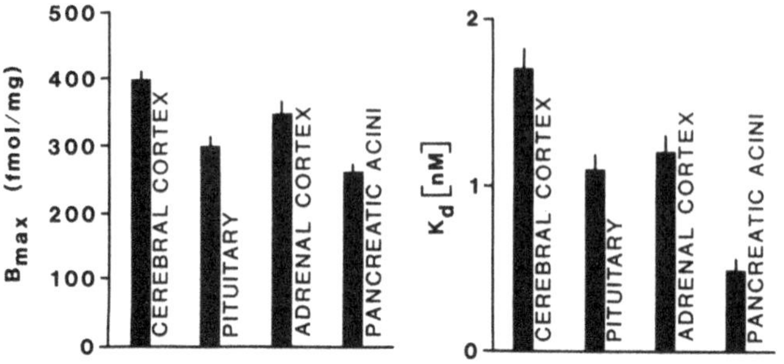

Fig. 2. Comparison of the binding capacity (B_{max}) and affinity (K_d) of S-14 receptors in normal rat tissues.

receptor binding. The same structural region constitutes the active site for biological action (27, 34). S-14 analogs such as [D-Trp^8] S-14 exhibiting greater potency than S-14 bound to S-14 receptors with greater affinity than S-14 (Table 2) in all the tissues tested thus far. Halogenated [Trp^8]S-14 analogs (containing F or Br) were more potent than [D-Trp^8]S-14. However, the binding affinities of some of these peptides were found to differ between tissues.

The affinity of [D-Trp^8]S-14 for binding to S-14 receptors in adrenal cortex was 2-5 fold lower than in pituitary and brain. [D-F_5-Trp^8] S-14 was the most potent analog in all these tissues whreas [L-F_5-Trp^8]S-14 was 2-3 times more potent in the brain and pituitary than in adrenal cortex. Likewise [D-Br_5-Trp^8]S-14 bound to S-14 receptors in pituitary with 2-fold greater affinity than in brain and adrenal cortex while [L-Br_5-Trp^8]S-14 exhibited 3-fold greater affinity for receptor binding in adrenal cortex compared to brain and pituitary. A striking dissociation in the potency of [oligo D-Trp^8]S-14 ([des AA^{1,2,4,5,12,13},D-Trp^8] S-14) was also observed in that its affinity for S-14 receptor binding was 2.5-fold lower than that of S-14 in the adrenal cortex whereas in the brain and pituitary it was more potent than S-14. Replacement of Lys^4 by Phe with or without introduction of basic groups in the Phe residue resulted in a pronounced generalized increase in binding (31) as well as biological potencies (35) but did not lead to dissociated affinities for binding to S-14 receptors in different tissues.

These data indicate that basic differences exist between S-14 receptors in different tissues. It is likely that alterations in the metabolism of the analogs may account, at least in part, for their variable _in vivo_ potencies. This could apply especially to [D-Trp^8]substituted analogs which are known to be relatively more resistant to enzymatic degradation than S-14 (27, 28, 34). The high _in vivo_ potency of intracisternally administered [oligo D-Trp^8]S-14

Table 2. Relative Affinities of S-14 and S-28 Analogs for Binding to S-14 Receptors in Normal Rat Tissues*

Peptide	Adrenal cortex	Pituitary	Cerebral cortex
S-14	1	1	1
[des ala^{1}] S-14	0.6	0.8	0.9
[Tyr^{11}] S-14	0.2	0.8	1.0
[Phe^{4}] S-14	1.5	3.5	1.5
[D-Trp^{8}] S-14	1.9	9.6	5.0
[D-Br_5-Trp^{8}] S-14	3.6	9.6	4.2
[L-Br_5-Trp^{8}] S-14	21.5	6.9	6.5
[D-F_5-Trp^{8}] S-14	46.2	31.3	32.2
[L-F_5-Trp^{8}] S-14	18.2	13.9	6.1
[des AA^{1,2,4,5,12,13}, D-Trp^{8}]S-14	0.4	3.0	2.6

*The relative binding affinities compared to that of S-14 taken as 1 were calculated from the concentration (IC_{50}) of the peptide required to produce half maximal inhibition of [^{125}I-Tyr^{11}] S-14 binding.

has similarly been suggested to be due to its increased penetration and distribution in the brain favoured by its greater lipophilicity and/or reduced size (36). However metabolism alone cannot explain the 3-fold differences in the receptor binding affinity of [L-Br_5-Trp^{8}]S-14 in the adrenal cortex compared to brain and pituitary or the striking differences in the in vivo brain potency of [oligo D-Trp^{8}]S-14 compared to its in vitro brain and pituitary receptor binding suggesting that such differences may arise at least in part from differences in the ligand specificity requirement of S-14 receptors in these tissues.

Receptor Binding of Somatostatin-28

Somatostatin-28 (S-28, a twenty-eight amino acid naturally occurring peptide which contains the S-14 moiety at the C-terminal end of the molecule) has been recognized to exhibit greater biological potency than S-14 in some tissues such as pituitary (for GH inhibition) and pancreas (for inhibiting insulin secretion and exocrine function) (37-39). S-28 was found to inhibit the binding of [^{125}I-Tyr^{11}]S-14 in all tissues tested and the displacement curves obtained with S-28 and S-14 were parallel (30, 40) (Fig. 3). The relative affinities of S-28 and S-14 for binding to S-14 receptors however revealed significant differences between tissues. S-28 bound to S-14 receptors with greater affinity than S-14 in the pituitary, but not in brain and in exocrine pancreas whereas both peptides interacted with comparable potencies with S-14 receptors in

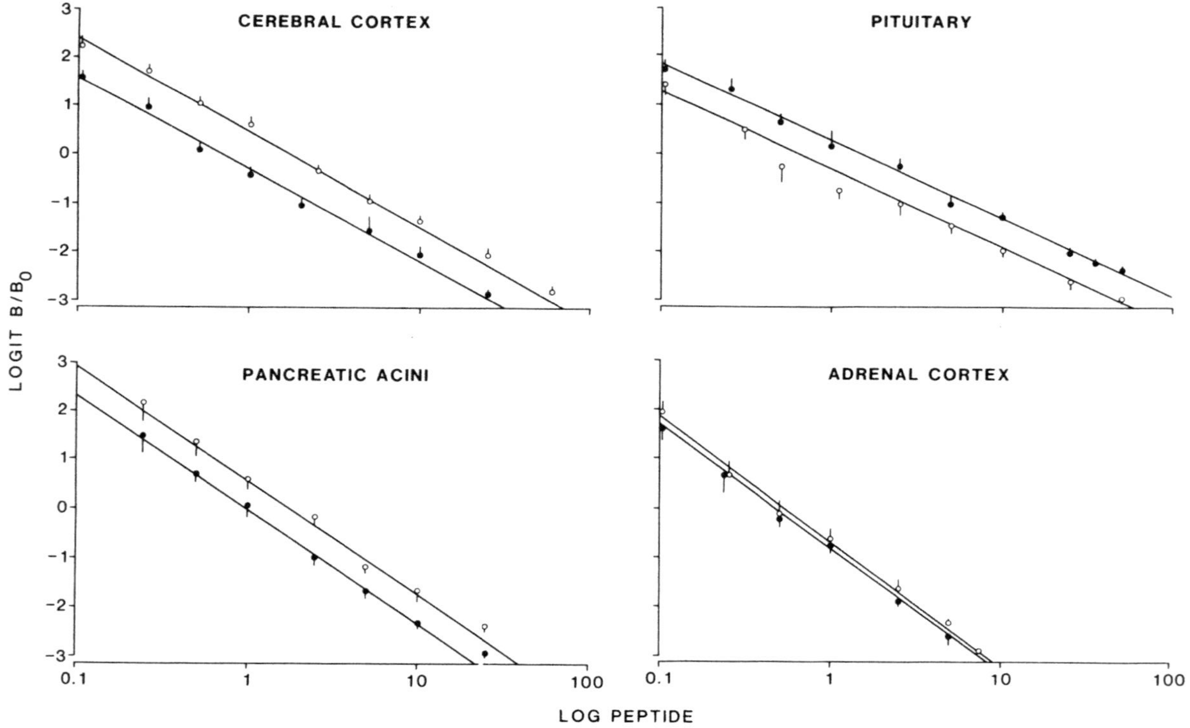

Fig. 3. Inhibition by S-14 (●--●) and S-28 (o--o) of the specific binding of [^{125}I-Tyr^{11}]S-14 to S-14 receptors in rat cerebral cortex, pituitary, exocrine pancreas and adrenal cortex. Competitive inhibition data obtained from equilibrium binding studies are expressed as Logit B/B_O (where B and B_O represent the amounts of radioligand specifically bound in the presence and absence of unlabelled peptide respectively) as a function of the peptide concentration. The curves for the two peptides in each tissue generated using a computer program were tested for parallelism by a t-test and the residual variances of the curves were tested for homogeneity using an f-test.

the adrenal cortex. In a clonal strain of mouse pituitary tumor cells (AtT-20/D16-16) also S-28 bound to S-14 receptors with greater affinity than did S-14 (41). Other groups however have reported that S-28 exhibits either slightly greater affinity (11) or reduced affinity in rat pituitary (6) and in GH_4C_1 cells (32). The reasons for these discrepancies are not clear and could be due to methodological differences and/or to different degrees of competition between S-28 and the various radioligands used in these studies.

The dissociated affinities of S-28 binding to S-14 receptors in different tissues further highlight the heterogeneity of S-14 receptors. Reubi et al. (42) have reported that S-28 bound with greater affinity than S-14 to receptor sites in rat brain quantitated using [Leu^8, D-Trp^{22}, ^{125}I-Tyr^{25}]S-28. In addition, S-28 was reported to be more potent than S-14 in inhibiting centrally mediated bombesin-induced hyperglycemia (36). These observations led us to speculate about the existence of separate S-28 receptors distinct from those of S-14 (40). Cerebrocortical synaptosomal membrane receptors were found to interact with comparable affinity and capacity with both [^{125}I-Tyr^{11}]S-14 and [Leu^8, D-Trp^{22}, ^{125}I-Tyr^{25}]S-28. The estimates of binding sites determined using these radioligands were comparable not only in the brain but also in other tissues (Table 3). Futhermore, S-28 exhibited greater ability than S-14 to inhibit [Leu^8, D-Trp^{22}, ^{125}I-Tyr^{25}]S-28 in the pituitary but not in brain similar to that observed for [^{125}I-Tyr^{11}]S-14 binding sites in these tissues (Table 4). [D-Trp^{22}]S-28 exhibited the highest potency for inhibiting the binding of these two radioligands to both pituitary and brain receptors and its binding affinity was comparable to that of [D-Trp^8]S-14. By contrast, [Leu^8, D-Trp^{22}, Tyr^{25}]S-28 exhibited only about 50% potency compared to [D-Trp^{22}] S-28 against both radioligands suggesting that the additional structural modification in

Table 3. Comparison of [^{125}I-Tyr^{11}]S-14 and [Leu^8, D-Trp^{22}, ^{125}I-Tyr^{25}]S-28 Binding Sites in Normal Rat Tissues

	[^{125}I-Tyr^{11}]S-14 Binding sites		[Leu^8, D-Trp^{22}, ^{125}I-Tyr^{25}]S-28 Binding sites	
	B_{max} (pmol/mg)	K_d(nM)	B_{max} (pmol/mg)	K_d(nM)
Cerebral cortex	400	1.7	360	1.5
Pituitary	305	1.1	320	1.1
Adrenal cortex	350	1.2	210	1.1
Exocrine pancreas	266	0.5	222	1.2

Table 4, Relative Binding Affinities of D-Trp Substituted S-14 and S-28 Analogs

	Relative affinity	
	Cortex	Pituitary
S-14	1	1
S-28	0.2	3.2
[D-Trp^{8}]S-14	5.0	9.6
[D-Trp^{22}]S-28	2.9	9.1
[Leu^{8}, D-Trp^{22}, Tyr^{25}]S-28	1.2	5.5

position 8 (substitution of Met by Leu) in [D-Trp^{22}]S-28 could not only have resulted in the reduced potency but also have conferred more S-14 like properties on the molecule. The use of these two radioligands thus do not appear to permit differentiation of distinct S-14 and S-28 receptors in direct binding studies in the tissues so far tested. Furthermore, the regional distribution of the binding sites in rat CNS quantitated with these two radioligands were similar except in striatum where [Leu^{8}, D-Trp^{22}, ^{125}I-Tyr^{25}] S-28 binding sites appeared to be 1.8 times lower than [^{125}I-Tyr^{11}] S-14 binding sites (Table 5). The highest concentration of receptor sites for both ligands was in the cerebral cortex. The thalamus, hypothalamus, amygdala and hippocampus contained intermediate

Table 5. Regional Distribution of [^{125}I-Tyr^{11}]S-14 and [Leu^{8}, D-Trp^{22}, ^{125}I-Tyr^{25}]S-28 Binding Sites in Rat Brain

Region	[^{125}I-Tyr^{11}] S-14 binding sites	[Leu^{8},D-Trp^{22}, ^{125}I-Tyr^{25}]S-28 binding sites
	(fmol/mg protein)	
Cortex	410 ± 40	360 ± 34.0
Hypothalamus	79 ± 4.3	88 ± 12.0
Thalamus	90 ± 6.0	126 ± 8.6
Hippocampus	34 ± 1.5	40 ± 4.0
Striatum	62 ± 4.8	35 ± 7.0
Amygdala	48 ± 5.7	52 ± 3.8
Midbrain	22 ± 4	15 ± 2.5
Medulla/pons	1.8±0.2	<1
Cerebellum	<1	<1

(N = 10)

receptor densities. Medulla-pons, midbrain, cerebellum and spinal cord exhibited poor binding.

Recently using in vivo autoradiographic labelling techniques we have observed that [Leu^{8}, D-Trp^{22}, ^{125}I-Tyr^{25}]S-28 preferentially labels binding sites in median eminence which interact poorly with [^{125}I-Tyr^{11}]S-14 (43). Thus, the presence of distinct S-28 and S-14 receptors at least in distinct areas of rat brain appears likely. These, however, could not be identified in direct binding studies using these radioligands and perhaps will have to wait development of more selective analogs of S-28.

Regulation of S-14 Receptors

Reisine and Axelrod showed that prolonged pretreatment of ACTH producing mouse pituitary tumor cell (AtT-20) with S-14 led to enhanced biological response of the cells to forskolin stimulation suggesting possible down-regulation of S-14 receptors (44). We have recently observed that pre-exposure of AtT-20 cells to S-14 and/or S-28 down-regulates S-14 receptors (41). Such down-regulation of S-14 receptors in normal tissues may also occur in pathophysiological situations such as stress, diabetes, conditions in which significant elevation in both tissue and plasma somtostatin levels are found (45, 46) but remains to be demonstrated by direct binding studies. Up-regulation of S-14 receptors resulting in increased binding due to decrease in tissue somatostatin was also observed following a depletion of endogenous hormone by cysteamine administration (47). Schonbrunn and Tashjian reported heterologous regulation of S-14 receptors by TRH (48) and glucocorticoids (49) in GH_4C_1 cells but such an heterologous regulation of somatostatin receptors was not observed in normal rat pituitary (4).

REFERENCES

1. Schonbrunn A, Tashjian A Jr 1978 Characterization of functional receptors for somatostatin in rat pituitary cells in culture. J Biol Chem 253:6473.
2. Srikant CB, Patel YC, Specific receptors for somatostatin in rat brain synaptosomal membranes. Program of the 62nd Annual Meeting of the US Endocrine Society, Washington DC 1980, p. 174 (Abstract).
3. Srikant CB, Patel YC 1981 Identification and characterization of somatostatin receptors in rat brain synaptosomal membranes. Proc Natl Acad Sci (USA) 78:3930.
4. Srikant CB, Patel YC 1982 Characterization of pituitary membrane receptors for somatostatin in the rat. Endocrinology 110:2138.
5. Enjalbert A, Tapia-Arancibia L, Rieutort M, Brazeau P, Kordon C, Epelbaum J 1982 Somatostatin receptors in rat anterior pituitary membranes. Endocrinology 110:1634.

6. Reubi J-C, Rivier J, Perrin M, Brown M, Vale W 1982 High affinity binding sites for somatostatin to rat pituitary. Biochem Biophys Res Commun 105:1538.
7. Aguilera G, Parker DS 1982 Pituitary somatostatin receptors: Characterization by binding with a non-degradable peptide analogue. J Biol Chem 257:1134.
8. Taparel D, Esteve JP, Sussini C, Vaysse N, Balas D, Berthon G, Wunsch E, Ribet A 1983 Binding of somatostatin to guinea pig pancreatic membranes: regulation by ions. Biochem Biophys Res Commun 115:827.
9. Esteve JP, Sussini C, Vaysse N, Antoniotti H, Wunsch E, Berthon G, Ribet A 1984 Binding of somatostatin to pancreatic acinar cells. Am J Physiol 247:G62.
10. Srikant CB, Lowden D, Patel YC 1984 Somatostatin receptors in rat pancreatic acini. (Manuscript in preparation).
11. Aguilera G, Parker DS, Catt KJ 1982 Characterization of somatostatin receptors in the rat adrenal glomerulosa zone. Endocrinology 111:1376.
12. Srikant CB, Lowden D, Patel YC, Characterization of rat adrenocortical somatostatin receptors. Program 7th International Congress of Endocrinology, Quebec City, June 1984, Excerpta Medica International Congress Series, p 1424 (Abstract).
13. Srikant CB, Patel YC 1985 Somatostatin receptors in rat adrenal cortex: Characterization and comparison with brain and pituitary receptors. Endocrinology,(in press).
14. Sakamoto C, Goldfine ID, Williams JP 1984 The somatostatin receptors on isolated pancreatic acinar cell plasma membranes: identification of subunit structure and direct regulation by cholecystokinin. J Biol Chem 259:9623.
15. Leitner JW, Rifkin RM, Maman A, Sussman KE 1979 Somatostatin binding to pituitary plasma membranes. Biochem Biophys Res Commun 87:919.
16. Mehler PS, Sussman AL, Maman A, Sussman KE 1980 Role of insulin secretagogues in the regulation of somatostatin binding by isolated rat islets. J Clin Invest 66:1334.
17. Bhathena S, Recant L 1980 Somatostatin receptors in circulating human blood cells. Horm Metab Res 12:277.
18. Marks N, Stern F, Benuck M 1976 Correlation between biological potency and biodegradation of a somatostatin analog. Nature 261:511.
19. Epelbaum J, Tapia-Arancibia L, Kordon E, Enjalbert A 1982 Characterization, regional and subcellular distribution of ^{125}I-Tyr^{1} somatostatin binding sites in rat brain. J Neurochem 38:1515.
20. Richardson UI, Schonbrunn A 1981 Inhibition of adrenocorticotropin secretion by somatostatin in pituitary cells in culture. Endocrinology 108:281.
21. Czernik AJ, Petrack B 1983 Somatostatin receptor binding in rat cerebral cortex: Characterization using a non-reducible somatostatin analog. J Biol Chem 258:5525.

22. Patel YC, Amherdt M, Orci L 1982 Quantitative electron microscopic autoradiography of insulin, glucagon and somatostatin binding sites on islets. Science 217:1155.
23. Ogawa N, Thompson J, Friesen HG, Martin JB, Brazeau P 1977 Properties of soluble somatostatin binding protein. Biochem J 165:155.
24. Sussman KE, Mehler PS, Leitner JW, Draznin B 1982 Role of secretion vesicles in the transport of receptors: Modulation of somatostatin binding to pancreatic islets. Endocrinology 111:316.
25. Reyl FJ, Lewin MGM 1982 Evidence for an intracellular somatostatin receptor in pancreas: A comparative study with reference to gastric mucosa. Biochem Biophys Res Commun 109:1324.
26. Reyl FJ, Lewin MGM 1982 Intracellular receptor for somatostatin in gastric mucosal cells: Decomposition and reconstitution of somatostatin stimulated phosphoprotein phosphatase. Proc Natl Acad Sci (USA) 79:978.
27. Vale W, Rivier J, Ling N, Brown M 1978 Biologic and immunologic activities and applications of somatostatin analogs. Metabolism 27 (Suppl. 1):1391.
28. Meyers CA, Coy DH, Huang WY, Schally AV, Redding TW 1978 Higher active position 8 analogues of somatostatin and separation of peptide diasterioisomers by partition chromatography. Biochemistry 17:2326.
29. Veber DF, Holly FW, Nutt RF, Bergstrand SJ, Brady SF, Hirschman R, Glitzer MS, Sapperstein R 1979 Highly active cyclic and bicyclic analogues of reduced ring size. Nature 280:512.
30. Srikant CB, Patel YC 1981 Somatostatin analogs: Dissociation of brain receptor binding affinities and pituitary actions in the rat. Endocrinology 108:341.
31. Srikant CB, Coy D, Patel YC 1983 Position 4 substituted somatostatin analogs: Increased binding to somatostatin receptors in pituitary and brain. Life Sci 33:201.
32. Schonbrunn A, Rorstad OP, Westendorf JM, Martin JB 1983 Somatostatin analogs: Correlation between receptor binding affinity and biological potency in GH pituitary cells. Endocrinology 113:1559.
33. Reubi J-C, Peerin M, Rivier J, Vale W 1982 Pituitary somatostatin receptors: dissociation at the pituitary level of receptor affinity and biological activity for selective somatostatin analogs. Regul Peptides 4:141.
34. Coy DH, Meyers CA, Arimura A, Schally AV, Redding TW 1978 Observations on the growth hormone, insulin and glucagon release-inhibiting activities of somatostatin analogues. Metabolism 27 (Suppl. 1):1407.
35. Meyers CA, Coy DH, Murphy WA, Redding TW, Arimura A, Schally AV 1980 [Phe^4]somatostatin: A potent selective inhibitor of growth hormone release. Proc Natl Acad Sci (USA) 77:577.
36. Brown M, Rivier J, Vale W 1979 Somatostatin: Central nervous system actions on glucoregulation. Endocrinology 104:1709.

37. Böhlen P, Brazeau P, Benoit R, Ling N, Esch F, Guillemin R 1980 Isolation and aminoacid composition of two somatostatin-like peptides from ovine hypothalamus: somatostatin-28 and somatostatin-25. Biochem Biophys Res Commun 96:725.
38. Brazeau P, Ling N, Esch F, Böhlen P, Benoit R, Guillemin R 1981 High biological activities of synthetic replicates of somatostatin-28 and somatostatin-25. Regul Peptides 1:255.
39. Sussini C, Esteve JP, Vaysse N, Pradayrol L, Ribet A 1980 Somatostatin-28: Effects on exocrine pancreatic secretion in conscious dogs. Gastroenterology 79:720.
40. Srikant CB, Patel YC 1981 Receptor binding of somatostatin-28 is tissue specific. Nature 294:259.
41. Srikant CB, Heisler S 1984 Relationship between receptor binding and biopotency of somatostatin-14 and somatostatin-28 in mouse pituitary tumor cells. Endocrinology (submitted).
42. Reubi J-C, Perrin M, Rivier J, Vale W 1981 High affinity binding sites for a somatostatin-28 analog in rat brain. Life Sciences 28:2191.
43. Patel YC, Baquiran G, Srikant CB, Posner BI, Localization of [^{125}I-Tyr^{11}] somatostatin-14 and [Leu^{8}, D-Trp^{22}, ^{125}I-Tyr^{25}] S-28 binding sites in the rat brain by in vivo autoradiography. Program Somatostatin Symposium, Montreal, June 1984, Abstract #25.
44. Reisine T, Axelrod J 1983 Prolonged somatostatin pretreatment desensitizes somatostatin's inhibition of receptor-mediated release of adrenocorticotropin hormone and sensitizes adenylate cyclase. Endocrinology 113:811.
45. Berelowitz M, Kronheim S, Pimstone B, Shapiro B 1978 Somatostatin-like immunoreactivity in rat blood. J Clin Invest 61:1410.
46. Orci L, Baetens D, Dubois MP, Rufener C 1975 Evidence for the D-cell of the pancreas secreting somatostatin. Horm Metab Res 7:400.
47. Srikant CB, Patel YC 1984 Cysteamine-induced depletion of brain somatostatin is associated with upregulation of cerebrocortical somatostatin receptors. Endocrinology 115:990.
48. Schonbrunn A, Tashjian A Jr 1980 Modulation of somatostatin receptors by thyrotropin-releasing hormone in a clonal pituitary cell strain. J Biol Chem 255:190.
49. Schonbrunn A 1982 Glucocorticoids down-regulate somatostatin receptors on pituitary cells in culture. Endocrinology 110:1147.

17

MECHANISMS OF SOMATOSTATIN ACTION IN PITUITARY CELLS*

AGNES SCHONBRUNN, LANETA J. DORFLINGER** AND BRUCE D. KOCH

Laboratory of Toxicology
Harvard School of Public Health
Boston, Massachusetts 02115

INTRODUCTION

Tetradecapeptide somatostatin (S-14, SRIF) inhibits secretion by a large number of different target cells, and therefore studies probing its mechanism of action have focused on the involvement of two intracellular messengers known to regulate secretory processes: cyclic AMP and calcium (for reviews see references 1-5). However, the results from mechanistic studies have been complex and, at times, contradictory. Thus, the biochemical events which mediate the inhibitory actions of S-14 are still not well understood. In fact, S-14 has been proposed to act at all possible sites: it has been hypothesized to regulate the concentrations of both cyclic AMP and calcium, as well as the effectiveness of a given concentration of each of these intracellular messengers. This review summarizes our studies on the role of cyclic AMP in S-14 inhibition of hormone secretion by a clonal pituitary-tumor cell line (GH_4C_1) and relates our observations to those reported by other investigators in the more complex mixed population present in primary cultures of pituitary cells.

Effect of S-14 on Cyclic AMP Levels

Three types of studies originally supported the hypothesis that inhibition of pituitary hormone release by S-14 resulted from

*The experiments described in this review were supported by a research grant from the NIADDK (AM-32234).
**Current address: Office of Population, Agency for International Development, Washington, D.C. 20523.

its depression of intracellular cyclic AMP levels. First, cyclic AMP analogs and inhibitors of cyclic nucleotide phosphodiesterases were found to stimulate the release of GH, TSH and PRL by primary cultures of pituitary cells (4, 5), whereas S-14 inhibited the secretion of these hormones (4-9). Second, under some conditions, S-14 was found to inhibit basal (10, 11) and stimulated (5, 10-14) cyclic AMP levels in pituitary tissue or dispersed pituitary cells. Finally, S-14 inhibited prostaglandin E_1-stimulated adenylate cyclase activity in rat pituitary membranes (15, 16) and basal and chlorpromazine-stimulated adenylate cyclase activity in membranes prepared from the GH_1 clonal rat pituitary cell line (17). However, other results were not consistent with the hypothesis that S-14 elicited its effects by decreasing intracellular cyclic AMP levels. Some investigators were unable to demonstrate an effect of S-14 on basal (12-14) or stimulated (18) cyclic AMP accumulation under conditions in which hormone secretion was inhibited. Furthermore, S-14 did not inhibit basal adenylate cyclase activity in rat pituitary membranes (15,16).

The conflicting observations regarding the requirement for reduced cyclic AMP levels in S-14 action may have resulted from the presence of several different cell types responsive to S-14 in the pituitary preparations used. This heterogeneity in the cell population precludes correlation of general intracellular metabolic events with the secretion of a specific hormone by a single cell type. To avoid such ambiguity, we have used a clonal cell line (GH_4C_1) derived from a rat pituitary tumor to examine the mechanisms of S-14 action in a homogeneous pituitary cell population.

GH_4C_1 cells synthesize and secrete GH and PRL and respond in culture to many of the same regulatory hormones as normal pituitary cells do <u>in situ</u> (19-21). Somatostatin-14 inhibits the secretion of PRL and GH by GH_4C_1 cells in a parallel manner (22, 23). The action of S-14 is rapid: maximal inhibition of hormone secretion is observed by 5 minutess, the earliest time examined (Koch and Schonbrunn, unpublished observations). Furthermore, S-14 inhibits both basal (22) and hormone-stimulated (23, 24) secretion by GH_4C_1 cells and all the biological actions of S-14 appear to be initiated by a single class of specific, high-affinity receptors (22, 25). Although S-14 receptors have not yet been characterized in intact normal pituitary cells, the analog specificity and affinity of the S-14 receptor in GH_4C_1 cells appear to be very similar, although not identical, to that described for rat pituitary membranes (22, 25, 26). Furthermore, the effects of S-14 on hormone secretion in GH_4C_1 cells mimic those observed in primary cultures of rat pituitary cells (22-24, 27-30).

To determine whether changes in cyclic AMP concentrations are involved in S-14 action, we first examined the ability of S-14 to inhibit cyclic AMP accumulation by GH_4C_1 cells. Although S-14 sometimes caused a small decrease in basal cyclic AMP levels, in most experiments it did not significantly inhibit basal cyclic AMP accumulation (93 ± 3% of control, n = 13) (31). In contrast, S-14 consistently inhibited stimulation of cyclic AMP accumulation by the secretagogue vasoactive intestinal peptide (VIP) (31). The inhibition of VIP-stimulated cyclic AMP accumulation by S-14 was maximal by 15 seconds, the earliest time tested and therefore appeared to be sufficiently rapid to initiate inhibition by S-14 of VIP-stimulated hormone release (31).

Several lines of evidence indicated that the inhibition of VIP-stimulated cyclic AMP accumulation by S-14 was mediated by the previously characterized high-affinity S-14 receptors. Half-maximal inhibition of VIP-stimulated cyclic AMP accumulation occurred with a concentration of S-14 (1.2 nM) close to its apparent equilibrium dissociation constant for binding to the cellular S-14 receptor K_d = 0.6 nM) (22, 31). The potencies of a series of S-14 analogs for inhibition of VIP-stimulated cyclic AMP accumulation correlated closely with the affinity of each analog for the S-14 receptor (25, 31). Finally, S-14 had no effect on VIP-stimulated cyclic AMP accumulation in GH_2C_1 cells, a closely related cell line which lacks S-14 receptors (22, 31).

The conclusion that inhibition of stimulated cyclic AMP accumulation by S-14 was a receptor-mediated process raised two related questions: 1) What was the mechanism by which S-14 receptor occupancy lowered cyclic AMP concentrations, and 2) What was the role of the induced changes in cyclic AMP levels in eliciting the biological effects of S-14?

How Does S-14 Inhibit Cyclic AMP Accumulation?

To determine whether the primary site of S-14 action was to stimulate phosphodiesterase activity or to inhibit adenylate cyclase, we measured the degree to which S-14 inhibited VIP-stimulated cyclic AMP accumulation in the presence of varying concentrations of the phosphodiesterase inhibitor 3-isobutyl-1-methylxanthine (IBMX). We reasoned that if S-14 acted to stimulate phosphodiesterase, pharmacological inhibition of this enzyme should block the effects of S-14 on cyclic AMP levels. As expected, increasing concentrations of IBMX (0-1 mM) markedly increased cyclic AMP levels. However, neither the stimulatory effect of VIP (1140 ± 40% of control), nor the degree to which S-14 inhibited VIP-stimulation (56 ± 3%), was altered at any concentration of IBMX (31). Therefore, both VIP and S-14 appeared to act primarily by modulating adenylate cyclase and not by inhibiting phosphodiesterase activity.

We then examined the effect of S-14 on adenylate cyclase activity in GH_4C_1 cell membranes to determine whether the S-14 receptor was directly coupled to adenylate cyclase (32). As in intact cells, maximal concentrations of S-14 (100 nM) had no significant effect on unstimulated adenylate cyclase activity (99.6 ± 7.3% of control). The results in Fig. 1 compare the effects of S-14 on VIP-stimulated cyclic AMP accumulation in intact GH_4C_1 cells and on VIP-stimulated adenylate cyclase activity in membrane preparations. VIP increased both membrane adenylate cyclase activity and cellular cyclic AMP levels in a concentration-dependent manner, with ED_{50} values of 1 and 3 nM, respectively (Fig. 1). Both in membranes and cells, 100 nM S-14 partially decreased the maximal stimulatory effect of VIP, but did not significantly change its ED_{50} value (Fig. 1). Half-maximal inhibition of adenylate cyclase was produced by 2.3 nM S-14, in good agreement with its potency as an inhibitor of cyclic AMP accumulation in intact cells (ED_{50} = 1.2 nM) (31, 32). Furthermore, the rank orders of potencies for several S-14 analogs as inhibitors of cyclic AMP production in cells and adenylate cyclase activity in membrane preparations were the same (31, 32).

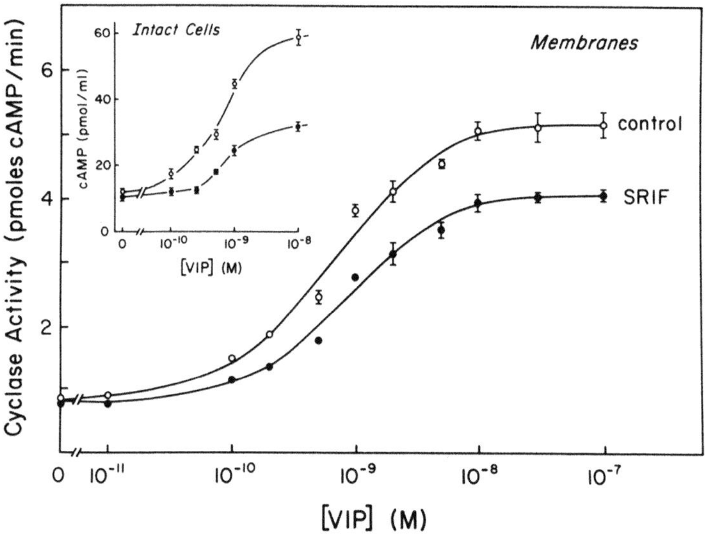

Fig. 1 Concentration dependence of VIP-stimulated adenylate cyclase activity and cyclic AMP accumulation in the absence and presence of S-14 (shown as SRIF). Adenylate cyclase activity was measured in GH_4C_1 cell membranes as previously described (32). Incubations were carried out for 10 min in the presence of the indicated concentrations of VIP in the absence (o) or presence (•) of 100 nM S-14. Each point represents the mean±SD of quadruplicate determinations. The inset shows the effect of various concentrations of VIP on cyclic AMP accumulation in intact GH_4C_1 cells during a 20-min incubation (31). Each point represents the mean ± SE of triplicate incubations.

The similarity between the effects of S-14 on cyclic AMP accumulation in intact cells and on adenylate cyclase activity in membranes further supported the conclusion that the observed changes in cyclic AMP levels were due to modulation of adenylate cyclase activity.

Other receptors which regulate adenylate cyclase do not interact directly with the enzyme. Rather, GTP is required for the hormonal modulation of enzyme activity and guanine nucleotides alter the binding properties of other cyclase-linked receptors (33-35). Regulation of both adenylate cyclase activity and agonist binding are mediated by subunits of adenylate cyclase which bind GTP. Therefore, to determine whether S-14 inhibited adenylate cyclase via a guanine-nucleotide binding protein, we examined the effects of various nucleotides on the binding of $[^{125}I\text{-}Tyr^1]$ S-14 to GH_4C_1 cell membranes.

At a concentration of 0.1 mM, the nonhydrolyzable GTP analog, Gpp(NH)p, decreased saturable $[^{125}I\text{-}Tyr^1]$ S-14 binding to GH_4C_1 cell membranes to 13% of the control value (32). The effect of Gpp(NH)p on $[^{125}I\text{-}Tyr^1]$ S-14 binding was concentration-dependent, with an ED_{50} of 0.3 μM. In contrast, the nonhydrolyzable ATP analog, App(NH)p, had no effect on $[^{125}I\text{-}Tyr^1]$ S-14 binding at a concentration of 0.1 mM (102 ± 7% of control values). In the presence of 0.1 mM App(NH)p, which acts as an inhibitor of nonspecific nucleotidases, 0.15 mM GTP decreased saturable $[^{125}I\text{-}Tyr^1]$ S-14 binding to 30% of the control value (32). Thus, the binding of $[^{125}I\text{-}Tyr^1]$ S-14 to its membrane receptor was decreased specifically by guanine nucleotides.

To determine whether guanine nucleotides altered receptor affinity or receptor number, we examined the effect of a submaximal concentration (0.15 mM) of GTP on the equilibrium binding of S-14 to GH_4C_1 cell membranes (32). Nonlinear regression analysis of these data showed that both in the presence and absence of GTP, the data were fit by an equation describing binding to a single class of saturable receptor sites. Furthermore, the B_{max} values in the absence (0.21 pmol/mg) and presence (0.23 pmol / mg) of GTP were not significantly different ($p > 0.9$, $n = 3$). In contrast, receptor affinity for S-14 was significantly reduced by GTP ($p < 0.001$). The equilibrium dissociation constant for S-14 was 0.11 nM in the absence of GTP and 0.40 nM in the presence of 0.15 mM GTP (32). Therefore, GTP did not alter the total number of S-14 binding sites in GH_4C_1 cell membranes, but it did reduce the affinity of these sites for the agonist S-14. The observation that guanine nucleotides decreased the apparent affinity of the S-14 receptor supported the involvement of a guanine nucleotide binding protein in S-14 inhibition of adenylate cyclase.

The results in Fig. 2 demonstrate that the decrease in binding affinity induced by guanine nucleotides can be explained by an increase in the rate constant for S-14 dissociation. In the absence of guanine nucleotides, [^{125}I-Tyr^{1}] S-14 dissociation followed first order kinetics ($t_{\frac{1}{2}}$ = 180 min) indicating that all occupied receptors were in the same affinity state. In contrast, in the presence of a half-maximal concentration of Gpp(NH)p, [^{125}I-Tyr^{1}] S-14 dissociation kinetics were more complex and could be resolved into the sum of two first order rates. Fifty percent of the specifically bound [^{125}I-Tyr^{1}] S-14 dissociated at a rate ($t_{\frac{1}{2}}$ = 150 min) not significantly different from that observed in the absence of nucleotide ($p > 0.2$), whereas the remainder dissociated 15 times more rapidly ($t_{\frac{1}{2}}$ =10 min). These results indicate the existence of two freely interconvertible forms of the S-14 receptor: a half-maximal concentration of Gpp(NH)p converted 50% of a slowly dissociating form of the receptor into a rapidly dissociating form.

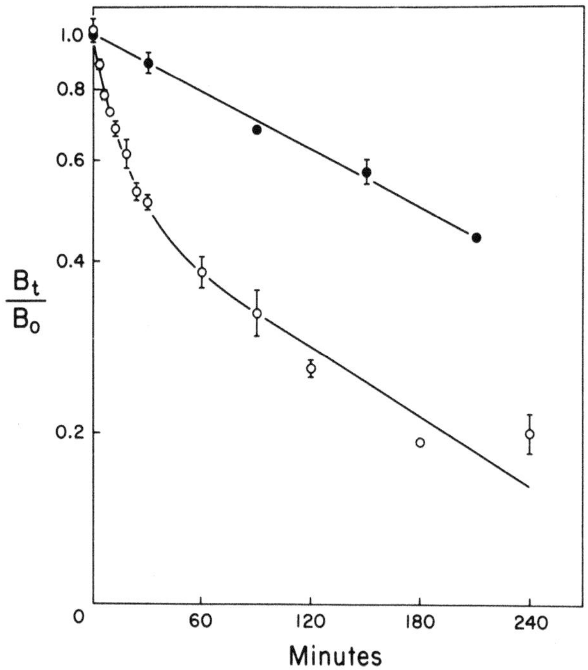

Fig. 2. Effect of 0.3 μM Gpp(NH)p on [^{125}I-Tyr^{1}] S-14 dissociation. [^{125}I-Tyr^{1}]S-14 was incubated for 90 min at 37 C in the absence (•) or presence (o) of 0.3 μM Gpp(NH)p as previously described (32). The reaction mixture was then diluted into 2 volumes of buffer containing 150 nM S-14 with or without 0.3 μM Gpp(NH)p. Saturable [^{125}I-Tyr^{1}] S-14 binding was determined at the times shown. Each point represents the mean ± SE of triplicate determinations, and the lines are the computer-fitted regression lines (32).

The ability of guanine nucleotides to alter the affinity of β-adrenergic receptors, which stimulate adenylate cyclase, has been explained by proposing an equilibrium between two interconvertible receptor forms with different affinities for agonists (36). In this model, hormone (H), receptor (R), and a guanine nucleotide binding protein (N) interact according to Equation I:

$$\begin{array}{lcccl} H + R & \rightleftharpoons & H.R & & \text{Low Affinity} \\ \quad\ \ \updownarrow N & & \updownarrow N & & \qquad\qquad (I) \\ H + R.N & & H.R.N & & \text{High Affinity} \end{array}$$

Binding of GTP or Gpp(NH)p to N results in destabilization of the ternary complex and a shift in the equilibrium from the high affinity form (H.R.N.) to the low affinity form of the receptor (H.R).

Our results with the S-14 receptor in GH_4C_1 cell membranes are consistent with the model shown in Equation I if the concentration of the guanine nucleotide-binding protein (N) substantially exceeds the receptor (R) concentration (37). Guanine nucleotides do regulate the interconversion of the S-14 receptor between a slowly dissociating, high affinity form and a rapidly dissociating, low affinity form. Thus, according to the model, the linear Scatchard plots observed both in the presence and absence of guanine nucleotides provide binding affinities which represent a weighted average of the affinities of the two states of the receptor (37, 38).

In contrast to our results, Enjalbert et al. (39) reported that guanine nucleotides reduce the number, but not the affinity, of S-14 receptors in rat pituitary membranes. In their experiments, equilibrium binding parameters were determined by increasing the concentration of the radioligand [^{125}I -Tyr]-S-14, whereas in our experiments increasing amounts of native S-14 were used to compete for the binding of nonsaturating concentrations of [^{125}I-Tyr^{1}] S-14. The different technical limitations of these methods could explain the discrepant results obtained in equilibrium binding studies with the two systems. Therefore, analysis of the kinetics of S-14 binding to normal rat pituitary membranes in the presence and absence of guanine nucleotides will be necessary to conclude that the coupling mechanisms in the two systems are indeed different. Nevertheless, our observations that guanine nucleotides increased the rate of [^{125}I-Tyr^{1}] S-14 dissociation and decreased the apparent affinity of the S-14 receptor in GH_4C_1 cells supported the conclusion that a guanine nucleotide-binding protein could mediate inhibition of adenylate cyclase by S-14 in a manner analogous to the action of stimulatory ligands.

We next utilized the Bordetella pertussis toxin, islets-activating protein (IAP), to determine whether the guanine nucleotide binding protein which couples the GH_4C_1 cell S-14 receptor to adenylate cyclase is related to that which mediates inhibition of adenylate cyclase by other receptors. Islets activating protein catalyzes the ADP-ribosylation of a membrane-associated guanine nucleotide binding protein (N_i) and thereby reduces the inhibition of adenylate cyclase by a variety of hormones and neurotransmitters (40, 41). Pretreatment of GH_4C_1 cells with IAP blocked S-14 inhibition of VIP-stimulated cyclic AMP accumulation (42). In membranes prepared from IAP pretreated cells, S-14 inhibition of VIP-stimulated adenylate cyclase activity was reduced and [^{125}I-Tyr^{1}] S-14 binding was decreased by over 90% (42). These results indicate that ADP-ribosylated N_i is unable to form a high affinity complex with the occupied S-14 receptor and suggest that S-14 inhibition of VIP-stimulated adenylate cyclase occurs by interaction with the S-14 receptor via this inhibitory guanine nucleotide binding protein.

Observations in other systems have also supported the conclusion that N_i participates in S-14 inhibition of adenylate cyclase activity. Using cyc^-S49 lymphoma cell membranes, Jakobs et al. (43, 44) showed that GTP is required for S-14 inhibition of forskolin-stimulated adenylate cyclase activity and that S-14 stimulates the hydrolysis of GTP. Furthermore, IAP prevented both of these actions of S-14 (45). Thus, S-14 appears to belong to a class of agents, including muscarinic agonists, adenosine, dopamine and certain opiates, which inhibit adenylate cyclase by interaction with the guanine nucleotide-binding regulatory subunit, N_i.

Does Inhibition of Cyclic AMP Production Elicit the Biological Actions of S-14?

Two approaches were used to determine the importance of changes in adenylate cyclase activity and cyclic AMP concentrations in the mechanism of S-14 action in GH_4C_1 cells (23). First, we quantitatively compared the effects of S-14 and VIP on hormone release and cyclic AMP production. Second, we determined the effects of S-14 on hormone release stimulated by two other secretagogues which increase effective intracellular cyclic AMP concentrations: forskolin, which increases intracellular cyclic AMP levels by activating adenylate cyclase, and 8-Br-cyclic AMP which mimics cyclic AMP action.

The results in Fig. 1 (insert) showed that S-14 inhibited VIP-stimulated cyclic AMP production in a non-competitive manner, but did not alter basal cyclic AMP accumulation. A parallel experiment showing the effects of S-14 on hormone secretion is shown in Fig. 3. VIP increased both GH and PRL release to the same extent (220% of control) and the concentrations of VIP required to produce half-maximal stimulation of GH and PRL secretion were the same (0.4 nM).

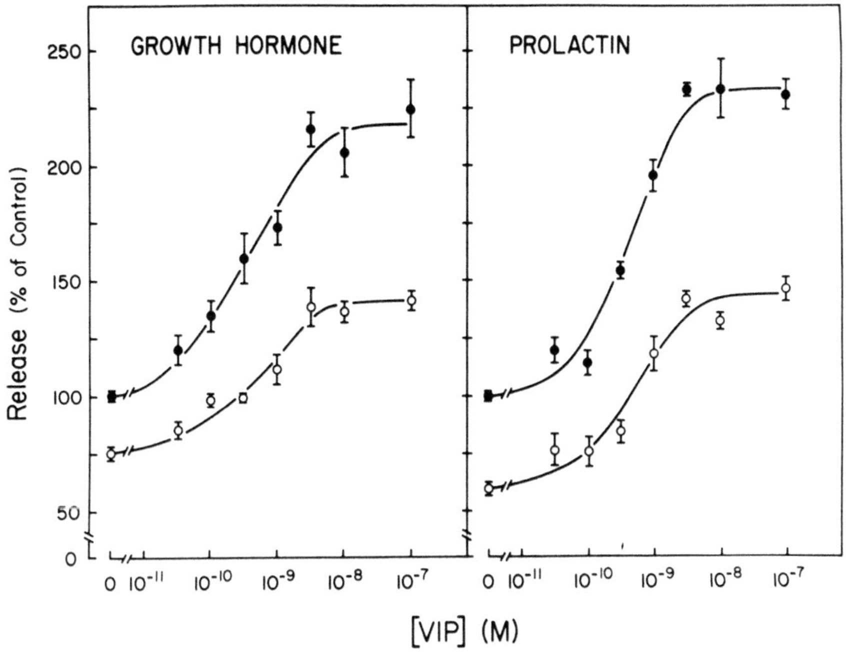

Fig. 3. Concentration dependence of VIP-stimulated hormone release in the absence and presence of S-14. Hormone release was determined during a 30-min incubation with the concentrations of VIP shown both in the absence (●) and presence (o) of 100 nM S-14 (23). The amounts of GH and PRL in the media were determined by RIA. Each value is expressed as a percent of the amount of hormone released in the absence of any added peptides in the same experiment and represents the mean ± SE of triplicate dishes in either two (left panel) or three (right panel) independent experiments.

In the presence of 100 nM S-14, both basal and VIP-stimulated hormone secretion were inhibited. Somatostatin-14 reduced maximal VIP-stimulated hormone secretion, but it did not significantly alter the dose-response characteristics of VIP. Therefore, the action of S-14 to noncompetitively inhibit VIP stimulation of hormone release paralleled its effects on VIP-stimulated cyclic AMP accumulation. However, there was a clear distinction between the inhibition of basal hormone secretion by S-14 and its lack of effect on basal cyclic AMP levels. Thus, if the effect of S-14 on VIP-stimulated cyclic AMP production is of biological significance, it is necessary to postulate two mechanisms for S-14 action. Inhibition of VIP-stimulated hormone release could be mediated by alterations in cyclic AMP levels, but inhibition of basal hormone release had to occur independently of changes in cyclic AMP concentrations. To test this hypothesis, we examined the effects of S-14 on hormone secretion stimulated by 8-Br-cyclic AMP and forskolin.

8-Br-cyclic AMP directly stimulates cyclic AMP-dependent protein kinases and therefore elicits cyclic AMP inducible effects at a site distal to the activation of adenylate cyclase (46). Concentrations of 8-Br-cyclic AMP from 1 to 20 mM produced a dose-dependent stimulation of PRL release in GH_4C_1 cells (Fig. 4). At each concentration of 8-Br-cyclic AMP, S-14 decreased PRL secretion by the same amount that it reduced basal release. Therefore, S-14 inhibition of this increment of hormone secretion appears to proceed by a mechanism which is unaffected by the concentration of intracellular cyclic AMP.

To determine the effect of S-14 on stimulation of hormone secretion by VIP and 8-Br-cyclic AMP, the difference between the amount of PRL secreted in the presence and absence of each secretagogue was calculated from the data in Figs. 3 and 4. The net effect of this calculation was to subtract the amount that S-14 inhibited basal hormone secretion (Fig. 5). The calculated data showed that 8-Br-cyclic AMP increased PRL release above the appropriate basal

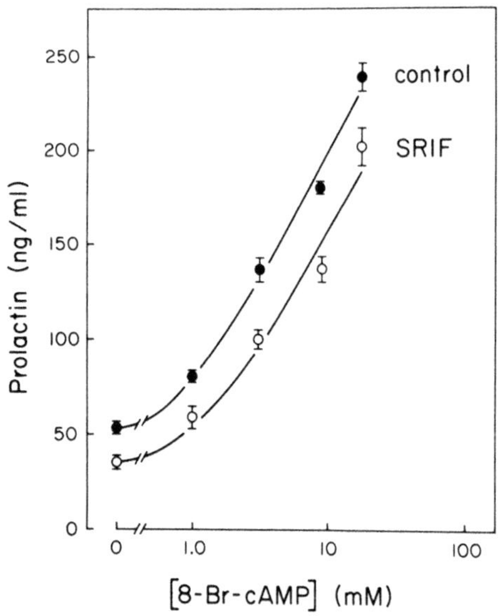

Fig. 4. Concentration dependence of 8-Br-cyclic AMP-stimulated PRL secretion in the absence and presence of S-14 (shown as SRIF). PRL release was determined during a 30-min incubation with the concentrations of 8-Br-cyclic AMP shown both in the absence (•) and presence (o) of 100 nM S-14 as previously described (23). Each point represents the mean ± SE of triplicate dishes in one of two independent experiments.

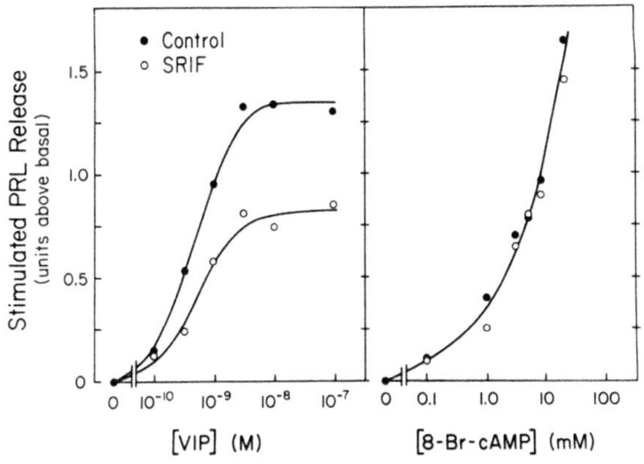

Fig. 5. Effect of S-14 (shown as SRIF) on the stimulatory action of VIP and 8-Br-cyclic AMP on PRL secretion. Within each experiment, the amount of PRL released in the absence of any secretagogue was assigned the control value of 1 both in the absence (•) and presence (o) of 100 nM S-14. The amount of PRL secreted at each concentration of secretagogue was then expressed as units above the corresponding control value. Each point represents the average of values from three independent experiments with VIP or two independent experiments with 8-Br-cyclic AMP. Error bars are omitted for clarity in this figure but are shown for the untransformed data in Figs. 3 and 4.

value by the same amount whether or not S-14 was present (Fig. 5, right panel). The inability of S-14 to inhibit the stimulatory effect of 8-Br-cyclic AMP, which acts distal to adenylate cyclase, was in marked contrast to its action to decrease VIP stimulation of hormone secretion (Fig. 5, left panel). In fact, the parallel inhibition of VIP-stimulated cyclic AMP accumulation and VIP-stimulated hormone secretion supported the conclusion that these two actions of S-14 were related.

The diterpene forskolin stimulates cyclic AMP accumulation in intact cells and activates adenylate cyclase in membrane preparations from several different tissues (47). Therefore, forskolin offered an alternate agent for manipulating cyclic AMP levels in GH_4C_1 cells and provided an advantage over 8-Br-cyclic AMP in that its effect on cyclic AMP concentrations, as well as on hormone secretion, could be evaluated.

Forskolin increased cyclic AMP levels in a concentration-dependent manner (ED_{50} of 2.4 μM) (23). Although 0.1 mM forskolin stimulated cyclic AMP levels to a much greater extent (35-fold) than did 100 nM VIP (10-fold), the two agents increased PRL secretion by the same amount (Fig. 6). Therefore the 10-fold increase in cyclic AMP concentrations induced by VIP must be sufficient to fully stimulate PRL release by a cyclic AMP dependent mechanism. Not unexpectedly, although forskolin and VIP added together caused an even greater increase in cyclic AMP levels than either agent alone, the combined effect of the two secretagogues on PRL secretion was not additive (Fig. 6).

We took advantage of the effect of forskolin to elicit supramaximal cyclic AMP levels in order to test whether inhibition of VIP-stimulated cyclic AMP accumulation was indeed required for S-14 inhibition of VIP-stimulated hormone release. Somatostatin-14 decreased forskolin (0.1 mM) stimulation of cyclic AMP accumulation from 35-fold to 25-fold (Fig. 6, top panel). As with 8-Br-cyclic AMP, S-14 inhibited PRL secretion in the presence of forskolin by about the same amount as in its absence (Fig. 6, bottom panel). In

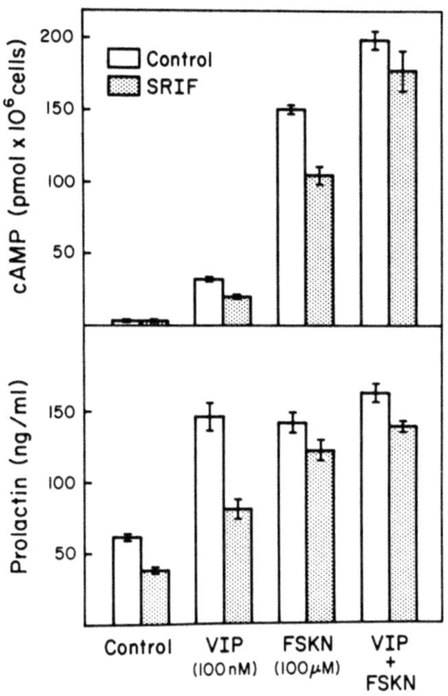

Fig. 6. The effect of S-14 (shown as SRIF) on VIP-stimulated cyclic AMP accumulation and PRL secretion in the absence and presence of forskolin. The effects of VIP and forskolin on cyclic AMP accumulation (top panel) were determined both in the absence and presence of 100 nM S-14 during a 20-min incubation (23). The effects of the same agents on PRL release (bottom panel) were determined during a 30-min incubation (23). Each point represents the mean ± SE of triplicate incubations.

contrast, S-14 reduced VIP-stimulated PRL release more than basal secretion. The inability of S-14 to decrease the stimulation of PRL release by forskolin was consistent with the observation that cyclic AMP levels achieved in the presence of forskolin plus S-14 exceeded those produced by 100 nM VIP.

Although S-14 slightly reduced the stimulation of cyclic AMP levels produced by forskolin plus VIP, the concentrations of cyclic AMP achieved still exceeded those produced by VIP alone. In the presence of both VIP and forskolin, S-14 decreased PRL secretion only the same amount as it did basal PRL release. Thus, forskolin prevented the inhibition of VIP-stimulated PRL release by S-14, but it did not appear to block the inhibition by S-14 of basal PRL release. The results with 8-Br-cyclic AMP and forskolin strongly support the hypothesis that inhibition of VIP-stimulated cyclic AMP accumulation by S-14 is causally linked to inhibition of VIP-stimulated hormone secretion, whereas inhibition of basal hormone secretion is independent of cyclic AMP concentrations.

Does the Same Receptor Initiate Both Mechanisms of S-14 Action?

Equilibrium binding studies with [^{125}I-Tyr^{1}] S-14 have shown that GH_4C_1 cells contain a single class of high-affinity binding sites for S-14 (22). To determine whether the receptors characterized by [^{125}I-Tyr^{1}] S-14 binding initiate one or both mechanisms of S-14 action, we determined the potencies of a series of S-14 analogs to inhibit VIP-stimulated cyclic AMP production (the cyclic-AMP mediated mechanism) and to inhibit basal PRL secretion (the cyclic AMP independent mechanism). The potencies in these two biological assays were then compared to the respective affinities for binding of the analogs to the cellular S-14 receptor measured under the same conditions (25). The relationship between the relative affinity of each S-14 analog for binding to GH_4C_1 cell receptors and its relative biological potency is plotted on a logarithmic scale in Fig. 7. A linear relationship was found over a 10,000-fold range in activities (correlation coefficient, r = 0.96; slope = 0.95). The excellent correlation observed between the biological activities and binding affinities of S-14 analogs supports the conclusion that the high affinity binding sites characterized in GH_4C_1 cells represent the biologically relevant receptors that mediate the actions of S-14 by both the cyclic AMP dependent and independent mechanisms.

Is a Functional N_i Required for Both Mechanisms of S-14 Action?

We utilized the Bordetella pertussis toxin IAP to determine whether a functional N_i was required for S-14 action by the cyclic AMP-mediated as well as by the cyclic AMP-independent mechanisms (42). Pretreatment of GH_4C_1 cells with IAP blocked both the inhibition of VIP-stimulated cyclic AMP accumulation and the inhibition of VIP-stimulated PRL secretion by S-14 (42). More

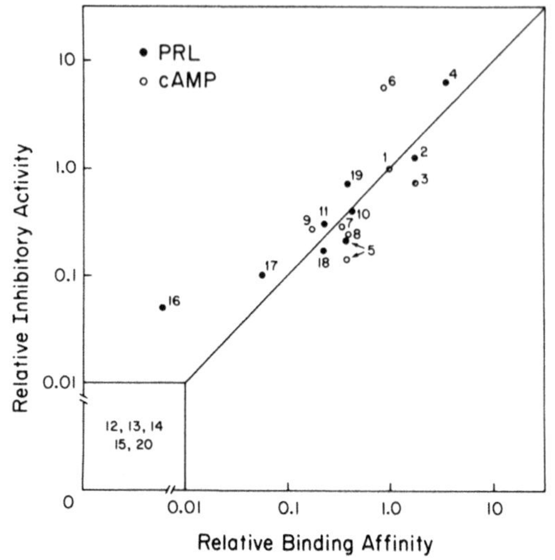

Fig. 7. Comparison of the relative biological potencies and receptor binding affinities of S-14 analogs. Relative biological activity was expressed as the ratio of the concentration of S-14 to analog required to give half-maximal inhibition of basal PRL release (●) or VIP-stimulated cyclic AMP accumulation (o). Relative affinity for the S-14 receptor was expressed as the ratio of the concentration of S-14 to analog required to elicit 50% inhibition of [^{125}I-Tyr^{1}] S-14 binding to GH_4C_1 cells. Each analog is identified by a number and its structure as well as the values for its potency and receptor affinity have been reported (25). The box in the left-hand corner shows peptides that have undetectable biological and binding activities.

interestingly, IAP pretreatment antagonized the inhibitory effect of S-14 on both basal PRL secretion and on PRL secretion stimulated by thyrotropin releasing hormone (TRH) (42). These results indicated that a functional N_i was required for the effects of S-14 which were mediated by inhibition of adenylate cyclase as well as those which were not.

SUMMARY

We have examined the mechanisms by which S-14 inhibits pituitary hormone secretion in a homogeneous cell population: the clonal GH_4C_1 cell line. The S-14 receptor in GH_4C_1 cells is coupled to N_i, a guanine nucleotide binding protein which mediates S-14-induced inhibitin of VIP-stimulated adenylate cyclase activity, cyclic AMP production and hormone secretion. In addition, a functional N_i is required for S-14 to inhibit basal hormone secretion, an action which appears to be independent of cyclic AMP concentrations.

Accumulating evidence indicates that the mechanism of S-14 action in somatotrophs is similar to that in GH_4C_1 cells. Although S-14 consistently inhibits basal GH secretion, its effects on basal cyclic AMP levels in normal pituitary cells are variable and often not significant (10-14). In contrast, S-14 inhibits prostaglandin and growth hormone releasing factor (GRF) stimulated cyclic AMP accumulation and GH release in parallel (5, 48, 49). Furthermore, S-14 partially blocks prostaglandin and GRF stimulation of adenylate cyclase activity in rat anterior pituitary membranes (16, 50, 51). Finally, pretreatment of primary cultures of rat pituitary cells with IAP antagonizes S-14 inhibition of both basal and GRF-stimulated GH release (52).

In summary, results in both normal pituitary cells and GH_4C_1 cells support the conclusion that the S-14 receptor is coupled to

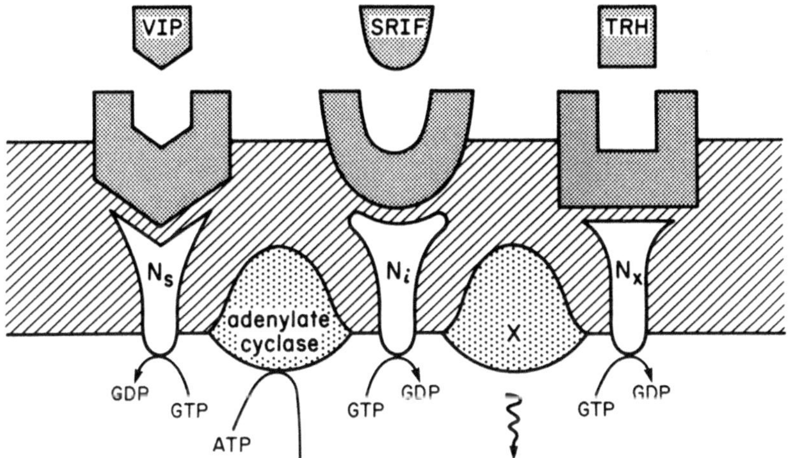

Fig. 8. Mechanisms for S-14 (shown as SRIF) inhibition of hormone release in GH_4C_1 cells. The receptors for VIP, S-14 and TRH are coupled to three different guanyl nucleotide binding proteins. N_s and N_i are the guanine nucleotide regulatory subunits which couple adenylate cyclase to stimulatory (VIP) and inhibitory (S-14) receptors, respectively. A yet-to-be named guanyl nucleotide binding protein (N_x) has been proposed to interact with the TRH receptor and may mediate the effects of TRH to increase intracellular free calcium and the hydrolysis of phosphotidylinositol 4,5 diphosphate (TPI) (55). The coupling of N_i is an intriguing possibility but is purely conjectural at this time.

the guanine nucleotide binding protein, N_i, and that a functional N_i is necessary for S-14 to elicit its biological effects (Fig. 8). In both systems, at least some of the actions of S-14 appear to result from inhibition of stimulated adenylate cyclase. The manner in which N_i antagonizes stimulation of adenylate cyclase is still incompletely understood, but is under intense investigation in highly purified systems (35). However, the manner in which N_i elicits effects independent of changes in adenylate cyclase is much less clear. Many investigators have postulated that intracellular calcium plays an important role in S-14 action (1-4) and recently, Schleger et al. have shown that S-14 transiently reduces cytosolic free calcium concentrations in GH_3 cells (53). These findings, combined with a recent report showing that calcium channels can be regulated by guanine nucleotides (54) certainly raise the interesting possibility that N_i may function in such a manner. Clearly this, as well as other, previously proposed mechanisms of S-14 action (1-4) provide ample opportunity for further experimentation.

REFERENCES

1. Arimura A 1981 Recent progress in somatostatin research. Biomed Res 2:233.
2. Pace CS 1980 Somatostatin: Control of stimulus-secretion coupling in pancreatic islet cells. In: Bloom FE (ed) Peptides: Integrators of Cell and Tissue Function. Raven Press, New York, p 163.
3. Gottesman IS, Mandarino LJ, Gerich JE 1982 Somatostatin: its role in health and disease. In: Cohen MP, Foa PP (eds) Special Topics in Endocrinology and Metabolism. Alan R Liss Inc, New York, vol 4:177.
4. Reichlin S 1983 Somatostatin. New Eng J Med 309:1495 & 1556.
5. Labrie F, Borgeat P, Barden N, Godbout M, Beaulieu M, Ferland L, Lavoie M 1980 Mechanisms of action of hypothalamic hormones in the anterior pituitary. In: Beers RF Jr, Bassett EG (eds) Polypeptide Hormones. Raven Press, New York, p 235.
6. Brazeau P, Vale W, Burgus R, Ling N, Butcher M, Rivier J, Guillemin R 1973 Hypothalamic polypeptide that inhibits the secretion of immunoreactive pituitary growth hormone. Science 179:77.
7. Vale W, Rivier C, Brazeau P, Guillemin R 1974 Effects of somatostatin on the secretion of thyrotropin and prolactin. Endocrinology 95:968.
8. Belanger A, Labrie F, Borgeat P, Savary M, Cote J, Drouin J, Schally AV, Coy DH, Coy EJ, Immer H, Sestang K, Nelson V, Gotz M 1974 Inhibition of growth hormone and thyrotropin release by growth hormone-release-inhibiting hormone. Molec Cell Endocrinol 1:329.

9. Drouin J, DeLean A, Rainville D, Lachance R, Labrie F 1976 Characteristics of the interaction between thyrotropin-releasing-hormone and somatostatin for thyrotropin and prolactin release. Endocrinology 98:514.
10. Borgeat P, Labrie F, Drouin J, Belanger A, Immer H, Sestanj K, Nelson V, Gatz M, Schally AV, Coy DH, Coy EJ 1974 Inhibition of adenosine 3',5'-monophosphate accumulation in anterior pituitary gland in vitro by growth-hormone-release-inhibiting hormone. Biochem Biophys Res Commun 56:1052.
11. Kaneko T, Oka H, Munemura M, Suzuki S, Yasuda H, Oda T 1974 Stimulation of guanosine 3',5'-cyclic monophosphate accumulation in rat anterior pituitary gland in vitro by synthetic somatostatin. Biochem Biophys Res Commun 61:53.
12. Schofield JG, Mira-Moser F, Schorderet M, Orci L 1974 Somatostatin inhibition of rat growth hormone release in vitro in the presence of $BaCl_2$ or 3-isobutyl-1-methylxanthine. FEBS Lett 46:171.
13. Lippmann W, Sestanj J, Nelson VR, Immer HU 1976 Antagonism of prostaglandin-induced cyclic AMP accumulation in the rat anterior pituitary in vitro by somatostatin analogs. Experientia 32:1034.
14. Sheppard MS, Spence JW, Kraicer J 1979 Release of growth hormone from purified somatotrophs: Role of adenosine 3',5'-monophosphate and guanosine 3', 5'-monophosphate. Endocrinology 105:261.
15. Labrie F, Borgeat P, Godbout M, Barden N, Beaulieu M, Lagace L, Massicotte J, Veilleux R 1978 Mechanism of action of hypothalamic hormones and interactions with sex steroids in the anterior pituitary gland. In: Justisz M, McKerns KW (eds) Synthesis and Release of Adenohypophyseal Hormones. Plenum Press, New York, p 415.
16. Rouleau D, Barden N 1981 Inhibition of anterior pituitary prostaglandin-stimulated adenylate cyclase activity by somatostatin. Can J Biochem 59:307.
17. Heindel JJ, Williams E, Robison GA, Strada SJ 1978 Inhibition of GH_1 at pituitary tumor cell adenylyl cyclase activity by somatostatin. J Cyclic Nuc Res 4:453.
18. Bicknell RJ, Schofield JG 1981 Role of cyclic nucleotides in the inhibition of growth hormone secretion by somatostatin. Molec Cell Endocrinol 22:85.
19. Tashjian AH Jr 1979 Clonal strains of hormone producing pituitary cells. Methods in Enzymol 58:527.
20. Bancroft FC 1981 GH cells: functional clonal lines of rat pituitary tumor cells. In: Sato G (ed) Functionally Differentiated Cell Lines. Alan R Liss Inc, New York, p 47.
21. Gourdji D, Tougard C, Tixier-Vidal A 1982 Clonal prolactin strains as a tool in neuroendocrinology. In: Ganong WF, Martini L (eds) Frontiers in Neuroendocrinology. Raven Press, New York, vol 7:317.

22. Schonbrunn A, Tashjian AH Jr 1978 Characterization of functional receptors for somatostatin in rat pituitary cells in culture. J Biol Chem 253:6473.
23. Dorflinger LJ, Schonbrunn A 1983 Somatostatin inhibits basal and vasoactive intestinal peptide-stimulated hormone release by different mechanisms in GH pituitary cells. Endocrinology 113:1551.
24. Westendorf JM, Schonbrunn A 1982 Bombesin stimulates prolactin and growth hormone release by pituitary cells in culture. Endocrinology 110:352.
25. Schonbrunn A, Rorstad OP, Westendorf JM, Martin JB 1983 Somatostatin analogs: correlation between receptor binding affinity and biological potency in GH pituitary cells. Endocrinology 113:1559.
26. Reubi JC, Perrin M, Rivier J, Vale W 1982 Pituitary somatostatin receptors: dissociation at the pituitary level of receptor affinity and biological activity for selective somatostatin analogs. Regulatory Peptides 4:141.
27. Vale W, Rivier C, Brazeau P, Guillemin R 1974 Effects of somatostatin on the secretion of thyrotropin and prolactin. Endocrinology 95:968.
28. Drouin J, De Lean A, Rainville D, Lachance R, Labrie F 1976 Characteristics of the interaction between thyrotropin-releasing hormone and somatostatin for thyrotropin and prolactin release. Endocrinology 98:514.
29. Enjalbert A, Epelbaum J, Arancibia S, Tapia-Arancibia L, Bluet-Pajot M-T, Kordon C 1982 Reciprocal interactions of somatostatin with thyrotropin-releasing hormone and vasoactive intestinal peptide on prolactin and growth hormone section in vitro. Endocrinology 111:42.
30. Rostene WH, Dussaillant M, Rosselin G 1982 Rapid inhibition by somatostatin of vasoactive intestinal peptide-induced prolactin secretion by rat pituitary cells. FEBS Lett 146:213.
31. Dorflinger LJ, Schonbrunn A 1983 Somatostatin inhibits vasoactive intestinal peptide-stimulated cyclic adenosine monophosphate accumulation in GH pituitary cells. Endocrinology 113:1541.
32. Koch BD, Schonbrunn A 1984 The somatostatin receptor is directly coupled to adenylate cyclase in GH_4C_1 cell membranes. Endocrinology 114:1784.
33. Cooper DMF 1982 Bimodal regulation of adenylate cyclase. FEBS Lett 138:157.
34. Spiegel AM, Downs RW Jr 1981 Guanine nucleotides: key regulators of hormone receptor-adenylate cyclase interaction. Endocrine Rev 2:275.
35. Gilman AG 1984 G proteins and dual control of adenylate cyclase. Cell 36:577.
36. De Lean A, Stadel JM, Lefkowitz RJ 1980 A ternary complex model explains the agonist-specific binding properties of the adenylate cyclase-coupled β-adrenergic receptor. J Biol Chem 255:7108.

37. Weber G 1975 Energetics of ligand binding proteins. Adv Protein Chem 29:1.
38. Ross EM, Maguire ME, Sturgill TW, Biltonen RL, Gilman AG 1977 Relationship between the β-adrenergic receptor and adenylate cyclase: studies of ligand binding and enzyme activity in purified membranes of S49 lymphoma cells. J Biol Chem 252:5761.
39. Enjalbert A, Rasolonjanahary R, Moyse E, Kordon C, Epelbaum J 1983 Guanine nucleotide sensitivity of [^{125}I]-iodo-N-Tyr-somatostatin binding in rat adenohypophysis and cerebral cortex. Endocrinology 113:822.
40. Ui M, Katada T, Murayama T, Kurose H, Yajima M, Tamura M, Nakamura T, Nogimori K 1984 Islet-Activating Protein, Pertussis Toxin: a specific uncoupler of receptor-mediated inhibition of adenylate cyclase. In: Greengard P (ed) Advances in Cyclic Nucleotide and Protein Phosphorylation Research. Raven Press, New York, vol 17:145.
41. Hewlett EL, Cronin MJ, Moss J, Anderson H, Myers GA, Pearson RD 1984 Pertussis toxin: lessons from biological and biochemical effects in different cells. In: Greengard P (ed) Advances in Cyclic Nucleotide and Protein Phosphorylation Research. Raven Press, New York, vol 17:173.
42. Koch BD, Dorflinger LJ, Hewlett E, Schonbrunn A 1984 Pituitary somatostatin receptors are coupled to the inhibitory guanine nucleotide binding subunit of adenylate cyclase. Proceedings of the Fourth International Congress on Prolactin, Charlottesville, Virginia, p 67.
43. Jakobs KH, Aktories K, Schultz G 1983 A nucleotide regulatory site for somatostatin inhibition of adenylate cyclase in S49 lymphoma cells. Nature 303:177.
44. Jakobs KH, Schultz G 1983 Occurrence of a hormone-sensitive inhibitory coupling component of the adenylate cyclase in S49 lymphoma cyc$^-$ variants. Proc Natl Acad Sci USA 80:3899.
45. Aktories A, Schultz G, Jakobs KH 1983 Adenylate cyclase inhibition and GTPase stimulation by somatostatin in S49 lymphoma cyc$^-$ variants are prevented by islet-activating protein. FEBS Lett 158:169.
46. Miller JP 1977 Cyclic nucleotide analogues. In: Cramer H, Schultz J (eds) Cyclic 3'5' nucleotides: mechanism of action. John Wiley and Sons, New York, p 77.
47. Seamon KB, Daly JW 1981 Forskolin: a unique diterpene activator of cyclic AMP generating systems. J Cyclic Nucleotide Res 7:201.
48. Bilezikjian LM, Vale WW 1983 Stimulation of adenosine 3', 5'-monophosphate production by growth hormone-releasing factor and its inhibition by somatostatin in anterior pituitary cells in vitro. Endocrinology 113:1726.
49. Michel D, Lefebvre G, Labrie F 1983 Interactions between growth hormone-releasing factor, prostaglandin E_2. and somatostatin on cyclic AMP accumulation in rat adenohypophyseal cells in culture. Mol Cell Endocrinol 33:255.

50. Harwood JP, Grewe C Actions of growth hormone releasing factor (GRF) and somatostatin (SRIF) on growth hormone and cyclic AMP production in cultured anterior pituitary cells. Program of the 66th Annual Meeting of the Endocrine Society, San Antonio, 1983, p 83 (Abstract 10).
51. Michel D, Gagne B, Coy DH GTP dependent stimulation of adenohypophyseal adenylate cyclase activity by GRF. Program of the 66th Annual Meeting of the Endocrine Society, San Antonio, 1983, p 309 (Abstract 915).
52. Cronin MJ, Rogol AD, Myers GA, Hewlett EL 1983 Pertussis toxin blocks the somatostatin-induced inhibition of growth hormone release and adenosine 3', 5'-monophosphate accumulation. Endocrinology 113:209.
53. Schlegel W, Wuarin F, Wollheim CB, Zahnd GR 1984 Somatostatin lowers the cytosolic free Ca^{2+} concentration in clonal rat pituitary cells (GH_3 cells). Cell Calcium 5:223.
54. Gomperts BD 1983 Involvement of guanine nucleotide-binding protein in the gating of CA^{2+} by receptors. Nature 306:64.
55. Hinkle PM, Kinsella PA 1984 Regulation of thyrotropin-releasing hormone binding by monovalent cations and guanyl nucleotides. J Biol Chem 259:3445.

18

SOMATOSTATIN AGONISTS AND ANTAGONISTS - PEPTIDE CONTROL OF GROWTH HORMONE SECRETION

DAVID H. COY, WILLIAM A. MURPHY, VALENTINE A. LANCE, SIMON J. HOCART, JAVIER SUEIRAS-DIAZ AND IRME MEZO

Section of Endocrinology and Metabolism
Department of Medicine
Tulane University School of Medicine
New Orleans, LA 70112

INTRODUCTION

Although somatostatin itself has numerous inhibitory activities which individually are of no little therapeutic interest, there are also several types of physiological effects where it might be of even greater basic and medical value to block activity instead. Perhaps principal among these would be an ability to block the inhibitory effects of somatostatin on growth hormone (GH) release. Antibody experiments (1) have clearly shown that basal GH levels are elevated when somatostatin is neutralized. There is also an unwanted negative participation of somatostatin when GH levels are stimulated with the GH-releasing factor, GRF. In fact, one group has actually been able to demonstrate that GRF(1-44) stimulates somatostatin release from hypothalamic cells in culture (2). It should also be mentioned that both GH (3) and somatostatin (4) can alter somatostatin levels. Somatomedin C has also been implicated in the negative feedback regulation of GH, at least partially by stimulating release of somatostatin (5). Given the successes which have been achieved in the development of very potent competitive antagonists of other peptides, notably in our own experience with LH-RH, there appears to be no reason to neglect the development of a somatostatin antagonist any longer.

Somatostatin Antagonists

Usually, the development of peptide competitive antagonists is a slow process; just coming up with an initial modification which gives a weak antagonist which can then be worked on to increase receptor binding affinity is not easy. Several years ago, we thought that in the case of somatostatin, there might be a short cut to this by utilizing the simplified, highly active analogs then being developed by a group at Merck.

Briefly, Veber et al. (6) found that conformational restriction produced by bridging positions 6 and 11 in the somatostatin ring enabled them to produce analogs which were not only much shorter than the 14 residues of somatostatin but also fully active. Simplest among these, although not least in terms of ease of synthesis, was a heptapeptide (6) (Fig. 1,A) which we picked as a base structure on which to try and produce a competitive antagonist. As we have reported previously (7), it was during synthetic studies with this peptide, and particularly shorter versions, that we made a chance observation on a partially protected pentapeptide analog (Fig. 1,B).

Attempts to make this pentapeptide by a normal solid-phase procedure (7) followed by removal of the side-chain protecting groups from the cyclic peptide by the method of choice, which is catalytic hydrogenation, unexpectedly gave a peptide which still contained the benzyl group on Thr even after prolonged reaction. Complete deprotection could only be achieved by resorting to HF treatment. It took us some time to become aware of this and, in the meantime, a variety of assays were performed on the pentapeptide with surprising results.

One would assume that a peptide shortened so much even in comparison to the original Merck structure would at best be a weak somatostatin agonist. Our standard bioassay system for measuring the inhibitory effects of somatostatin or its analogs on GH release utilizes the sodium pentobarbital-anesthetized rat in which plasma GH levels are stabilized at around 400 ng/ml. Somatostatin then readily gives a dose-related inhibition of GH release, at doses of 0.4 and 2.0 μg/ 100g bw, as shown in Fig. 2. If larger doses of the pentapeptide analog are used in this system, then it does indeed behave like a weak somatostatin agonist. However, at doses similar

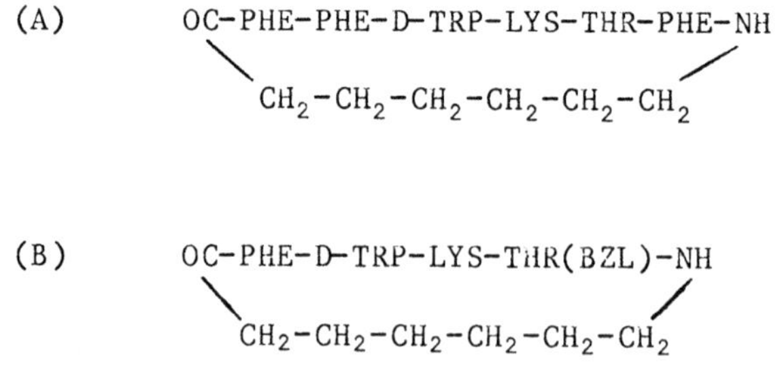

Fig. 1. Short chain aminoheptanoyl superagonist (A) and corresponding pentapeptide antagonist (B).

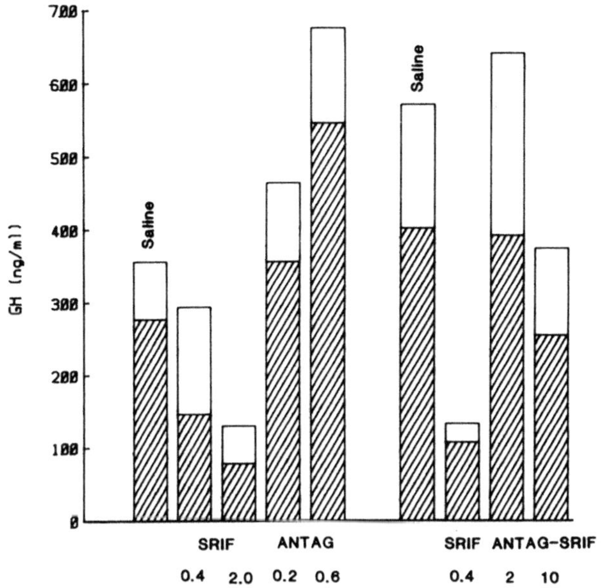

Fig. 2. Effects of c[Ahep-Phe-D-Trp-Lys-Thr(Bzl)] on GH release in nembutal-anesthetized rats.

to those used for somatostatin, in this instance 0.2 and 0.8 μg, an actual stimulation of plasma GH levels was observed (Fig. 2). Furthermore, simultaneous administration of 2 and 10 μg of the pentapeptide completely blocked the inhibitory effects of a 0.4 μg dose of somatostatin and, in fact, again resulted in an elevation of GH levels above basal. Note, however, that the higher dose of the pentapeptide was less effective than the low dose.

A similar experiment was carried out on the pancreatic effects of the Thr benzyl peptide. Fig. 3 illustrates insulin levels in rat hepatic portal blood. Again, there was a normal dose response inhibition produced by 0.4 and 2 μg of somatostatin. Once more, the analog resulted in a stimulation above basal, although not as dramatic as in the case of GH. Also, a 2:1 dose of antagonist blocked the effect of somatostatin, although on a molar basis this would be a ratio of about 6:1. The situation with respect to hepatic portal glucagon was also similar (Fig. 4) in that the pentapeptide was again able to stimulate glucagon to well over basal concentrations even in the presence of an inhibitory dose of somatostatin.

These experiments indicate that basal GH, insulin, and glucagon release, at least in normal rats, appear to be under the control of endogenous somatostatin. These observations appear to fit well with experiments in which endogenous somatostatin is neutralized with

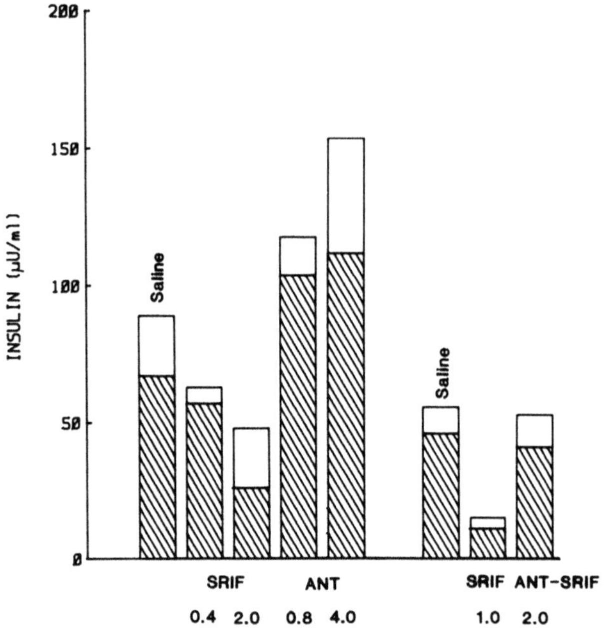

Fig. 3. Effects of c[Ahep-Phe-D-Trp-Lys-Thr(Bzl)] on hepatic portal insulin release in rats.

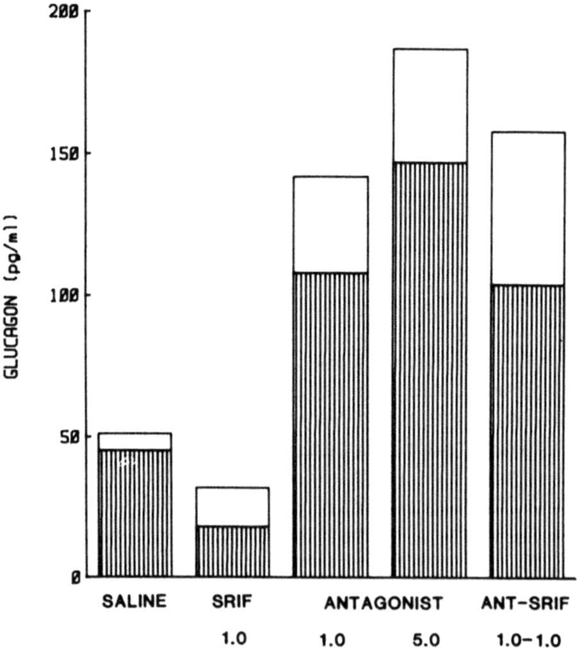

Fig. 4. Effects of c[Ahep-Phe-D-Trp-Lys-Thr(Bzl)] on hepatic portal glucagon release in rats.

antiserum. Therefore, on the face of it we have an analog which could be of enormous value in elucidating the physiological effects of somatostatin. The residual agonist activity of the analog coupled with low receptor affinity (Dr. Y. Patel, personal communication), however, makes it very difficult to use on a routine basis. Work has, therefore, continued on the development of more powerful compounds. In terms of improving binding affinity, there are, for instance, other analogs which the Merck group has since developed (8) which have even greater somatostatin activity, such as the analog in Fig. 5. This analog is an hexapeptide in which the aminoheptanoic acid bridge and one Phe have been replaced by Pro. Activity is increased by about a factor of 3 or 4. We have made the Phe deleted, Thr benzyl pentapeptide analog of this and, in the GH bioassay (Fig. 6), achieved strong stimulation of GH release at the 0.2 μg dose. The effect dropped off rapidly with increasing doses and was already much diminished at 0.6 μg. Thus, although this is probably a more active antagonist in terms of minimum effective dose levels, it also seems to have increased agonist activity also.

We have made many variations on the pentapeptide structure including the analogs shown in Table 1. The Thr benzyl residue, as might be expected, was very critical to inhibitory activity. Its removal or replacement with a somewhat similar aromatic side-chain, such as that present in Phe, destroyed activity. The Ser benzyl

Table 1. Pentapeptide Antagonist Analogs

Cyclo [	Ahp	- Phe -	D - Trp - Lys -	Thr(Bzl)]	Antagonist activity
				Thr	inactive
				Phe	inactive
				Ser(Bzl)	+
	Ahx				inactive
	Aoc				inactive
	Pro				+ + +
	Pro			Thr	inactive
	Pro	D-Phe			inactive

Ahp = aminoheptanoyl; Ahx = aminohexanoyl; Aoc = aminooctanoyl

(A) PRO-PHE-D-TRP-LYS-THR-PHE

(B) PRO-PHE-D-TRP-LYS-THR(BZL)

Fig. 5. Proline-bridged superagonist (A) and corresponding pentapeptide antagonist(B).

analog had very weak antagonist activity. We have also tried bridging groups other than aminoheptanoic acid and Pro. Neither the shorter hexanoic nor the longer octanoic acid chains preserved activity. We have also begun to look at analogs of the whole hexapeptide. Here at least we are beginning with a compound which has high binding affinity. Unfortunately, the Thr(Bzl) hexapeptide has no significant stimulating activity and enhances rather than blocks somatostatin effects at high doses (Fig. 7). However, the corresponding D-Lys analog at a 1 mg dose, which is a 1000:1 ratio, produced a slight blockade of somatostatin effects. This result, while not too spectacular, is something which perhaps can be built upon to produce some pure antagonists of greater activity.

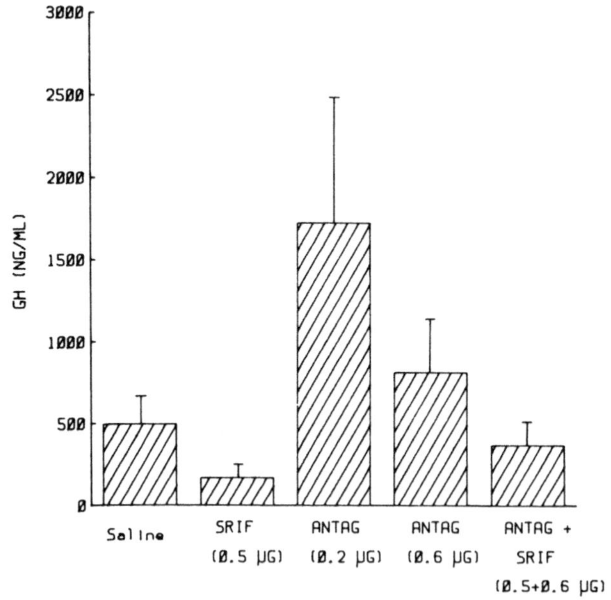

Fig. 6. Effects of c[Pro-Phe-D-Trp-Lys-Thr(Bzl)]on GH release in nembutal-anesthetized rats.

Table 2. Amidated Somatostatin Analog Effects on Plasma GH in Nembutal-Stimulated Rats

Analog	% GH inhibiting activity
SS	100
SS-amide	63 (35-122)
SS-amide (Rivier, 1976)	30
SS-ethylamide	45 (78-345)
Ac-D-Trp-8-SS_r-NH_2	582 (341-994)

SS_r = desAla-1,Gly-2-somatostatin (i.e. ring portion)
Ac = N-acetyl

Table 3. Position 6 Halogenated Somatostatin Analog Effects on Plasma GH in Nembutal-Stimulated Rats and on Rat Hepatic Portal Insulin, and Cat Gastric Acid

Analog	% inhibitory effects on release of GH	insulin	gastric acid
SS	100	100	100
p-Cl-Phe-6	331 (137-795)	474 (114-1975)	274 ± 62
p-Br-Phe-6	164 (784-345)	-	-
F_5-Phe-6	47 (18-119)	-	-
F_5-Phe-11	121 (49-299)	-	-

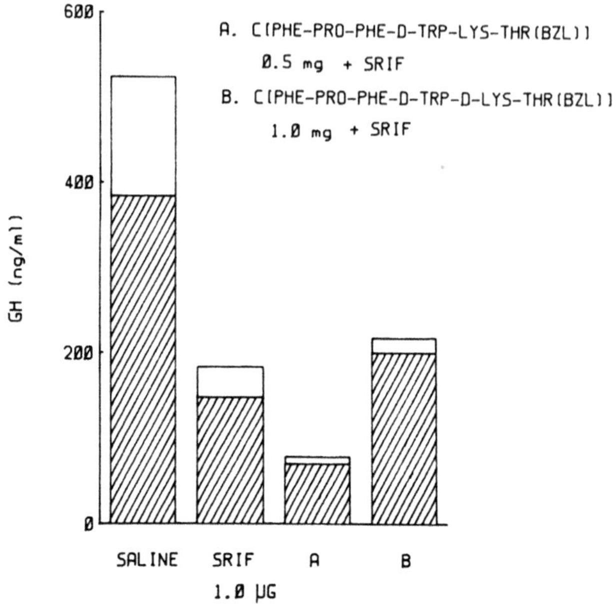

Fig. 7. Effects of c [Phe-Pro-Phe-D-Trp-Lys-Thr(Bzl)] and its D-Lys analog on somatostatin inhibition of GH release in nembutal-anesthetized rats.

Somatostastin Agonists

It could be of course, that our attempt to utilize these highly simplified Merck analogs in antagonist design is working against us. It is possible that more subtle manipulations of conformation and secondary binding sites might be, in fact, more easy in a parent molecule containing all amino acids. For instance, selectivity is much more readily built into analogs containing the whole ring portion of the chain. If we were to begin an antagonist design program based on the whole chain, then again, it would make sense to begin with the most active analogs available. Simultaneously, therefore, we have been continuing with structure-activity studies aimed at increasing the activity of the whole ring. These new compounds are based on several observations. Firstly, we have always been searching for ways in which to block the C-terminus, for instance, with an amide group. We were deterred by an early result of Rivier et al. (9) who reported only 30% *in vitro* activity for somatostatin amide. However, when this analog was synthesized and tested *in vivo* by us, the activity was found to be an acceptable 60% (Table 2). If the amide is combined with an acetylated ring N-terminus, the standard D-Trp-8 modification gives a dodecapeptide which is even more active than D-Trp-8 somatostatin itself (Table 2).

Another favorable approach has been to make use of a p-Cl-Phe-6 substitution which increased activity about 3-fold for GH, insulin, and also gastric acid inhibition (Table 3) (B.H. Hirst, personal communication). The Cl-substitution was superior to other halo substituents tried (Table 3). The combination of all of these alterations to give the first analog in Table 4 boosted activity to 15 or 20 times that of somatostatin for inhibition of all 3 hormones. This is the kind of potency seen with the Sandoz analogs reported elsewhere in this book and, until just recently, the best of the Merck analogs. The advantage of having almost the whole of the somatostatin sequence intact is now apparent for we can take advantage of other modifications which have previously resulted in selectivity. Perhaps the most well known of these is D-Cys-14 which has been reported (10) to increase inhibition of glucagon release. In the present analog family, the same effect was again achieved with about a 10-fold increase in the glucagon:GH ratio. This analog is the most potent that we have tested for inhibitory effects on glucagon. It should also be mentioned that these N- and C-terminally blocked analogs exhibit very prolonged activity compared to somatostatin in the rat.

Table 4. Somatostatin Analog Effects on Plasma GH in Nembutal-Stimulated Rats and on Rat Hepatic Portal Insulin and Glucagon

	% inhibitory effects on release of		
Analog	GH	Insulin	Glucagon
SS	100	100	100
Ac-p-Cl-p-Phe-6,D-Trp-8-SS_r-NH_2	1515 (224-10242)	1529 (588-3980)	1150 (258-5214)
Ac-p-NH_2-Phe-4,p-Cl-Phe-6-D-Trp-8-SS_r-NH_2	596 (371-959)	-	-
Ac-p-Cl-Phe-6,D-Trp-8,C-Cys-14-SS_r-NH_2	727 (555-952)	1152 (643-2066)	6624 (1208-3625)

SS_r = somatostatin ring portion; Ac = N-acetyl

Other Peptides and Analogs Involved in Control of GH Release

Our knowledge of mechanisms of control of GH release has increased so dramatically over the past few years that it cannot really be considered that somatostatin is the only possible means of blocking GH release any more than GRF is the sole means of stimulating GH release. Consider, for instance, the possibility of developing GRF antagonists. It is often the case that antagonists are discovered during the process of developing more active agonist analogs. This appears to be the case with GRF. We reported recently (11, 12) that, of six D-amino acid-substituted analogs of GRF (1-29) amide, several exhibited improved GH-releasing activities in the rat. The D-Ala-2 analog shown in Table 5 was 50 times more active in stimulating GH release in the rat and pig and also in terms of specific receptor affinity (13). In examining the function of the position 2 side-chain, we also synthesized D-Arg-2 and D-Phe-2 analogs which were found to have less than 1% GH-releasing activity (12). Christophe et al. (14) have examined these and many other analogs for effects on adenylate cyclase in several tissue types. The D-Arg-2 analog was devoid of adenylate cyclase effects in rat anterior pituitary preparations. It was, however, able to inhibit the effects of GRF(1-29) itself in a dose-dependent fashion, giving complete inhibition of GRF at a molar ratio of about 100:1. As a control, VIP was without inhibitory effects as was the D-Phe-2 analog. The latter did, however, inhibit the adenylate cyclase activity of GRF on rat pancreatic acinar membranes and also that of VIP (15). Secretin effects were not altered. The D-Arg-2 analog was devoid of effects in this system. How these adenylate cyclase observations will tie in with observations on, for instance, inhibition of GRF-stimulated GH release remains to be seen; however, the GRF antagonist approach is certainly probably practical and of undoubted little basic and therapeutic interest.

Table 5. Effect of D-Amino Acid Replacements on the GH-Releasing Activity of GRF(1-29)-Amide in the Anesthetized Rat

	1		2		3		4		% activity
H	- Tyr	-	Ala	-	Asp	-	Ala	-	100
	D-Tyr								993
			D-Ala						5146
					D-Asp				670
							D-Ala		110

Table 6. Effects of Bombesin on Plasma GH Levels in Nembutal-Anesthetized Rats

Time (min)	Saline	Bombesin (10 μg/100 g bw)
5	428 ± 110	319 ± 69
15	361 ± 51	95 ± 14
30	-	73 ± 9
45	-	86 ± 21
60	371 ± 47	52 ± 24
90	-	94 ± 27
120	477 ± 90	517 ± 127
150	301 ± 125	373 ± 175

5-6 animals per group

Many other peptides also affect GH release one way or another. Recent data (Table 6) concerning their effects on GH release in the anesthetized rat model indicate that bombesin and GRP should be added to the top of this list. Bombesin is remarkable in terms of its potency and the length of the inhibitory response after simple peripheral injection. The 10 μg ip dose of the peptide gives inhibition of GH release for about 6 times longer than an equivalent amount of somatostatin. A dose as low as 1 μg/100 g bw also gave prolonged inhibition. Whether this inhibitory effect is mediated by somatostatin release remains to be evaluated.

CONCLUSIONS

Many classes of super-active somatostatin agonists have now been discovered. These not only offer improved biological properties of therapeutic interest but also starting points for the design of more active competitive inhibitors of somatostatin. The numerous negative feedback controls contributing to the difficulty of producing and sustaining high GH levels would seem to make it essential to develop powerful somatostatin antagonists if these processes are to be studied and if optimum growth rates are to be achieved by GRF and GH administration. Additional analog research on GRF and other peptides such as bombesin and GRP appear to offer further powerful potential methods of manipulating GH levels.

ACKNOWLEDGMENT

This work was supported by NIH grants AM-18370, AM-30167, and AM-32476.

REFERENCES

1. Oliver C, Giraud P, Lissitzky JC, Cote J, Boudouresque F, Gillioz P, Conte-Devolx B 1982 Influence of endogenous somatostatin on GH and TSH secretion in neonatal rats. Endocrinology 110:1018.
2. Iwasaki K, Arimura A, Stimulation of somatostatin release by hpGRF-44 from rat hypothalamic cells and fragments in vitro. Program of the 7th International Congress of Endocrinology. Quebec City, July 1984, A963 (Abstract).
3. Berelowitz M, Firestone SL, Frohman LA 1981 Effects of GH excess and deficiency on hypothalamic somatostatin content and release and on tissue somatostatin distribution. Endocrinology 109:714.
4. Lumpkin MD, Negro-Vilar A, McCann SM 1981 Paradoxical elevation of GH by intraventricular somatostatin: possible ultra short-loop feedback. Science 211:1072.
5. Abe A, Molitch ME, Van Wyk JJ, Underwood LE 1983 Human GH and somatomedin C suppress the spontaneous release of GH in unanesthetized rats. Endocrinology 113:1319.
6. Veber DF, Holly FW, Nutt RF, Bergstrand SJ, Brady SF, Hirschmann R, Glitzer MS, Saperstein RS 1979 Highly active cyclic and bicyclic somatostatin analogues of reduced ring size. Nature 280:512.
7. Fries JL, Murphy WA, Sueiras-Diaz JA, Coy DH 1982 Somatostatin antagonist analog increases GH, insulin and glucagon release in the rat. Peptides 3:811.
8. Veber DF, Friedinger RM, Perlow DS, Palaveda WJ, Holly FW, Strachan RG, Nutt RF, Arison BH, Homnick C, Randall WC, Glitzer MS, Saperstein R, Hirschmann R 1981 A potent cyclic hexapeptide analogue of somatostatin. Nature 292:55.
9. Rivier J, Brown M, Rivier C, Ling N, Vale W 1976 Hypothalamic hypophysiotropic hormones. In: Loffet A (ed) Peptides. Editions de l'Université de Bruxelles, Brussels, p 427.
10. Meyers C, Arimura A, Gordon A, Fernandez R, Coy DH, Schally AV, Drouin L, Ferland M, Beaulieu M, Labrie F 1977 Somatostatin analogs which inhibit glucagon and GH more than insulin release. Biochem Biophys Res Commun 74:630.
11. Lance VA, Murphy WA, Sueiras-Diaz JA, Coy DH 1984 Super-active analogs of growth hormone-releasing factor(1-29) amide. Biochem Biophys Res Commun 119:265.
12. Coy DH, Murphy WA, Sueiras-Diaz JA, Coy EJ, Lance VA 1984 Structure-activity studies on the N-terminal region of growth hormone releasing factor. J Med Chem, in press.
13. Heiman ML, Nekola MV, Lance VA, Murphy WA, Coy DH, Potency of GRF agonists stimulating GH release from cultured pituitary cells correlates with binding to a putative GRF receptor. Program of the 7th International Congress of Endocrinology. Quebec City, July 1984, A956 (Abstract).

14. Robberecht P, Coy DH, Waelbroeck M, de Neef P, Camus J-C, Christophe J 1984 Structural requirements for the activation of rat anterior pituitary adenylate cyclase by GRF - discovery of [N-Ac-Tyr-1, D-Arg-2]-GRF(1-29)NH_2 as a GRF antagonist. Endocrinology, in press.
15. Waelbroeck M, Robberecht P, Coy DH, Camus J-C, de Neef P, Christophe J 1985 Interaction of GRF and 14 GRF analogs with rat pancreatic VIP receptors. Discovery of [N-Ac-Tyr-1,D-Phe-2]-GRF(1-29)NH_2 as a VIP antagonist. Endocrinology (in press).

19

CLINICAL APPLICATIONS OF SOMATOSTATIN ANALOGS

PETER MARBACH, MICHAEL NEUFELD AND JANOS PLESS

Preclinical and Clinical Research Dept.
Sandoz Ltd.
CH-4002 Basel, Switzerland

INTRODUCTION

It has often been shown that tetradecapeptide somatostatin (S-14), discovered in 1973 by Brazeau et al. (1), is effective in the treatment of acromegaly, as adjunct to insulin therapy of type I diabetes, in stopping gastrointestinal bleeding, in treatment of carcinoid syndrome, etc. But S-14 has always had to be given as an iv infusion, which has severely limited its practical application. It was therefore an important exercise of peptide chemists to improve the metabolic stability of the molecule, i.e. to synthesize analogs with a longer duration of action. However, until quite recently, little progress had been made in providing clinically useful compounds.

The synthesis and biological characterization of SMS 201-995 (SMS: DPhe-Cys-Phe-DTrp-Lys-Thr-Cys-Thr-ol) by Bauer et al. (2) represents a genuine breakthrough in the field. The high potency and remarkable stability against enzymatic degradation of this compound have enabled its use in clinical studies without the need for immobilizing the patient. This chapter gives a brief summary of all published data on clinical application of analogs of S-14 with special emphasis on SMS.

Clinical Applications: Literature Review

Table 1 lists all publications found by means of a computer-aided literature research during May 1984. As early as 1975, reports from Brazeau et al. (3) that N-acylation of [DesAA^{1,2}] S-14 renders the molecule less soluble and prolongs its duration of action in rats prompted clinicians to treat an acromegalic patient

Table 1. Clinical Applications of Somatostatin Analogs

Modification	Indication	N	Reference
N-Acetyl-$DesAA^{1,2}$	Acromegaly	1	4
N-Benzoyl-$DesAA^{1,2}$	Acromegaly	1	4
$DTrp^{8}$, $DCys^{14}$	Diabetes type I	6	5, 6
	Acromegaly	4	7
	Mild diabetics	4	7
	Glucagonoma	1	8
	Pancreatic tumors	7	9
$DesAA^{1,2,4,5,12,13}$	Pancreatic tumors	8	10, 11
		7	9
$DTrp^{8}$	Cirrhosis	8	12
	Glucagonoma	1	8
	Pancreatic tumors	7	9
$DesAA^{1,2,4,5,12}$,$DTrp^{8}$	Carcinoid syndrome	1	13, 14
Protamine-Zn-	Nesidioblastosis	1	15
$DVal^{1}$,$DTrp^{8}$-	Relaxation of GI-tract	7	16
$DCys^{14}$-	Glucagonoma	1	8
	Pancreatic tumors	7	9
$DesAsn^{5}$,$DTrp^{8}$,$DSer^{13}$-	Pancreatic tumors	7	9
$DAla^{2}$,$DTrp^{8}$,$DCys^{14}$-	Acromegaly	4	17
5-F-$LTrp^{8}$	Acromegaly	4	17
$DesAA^{1,2}$,$His^{4,5}$,$DTrp^{8}$-	Diabetes type I	7	18

with two analogs of that type (4). Subcutaneous injection of 0.5 mg of either [N-Acetyl-DesAA^{1,2}] S-14 or [N-Benzoyl-DesAA^{1,2}] S-14 inhibited GH levels by 50% but the duration of action was not prolonged.

Strong emphasis has been put on the synthesis of analogs with more selective actions. In view of the great potential of S-14 in the therapy of diabetes, it would have been advantageous to have analogs with preferential actions on glucagon and GH release but not on insulin release. Among a series of peptides which had been described to exhibit this kind of biological profile, the analog [DTrp^{8}, DCys^{14}] S-14 has been investigated most (see Table 1 for references). However, the substance had to be given as intravenous infusions and its practical use was therefore quite limited. Moreover, it has been shown with a series of analogs (9) that all kinds of specificity which had been predicted from preclinical characterizations, did not hold in patients with pancreatic and gastrointestinal tumors. It is most probable that this was the case because the analogs had been tested in different kinds of animal models, e.g. GH *in vitro* but insulin and glucagon *in vivo*.

A potential use of a long acting S-14 analog would be as an adjunct to insulin in the treatment of type I diabetes mellitus. Because of the dependence on exogenous insulin, the suppression of endogenous insulin by the drug would hardly be harmful to the patient. On the other hand, the delay in gastrointestinal absorption, the suppression of glucagon and GH and possibly of other hormones of the GI tract by S-14 and analogs had been demonstrated to lead to an overall reduction in the amount of insulin required and to an inhibition of the post-prandial elevation of serum glucose concentrations. A recent report (18) described the use of WY-41474 as an adjunct to subcutaneously infused insulin in the management of type I diabetes. About 1 mg of the analog was infused sc during 30 minutes either before or at meal-time. The inhibition of postprandial hyperglycaemia was clearcut as was the inhibition of glucagon and triglycerides and the delay in xylose absorption. The authors concluded that "such an agent may prove useful as an adjunct to insulin in the management of diabetes mellitus".

The inhibitory effects of S-14 on a wide variety of hormones suggested its use as a treatment in endocrine diseases characterized by excess production of one or more of these hormones. However, only analogs with a markedly prolonged duration of action, which would be applicable without the need to immobilize the patient, would be of potential use in these indications, The early findings, that the S-14 molecule was open to a wide range of chemical modifications which included substitutions, deletions and/or modifications of the amino acid residues, allowed the synthesis of oligosomatostatins with enhanced metabolic stability. Two of them, the octapeptide [DesAA^{1,2,4,5,12,13}-DTrp^{8}] S-14 (9, 10, 11) and the nonapeptide

[DesAA[1,2,4,15,12]-DTrp[8]] S-14 (13, 14) have been tested in patients with pancreatic tumors and tumors of the gastrointestinal tract or in the carcinoid syndrome. 2-10 mg was injected subcutaneously and the effect was followed by measuring the hormone levels or the number of flushing episodes. Both oligopeptides proved to be effective over a period of up to 12 h. Since no prolongation of action had been observed after iv infusion of the octapeptide, it has to be concluded that the oligopeptide is slowly absorbed from a depot at the injection site.

Another class of oligosomatostatin analogs has been synthesized by Veber et al. at Merck (19). Cyclic hexapeptides without the disulfide bridge of the parent molecule showed promising biological activities in rats and dogs. However, to our knowledge, no data have been published on clinical trials with one or other of these peptides.

In summary, it can be concluded that up to very recent times, somatostatin analogs have only sporadically been used in the clinic. The lack of specificity with iv infusions, together with the need to immobililize the patient have excluded the metabolically unstable analogs from practical applications. The low activity of the oligosomatostatins required the sc application of rather high doses which makes them less attractive despite their striking clinical effectiveness.

Clinical Applications of SMS 201-995 in Normal Volunteers

It has been shown in animal studies in rats and rhesus monkeys (2), that SMS is a very potent and stable octapeptide anlog of S-14. It proved to be more potent in inhibiting GH relative to insulin, and it demonstrated a clearly prolonged duration of action, especially after sc applications. Excellent results from local tolerance and toxicological studies in rats and dogs allowed its clinical investigation. Tolerance studies in healthy volunteers established the preclinical results. No side effects or changes of vital signs, routine blood, biochemical, hematological and electrocardiographic parameters were reported.

Pharmacokinetic studies with SMS 201-995

SMS plasma levels were measured by means of a specific radioimmunoassay (RIA). The antiserum originated from a rabbit which had been immunized with a conjugate of SMS with bovine serum albumin (BSA) in complete Freunds adjuvant. The RIA is set up in 0.05 M phosphate buffer pH 7.6 with 0.9% NaCl, 0.025 M EDTA, 0.01% NaN_3 and 0.5% BSA. The [DTyr[1]] SMS analog is used for radioiodination. The iodination is done according to a standard chloramine T method or to an indirect iodogen procedure. This was worked out thanks to a personal communication of P. Lowry.

The RIA is routinely sensitive to 1 pg/tube. The intraassay and interassay coefficients of variation are below 10%. The specificity of the antiserum is directed against positions 4-6 as could be shown by testing the cross-reactivity of a number of structurally related analogs of SMS. Natural S-14 cross-reacts to the extent of 0.01%. No other naturally occurring peptide demonstrated any interference with the assay.

SMS plasma levels were measured to assess elimination rate constants, plasma elimination half-life, volume of distribution, and clearance after a two-hour iv infusion with various concentrations, and after single injections of 50 and 100 µg SMS. During the iv infusion (Fig. 1), SMS plasma levels rose continually and started to plateau at about 70-90 min. The height of the plateau was proportional to the dose. After stopping the infusion, the compound disappeared with an elimination half-life of 41-58 min. The half-lives seemed to increase with increasing infusion rates. The volume of distribution was between 12.3-14.2 litres and seemed to decrease with increasing infusion rates, as did the clearance, which was between 148 and 240 ml/min. These results are interesting in comparison to a very recent paper by Skamene and Patel (20) on the pharmacokinetic behaviour of natural S-14.

After single sc injections, peak values of 1.9 and 2.9 ng/ml SMS were measured in the plasma after 50 and 100 µg SMS respectively.

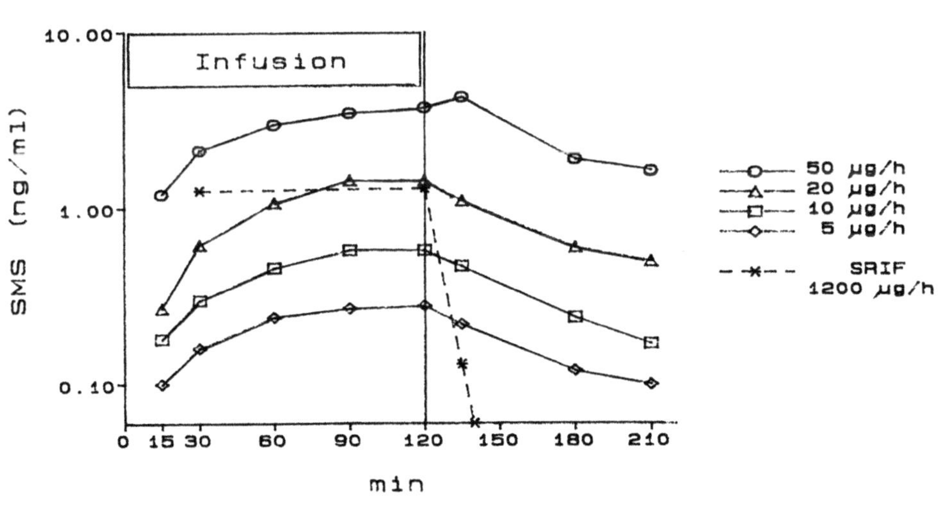

Fig. 1. Plasma levels of SMS in normal volunteers after constant infusion for two hours (N = 2,5,5 and 4 at infusion rates of 5, 10, 20 and 50 µg/h respectively). The curve for S-14 (shown as SRIF) is reproduced from the literature (9).

The level peaked after 15 to 30 min and the elimination half-life was 113 minutes, which was 2-3 times longer than that found after the iv. infusion. The area under the plasma concentration-time curve (AUC) after the sc injection of 50 µg SMS was almost 100% of the same iv dose, demonstrating its very high absolute bio-availability.

Specific endocrine actions of SMS

When SMS was given to normal volunteers as iv infusions, the minimal effective dose in inhibiting arginine-stimulated GH release was 5 µg/hr (Fig. 2). The AUC was diminished by 73% relative to placebo. At the same infusion rate, the steady state plasma level of SMS was 300 pg/ml. Insulin and glucagon release were only affected at 10 µg/h by 43% and 38% respectively. The study demonstrated the very high absolute potency of SMS and seemed to reveal a certain degree of specificity toward the inhibition of GH release.

More physiological stimuli were also applied togetner with iv infusions of SMS.

To assess the efficacy of SMS in inhibiting sleep-related GH increase, 10 µg/h of the drug were infused from one hour before the expected time for onset of sleep for about 5 hours. There was a significant 70% suppression of the AUC compared to a control night. No rebound phenomenon was observed after stopping the infusion.

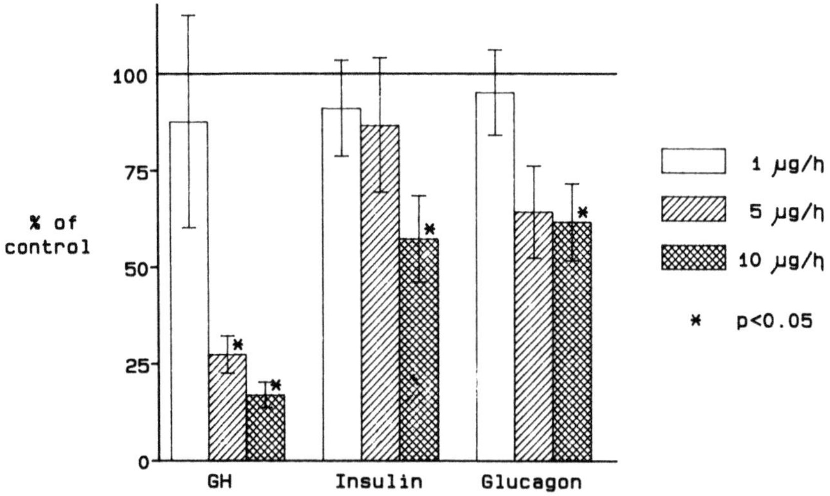

Fig. 2. Areas under the GH, insulin and glucagon plasma concentration time curves (AUC 80'-180') during 2-h infusions of SMS with arginine stimulation in 10 normal volunteers (mean ± SE). Arginine (0.5 g/kg body weight) was infused between the 75th and 105th min after the onset of SMS infusion.

To assess the effect and length of action in inhibiting exercise-stimulated GH secretion, a total of 19 healthy volunteers were studied by ergometry, either immediately or one hour after the end of a 60 min iv infusion of 20 µg/h SMS. GH release was significantly inhibited even 1 hour after the end of the infusion, demonstrating the prolonged duration of action after this kind of application.

The effects of SMS after sc injection in normal volunteers were studied after arginine and standard mixed meal stimulation.

When 50 ug SMS were injected sc and arginine was infused after 15 and 180 min respectively at a rate of 0.5 g/kg for 1/2 h, the GH release was significantly inhibited by 89% and 82% respectively (Fig. 3). On the other hand, the insulin release was inhibited by 80% ($p < 0.05$) only after 15 min but not at all after 3 h. The same profile emerged with C-peptide whereas glucagon release was not affected by SMS at either time (data not shown). It can be concluded that SMS inhibited GH for a markedly longer period of time than insulin, demonstrating a kind of pharmacodynamic specificity.

In a further investigation, a standard mixed meal, which is a more physiological hormonal stimulation of insulin release than arginine, was given during the morning to 6 healthy volunteers who had fasted from midnight. The meal contained 26 g protein, 50 g fat and 75 g carbohydrates and was ingested either immediately (study A) or 3 h after (study B) the injection of SMS (Fig. 4). Insulin, glucose, glucagon and gastrin levels were followed for up to 6 1/2 h.

In study A, SMS induced a 50% fall in basal insulin levels and completely abolished the meal-stimulated rise of this hormone. Glucose levels were elevated to 184 mg% and the peak level was retarded by 1 hour relative to the placebo control group. The post-prandial rises in glucagon and gastrin levels were also completely inhibited (not shown). In study B, basal insulin was again inhibited by 50% for half an hour. However, the AUC of the meal-stimulated hormone secretion was not significantly different from that of the placebo group. Glucose levels were elevated to 105 mg% two hours after injection of SMS, presumably because of the suppression of insulin secretion. The post-prandial peak of plasma glucose, occurring 90 minutes after the meal, was within normal limits of glucose tolerance (128 mg%). This peak was also delayed by one hour when compared with that of the placebo-injected group. With glucagon there was only a tendency towards inhibition whereas gastrin secretion was unaffected 3 hours after the SMS injection.

To summarize the investigations in normal volunteers, it can be concluded that SMS is very well tolerated in clinically relevant dosages, that the absolute bioavailability after sc injections is almost 100% and that the biological half-life is substantially

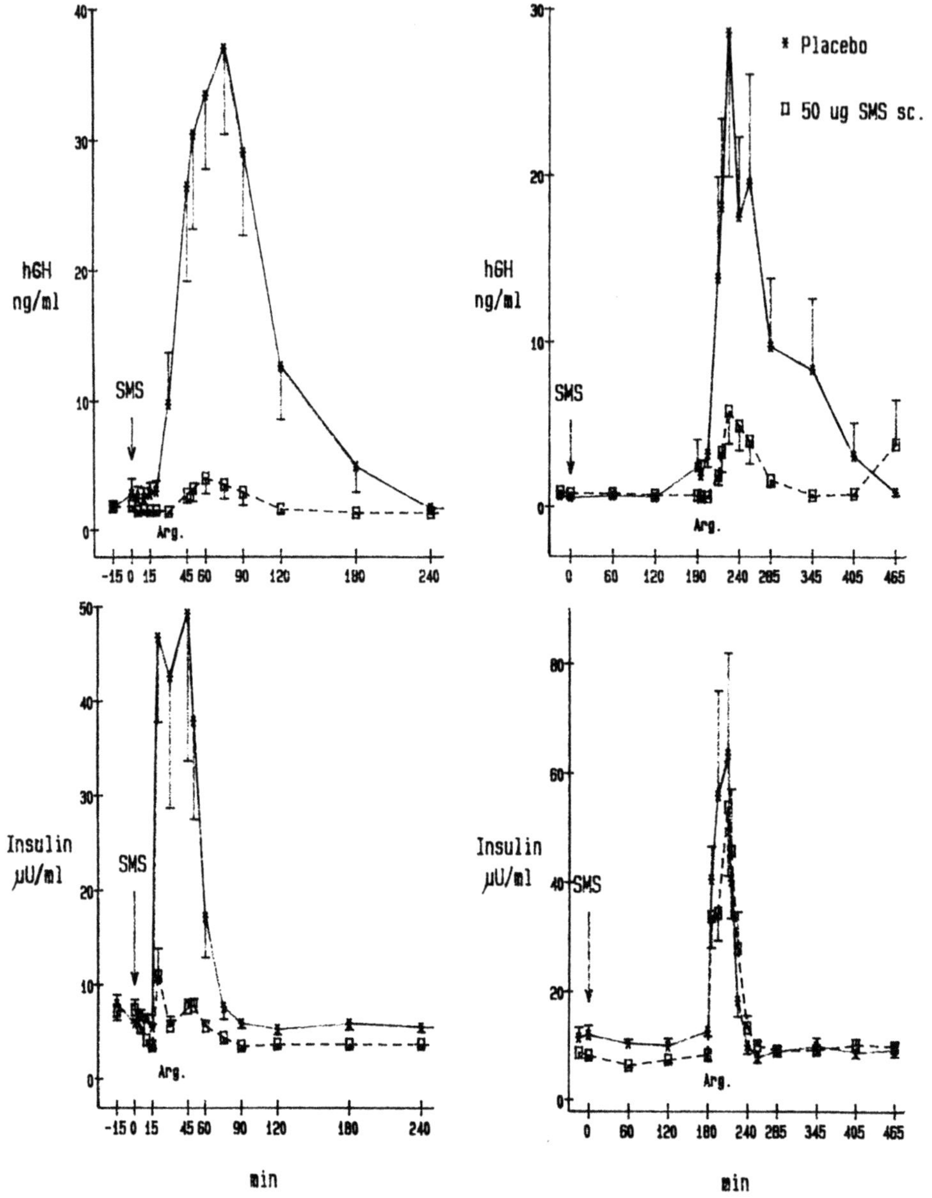

Fig. 3. Effect of a single sc injection of 50 µg SMS on arginine-stimulated growth hormone and insulin release in 6 healthy male volunteers (mean ± SEM). Arginine was infused from 15'-45' (left) and from 180'-210' (right) after the injection of SMS.

prolonged in comparison to S-14, especially after sc applications. The length of action is consequently markedly prolonged and no signs of rebound phenomena have ever been observed for any of the hormones measured. However, the length of action depends on the hormone which is determined. SMS is particularly potent and long-acting with regard to GH inhibition whereas the effect on insulin is less pronounced and more transient.

Clinical Applications of SMS 201-995 in Patients

The very favourable results with SMS in normal volunteers were the basis for starting clinical trials in patients. Out of many studies, we will review in the following chapter, a few representative ones which have been performed for the most promising indications. We will focus on the sc route of administration because this would most probably be the preferential application for long term treatment of outpatients.

Applications of SMS in diabetic patients

Spinas et al. (21) treated ten nonobese patients with type I diabetes with a single sc injection of 100 μg SMS, concomitantly with their insulin injection and 15 min before the ingestion of a standard mixed meal. The insulin dose was reduced by one third. Blood samples were taken at 15-30 min intervals for 180 min. After SMS, post-prandial blood glucose decreased slightly from 8.9 ± 0.7 to 7.8 ± 0.6 mM within 30 min and remained at a similar level until the end of the study (Fig. 5). In contrast, after placebo injection, blood glucose concentration rose post-prandially from 9.6 ± 0.8 to 13.8 ± 0.9 mM. Plasma glucagon decreased within 15 min after the SMS injection from 115 pg/ml to less than 50 pg/ml until 180 min but increased after placebo significantly to 215 pg/ml (data not shown). Preliminary studies with only 50 μg SMS show a similar effectiveness. In summary, this study shows that a single sc injection of 100 μg SMS is able to markedly decrease post-prandial hyperglycemia, even in the presence of a reduced insulin dose. The mechanism of action is not completely understood at present. The inhibition of glucagon release is certainly one of the factors, eventually along with a decreased glucose absorption rate secondary to delayed gastric emptying (18). SMS may improve glycemic stability and decrease insulin requirements in unstable diabetics.

Application of SMS in acromegalic patients

In a study by Plewe et al. (22), six acromegalic patients were treated with single sc injections of 50 μg SMS, 2 h after having breakfast. A rapid fall in plasma GH levels was induced in all cases, reaching a nadir of 1.4 ± 0.4 ng/ml three hours after the administration (Fig. 6). The hormone level returned to preinjection levels after 9 h. Insulin levels fell immediately after the

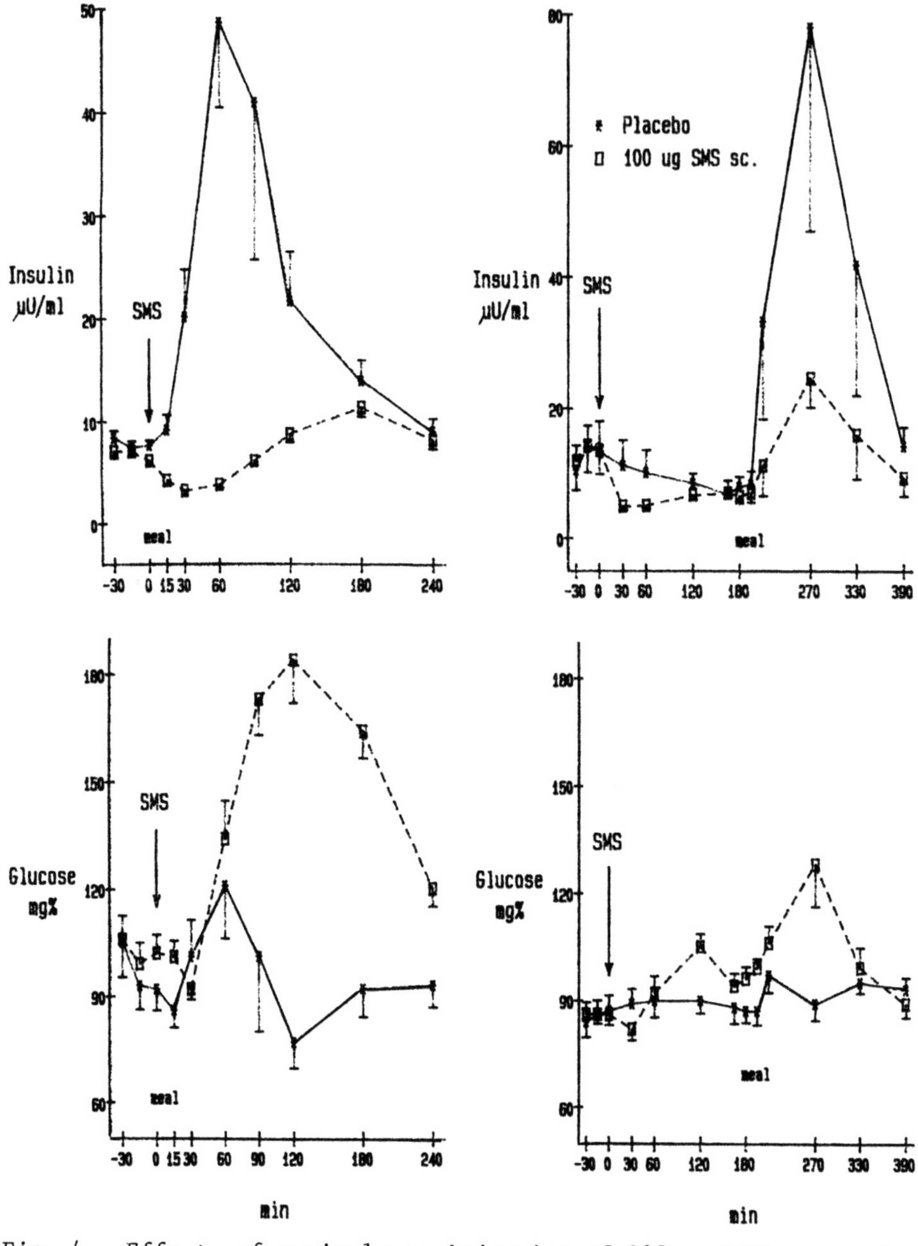

Fig. 4. Effects of a single sc injection of 100 µg SMS on standard mixed-meal-stimulated insulin and glucose release in 6 healthy male volunteers (mean ± SEM). The meal was ingested immediately (left) or 3 h after (right) the injection of SMS.

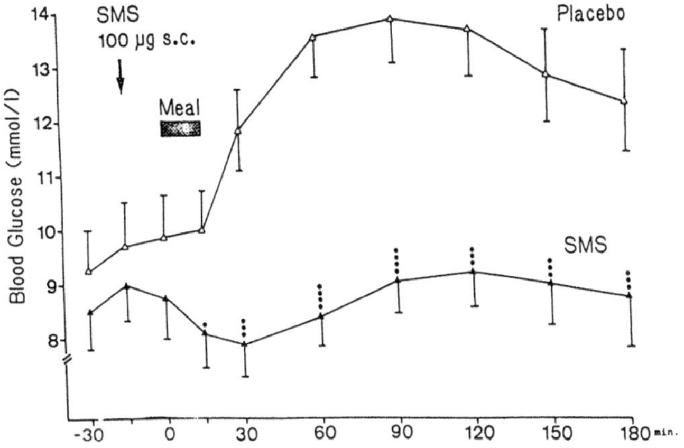

Fig. 5. Effect of a single sc injection of SMS and placebo on post-prandial blood glucose levels in type I diabetics (N = 10). *, $p < 0.05$; ***, $p < 0.001$ relative to placebo.

injection from 86 ± 31 to 8.3 ± 2.6 μU/ml. When the patients received a standard meal of 10 Kcal/kg body wt 2 h after SMS, the insulin release was distincly stimulated to 36 ± 11 μl/ml, which was somewhat lower than in the control period. Post-prandial glycemia was raised to 130 mg% which can be considered as being at the upper limit of the normal range. Plasma TSH, T3, cortisol, LH, FSH and PRL were not altered by SMS. It can be concluded that SMS represents a new option in the medical treatment of acromegaly. This anticipation is further substantiated by two interesting findings (personal communications by A. Gomez Pan and M. Besser respectively). The first observation deals with multiple injections of SMS. In a patient who received 3 times 50 μg SMS sc every 8 h, glucose tolerance became normal after the second injection, suggesting tachyphylaxis with respect to insulin inhibition. The second finding was in acromegalic patients who had been resistant to bromocriptine. 50-100 μg SMS was able to normalize GH release even in these cases. Therefore, SMS could be used in the treatment of acromegalic patients either alone, or in a combined therapy with dopamine agonists.

Application of SMS in endocrine tumors

Somatostatin-14 is known for its inhibitory effects on many different peptides. On the other hand, it has been recognized that the clinical and the biochemical manifestations of gut and pancreatic endocrine tumors are determined by the peptides and amines secreted by these tumors (23, 24) and that suppression of tumor-related peptides and amine secretion can produce relatively prolonged symptomatic remission. Somatostatin-14, even more so, SMS, should therefore be of value in treating peptide hypersecreting endocrine tumors. This has indeed been shown with S-14 (25, 26, 27) and analog (see Table 1 for references). SMS, thanks to its metabolic stability and its high potency, can be applied sc, as insulin is routinely self-administered in diabetics. It could thus be tested in different endocrine tumors on an outpatient basis.

Most of the patients have been treated by the group of S. Bloom at the Hammersmith Hospital in London: two glucagonomas (both also secreting gastrin), two VIPomas (both also secreting neurotensin and peptide histidine isoleucine), three gastrinomas, one insulinoma and one carcinoid syndrome (28). The patients received 50 g SMS sc twice daily which produced at least a 50% fall in basal concentrations of all secreted peptides except glucagon which fell by only 15-20%, associated with a marked improvement in all peptide related

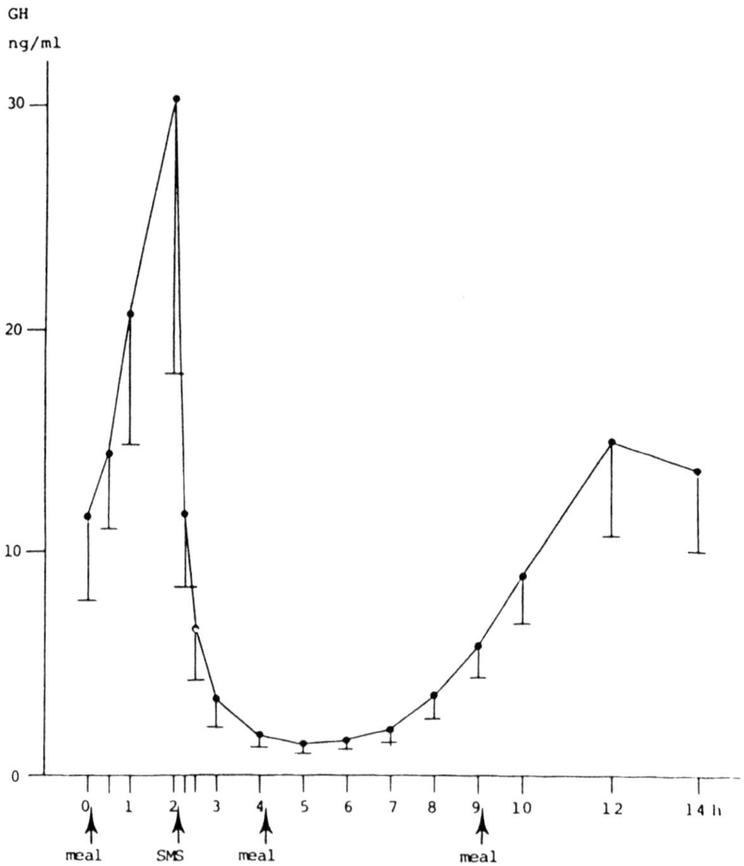

Fig. 6. Plasma GH levels (mean ± SE) after a single sc injection of 50 μg SMS in 6 acromegalic patients.

symptoms. Some of the patients have been treated for periods up to one year and in these cases prolonged relief of symptoms and suppression of hormone levels were seen. No patients had problems with self-administration of the drug and essentially no side effects were reported with the exception of mild nausea (1 case) and worsening of postural hypotension (1 case with diabetic autonomic neuropathy).

Maybe the most demonstrative case of the clinical usefulness of SMS is a VIPoma patient, treated also by S. Bloom (29). This 43 year old man with a malignant VIP secreting tumor developed recurrence of severe watery-diarrhea and hypokalaemia having been in total symptomatic and biochemical remission following chemotherapy with steptozotocin. Neither streptozotocin and 5-fluorouracil, nor hepatic artery embolization could induce a second remission. The patient had to be replaced with continuous intravenous fluid and electrolytes. Treatment with twice daily 50 μg SMS subcutaneously resulted in a marked improvement of diarrhoea from 8 stools/day to 2 stools/day. Withdrawal of SMS led to recurrence of severe symptoms. The patient has now been treated with SMS for one year as an outpatient. He has had no recurrence of diarrhea and has been able to return to full time work and to his hobby of marathon running. Exciting is the finding with CT scans that hepatic metastases show considerable reduction in size during this prolonged treatment (29). SMS may not only offer a palliative treatment but also have a future place as a tumor shrinking agent in the treatment of endocrine tumors.

ACKNOWLEDGMENT

The authors are well aware of the fact that the development of SMS 201-995 to the clinical phase has been dependent on excellent contributions of many colleagues, as has been the clinical testing in normal volunteers and in patients. We would like to express our thanks to all of them, especially to W. Bauer, U. Briner, W. Doepfner and T.J. Petcher from our Preclinical and to W. Kutz and E. del Pozo from the Clinical Research Department. We thank also the many clinicians who have been involved, especially K. Schluter at the University Hospital in Freiburg, U. Keller at the University Clinic in Basel and G. Plewe at the University of Mainz.

REFERENCES

1. Brazeau P, Vale W, Burgus R, Ling N, Butcher M, Rivier J, Guillemin R 1973 Hypothalamic polypeptide that inhibits the secretion of immunoreactive pituitary growth hormone. Science 179:77.
2. Bauer W, Briner U, Doepfner W, Haller R, Huguenin R, Marbach P, Petcher TJ, Pless J 1982 SMS 201-995: A very potent and selective octapeptide analogue of somatostatin with prolonged action. Life Sci 31:1133.

3. Brazeau P, Vale W, Rivier J, Guillemin R 1974 Acylated Des-[Ala_1-Gly_2]-somatostatin analogs: prolonged inhibition of growth hormone secretion. Biochem Biophys Res Commun 60:1202.
4. Evered DC, Gomez Pan A, Tunbridge WMG, Hall R, Lind T, Besser GM, Mortimer CH, Thorner MO, Schally AV, Kastin AJ, Coy DH 1975 Analogues of growth hormone release inhibiting hormone. Lancet 1:1250.
5. Raptis S, Zoupas CH, Mallas E, Moulopoulos S 1978 Effects of a new somatostatin analogue in insulin dependent diabetics. Diabetologia 15:264.
6. Lenti G, Trovati M, Lorenzati R, Vitelli F, Tagliaferro V, Marocco A, Pagano GF 1980 Effect of a somatostatin analog on insulin requirement and hormone levels in 6 insulin-dependent juvenile-onset diabetics subjected to artificial pancreas. Acta Diabetologica Lat 17:9.
7. Trovati M, Massara F, Camanni F, Molinatti GM, Lorenzati R, Pagano GF 1980 Effect of the somatostatin analog D-Trp^8, D-Cys^{14} on glucose, insulin, pancreatic glucagon and growth hormone plasma levels in acromegalics and mild diabetics. J Endocrinol Invest 3:189.
8. Kahn R, Bhathena SJ, Recant L, Rivier J 1981 Use of somatostatin and somatostatin analogs in a patient with a glucagonoma. J Clin Endocrinol Metab 53:543.
9. Adrian TE, Barnes AJ, Long RG, O'Shaughnessy DJ, Brown MR, Rivier J, Vale W, Blackburn AM, Bloom SR 1981 The effect of somatostatin analogs on secretion of growth, pancreatic, and gastrointestinal hormones in man. J Clin Endocrinol Metab 53:675.
10. Long RG, Adrian TE, Brown MR, Rivier JE, Barnes AJ, Mallinson CN, Vale W, Christofides ND, Bloom SR 1979 Suppression of pancreatic endocrine tumour secretion by long-acting somatostatin analogue. Lancet 2:764.
11. Barnes AJ, Long RG, Adrian TE, Vale W, Brown MR, Rivier JE, Hanley J, Ghatei MA, Sarson DL, Bloom SSR 1981 Effect of a long-acting octapeptide analogue of somatostatin on growth hormone and pancreatic and gastrointestinal hormones in man. Clin Sci 61:653.
12. Reding P, Naeije R, Melot C, Hallemans R, Mols P 1980 Action de deux types de somatostatine sur l'hémodynamique portale, pulmonaire et systémique du patient cirrhotique. Gastroentérologie Clin Biol (France) 4:928.
13. Long RG, Peters JR, Grahame-Smith DG, O'Shaughnessy DJ, Vale W, Rivier JE, Brown MR, Bloom SR 1980 Effects of somatostatin on flushing and plasma gastrointestinal peptides in the carcinoid syndrome. Clin Sci 59:9P.
14. Long RG, Peters JR, Bloom SR, Brown MR, Vale W, Rivier JE, Grahame-Smith DG 1981 Somatostatin, gastrointestinal peptides and the carcinoid syndrome. Gut 22:549.

15. Roti E, Ghinelli C, Baudini P, Del Rossi C, Emanuele R, Robuschi G, Gundi A 1981 Effects of somatostatin in a case of severe hypoglycemia due to nesidioblastosis. J Endocrinol Invest 4:209.
16. Chernish STM, Miller RE, Rosenak BD, Brunelle RL 1981 Effect of D-Val^{1},D-Trp^{8} -somatostatin on the motility of the stomach, duodenum and jejunum. Am J Gastroenterol 75:36.
17. Wajchenberg BL, Cesar FP, Leme CE, Borghi VC, Souza ITT, Neto DG, Germek OA, Coy DH, Comaru-Schally AM, Schally AV 1983 1983 Dissociated effects of somatostatin analogs on arginine-induced insulin, glucagon and growth hormone release in acromegalic patients. Horm Metab Res 15:471.
18. Dimitriadis G, Tessari P, Gerich J 1983 Effects of a long-acting somatostatin analogue on postprandial hyperglycemia in insulin-dependent diabetes mellitus. Metabolism 32:987.
19. Veber DF, Freidinger RM, Perlow DS, Paleveda WJ, Holly FW, Strachan RG, Nutt RG, Arison BH, Homnick C, Randall WC, Glitzer MS, Saperstein R, Hirschmann R 1981 A potent cyclic hexapeptide analogue of somatostatin. Nature 292:55.
20. Skamene A, Patel YC 1984 Infusion of graded concentrations of somatostatin in man: pharmacokinetics and differential inhibitory effects on pituitary and islet hormones. Clin Endocrinol 20:555.
21. Spinas GA, Keller U, Varga L, Neufeld M 1984 Reduction of postprandial hyperglycemia and suppression of gastrointestinal hormones after s.c. administration of a new somatotatin analogue in type 1 diabetics. Eur J Clin Invest 14:24.
22. Plewe G, Beyer J, Krause U, Neufeld M, del Pozo E, Program of the 7th International Congress of Endocrinology, Quebec City 1984 (Abstract).
23. Friesen SR 1982 Tumours of the endocrine pancreas. New Engl J Med 306:580.
24. Wood SM, Polak JM, Bloom SR 1983 Gut hormone secreting tumours. Scand J Gastroenterol 18 (Suppl 82):165.
25. Bonfils S, Rene E, Piginal F, Rambaud JC 1979 Rebound effect after somatostatin treatment in Verner Morrison syndrome. Lancet 2:476.
26. Sohier, J, Jeanmougin M, Lombrail P, Passa PH 1980 Rapid improvement of skin lesions in glucagonomas with intravenous somatostatin infusion. Lancet 1:40.
27. Dharmsathaphron K, Sherwin RS, Cataland S, Jaffe B, Dobbins J 1980 Somatostatin inhibits diarrhoea in the carcinoid syndrome. Am Int Med 92:68.
28. Wood SM, Kraenzlin ME, Bloom SR 1983 New Somatostatin Analogue for home treatment of endocrine tumours. Gut 24:A984.
29. Kraenzlin ME, Ch'ng JLC, Wood SM, Bloom SR 1984 Remission of symptoms and shrinkage of metastasis with long term treatment with somatostatin analogue. Gut 25:A576.

20

THE EFFECTS OF SOMATOSTATIN AND SELECTED ANALOGS ON LIPID ABSORPTION IN ANIMALS

EVE E. SLATER, HOWARD M. KATZEN, RUTH F. NUTT, RICHARD SAPERSTEIN AND SANFORD L. STEELMAN

Merck Institute for Therapeutic Research
Rahway, New Jersey 07065

ABSTRACT

Based upon the clinical finding that a Merck somatostatin-14 (S-14) analog (1) induced steatorrhea in man, we sought to develop animal models to study the effects of S-14 and a series of synthetic analogs on absorption.

Rats were trained to eat a diet (preweighed) containing 15% fat. Following the feeding period, the remaining diet was removed and the amount consumed recorded. This food conditioning of the rats was continued until the rats consumed approximately 15 g of the diet per day. Feces were collected and weighed prior to feeding periods. On test days, S-14 or analogs were administered sc to rats immediately prior to feeding. For each compound tested, fat absorption decreased in dose-dependent fashion. For example, S-14 at 0.5 mg/kg did not increase % of dietary fat in feces (% DFF). At 1.0 mg/kg, S-14 increased % DFF from 7.9 to 10.2 ($p < 0.01$, pretest day vs test day), and at 10 mg/kg S-14, % DFF increased from 9.1 to 12.8 ($p < 0.001$).

For each analog, the subcutaneous dose required to decrease fat absorption in rats was several orders of magnitude higher than the intravenous dose required to inhibit insulin and glucagon. Moreover, the threshold for production of statistically significant increases in fecal fat differed among analogs when compared to their endocrine potencies. One analog administered in the model for 14 days was shown to produce consistent fat malabsorption throughout the entire test period; however, this lipid malabsorption was substantially more pronounced on the first three days of the treatment period. When the compound was not administered on day 15, the % DFF significantly decreased.

In an attempt to develop a system more suitable for rapid screening, pancreatic secretagogues such as secretin or cholecystokinin, were administered intravenously to anesthetized rats whose duodena had been cannulated and perfused to enable collection of pancreatic secretions. Total amylase, lipase, and protein were determined in single animals in response to a secretagogue, both before and after iv pretreatment by S-14 or an analog. Pancreatic enzyme secretion in response to sequential secretagogue-stimulation was found to be reproducible for up to three injections and behaved in a dose-dependent fashion. In general, secretagogue-induced increases in amylase, lipase, and total protein were comparable.

Pretreatment with the S-14 analogs substantially inhibited secretagogue-induced pancreatic exocrine secretion and was dose-dependent. Individual potencies correlated well with the ability to inhibit endocrine hormone release (glucagon, insulin, and growth hormone), although one compound with significantly less exocrine inhibitory effect was noted.

Our experience demonstrates that it is possible to produce S-14-induced fat malabsorption in rats, when fed a lipid rich diet. The animal models described herein show that S-14 and selected S-14 analogs have different potencies to induce fat malabsorption in rat and to inhibit exogenously stimulated pancreatic enzyme release. Nonetheless, the potential clinical significance of these separations is difficult to predict.

INTRODUCTION

Veber et al. (1) have reported the synthesis of a cyclic hexapeptide analog of somatostatin, cyclo(N-Me-Ala-Tyr-D-Trp-Lys-Val-Phe) (Merck-I). In various experimental systems, this analog was 50-100 times more potent than S-14 in inhibiting the release of insulin, glucagon, and growth hormone. In insulin-deficient diabetic animals, Merck-I administered with insulin, improved postprandial glycemic control. This analog was metabolically stable in the gastrointestinal tract and blood, but had limited oral bioavailability.

Recently, Merck-I was given to normal and Type I diabetic subjects by both the intravenous and intranasal routes. The desired effects on blood sugar were obtained and the drug was well tolerated. Nevertheless, in certain subjects, an increase in stool fat content was observed (Gerich JE et al., unpublished results).

Thus, we sought to develop model systems in animals for the evaluation of this side effect and to screen additional analogs for possible selectivity. Our results in animals will be described below. The clinical experience will be reported separately.

MATERIALS AND METHODS

The cyclic hexapeptide somatostatin analogs, Merck-I, II, III, and IV, were synthesized using the solid phase method to prepare linear intermediates which were removed from the resin as acylhydrazides with hydrazine and cyclized via the azide method. Cyclization points were the Tyr-D/L-Trp and the Lys-Ser amide bonds. These procedures have been detailed for related cyclic structures (2). For the synthesis of Merck-III, the linear intermediate Boc-D-Phe-Cys(Acm)-Phe-D-Trp-Lys(2-Cl-Cbz)-Thr(Bzl)-Cys(Acm)-Thr(Bzl)-O-® was prepared. Removal from the resin as carboxy-terminal threoninol peptide was carried out with $NaBH_4$ in THF (3). Stepwise removal of protecting groups with HCl/ETOAc and HF and subsequent disulfide formation by treatment with iodine gave Merck-III. All analogs were at least 97% pure as measured by HPLC, and were further characterized by amino acid analysis, TLC, NMR, and FABMS. Somatostatin-14 (Merck-V) was obtained from Bachem Co., Torrance, CA.

In the in vivo model, male Sprague Dawley rats (approximately 200 g) were trained to eat a preweighed diet containing 15% lard. Following this feeding period, the remaining diet was removed and the amount consumed recorded. This food conditioning was continued until the rats consumed approximately 15 g of the diet per day. Feces were collected and weighed prior to each feeding period and on subsequent days thereafter. Fat extraction was performed using the method of Folch et al. (4) and % dietary fat in feces (% DFF) recorded. On test days, S-14 or analogs were administered sc to rats (n = 5/group) prior to feeding.

In a separate series of experiments, adult male Beagle dogs were trained to eat a similar diet and fecal fat excretion determined.

In the in situ model (5), male Sprague Dawley rats were allowed free access to Purina Chow and water until 1 h prior to selection for study. Anesthesia consisted of two sequential ip injections of urethane (1.5 mg/kg), after which the peritoneal cavity was entered and the duodenum incised approximately 1 cm proximal to the entrance of the bile duct. The duodenum was then cannulated by a 2 mm polyethylene catheter and ligated. A similar duodenal incision, cannulation and ligation was performed 1 cm distal to the bile duct. Perfusion of 0.15 M saline from a reservoir through the proximal tube was begun and after a 5 min wash period, basal secretions were collected from the distal tube at a perfusion rate of 0.25 ml/min.

Secretagogues or analogs were administered by iv injection into the jugular vein in a 100 µl volume. For the experiments described below, saline or analogs were administered 20 min prior to 0.5 U secretin (Chemalog and Sigma). Pancreatic enzyme secretion in response to sequential stimulation was found to be reproducible for up to three injections and behaved in a dose-dependent fashion. In general, secretagogue-induced increases in amylase, lipase, and total protein were comparable. α-Amylase, lipase and protein assays were conducted as previously described (5).

RESULTS

In the *in vivo* model, rats received varying doses of S-14 or analogs subcutaneously. In response to S-14 at 0.5 mg/kg, the % DFF was not changed significantly (9.6 ± 0.7 to 11.0 ± 0.8). At 5 mg/kg S-14, the % DFF increased significantly from a pretest value of 6.9 ± 0.4 to 11.6 ± 1.0 ($p < 0.005$) after treatment (Fig. 1). Note that in Fig. 1 through Fig. 4 each point represents the mean ± SE of 5 rats. In another experiment, S-14 was administered at 1.0 and 10.0 mg/kg. The % DFF rose from a pretest value of 7.9 ± 0.2 to 10.2 ± 0.7 ($p < 0.02$) and 9.1 ± 0.5 to 12.8 ± 0.6 ($p < 0.02$), respectively (Fig. 2). The iv dose of S-14 necessary to completely inhibit insulin and glucagon secretion is approximately 250 μg/kg.

When Merck-I was administered in graded doses, significant increases in % DFF from pretest values were noted at 0.5 and 2 mg/kg (9.8 ± 0.9 to 14.6 ± 1.1, ($p < 0.01$) and 9.9 ± 0.4 to 18.3 ± 1.2, ($p < 0.001$), respectively) (Fig. 3). The iv dose of Merck-I which completely inhibits insulin and glucagon secretion is 5 μg/kg.

In order to determine whether tachyphylaxis would result after prolonged administration to rats, Merck-I (2 mg/kg, sc) was given each day for 14 days and the % DFF calculated (Fig. 4). When vehicle alone was administered to a group of control rats, no significant change in % DFF was noted during the experiment. The administration of Merck-I resulted in a 250% increase in % DFF on the first day of treatment. From days 3 to 14, the observed increase in % DFF was approximately 65% of the pretest value ($p < 0.05$). The day following cessation of treatment, the % DFF significantly decreased ($p < 0.05$), but not to its pretest value.

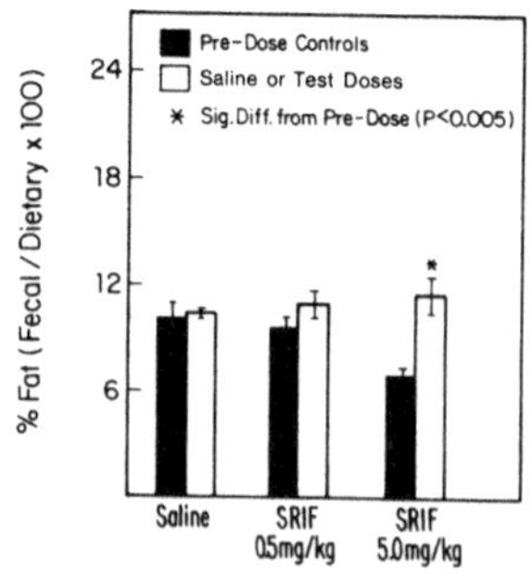

Fig. 1. Effect of somatostatin-14 (SRIF) on dietary fat accumulation in feces.

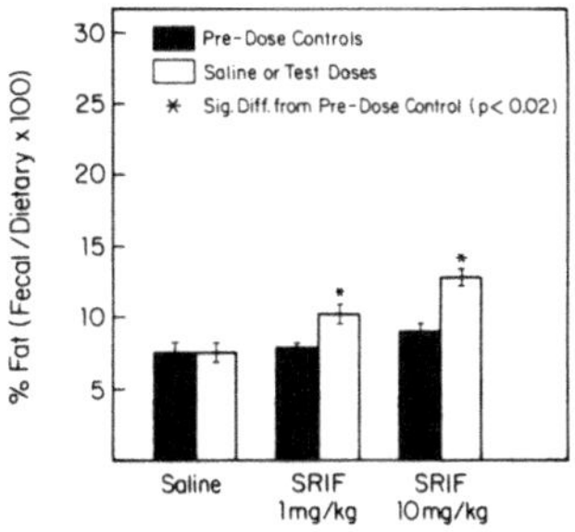

Fig. 2. Effect of somatostatin-14 (SRIF) on dietary fat accumulation in feces.

While Merck-I administered subcutaneously could be shown to produce a significant increase in fecal fat in dogs similarly trained to ingest a 15% fat diet, we were unable to demonstrate a clear-cut dose response relationship, as in the rat. At increasing doses, retardation in stool output occurred. Interestingly, no significant alterations in plasma triglyceride levels were demonstrable. Thus, this model was abandoned for further study.

In the *in situ* model, increasing iv doses of S-14 or analogs, quite unexpectedly caused an increase in amylase, lipase and, to a lesser extent, protein. Nonetheless, as predicted, pretreatment with S-14 or analogs resulted in marked reduction of the stimulation of amylase, lipase and total protein, by exogenously administered secretin (0.5 U) or other pancreatic secretagogues. Thus, treatment with Merck-I at 50 μg/kg, 20 min prior to secretin administration, resulted in an 80% inhibition of secretin-induced stimulation (6). The degree of inhibition was dependent upon timing of pretreatment and could be represented by a bell-shaped inhibitory response curve with maximal inhibition occurring between 20-30 minutes of pretreatment by S-14 or analogs, regardless of the analog tested. Thus, all further protocols were performed with analog administered 20-25

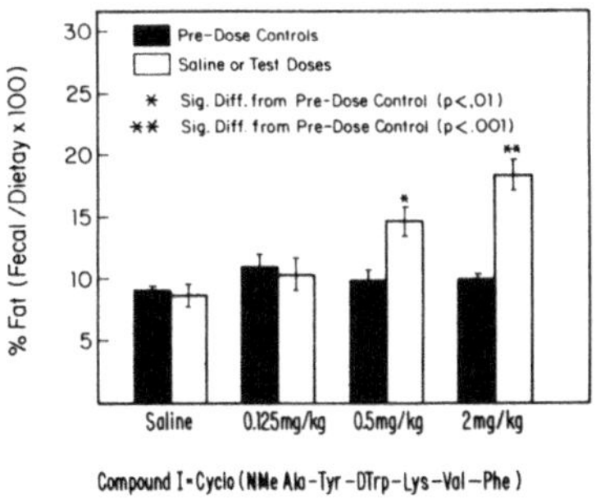

Fig. 3. Effect of compound I on fecal fat accumulation.

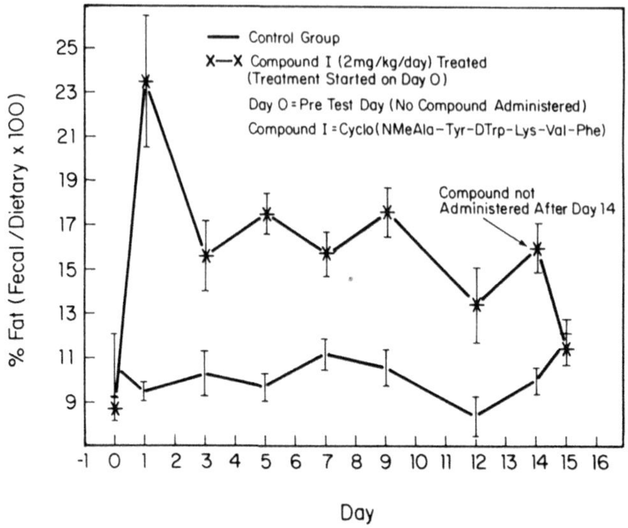

Fig. 4. Effect of compound I on fecal fat accumulation: 14 day treatment.

min prior to secretagogue injection. Results were calculated as % inhibition comparing the areas under the curves for amylase, lipase and protein in a single animal who first received a saline injection prior to secretagogue administration, and secondly an analog injection. In later experiments, secretions from each time period were pooled. For the most part, the responses of amylase, lipase and total protein to both stimulus and inhibition were comparable.

For S-14 and each analog tested, inhibition was dose-responsive, once again in a bell-shaped pattern. Thus, percent inhibition increased with increasing dosages to a maximum and then decreased, presumably due to the intrinsic stimulatory effect of S-14 and analogs at higher doses, as described above. Maximum amylase inhibition for S-14 iv was at 125 µg/kg and for Merck-I iv was at 50 µg/kg. It should be noted that the doses of test compounds which produced maximal exocrine inhibition were 2-10 fold higher than those required for glucagon inhibition.

For each compound, percent maximal inhibition of amylase and lipase at a dose of 50 µg/kg was compared to that for Merck-I, the reference compound, and this ratio termed exocrine inhibitory potency. Similarly, the dose which completely inhibited glucagon secretion was compared to Merck-I, and this ratio termed endocrine inhibitory potency. The results for S-14 and several analogs are presented in Table I. Compounds with ratios greater than 1 would be expected to have relatively more exocrine inhibitory potency than

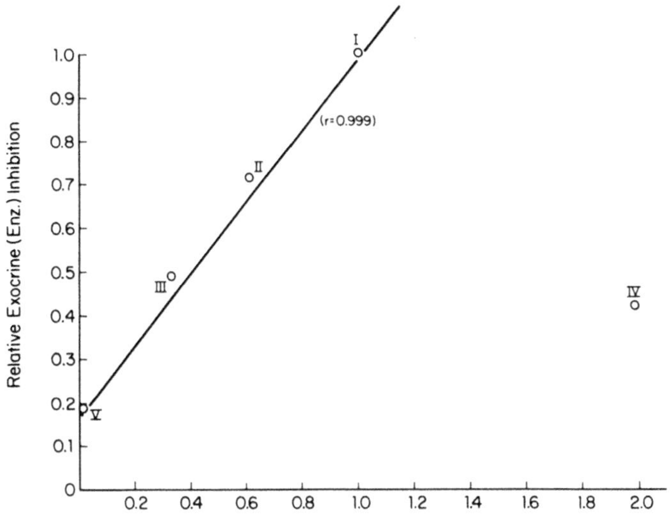

Fig. 5. Relationship between relative exocrine and endocrine inhibitory potency.

Merck-I and conversely compounds with ratios of less than 1 might be expected to inhibit exocrine pancreatic function less. One compound, Merck-IV, possessed a ratio of less than 1. The data of Table I are plotted in Fig. 5. As can be seen, a high degree of correlation between relative exocrine and endocrine inhibitory potency existed ($r = 0.999$) and has since been demonstrated for a larger series of analogs. While Merck-IV exhibited a degree of endocrine inhibitory potency comparable to Merck-I, its exocrine inhibitory effect was significantly less ($p < 0.05$).

DISCUSSION

The effects of S-14 on gastrointestinal function are multiple and complex (7). These are summarized in Table II. A fairly extensive literature describes the ability of S-14 to impair carbohydrate absorption (7, 8). In fact, endogenous S-14 is believed to perform a regulatory function for nutrient entry and metabolism (9, 10). In addition to these direct anti-absorptive effects, S-14 would be expected to inhibit the endocrine secretion of a host of gastrointestinal hormones, for example, cholecystokinin, gastrin, secretin and VIP; to inhibit exocrine secretion of gastric acid, pancreatic amylase and lipase; to inhibit gastric emptying, gall bladder contraction and small intestinal motility; and to decrease splanchnic blood flow. Thus, its effects on lipid absorption would be expected to be

Table I

Compounds tested	Relative inhibitory potency Exo	Relative inhibitory potency Endo	Exocrine/ endocrine ratio
I- Cyclo (N-Me-Ala-Tyr-D-Trp-Lys-Val-Phe)	1.00	1.00	1.00
II- Cyclo(N-Me-Ala-Tyr-Trp-Lys-Val-Phe)	0.71	0.61	1.16
III- D-Phe-Cys-Phe-D-Trp-Lys-Thr-Cys-Thr-OL*	0.49	0.34	1.14
IV- Cyclo(N-Me-Phe-His-D-Trp-Lys-Ser-Ala)	0.42	1.99	0.21
V- Somatostatin-14	0.19	0.01	19.0

* This compound is Sandoz SMS201-995.

substantial, and those reported cases of steatorrhea accompanying somatostatin-secreting tumors confirm this expectation (11-13).

Conversely, exogenously administered S-14 was not thought to be associated with significant lipid malabsorption until recently. In a 1981 review, Gerich (14) states, "Despite these numerous effects of somatostatin on gastrointestinal function, to date, no malabsorption has been reported during long-term infusions of somatostatin in man."

Table II. Effects of S-14 on Gastrointestinal Function

1. Gastric acid secretion
2. Gastric emptying
3. Duodenal motility
4. Bile flow
5. Gall bladder function
6. Hormone secretion inhibition: Pepsin, gastrin, secretin, CCK, etc.
7. Basal and stimulated pancreatic exocrine function
8. Glucose, xylose, triglyceride, amino acid absorption
9. Splanchnic blood flow

Paradoxically, S-14 infusions have been shown to decrease gastrointestinal motility and the diarrhea associated with either short bowel syndrome (15) or carcinoid (16). In these studies, S-14 treatment was associated with a modest increase in fecal fat in one of four patients with short bowel syndrome. Stool weight decreased in all. In the carcinoid patient, fecal fat increased four-fold with a modest increase in fecal weight. Since this patient's diarrhea diminished despite the above, it was postulated that S-14 blocked fatty acid-induced secretion of fluid and electrolytes in the colon.

In the pioneering studies of Gerich et al. (17), S-14 administered at doses of 100 μg/h (approximately 1.5 μg/kg/h) continuously for 3 days to seven diabetic subjects was associated with no adverse effects. The diet contained 2032 Kcal/day as 50% carbohydrate, 30% fat, and 20% protein.

In their classic study, Raskin and Unger (18) infused S-14 in diabetic patients fed relatively high fat diets (55-65% fat). No reference was made to fat malabsorption during S-14 infusion.

On the other hand, Hengl et al. (19) administered 100 g neutral fat orally to seven healthy subjects, followed by S-14 infusion (at approximately 1 μg/kg/min) over three hours with and without lipase in the test meal and reported an absence of the normal postprandial increase in serum triglyceride levels. Stool fat content was not reported in this study.

Hengl and colleagues (20) did, however, quantitate twenty-four hour stool fats in three nondiabetic subjects after Billroth II hemigastrectomy. These patients received a 100 g fat meal with an iv bolus injection of S-14 (1000 μg) followed by a continuous infusion of 1000 μg/h for 3 hours (approximately 0.2 μg/kg/min). As expected, postprandial triglyceride elevation was completely blocked by the S-14. Stool fat was measured in three patients and elevated to levels between 5 and 15 g/day.

Studies demonstrating lipid malabsorption in animals are few. The rigorous studies of Sakurai et al. (21) in conscious dogs in which S-14 was administered at 3.3 μg/min over 1.5 to 2.5 h showed no statistically significant differences between mean triglyceride levels in treated and control groups at any point, although mean maximal triglyceride increment was significantly greater in the latter group.

Schusdziarra et al. (22) administered several S-14 analogs sc to alloxan diabetic dogs over three days using doses known to inhibit glucagon and to control blood sugar with insulin. While decreases in serum triglycerides were noted, no overt evidence of steatorrhea or weight loss was reported. Details of dietary intake were not recorded.

Using anesthetized rats, Daumerie and Henquin (23) reported no significant effect of S-14 at substantial doses (approximately 5 µg/kg/min) in palmitate, leucine, galactose, or sucrose absorption from a "tied duodenojejunal loop".

Two studies, one in dogs and the other in primates, do, however, demonstrate fat malabsorption when animals were challenged by meals containing a high content of lipid (24, 25). An additional study, reported in abstract form demonstrated decreased oleic acid absorption from duodenal loops in dogs in response to S-14 (26).

Schusdziarra et al. (24), using conscious dogs, reported that "physiologic" doses (approximately 2-3 ng/kg/min) of S-14, infused intraportally, decreased the postprandial rise in peripheral venous triglyceride after administration of a fat-protein meal consisting of 80 g fat and 80 g protein. Somatostatin-14 infusion was begun 30 min prior to eating and was continued for 6 h. Triglyceride levels were substantially blunted for approximately 3 h (75 to 270 min postprandially). Fecal fat content was not assessed. Immunization of dogs against S-14 resulted in increased postprandial serum triglycerides (27). This experiment, however, did not attempt to predict the effects of exogenous S-14 on fat absorption in dogs. It simply demonstrated the importance of endogenous S-14 in lipid absorption.

Koerker and Hansen (25) studied the effects of S-14 on gastric motility and absorption of [3-^{3}H] glucose and [9,10-^{3}H]triolein in rhesus monkeys. Continuous S-14 infusion at 0.8 µg/kg/min following administration of a liquid diet, containing the above, resulted in marked impairment of lipid absorption without effects on gastric motility or rate of glucose absorption.

In an <u>in situ</u> preparation of isolated proximal small bowel loops in dogs, absorption of micellar oleic acid containing a tritium label was decreased by 80% after continuous iv S-14 (0.16 µg/kg/min) (26).

When it became apparent that Merck-I administered intravenously or intranasally with meals was capable of inducing steatorrhea in both normal and diabetic subjects, we sought to assess this "side effect" in an animal model.

Our attempts to develop a canine model for fat malabsorption were unsuccessful. Unlike the experience of Schusdziarra et al. (24) who administered S-14 by continuous intraportal infusion, multiple subcutaneous injections of Merck-I to dogs trained to eat a high fat diet failed to significantly alter serum triglyceride levels. While increases in fecal fat were observed, no definite dose-response relationship could be demonstrated. This, coupled with the observation of others, may indicate that the dog is particularly resistant to the development of S-14-induced lipid malabsorption (28).

Conversely, the rat model described herein provides a reliable and effective means to demonstrate the effects of S-14 and analogs on fat malabsorption in relatively large numbers of animals. While we noted that the threshold for production of statistically significant increases in fecal fat varied among compounds when compared to the minimally effective endocrine inhibitory dose, it is difficult to know whether these same differences might pertain to man. Such extrapolation is especially difficult given the relative resistance of the rat to develop fat malabsorption at S-14 or analog doses well above those iv doses required to produce the desired endocrine effects.

This model has proved useful to assess whether tachyphylaxis developed due to the administration of Merck-I. While our results show statistically significant fat malabsorption over a two-week period, this effect was clearly more pronounced on the first several days of the study.

Similarly, the _in situ_ test system described above has been valuable for the rapid screening of a number of compounds. Unlike the _in vivo_ model, however, this system is not amenable to the use of large numbers of animals. Nonetheless, it has raised several interesting physiologic questions. The apparent stimulatory effect by higher doses of S-14 and analogs on basal pancreatic enzyme secretion is an unexpected observation. The requirement of a pretreatment period to effect maximal inhibition of pancreatic exocrine function suggests that the effect of S-14 is not direct. While prostaglandins have been implicated in mediating the inhibitory effect of S-14 on gastric acid secretion (29), preliminary data from our laboratory do not indicate that indomethacin alters the observed results.

Moreover, the _in situ_ system assesses only one aspect of the multiple effects of S-14 on gastrointestinal function. Thus, gastrointestinal motility, bile flow and gall bladder emptying are not tested in this system (30, 31). The relative resistance of animals to steatorrhea as compared to man suggests that differing mechanisms may be responsible, depending upon the species.

For the above reasons, the apparent differences among analogs in their ability to affect stimulated pancreatic enzyme secretion is difficult to interpret. Nevertheless, we hope to determine whether compounds with a significant negative correlation between exocrine and endocrine effects do indeed possess a lesser potential for the production of steatorrhea in man. Such separation, if it extends to the human experience, would provide even greater impetus for the long awaited use of S-14 analogs as adjuncts in the treatment of Type I diabetes mellitus.

ACKNOWLEDGMENT

We are grateful to Drs. G. Kuron and J. Huff for their advice regarding animal diets and fat extraction. Dr. S.F. Brady synthesized Merck-III. We thank E. Brady, E. Chapin, G. Chicchi, B. Green, E. Morgan, M. Pastor and P. Vicario for technical assistance and M. Spencer for typing this manuscript. We thank Drs. E.H. Cordes, R.F. Hirschmann and D.F. Veber for their support during these studies.

REFERENCES

1. Veber DF, Saperstein R, Nutt RF, Freidinger RM, Brady SF, Curley P, Perlow DS, Paleveda WJ, Colton CD, Zacchei AG, Tocco DJ, Holt DR, Vandlen RL, Gerich JE, Hall L, Mandarino L, Cordes EH, Anderson PS, Hirschmann R 1984 A superactive cyclic hexapeptide analog of somatostatin. Life Sci 34:1371.
2. Nutt RF, Veber DF, Curley PE, Saperstein R, Hirschmann R 1983 Somatostatin analogs which define the role of the lysine-9 amino group. Int J Peptide Protein Res 21:66.
3. Stewart JM, Morris DH Peptide alcohols. 1981. U.S. Pat. 4,254,023, 3/3/1981.
4. Folch J, Lees M, Sloane-Stanley GH 1957 A simple method for the isolation and purification of total lipids from animal tissues. J Biol Chem 226:497.
5. Katzen HM, Vicario PP, Green BG 1984 Characteristics of secretory responses of the rat exocrine pancreas in vivo to various secretagogues. (submitted for publication).
6. Katzen HM, Vicario PP, Green BG 1984 Inhibition of secretagogue induced, and stimulation of basal, enzyme secretions from rat exocrine pancreas by somatostatin and a hexapeptide analog. (submitted for publication).
7. Gerich JE 1981 Somatostatin. In: Brownlee M (ed) Handbook of Diabetes Mellitus. Garland STPM Press, New York, 1:297.
8. Wahren J, Felig P 1976 Influence of somatostatin in carbohydrate disposal and absorption in diabetes mellitus. Lancet 2:1213.
9. Schusdziarra V 1980 Somatostatin - a regulatory modulator connecting nutrient entry and metabolism. Horm Metab Res 12:563.
10. Schusdziarra V 1983 Somatostatin - physiological and pathophysiological aspects. Scand J Gastroenterol 18:69.
11. Krejs GJ, Orci L, Conlon JM, Ravazzola M, Davis GR, Raskin P, Collins SM, McCarthy DM, Baetens D, Rubenstein A, Aldor AM, Unger RH 1979 Somatostatinoma syndrome - biochemical, morphologic and clinical features. N Engl J Med 301:285.

12. Pipeleers D, Somers G, Gepts W, De Nutte N, De Vroede M 1979 Plasma pancreatic hormone levels in a case of somatostatinoma - diagnostic and therapeutic implications. J Clin Endocrinol Metab 49:572.
13. Larsson LI, Hirsch MA, Holst JJ, Ingemansson S, Kuhl C, Jensen SL, Lundqvist G, Rehfeld JF, Schwartz TW 1977 Pancreatic somatostatinoma - clinical features and physiological implications. Lancet 1:666.
14. Gerich JE 1981 Somatostatin. In: Brownlee M (ed) Handbook of Diabetes Mellitus. Garland STPM Press, New York, vol. 1:302.
15. Dharmsathaphorn K, Gorelick FS, Sherwin RS, Cataland S, Dobbins JW 1982 Somatostatin decreases diarrhea in patients with the short bowel syndrome. J Clin Gastroenterol 4:521.
16. Dharmsathaphorn K, Sherwin RS, Cataland S, Jaffe B, Dobbins J 1980 Somatostatin inhibits diarrhea in the carcinoid syndrome. Ann Int Med 92:68.
17. Gerich JE, Schultz TA, Lewis SB, Karam JH 1977 Clinical evaluation of somatostatin as a potential adjunct to insulin in the management of diabetes mellitus. Diabetologia 13:537.
18. Raskin P, Unger RH 1978 Hyperglucagonemia and its suppression-importance in the metabolic control of diabetes. N Engl J Med 299:433.
19. Hengl G, Prager J, Miorz R, Pointner H, Deutsch E 1980 Further examinations of the influence of somatostatin on triglyceride absorption. Wien Med Wochenschr 130:49.
20. Hengl G, Prager J, Pointner H 1979 The influence of somatostatin on the absorption of triglycerides in partially gastrectomized subjects. Acta Hepato-Gastroenterol 26:392.
21. Sakurai H, Dobbs RE, Unger RH 1975 The effect of somatostatin on the response of GLI to the intraduodenal administration of glucose, protein, and fat. Diabetologia 11:427.
22. Schusdziarra V, Rivier J, Dobbs R, Brown M, Vale W, Unger R 1978 Somatostatin analogs as glucagon suppressants in diabetes. Horm Metab Res 10:563.
23. Daumerie C, Henquin JC 1982 Somatostatin and the intestinal transport of glucose and other nutrients in the anaesthetized rat. Gut 23:140.
24. Schusdziarra V, Harris V, Arimura A, Unger RH 1979 Evidence for a role of splanchnic somatostatin in the homeostasis of ingested nutrients. Endocrinology 104:1705.
25. Koerker DJ, Hansen BC 1981 Influence of somatostatin on gastric motility and meal absorption in rhesus monkeys, Macaca Mulatta. Metabolism 30:335.
26. Ross SA, Shaffer EA 1981 Somatostatin suppresses glucose and fat absorption and gastric inhibitory polypeptide (GIP) secretion from the canine duodenum. Clin Res 29:311A.
27. Schusdziarra V, Zyznar E, Rouiller D, Boden G, Brown JC, Arimura A, Unger RH 1980 Splanchnic somatostatin: a hormonal regulator of nutrient homeostasis. Science 207:530.

28. Rizza RA, Gerich JE 1978 Somatostatin and diabetes. In: Podolsky S (ed) Med Clin N Amer, WB Saunders Company, Philadelphia, 62:735.
29. Ligumsky M, Goto Y, Debas H, Yamada T 1983 Prostaglandins mediate inhibition of gastric acid secretion by somatostatin in rat. Science 219:301.
30. Johansson C, Kollberg B, Efendic S, Uvnas-Wallensten K 1981 Effects of graded doses of somatostatin on gall bladder emptying and pancreatic enzyme output after oral glucose in man. Digestion 22:24.
31. Johansson C, Wisen O, Efendic S, Uvnas-Wallensten K 1981 Effects of graded doses of somatostatin on gastrointestinal propagation and absorption of oral glucose in man. Digestion 22:126.

MECHANISMS OF ACTION/ANALOGS OF SOMATOSTATIN

PANEL DISCUSSION

MODERATOR: J. GERICH

DR. J. GERICH (Rochester): Dr. Srikant presented evidence for heterogeneity of somatostatin receptors in different tissues suggesting that there may be separate receptors for somatostatin-28 and somatostatin-14, and I was wondering whether some of these differences might be due to differences in the degradation of the peptides in the binding studies. In looking at his data, it seemed to me that the Scatchard plot for somatostatin-28 might actually be curvilinear rather than linear and that perhaps what we're seeing there is binding of somatostatin-28 to somatostatin-14 receptors. Dr. Schonbrunn presented evidence for somatostatin working through inhibition of adenylate cyclase, and I was wondering how willing she would be to generalize her observations to the inhibitory effects of somatostatin in other tissues where, perhaps, it may actually be working through different mechanisms, let's say a calcium action. We heard from Dr. Coy about the development of antagonists which would be very useful tools for looking at the biologic role of endogenous somatostatin, and we saw progress towards selectivity in somatostatin analogs; perhaps we'd like some information on how the antagonists work. Do they work primarily by inhibiting binding of endogenous somatostatin to its receptors or perhaps distally to binding? Finally, we heard some very exciting data from Dr. Pless which seem to indicate that we have a somatostatin analog which appears very close to being clinically useful. It may have some anti-tumor effects and I was wondering whether he might comment later, on long-term side effects that may have been observed with the agent. And finally, we heard from Dr. Slater about the investigation of gastrointestinal side effects of some analogs. In my own experience, this seems perhaps to be the rate-limiting factor in tolerance to somatostatin, and I would pose to her whether she thinks that the Merck 6 compound might have a therapeutic window that might make it clinically applicable.

DR. P. BRAZEAU (La Jolla): My first question is addressed to David Coy. From all the data that you've presented this morning, most of your physiological studies are based on a sodium pentobarbital anesthetized animal. I have some doubt about the physiological validity of this model. Namely, that with sodium pentobarbital you are likely to inhibit, at least partially if not entirely, somatostatin secretion based on hypothalamic culture; and who knows what you are doing to GRF secretion. Wouldn't it be better to use the permanently cannulated animal as a model where you would be able to show that your antagonists counteract the endogenous somatostatin of the animal and therefore would render the animal responsive to a bolus injection of GRF, administered in an episodic fashion every 30 or 60 min? Wouldn't that be a better way to prove your point?

DR. D. COY (New Orleans): I think the drawbacks of the sodium pentobarbital system are well known among the people who use it. The fact remains that there really is not another convenient system which, to my mind, is any better. I think previous systems have used infusion of huge amounts of arginine and things like that, and to me that's not going to give you any more relevant physiological results than the pentobarbital method. With respect to the "somatostatin antagonist" that we have been talking about, which is producing a lot of questions in terms of how it's acting, as I said during the talk, I now feel that it is not a competitive antagonist, as Dr. Brazeau indicated, and that it probably is having some quite dramatic effects on hypothalamic somatostatin release in terms of actually inhibiting somatostatin release from the hypothalamus. Since it does also have pancreatic effects, then it must also be doing similar kinds of things on pancreatic cells. Obviously, we have to do some things to check that out. One of the things would be for somebody with a hypothalamic cell culture system to put this peptide in and measure just how potent it is in that system. We can't do it since we don't have the system. So, does that answer most of your questions?

DR. P. BRAZEAU: Partly. The main question is - is your antagonist capable of counteracting with the normally secreted endogenous somatostatin in the rat? In other words, to prove the point that your compound is an antagonist, you don't need a hypothalamic culture to do that, you just need the pituitary cell culture or a whole animal.

DR. D. COY: Yes, it is something that sounds lke a good thing to try. We'll do it.

DR. A. VINIK (Ann Arbor): Dr. Gerich, I just have a couple of questions which will elaborate a little on the questions that you have set to the panel. The first question I have is to Dr. Schonbrunn. I really thought that was gorgeous and the way you did that was absolutely magnificent, Dr. Schonbrunn. One of the questions that I have is along the lines of whether there's a universal system, because this afternoon, I'll show that it is not a universal system when applied to the gut. Are you excluding the fact that phosphodiesterase may be involved in the action because you used IBMX? One of the things we find with IBMX is that it is a potent antagonist of the adenosine receptor. You may be looking not only at a phosphodiesterase effect but a combined effect of inhibition of adenosine inhibition so that you are not neutralizing the one effect and seeing only the other and thus when you come out without any change you have not excluded an action through phosphodiesterase.

DR. A. SCHONBRUNN (Boston): We're worried about that. But the concentrations of IBMX which are required to act as an antagonist on adenosine receptors are very different from the concentrations which are required to act as a phosphodiesterase inhibitor. In fact, what you might expect if it was having a dual mechanism of action would be perhaps an alteration in the ratio of inhibition that you see for somatostatin. You could predict, based on which one it's acting at mostly, what might happen. And in fact, there is just absolutely no change. So that's most consistent with a single mechanism of action.

DR. A. VINIK: You haven't used a non-xanthine derivative in which you could exclude an adenosine effect?

DR. A. SCHONBRUNN: We haven't done as careful studies with that, but a rough preliminary kind of experiment indicates a parallel result.

DR. A. VINIK: Very good. Can I ask another question? Dr. Pless, I find it very interesting when I compare your results with Dr. Slater's results in terms of the reduction in number of stools. There is a reduction in diarrhea in patients with tumors, yet Dr. Slater was talking to us about the increase in the fat content of stools. What happens to these people, do they get reduced numbers of stools with more fat in them?

DR. J. PLESS (Basle): Well, what we know for the moment is that in some of these patients, Dr. Bloom carried out fat determinations and he has not seen a great amount of reduction, only a slight trend in one or two of these. It may be related to the dose he uses because we have seen that in this study, which are animal studies, the doses are extremely high. So with twice 50 µg subcutaneous injections, they didn't find any sign of that or only a slight trend in some of these patients.

DR. A. VINIK: Could I ask you the other question? One of the dominant symptoms that you have is the flush, which you see in patients with carcinoid, and as has been reported sometime back, you could eliminate the flush with somatostatin but you got the tremendous rebound. Did flushing improve?

DR. J. PLESS: Flushing, yes, definitely, immediately. After having stopped the SMS treatment, it came back slowly after one or two days.

DR. A. VINIK: That's a very useful addition because we have had problems with management of flush. Could I ask one more question, and that is to Dr. Srikant, and it's along the lines of the question you asked about degradation. Dr. Srikant, you didn't show us what happened to dissociation of the S-28 vs the S-14 tracer. With a number of partial antagonists, certainly for the insulin receptor, it is a question of dissociation of the antagonist, which is different from that of natural insulin, when you have a substituted molecule.

DR. C.B. SRIKANT (Montreal): Yes, we have looked at the dissociation of these radioligands from receptors in several tissues but we don't find any significant difference, and we really cannot rule out changes in dissociation rates which could point to differences in the binding sites. However, as Dr. Schonbrunn pointed out, the guanine nucleotides do seem to have certain effects and we have not completed the detailed study of the effect of guanine nucleotides to see if it differentiates the rate of dissociation of these ligands. We still have to check that out to assess the differences.

DR. J. WASS (London): I have some questions of Dr. Srikant. Firstly, I wanted to ask about somatostatin receptors in the adrenal medulla. I don't believe you mentioned this, however, I am sure you have studied them and I wonder if they are there? Certainly in man, you can find somatostatin in pheochromocytoma tissue sometimes. Secondly, I wondered if you have done any work on species difference in somatostatin receptors. And thirdly, I wonder whether you'd postulate as to why you have increased binding of S-28 receptors in the pituitary when, according to Dr. Patel yesterday, the one predominant form of somatostatin there is S-14. Have you done any studies on relative receptor density in the pituitary, S-28 vs S-14?

DR. C.B. SRIKANT: To answer the first question, we have not been able to identify any detectable binding of either S-28 or S-14 in the adrenal medullary preparations. The second question of species differences - we have not been able to complete any detailed studies so I cannot answer whether there is a species difference in somatostatin receptors. Finally, in the case of the pituitary, we have looked at the effect of S-14 and S-28 binding and we cannot pick up any differences. Of course, the relative distribution of S-14 and S-28, as shown by Dr. Patel yesterday, indicates that S-14 is about 3-4 times the concentration of S-28 in the hypophyseal portal circulation. Despite the fact that S-28 is low in concentration compared to S-14 the effect of S-28 is more potent than that of S-14, and this will be seen in one of the posters that is being preented by Dr. Jacovidou this morning. We cannot find a difference in the S-14 and S-28 binding, based on these things. It certainly indicates that S-28 is more potent than S-14 based on the in vitro binding studies as well as on the in vivo experiments.

DR. J. WASS: Dr. Pless, I have been involved with Dr. Michael Besser looking at acromegalics and we have now gone on to study 6 of these patients. The one thing I would like to emphasize, which I don't think came over, is that these are bromocryptine-responsive patients whose growth hormone levels have fallen on bromocryptine, but whose growth hormone levels haven't become normal on bromocryptine. In all these patients, the growth hormone levels have fallen further using this analog. The problem lies with its administration subcutaneously. In the slide you showed of our data, the growth hormone suppressive effect went on for about 6 hours. We have now gone on to study a small number of patients using double that dose of 100 μg and it appears that it lasts longer; clearly we need to do a dose-response study now to look at that effect further. But the problem really relates to its subcutaneous administration and 6 hour duration of action. Clearly, subcutaneous administration, is not enough. I wonder whether you have done any work using other nonparenteral methods of administration, particularly intranasal administration, because I think that in order for it to be an acceptable long-term treatment of acromegaly, and there are certainly numbers of patients who don't respond to radiotherapy and surgery as is well known to all of us in that field, it needs to be administered nonparenterally.

DR. J. PLESS: Well, to answer your first question regarding 6 hours. It depends. Sometimes you have 6, 7, or 10 hours. Lamberts has seen, for instance, 12 hr inhibition with many patients, but I agree that it is not enough; it would be nice to have something which is more active than that. Concerning the nasal spray, of course, every small molecular weight peptide can more or less be used in the form of a nasal spray, and we have forms already available for nasal application, which could be a way out of this unpleasant situation sometimes. So it will be available very soon.

DR. J. WASS: Is it absorbed orally?

DR. J. PLESS: Oral, yes. You know that all peptides are poorly active orally when compared to parenteral administration, but what we can say is that the SMS analog is active orally to inhibit growth hormone in a dose of 3 to 5 mg per man. The duration of action is interestingly rather long, not so long as by the subcutaneous route but it's interesting.

DR. H. SACKS: Just one comment and one question. The comment relates to the adrenal cortex and receptors. There have been a few papers recently demonstrating that somatostatin infusion may blunt the aldosterone rise to provocative stimuli which suggests, perhaps, that if there is somatostatin in the adrenal medulla there may be short-loop vascular connections that may mediate intramedullary control of adrenocortical aldosterone secretion. The question is to Dr. Srikant. You've demonstrated clearly using labelled Tyr^{11} somatostatin that there is a good correlation between binding and biological activity. Have you looked at the ability of all these different analogs to inhibit the degradation of that labelled peptide by your membrane preparations?

DR. C.B. SRIKANT: Regarding the regulation of the presence of somatostatin in the adrenal medulla, although the initial study of Aguilera et al. reported very high levels of endogenous somatostatin, we have not been able to confirm the presence of somatostatin in the adrenal medullary gland. In fact, detailed studies in our laboratory indicate that the concentration of somatostatin is extremely low and perhaps undetectable (< 2-3 pg/mg protein) in adrenal medullary extracts. So, I don't think that realistically one can expect local regulation of aldosterone by the medullary levels of somatostatin that are present. This is also supported by the fact that in vivo injection of radiolabelled somatostatin is maximally taken up by the adrenal cortical glomerulosa cells compared to any other tissue which have high levels of endogenous hormone; so this suggests that there is no such regulation by the medullary or cortical somatostatin that is present endogenously. Also, the second question about the effect of these analogs on the degradation of the Tyr^{11} radioligand. We have not found any difference in the stability of Tyr^{11} radioligand in the presence of different analogs. In fact these analogs have been shown to be more stable and they have really no effect on the stability of radioligands in different membrane systems.

DR. S. HEISLER (Quebec City): I have two questions addressed to Dr. Schonbrunn. First, I would like to know a little bit more about your pertussis toxin experiments. You showed, although you didn't mention it in your talk, that there was about a 20-30% increase in the ability of TRH to stimulate the release of prolactin following the pertussis toxin experiment. My question relates to the effect of pertussis toxin on somatostatin; that is, its ability to attenuate the effect of somatostatin - have you confirmed, with calcium flux or calcium homeostasis studies, that these effects are indeed, both of them, related to changes in calcium.

DR. A. SCHONBRUNN: No, we don't have any information that the other mechanism is calcium-dependent at all. That's just a hypothesis that remains to be tested. We have no evidence. But, other people have tried to look at that. Katmi Tan Khan, in particular, in Armen Tashjian's laboratory, has done extensive work looking at the effects of TRH on calcium fluxes and in her experiments she didn't really find an effect of somatostatin. Now, she didn't look to see whether those cells responded biologically to somatostatin under the same conditions, so that negative result is tentative. But that's what's known.

DR. S. HEISLER: The second question relates to a comment that Dr. Srikant made with respect to the breakdown of [^{125}I Tyr^{1}] somatostatin. In your binding studies, would you care to compare your findings with his?

DR. A. SCHONBRUNN: We have looked very carefully at degradation and for reasons I don't understand, we have just been lucky. Membranes prepared from these cells, whether it's because they are a homogenous population or whatever, really don't seem to significantly degrade [^{125}I Tyr^{1}] somatostatin, or for that matter [^{125}I Tyr^{11}] somatostatin, during the course of the binding assay. In that experiment that I showed on the GMP-PNP effects for example, those are usually done at 37 C for 90 min, and during that time there is less than 5% degradation of iodinated [^{125}I Tyr^{1}] somatostatin.

DR. J. GERICH: Do you have any inhibitors of proteolysis in there that may explain the difference?

DR. A. SCHONBRUNN: We have inhibitors of proteolysis in there. We have bacitracin, but I don't think that that alone explains the difference.

DR. J. GERICH: Dr. Srikant, do you want to make a comment on this?

DR. C.B. SRIKANT: We have not really looked at these tumor cells except the AtT-20 cell membranes; in terms of the normal tissue receptor preparations we definitely see a difference in the stability of [Tyr^{1}] S-14 versus [Tyr^{11}] S-14. In our hands the N-terminally labelled somatostatin ligands are quite unstable compared to [Tyr^{11}] S-14. So I really cannot explain our differences. I am not sure what concentration of bacitracin Dr. Schonbrunn has used but definitely the higher concentration of bacitracin increases the stability; however, it also decreases the specific binding and I don't know what sort of results Dr. Schonbrunn has got.

DR. A. SCHONBRUNN: I don't remember the concentration of bacitracin, but we looked at a number of concentrations. Even when the concentrations are very, very low there is very little degradation and so we put it in there to get it down to virtually nothing. We did check at each concentration of bacitracin to determine whether or not there was an effect on binding, and up to the concentrations we used, there wasn't. I just can't figure it out.

DR. J. TABORSKY (Seattle): I have two comments. The first is to Dr. Srikant. We have used some nonimmunoreactive analogs of somatostatin to try to demonstrate that the receptors for somatostatin on the A, B, and D cells of the pancreas are in fact different. What we have not done are the classical binding studies with tagged somatostatin. I was wodering if you had a chance to do that kind of work on the A, B, and D cells of the pancreatic islet, and if you find any differences in their ability to bind various analogs and displace tracer.

DR. C.B. SRIKANT: No, as I mentioned in my talk, we have not so far performed direct binding studies using enriched fractions of A- , B- and D-cells, so we don't have any direct studies to report on the effect of different selective analogs on these islet cell receptors.

DR. J. TABORSKY: My other comment is to Dr. Coy. He mentioned with regard to his somatostatin antagonist that there was a problem trying to show antagonism. We have obtained this antagonist from Dr. Coy, and I think I have some comments which may help clarify it. First of all, I think that you have to look fairly hard. When we looked at the ability of this antagonist to reverse the inhibition of insulin secretion by a low dose of exogenous somatostatin, we indeed did antagonize the action of a submaximal dose of cyclic somatostatin. So in my opinion this analog really does work. The problem may be that, also in our hands, it did not seem to affect the inhibitory action of the higher dose of somatostatin, i.e. more toward the maximal end of the dose-response curve. So, I think a fair statement about it is that it is a weak competitive antagonist and I am encouraged that, in fact, it is a real antagonist. I think it is worthy of a lot of further work because, as Dr. Vale pointed out yesterday, we really need these kind of tools, particularly for brain function. The other comment is that we have looked at its effect on the release of endogenous somatostatin from the pancreas and find no effect there.

DR. S. GUTTMAN (Basle): I have a question to Dr. Slater and maybe to Dr. Gerich. Why are you especially concerned with the activity of somatostatin on fat absorption metabolism since, in your model you have shown that the doses necessary are about 100 times higher for the fat metabolism than for the endocrine effects. So the question is, how relevant is the animal model?

DR. E. SLATER (New Jersey): I think your last point is one that needs to be underscored since it's always impossible to know how directly comparable an animal model is. I neglected to mention, and I should have, that when we attempted a similar in vivo study in the dog, in which the dogs were trained to eat a diet containing high fat, we were not able to produce anything near a dose-response curve such as what you saw in the rat. So there are distinct differences in animal models. Thus it is difficult to know what to make of those, and which multiplex mechanisms are at play. In answer to the first part of your question as to what difference does it make, it is simply a fact that we have observed steatorrhea in certain patients when they are given relatively low doses of our 586, in amounts say, that do give us the desired endocrine effects. Dr. Gerich is the principal investigator in this work. Therefore, the interest in developing animal models was (a) to determine mechanism, and I am really not prepared to speak on that since the mechanism in the rat is probably, or possibly, different from the mechanism in man, and (b) to look at differences between compounds or among compounds revealing the differences that I showed, so that there is perhaps some selectivity, although that may be an overstatement.

DR. S. GUTTMAN: Dr. Schonbrunn, you have mentioned that intracellular calcium level is also decreased by somatostatin. Is there any interference between somatostatin and calcium channel blockers?

DR. A. SCHONBRUNN: And calcium channel blockers? I am not exactly sure what experiment you are referring to. Do you mean calcium channel blockers will decrease secretion in and of itself? Once secretion is decreased you can block it all the way down, so I am not sure how you would expect somatostatin to decrease that further. As far as I know, careful dose-response curves have not been done.

DR. C.B. SRIKANT: I have a comment and a question to Dr. Schonbrunn in this regard. The sensitivity of the GH_4C_1 cells to calcium appears to be different compared to normal pituitary cells based on the report by Priscilla Danies. Have you observed any differences in the role of calcium on the secretion of prolactin by these cells under stimulation by forskolin; and secondly, have you observed any differences or dependence on calcium for the effect of guanine nucleotides, especially GMP-PNP, on the dissociation or the binding of somatostatin to GH_4C_1 cells?

DR. A. SCHONBRUNN: The answer to both of those questions is no. We really haven't looked. But it is certainly true that the stimulation of hormone secretion in these cells by forskolin, as by just about every other secretagogue, eventually is calcium-dependent and it seems that the concentration of intracellular calcium pools in these cells is somewhat different from the concentrations in normal cells. So exactly how and to what extent that will determine how somatostatin inhibits hormone secretion in these cells, really remains to be seen, but we just don't have any data yet.

DR. S. SZABO (Boston): Dr. Srikant, I could easily follow your *in vivo* experiments with cysteamine in which you find a decrease in the somatostatin level already at 5 and 15 min, and an increase in the number of binding sites, but I could not follow the *in vitro* part. Was there any correlation also between the somatostatin level and the binding sites, and the parallel of this, did only the binding sites number change or was there any alteration in the affinity also?

DR. C.B. SRIKANT: In the *in vitro* system we used the intact synaptosomes which is really a subcellular fraction of the intact cell. There was a time-dependent decrease in endogenous somatostatin levels but such a decrease in somatostatin levels in the synaptosomes did not produce significant changes in binding for up to 30 min, whereas prolonged incubation with 1 mM concentration of cysteamine did decrease the affinity of receptors without significantly altering the number of sites.

DR. S. SZABO: So affinity was affected, not the number, *in vitro*.

DR. C.B. SRIKANT: Yes. And this effect is really opposite to what we saw in the *in vivo* situation. This suggests that this effect is probably an *in vivo* phenomenon or requires the intact cell. We really have to study the role of cysteamine on somatostatin levels and receptors in intact cells *in vitro* and we have to look at cultured brain cells to answer this question.

DR. S. SZABO: The minimal incubation time was how much?

DR. C.B. SRIKANT: For the synaptosomes?

DR. S. SZABO: Yes.

DR. C.B. SRIKANT: We studied them from 5 to 90 min.

DR. L. UCCIOLI (Rome): I have a question for Dr. Pless. You stated that your analog has very potent action on insulin, glucagon, and GH secretion, yet you didn't refer to side effects during long therapy with this analog. We know what when we use somatostatin normally, it causes nausea and gastrointestinal pain. Do you think this lack of side effects may be related to different receptors in the gastrointestinal tract for this analog, or perhaps it is related to the dose of the analog used?

DR. J. PLESS: Yes, it may be both, but what I can say about the tolerance studies is that if you increase the dose to a factor of 50 or 100 you have the same phenomenon as you described for natural somatostatin; that is, you have some nausea and gastrointestinal side effects, but about 50-100 times higher doses are necessary for that. Concerning the receptors, it might also be responsible for that; I can't say anything.

DR. L. UCCIOLI: Did you note a reduction in heart rate of the patients during the administration of your analog?

DR. J. PLESS: No, there was no such thing observed.

DR. Y.C. PATEL: Two points; first of all I would like Dr. Srikant to comment on some binding data that have looked directly at the effects of the Coy antagonist as a competitive antagonist of somatostatin binding to membrane receptors. Can you comment on that?

DR. C.B. SRIKANT: We did some studies on the binding of the two antagonists, the cyclic hexapeptide somatostatin analogs that Dr. Coy provided us, and in all the tissues that we have looked they appear to behave as very weak agonists for receptor binding. We really cannot pick up any antagonistic effects with direct binding studies.

DR. Y.C. PATEL: My question is to David Coy - In view of the fact that somatostatin is now known to downregulate its own receptors, how about the approach of using superagonists for downregulating receptors as a potential way of inducing antagonism. Your "antagonist" does not seem to be sufficiently strong as an agonist to really account for its in vivo effects, but perhaps other such agonists along the lines of LHRH superagonists, might be a potential way of getting some sort of antagonism. Can you comment on that?

DR. D. COY: Yes, to go back to the antagonist, you know, I think we feel that there is so much discrepancy in using that peptide that we prefer to devote as much effort as possible into coming out with something much better, a pure antagonist that could be used straight forwardly without any of these complicating factors. That is what we are really aiming at now. With repect to somatostatin downregulation of receptors, I think that probably some other people in this audience, or maybe on this panel, could answer that question much better. As far as I am aware there is no evidence that you can use a prolonged or acute somatostatin treatment to produce downregulation of somatostatin receptors in the same way that you can with LHRH superagonists, but maybe Dr. Pless could comment on that.

DR. J. PLESS: I think Dr. Patel's suggestion is very interesting, using the same procedure as with LHRH superagonists. We can say that with long-term treatment in animals, in studies of toxicity and in toxicology, we have seen that if you use an extremely high dose of the compound you have downregulation. There is no inhibition of growth hormone anymore, but then you have to use about 1000-10,000 times higher doses and you can wipe out the response. So what you propose is possible.

V

PERIPHERAL SOMATOSTATIN

21

DISTRIBUTION AND MORPHOLOGY OF SOMATOSTATIN CELLS

LARS-INGE LARSSON

Unit of Histochemistry
University Institute of Pathology
Frederik den V's vej 11
DK-2100 Copenhagen Ø, Denmark

INTRODUCTION

After its isolation from the hypothalamus as a neuroendocrine regulator of anterior pituitary growth hormone secretion, somatostatin was rapidly shown to possess many extrapituitary actions and to be widely distributed in the body. Somatostatin was, hence, found to be a potent inhibitor of the secretion of insulin, glucagon, gastrin and several other hormones as well as to inhibit exocrine secretion from the stomach and pancreas (see 1 for review). These actions correlated with the finding of somatostatin immunoreactants in endocrine-like D cells of the entire gastrointestinal tract and the pancreas (2-4). Additionally, somatostatin-like immunoreactivity was detected in a widespread system of central and peripheral nerves (2), in calcitonin-producing C cells of the thyroid (2, 5, 6), in the submandibular gland (7), placenta (8, 9) and urinary tract (10).

Its many and varied actions, paired with its extensive distribution, suggested that somatostatin did not act as a classical hormone but rather served distinct functions depending upon its localization. It, hence, appeared that this peptide could serve roles as a neuroendocrine, paracrine and neuronal regulator, actions which all depend upon local delivery of secretory material to neighboring cells. It seemed much more difficult to entertain the concept of somatostatin as a systemic hormone since its many and seemingly unrelated physiological actions would be impossible for the body to orchestrate.

After the immunocytochemical demonstration of somatostatin immunoreactivity in gastroenteropancreatic endocrine-like cells, these cells were rapidly identified as D (A_1) cells, characterized by a distinct ultramorphology and by a peculiar affinity for silver in the Hellerström-Hellman modification of the Davenport argyrophil staining technique (2-4). Ultrastructural immunocytochemistry revealed that somatostatin immunoreactivity resided within the secretory granules of these cells and, hence, probably represented a secretory molecule (11, 12). These observations correlated well with the demonstration of somatostatin-like bioactivity in an extract of the D-cell-rich lobe of the avian pancreas made by Lernmark and Hellman several years before (13). Soon the first two cases of pancreatic islet D cell tumors producing somatostatin were described (14, 15) and an extract of one of these, a pure somatostatinoma, was chromatographically fractionated and shown to inhibit the secretion of insulin and glucagon from the isolated perfused porcine pancreas (15).

Apart from the very early observations made by Lernmark and Hellman, the functions of the pancreatic D cells had been completely in the dark. Although previous immunocytochemical studies had reported the presence of gastrin immunoreactivity in the pancreatic D cells (16), these results could not be reproduced with antisera to synthetic forms of gastrin and most probably must be ascribed to antibodies to contaminants of the natural gastrin preparations used in these early studies (17). In addition, radioimmunoassay studies failed to detect significant quantities of gastrin in the adult pancreas; pancreatic gastrinomas were found not to be D-cell tumors and the transitory population of true gastrin cells occurring in the fetal and neonatal, but not in the adult, rat pancreas were G cells and not D cells (18). So far, convincing evidence for additional secretory peptides in the gastroenteropancreatic D cells is lacking.

In the thyroid gland of many species, however, solid biochemical and immunocytochemical evidence for the coexistence of somatostatin and calcitonin exists (2,5,6,19). Similarly, in the peripheral nervous system evidence for coexistence of somatostatin and biogenic amines has been presented (20).

This pattern of distribution represents an interesting challenge to our concept of the embryonic origin of regulatory peptide-producing cells.

D cells, like other gastroenteropancreatic endocrine-like cell types, thyroidal calcitonin cells, adrenal phaeochromocytes and several other cell types are included in Pearse's APUD (Amine content or amine Precursor Uptake and Decarboxylation) series (21). This important concept grouped together regulatory cells sharing a number of cytochemical characteristics with central and peripheral neurons and caused Pearse to suggest that such cells shared a common neuroectodermal origin (see ref. 21 for review). Embryologic studies by Le Douarin soon confirmed the neuroectodermal origin of the calcitonin cells from the neural crest (22). Pancreatic and gastrointestinal endocrine-like cells were, however, equally convincingly shown not to be derived from neuroectoderm and probably stem from endoderm (22,23). Apparently, then, cells derived from either ectoderm, like neurons and C cells, or from endoderm, like gastroenteropancreatic D cells, may express somatostatin synthesis.

It is now obvious that the embryonal origin of a cell type is not the only factor governing its choice of messenger molecule and this realization may have important implications for tumor pathology.

Gastric Mucosa

The somatostatin-producing D cells are found in both the antropyloric and in the oxyntic mucosa. In rat, mouse and man they possess a peculiar morphology, characterized by long cytoplasmic processes which travel between the base of the epithelium and the basement membrane and often end with one or two bulbous expansions (24). Occasionally, the processes branch and twist - a feature most marked in the rat oxyntic mucosa. Double-staining immunocytochemistry demonstrates that the processes come into close contact with cells that are affected by somatostatin. Thus, in the antropyloric mucosa, the somatostatin cell processes end on gastrin-producing G cells, and in the oxyntic mucosa, the processes often end in close vicinity to parietal cells (24) (Fig. 1). As somatostatin is known to decrease gastric acid secretion, both directly at the parietal cell level and indirectly by inhibiting secretion of the parietal cell-stimulating hormone, gastrin, the observed arrangement could have a direct physiological correlate. We thus suggested that somatostatin cells could regulate gastric acid secretion by delivering their secretory product through their nerve-like processes directly onto the membranes of the cells they contacted (24, 25). Evidence for such a directed paracrine secretion has come from studies exploiting the APUD properties of mouse gastric somatostatin cells (26). These cells take up and convert the amine precursors L-5-hydroxytryptophan (L-5-HTP) and L-3,4-dihydroxyphenylalanine (L-DOPA) to their corresponding biogenic amines, serotonin (5-HT) and dopamine, respectively. Evidence from both electron microscopic autoradiography, subcellular fractionation and ultracytochemistry shows that the amines formed are exclusively stored in the secretory granules of these cells (reviewed in ref. 26). By the Falck-Hillarp fluorescence cytochemical technique, the two amines, serotonin and dopamine, can be converted to yellow- and blue-fluorescent derivatives, respectively. By first administering one precursor (L-5-HTP), all secretory granules of the gastric somatostatin cells could be induced to fluoresce yellow. After 4-8 hours the second amine precursor, L-DOPA, was administered. While the "old" secretory

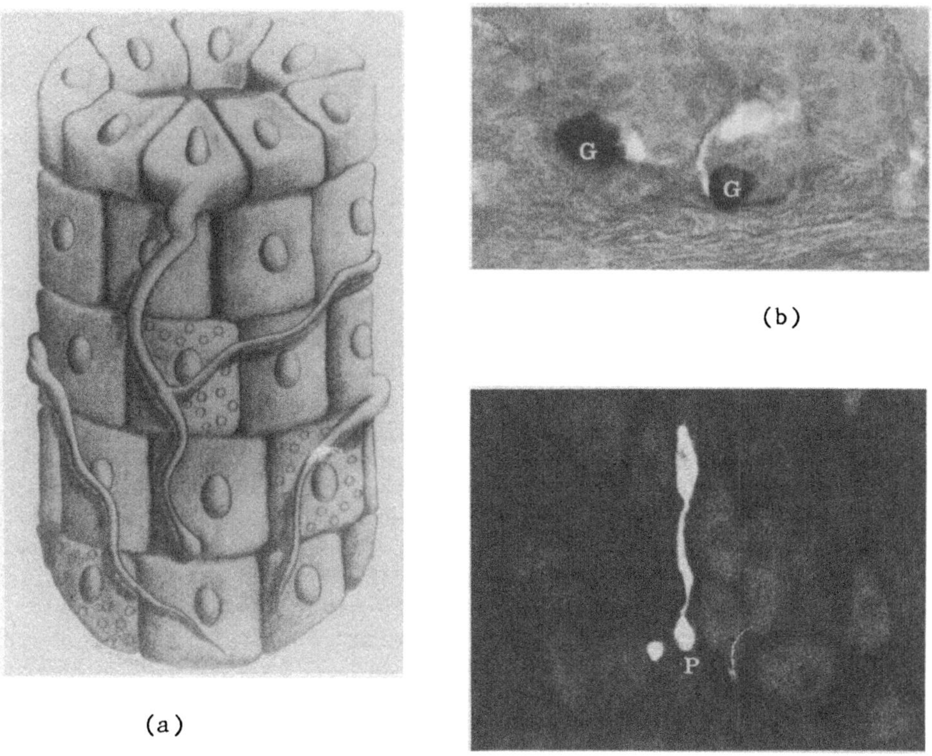

Fig. 1. Somatostatin cells in rat stomach. In (a) is shown a schematic drawing illustrating the three-dimensional arrangement of somatostatin cells in an antropyloric gland. In (b) gastrin (G) cells have been stained with an immunoperoxidase (PAP) technique, followed by indirect immunofluorescence staining for somatostatin. Somatostatin cells give off long processes that end on gastrin cells. In (c) is shown a section of rat oxyntic mucosa stained by immunofluorescence for somatostatin. A long somatostatin cell process ends in the vicinity of a parietal (P) cell (the parietal cells emit a weak reddish fluorescence due to counter-staining with Evans blue which aids in their identification. (Fig. 1(a) is reproduced from ref. 24 with permission).

granules that existed at the time of the first (L-5-HTP) injection retained their yellow fluorescence, new granules synthesized in the interval between the first and second injection were loaded with dopamine, producing a blue fluorescence. Hence, by this technique we could label new and old secretory granules in two different colors and show that the old secretory granules were transported in an anterograde fashion down the paracrine processes towards the terminal swellings (26). This axonal-like ("paraxonal") transport of secretory molecules forms additional evidence that gastric paracrine cells directly deliver their secretory products onto the membranes of cells they contact.

Studies with the isolated perfused rat stomach and the isolated antropyloric gland column have provided support for the concept that paracrine somatostatin secretion from gastric D cells controls gastrin secretion. Thus, in the effluent from both models, gastrin and somatostatin secretion are perfectly inversely correlated (27, 28). Infusion of somatostatin antiserum into the perfused stomach causes a rise in gastrin secretion (29). Moreover, stimulation of gastrin secretion by carbachol or metacholine is associated with a drop in somatostatin secretion (27, 28). Addition of somatostatin antiserum to cultured antropyloric mucosa also causes an increase in gastrin release, whereas intravenous injection of somatostatin antiserum to intact rats is reported to be ineffective in stimulating gastrin release, although potent in stimulating pituitary GH release (30). Very recently, in an organ-culture model it was shown that secretin is a potent stimulator of somatostatin release and that this hormone simultaneously inhibited gastrin release (31). The inhibition of gastrin release could be overcome by addition of somatostatin antiserum to the secretin.

Taken together, all these observations form strong support for the notion of a direct tonic control of gastrin secretion by somatostatin delivered through paracrine secretion and not via the bloodstream. So far, critical studies have yet to be carried out to see if similar mechanisms account for the action of somatostatin on oxyntic parietal cells.

Apart from their characteristic processes contacting gastrin cells and parietal cells, respectively, antropyloric and oxyntic somatostatin cells differ in their morphology. Thus, while antropyloric somatostatin cells have direct contacts with the gastric lumen via luminal processes endowed with microvilli, oxyntic somatostatin cells are devoid of luminal contacts (32). This morphological feature correlates well with observations made by Schusdziarra and colleagues showing that instillation of hydrochloric acid into the dog stomach was associated with increased secretion of somatostatin into the antropyloric venous effluent but caused no stimulation of somatostatin into the oxyntic venous effluent (33). These data, hence, indicate that a decrease of the intragastric pH is a stimulus for antropyloric, but not for oxyntic, somatostatin release.

It has long been known that a decrease in gatric pH results in inhibition of gastrin release. As both antropyloric somatostatin cells and gastrin cells contact the gastric lumen it is conceivable that low pH affects both cell types. Recent studies with the isolated perfused porcine stomach have however shown that the inhibiting effect of low intragastric pH on gastrin release can be abolished by arterial infusion of low concentrations of a hyperactive somatostatin analog (34). This hyperactive analog has been shown to inhibit the endogenous secretion of somatostatin at such very low doses (34). It, hence, seems possible that, at least in pigs, low pH acts primarily to stimulate paracrine D cell secretion, which secondarily inhibits gastrin cell secretion. As the apical portion of the gastrin cell may not be directly affected by low pH, it is possible that it may be affected by other components of the gastric juice, possibly factors known to stimulate, rather than inhibit, gastrin secretion. Whether such luminal gastrin-stimulatory molecules are inhibitory to somatostatin cells is not known.

Candidates for stimulating oxyntic somatostatin secretion include neural reflexes, distension and hormonal stimuli. Interestingly, Schusdziarra et al. (33) found that while decreased gastric pH did not stimulate oxyntic somatostatin secretion, decreased duodenal pH caused a potent stimulation. This could be ascribed to activation of duodenal endocrine cells and/or local neural reflexes that stimulated oxyntic somatostatin cells. Among possible humoral mediators of such a long feedback loop are secretin and the gastric inhibitory polypeptide (31, 35).

So far, the tentative model for somatostatin as a gastric secretory regulator involves, firstly, a short feedback loop whereby decreased gastric pH stimulates antropyloric somatostatin cell secretion. This leads to decreased gastrin secretion and, indirectly, to decreased parietal cell activity. Secondly, a long feedback loop activated only in the emergency situation of a lowered duodenal pH results in activation of oxyntic somatostatin cells which effect an immediate and efficient brake on further acid secretion (25).

While a wealth of data seem to confirm the validity of this theory in a wide variety of species it is important to note that the entire story has yet to be unraveled. Thus, while the somatostatin cell morphology described holds true for rat, mouse, dog and man, gastric somatostatin cells of pigs and cats do not possess cytoplasmic processes. In these latter species, however, there is a close juxtaposition between somatostatin cells and gastrin cells, which may substitute for the processes in terms of paracrine secretion (Fig. 2). Secondly, although it is possible under basal conditions to demonstrate a "paraxonal" transport of secretory material towards

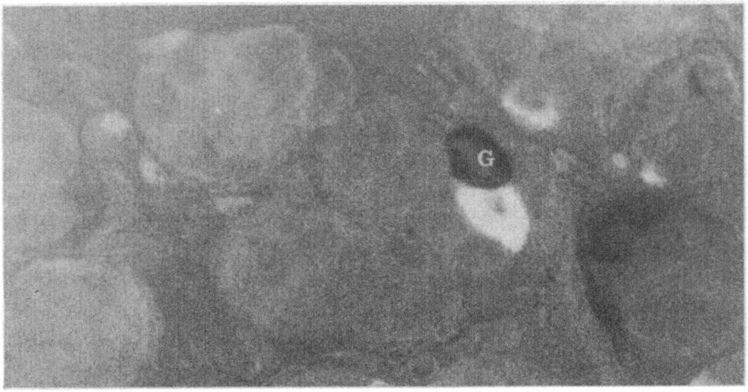

Fig. 2. Cat antropyloric mucosa double-stained for gastrin (G) with PAP technique and for somatostatin with indirect immunofluorescence. In the cat, processes from antropyloric somatostatin cells are almost never detected but double-staining experiments show that close juxtapositions between gastrin and somatostatin cell bodies are frequent.

somatostatin target cells (26), it is impossible to exclude that secretion from D cells also occurs in other directions. Possible additional targets may include excitatory/inhibitory nerve terminals in the lamina propria mucosae, the gastric lumen and the blood stream. It is, hence, possible that the directed paracrine secretion is important only for initiating the inhibitory events and that continued need for restraints on gastric acid secretion may be mediated via luminal, hormonal or nervous effects that would not be apparent in the *in vitro* models described above. In this context it seems of interest to determine the relative proportions of somatostatin-14 and somatostatin-28 secreted early and late during gastric D cell stimulation. Moreover, much data exists to indicate luminal secretion of gastrointestinal hormones including gastrin and somatostatin (36). It remains to be seen whether this represents active, directed secretion or passive overflow from other routes. With gastrin cells there is as yet little morphological evidence for an apical secretory route, as virtually all immunoreactive hormone is gathered at the base of the cell. With rat antropyloric somatostatin cells, however, we frequently observe that the luminal apical process is also filled with immunoreactivity. Continued ultramorphological studies on these cells are clearly needed.

Intestinal Tract

Somatostatin cells are, together with the enterochromaffin cells, unique in that they are represented all along the gastrointestinal tract from the cardia to the rectum. Although the intestinal somatostatin cells, by virtue of their argyrophilia and morphology of their secretory granules, are also classified as D cells, they differ from the gastric D cells of most species in that they rarely give off cytoplasmic processes (37). Thus, in the small intestine, somatostatin cells usually possess the triangular, flask-like shape of typical endocrine-like cells. This morphological appearance may suggest that they function as endocrine cells (Fig. 3). However, it is impossible to exclude that they, additionally or alternatively, work as paracrine cells releasing somatostatin to their immediate neighbors. In the cat and the guinea pig the duodenal mucosa also contains numerous somatostatin immunoreactive nerve terminals (37) (Fig. 3). These branch extensively in the lamina propria mucosae and come into close contact with a great number of epithelial cells, of which enterochromaffin cells and cholecystokinin cells have been identified by double-staining techniques (37) (Fig 4). Such nerves are scarce in other species, including the rat.

In the rat, studies by Patel and colleagues have shown that larger molecular-weight forms of somatostatin immunoreactants, including somatostatin-28, are much more predominant in the intestinal mucosa than in the intestinal muscle, stomach or pancreas (38). Hence, somatostatin-28 and larger somatostatin components are mainly associated with the triangular endocrine-like cells of the rat intestines whereas somatostatin-14 is mainly associated with the nerves and process-carrying, nerve-like D cells of the stomach and pancreas. This is interesting in view of the differences in terms of potency and selectivity of actions between somatostatin-14 and -28 (39, 40).

Pancreas

The pancreatic D cells were among the first cells shown to contain somatostatin (2-4, 11). The potent inhibitory actions of somatostatin on insulin and glucagon release rapidly led to speculations about an intra-islet regulatory role for somatostatin (41). In rat islets the somatostatin cells are distributed together with glucagon cells and PP cells in the peripheral mantle zone. In this species, very few somatostatin cells occupy extrainsular locations. This, however, is frequently observed in other species, including the dog (Larsson, unpublished data). In guinea pigs, islet somatostatin cells give off extremely long cytoplasmic processes that appear to permeate most of the islet like a network (Fig. 5). Mostly, these processes appear to end on intra-islet capillaries (37). In most other species, including the rat, processes of islet somatostatin cells are also observed, but these are generally shorter and much less extensively distributed than in the guinea pig (37).

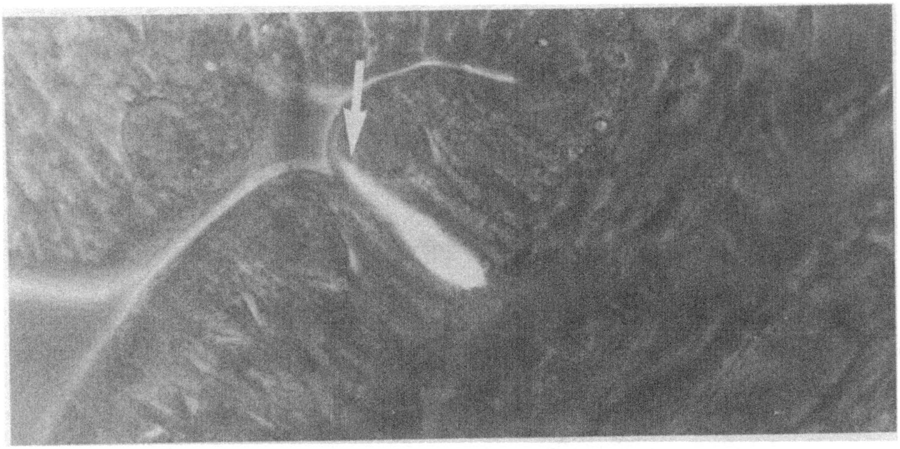

(a)

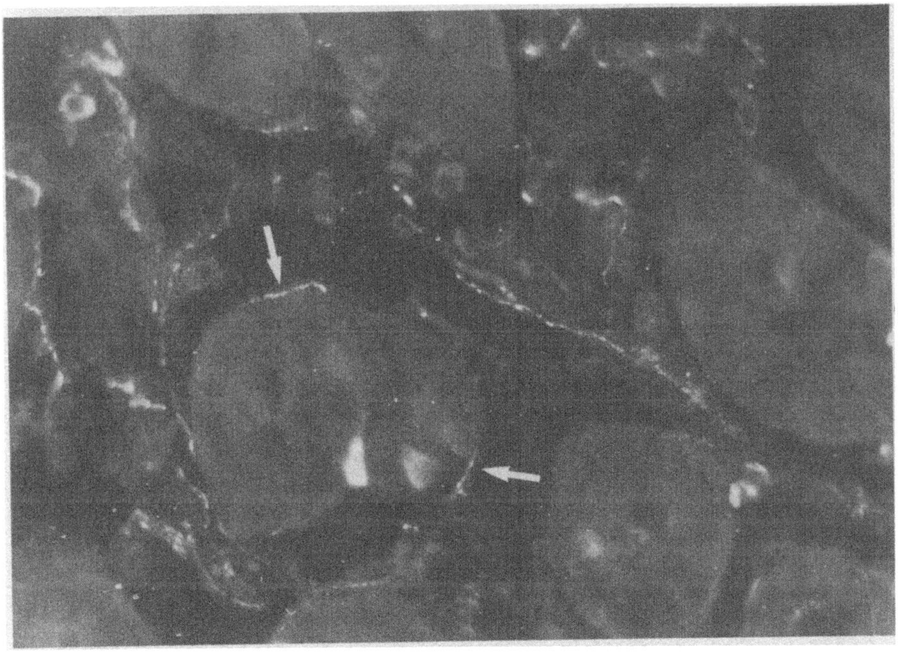

(b)

Fig. 3. (a) Duodenal somatostatin cell (cat) stained by indirect immunofluorescence and viewed in combined epifluorescence and transmitted light through Nomarski optics. Note the characteristic endocrine-like morphology of the flask-shaped somatostatin cell. Note also that its apical process (arrow), which seems to reach the lumen, is filled with somatostatin immunoreactivity. Normally, gut endocrine cells have their secretory material concentrated in their basal portions. (b) Duodenal mucosa of guinea pig. Note the presence of several immunofluorescent flask-shaped somatostatin cells as well as immunofluorescent somatostatin nerves which come into close contact with the epithelium (arrows).

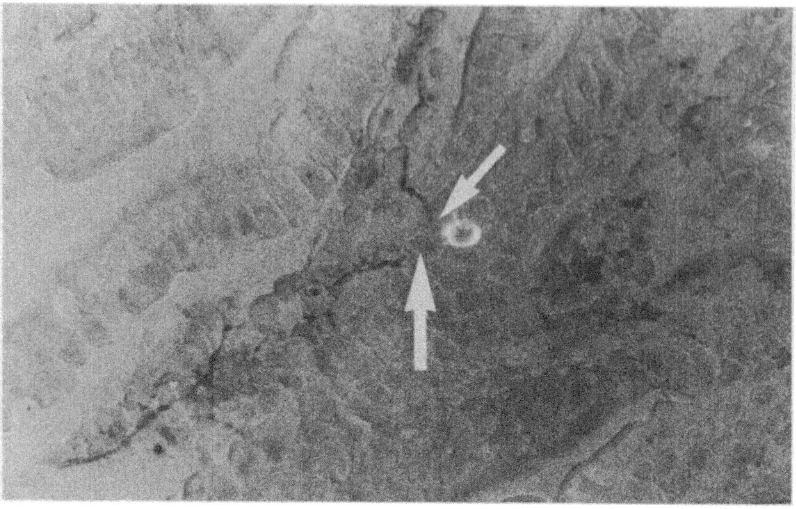

Fig. 4. Guinea pig duodenal mucosa double-stained for somatostatin nerves with the PAP technique and then stained with indirect immunofluorescence for CCK-33. Note that immunopositive somatostatin cells come into close contact with the epithelium containing an immunofluorescent CCK cell (arrows).

With such species variation it is perhaps understandable that a simple working hypothesis for the role of islet somatostatin is still lacking. This issue is further bedevilled by conflicting reports on the direction of the intra-islet blood flow (42, 43). Recent studies have documented that in the isolated perfused dog pancreas, very minute quantities of somatostatin have effects on insulin and glucagon secretion (44). As these quantities are lower than those measured in the venous effluent from the organ, one possible interpretation is that they reach a somatostatin-poor compartment of the islet (44). Such a compartment may occur if, in the dog, as reported for the rat, the islet blood flow goes from the insulin cells to the non-B cells of the islets (43) and/or if tight junctions could seal off a "receptor part" of the islet cells from a "releaser part". This must remain speculative so far since, indeed, it would be nearly impossible morphologically to demarcate such zones in the islets. A further complication of the dog studies is the presence of extrainsular somatostatin cells, making it difficult to determine how much somatostatin is secreted by the insular versus the extrainsular compartments (Fig. 6). Nevertheless, the results show that circulating somatostatin levels probably actively participate in regulating islet function although we are still in the dark concerning the function(s) of islet somatostatin cells.

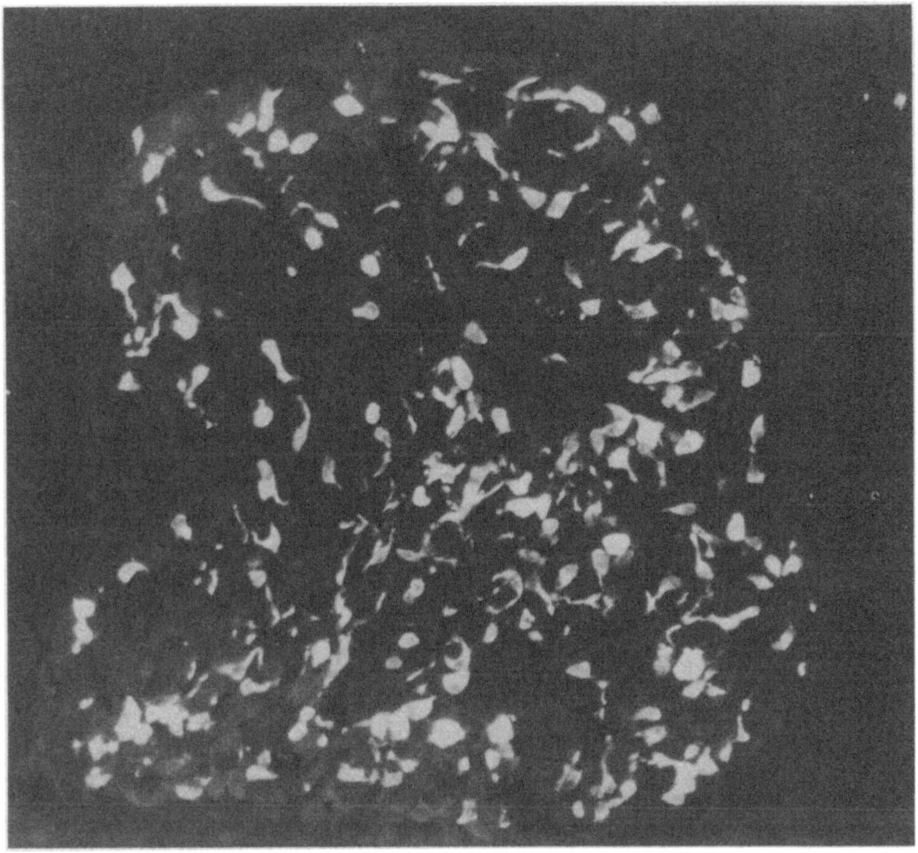

Fig. 5. Guinea pig pancreatic islet stained for somatostatin by indirect immunofluorescence. The somatostatin cells are numerous and give off long processes that seem to permeate the islet. Often the processes end on capillaries.

Thyroid

Somatostatin has been localized to parafollicular calcitonin (C) cells of the thyroid (2, 5, 6). However, much species variation has been noted (45). Thus, in the rabbit and guinea pig thyroid nearly all C cells store both calcitonin and somatostatin (6, 45) (Fig. 7), whereas in the adult rat and human thyroid only a small subpopulation of calcitonin cells are somatostatin immunoreactive (5, 45). Finally, in the cat thyroid, calcitonin cells are devoid of detectable somatostatin, but in this species somatostatin immunoreactivity can be detected in all parenchymal cells of the parathyroid - a localization which is negative for somatostatin in most other species studied (Larsson, unpublished data).

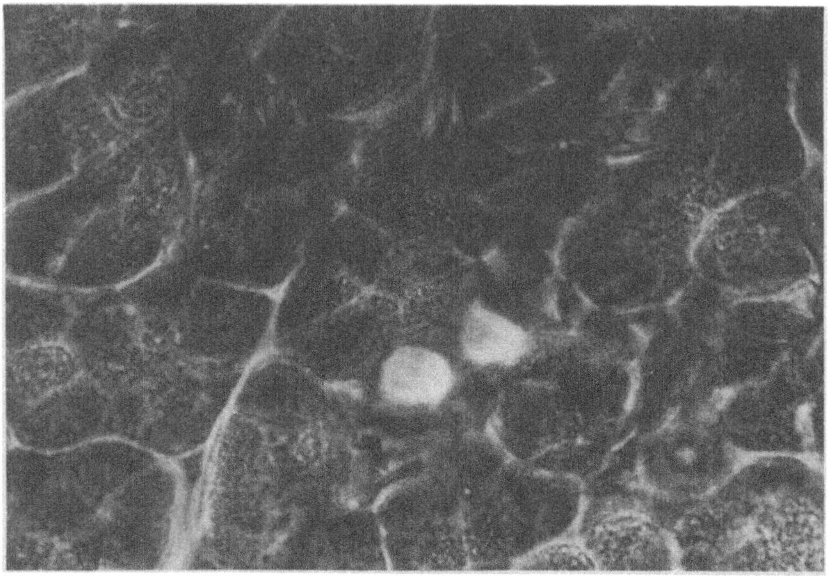

Fig. 6. Guinea pig exocrine pancreas stained for somatostatin witn immunofluorescence and viewed in combined epiillumination and transmitted light through Nomarski optics. Note the presence of two triangular somatostatin cells close to an exocrine acinus. In dog and guinea pig extrainsular somatostatin cells are relatively frequent. In many other species they are scarce or absent.

As shown by studies in rats and dogs, an ontogenetic sequence in the occurrence of thyroidal somatostatin immunoreactivity also takes place (46, 47). Recent double staining experiments show that in neonatal rats, from birth up to about 6-7 days postnatally, nearly all thyroidal C cells are immunopositive for both calcitonin and somatostatin (Larsson, unpublished data). At around day 7, somatostatin begins to disappear from the calcitonin cells leading to the situation seen in adult rats where less than 5 per cent of the calcitonin cells are somatostatin positive. Interestingly, in parallel with the disappearance of somatostatin from the calcitonin cells another antigen starts to appear. This antigen, detectable with some antibodies reading the COOH-terminal tetrapeptide region of gastrin/CCK, is present in extremely few calcitonin cells in the newborn rat, increases gradually in parallel with the disappearance of somatostatin immunoreactivity, and is present in over 80 per cent of the calcitonin cells of the adult rat (Larsson, unpublished data). The inverse relationship between the gastrin/CCK-like antigen and somatostatin holds true not only for the developing and adult rat but also occurs in other species. Hence, in guinea pigs,

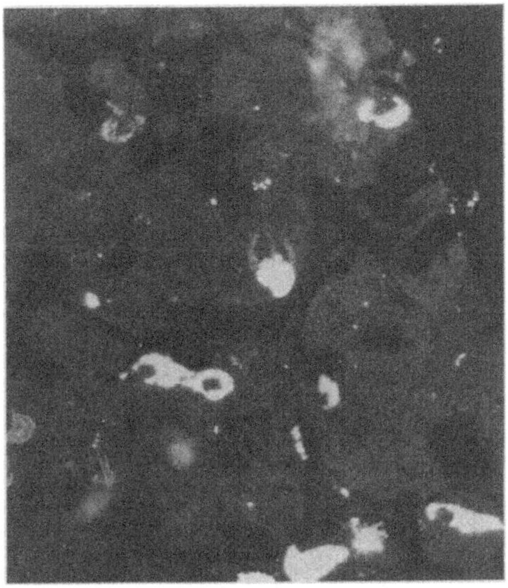

a

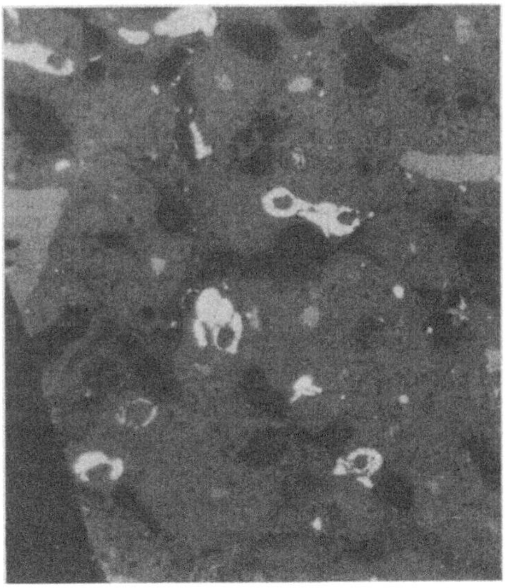

b

Fig. 7 a, b. Adjacent semithin plastic sections of rabbit thyroid stained by indirect immunofluorescence for somatostatin (a) and calcitonin (b). Note that virtually all somatostatin cells are also calcitonin-positive in this species.

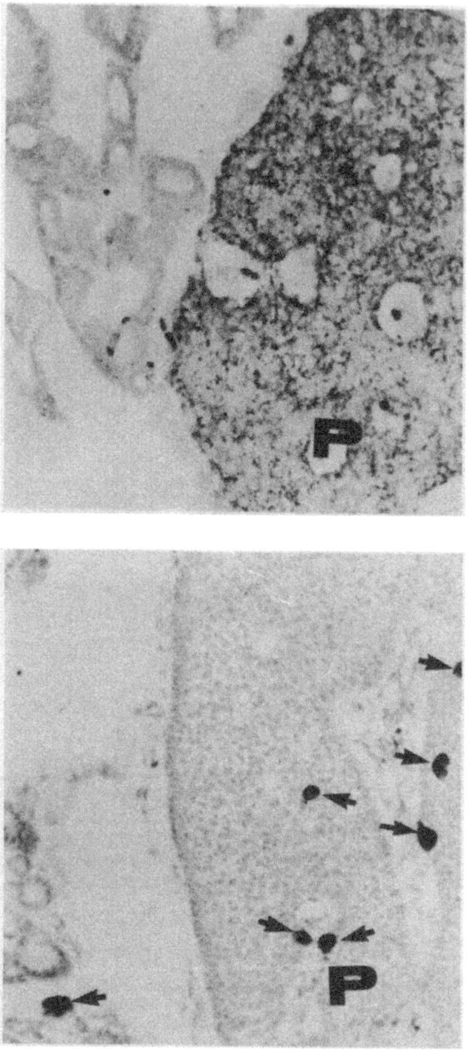

a

b

Fig. 7 c, d. Adjacent cryostat sections of cat thyroid-parathyroid, stained by immunoperoxidase for somatostatin (c) and calcitonin (d). Note that in the cat thyroid no cells positive for somatostatin are seen whereas the parathyroid (P) is intensely stained. Few calcitonin cells (d, arrows) occur scattered in the thyroid and parathyroid.

where all calcitonin cells also are positive for somatostatin, no gastrin/CCK-like immunoreactivity can be detected, whereas in the cat, virtually all calcitonin cells are negative for somatostatin and positive for the gastrin/CCK-like antigen.

So far, we are uncertain about the molecular identity of this new antigen. It is not detected by all antisera recognizing the C-terminal tetrapeptide of gastrin/CCK and CCK-specific antisera do not react with thyroidal C cells. As the immunoreactivity can be abolished by preabsorbing the antisera with the synthetic tetrapeptide amide of gastrin/CCK it is probable that a yet unknown molecule containing a sequence resembling this peptide is being detected. At the moment, however, we must refer to it as an interesting antigen that is expressed (or taken up) by the C cells when they stop expressing somatostatin immunoreactivity. Although recent studies have identified the occurrence of a mRNA coding for cholecystokinin (CCK) in a rat C cell tumor (48) we are at present unable to equate the immunoreactivity we observe with known forms of CCK.

In the gut and the pancreas similar transitory immunoreactivities have previously been noted, particularly with respect to pancreatic gastrin (17) and duodenal gastrin and secretin cells (49, 50). Interestingly, during their development and decline the duodenal gastrin and secretin cells in both rat and man also contain serotonin - a biogenic monoamine which is never detected in the adult counterparts of these cells (49). It is possible that the transitory expression of messenger molecules in developing animals may serve a functional, trophic or other role. Notably, in the neonatal rat pancreas, gut and thyroid these transitory messengers seem to peak at days 5-7 and thereafter decline.

The pronounced species variation in the occurrence of somatostatin in the thyroid makes it difficult to speculate about its role. As the peptide coexists with calcitonin in the same cells it is possible that it could work either as a paracrine (working on neighboring cells) or autocrine (regulating hormone release from its own cell of origin) messenger. Additionally, the thyroid parafollicular cells, as the name implies, have a most intimate relationship to the thyroid follicles (Fig. 8). This arrangement is, phylogenetically speaking, a recent invention as the C cells are gathered in the ultimobronchial bodies of submammalian vertebrates. Whether their colonization of the thyroid implies an interaction between the follicle cells and the C cells, and whether somatostatin participates in such a relationship remains to be seen.

Other Localizations

Apart from various neural localizations, dealt with elsewhere in this volume, somatostatin immunoreactivity has also been detected in the cytotrophoblasts of the human placenta (8, 9), in amacrine-

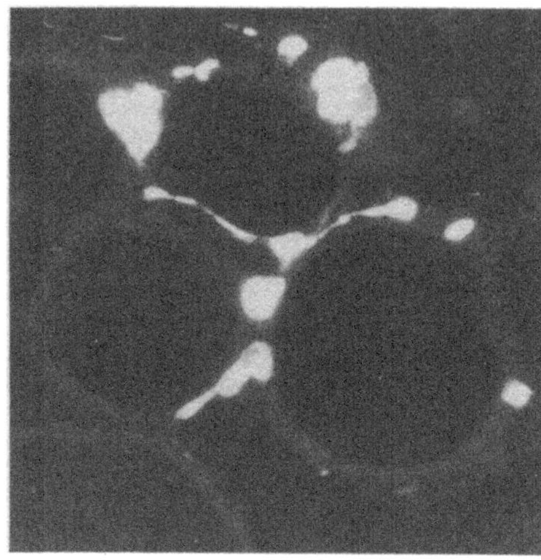

a

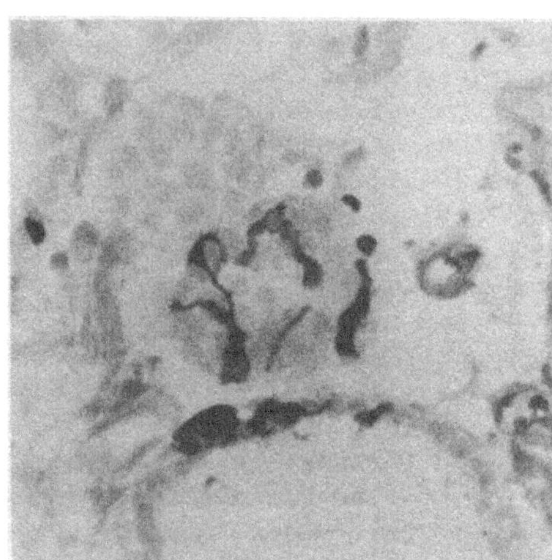

b

Fig. 8. Sections from guinea pig thyroid gland stained with immunofluorescence (a) or PAP method (b) for somatostatin immunoreactivity. Note that in this species the somatostatin-positive C cells branch extensively and give off numerous processes that come into intimate contact with the non-immunoreactive follicle cells. This arrangement is particularly striking in tangentially cut follicles (b).

like cells of the retina (51, 52), in the submandibular gland (7), and in the frog urinary tract (10). The possible functions of somatostatin in these localizations are uncertain.

ACKNOWLEDGMENTS

Studies by the author have over the years been supported by the Danish MRC and Cancer Foundation. I thank Mrs. A. Jakobsen for typing the manuscript and Mrs. K. Høgenhaven and B. Traasdahl for expert technical assistance.

REFERENCES

1. Patel YC, Zingg HH, Fitzpatrick D, Srikant CB 1981 Somatostatin: Some aspects of its physiology and patho-physiology. In: Bloom SR, Polak JM (eds) Gut Hormones. Churchill Livingstone, Edinburgh, p 339.
2. Hökfelt T, Efendic S, Hellerström C, Johansson O, Luft R, Arimura A 1975 Cellular localization of somatostatin in endocrine-like cells and neurons of the rat with special references to the A_1 cells of the pancreatic islets and the hypothalamus. Acta Endocrinol 80:1.
3. Polak JM, Pearse AGE, Grimelius L, Bloom SR, Arimura A 1975 Growth hormone-release inhibiting hormone in gastrointestinal and pancreatic D-cells. Lancet 1:1220.
4. Orci L, Baetens D, Dubois MP, Rufener C 1975 Evidence for the D-cell of the pancreas secreting somatostatin. Hormone Metab Res 7:400.
5. Van Noorden S, Polak JM, Pearse AGE 1977 Single cellular origin of somatostatin and calcitonin in the rat thyroid gland. Histochemistry 53:243.
6. Buffa R, Chayvialle JA, Fontana P, Usellini L, Capella C, Solcia E 1979 Parafollicular cells of rabbit thyroid store both calcitonin and somatostatin and resemble gut D cells ultrastructurally. Histochemistry 62:281.
7. Girod C, Dubois MP, Durand N 1980 Immunocytochemical evidence for the presence of somatostatin-like immunoreactivity in scattered cells of the duct system of the submandibular glands in the monkey, Macaca irus. Histochemistry 69:137.
8. Nishihira M, Yagihashi S 1979 Simultaneous detection of immunoreactive HCG- and somatostatin-containing cells and their gestational changes in the human placental villi and decidua. Acta Histochem Cytochem 12:434.
9. Watkins WB, Yen SSC 1980 Somatostatin in cytotrophoblast of the immature human placenta: localization by immunoperoxidase cytochemistry. J Clin Endocrinol Metab 50:969.

10. Bolaffi JL, Reichlin S, Goodman DBP, Forrest JN 1980 Somatostatin: occurrence in urinary bladder epithelium and renal tubules of the toad Bufo Marinus. Science 210:644.
11. Goldsmith PC, Rose JC, Arimura A, Ganong WF 1975 Ultrastructural localization of somatostatin in pancreatic islets of the rat. Endocrinology 97:1061.
12. Canese MG, Bussolati G 1977 Immunoelectron cytochemical localization of the somatostatin cells in the human antral mucosa. J Histochem Cytochem 15:1111.
13. Hellman B, Lernmark Å 1969 A possible role of the pancreatic α_1- and α_2-cells as local regulators of insulin secretion. In: Falkmer S, Hellman B, Täljedahl SB (eds) The Structure and Metabolism of the Pancreatic Islets. Pergamon Press, Oxford, p 453.
14. Ganda OP, Weir GC, Soeldner JS, Legg MA, Chick WL, Patel YC, Ebeid AM, Gabbay KH, Reichlin S 1977 Somatostatinoma - a somatostatin containing tumour of the endocrine pancreas. New Engl J Med 297:1352.
15. Larsson LI, Hirsch MA, Holst JJ, Ingemansson S, Kühl C, Lindkaer-Jensen S, Lundqvist G, Rehfeld JF, Schwartz TW 1977 Pancreatic somatostatinoma: clinical features and physiological implications. Lancet I:666.
16. Lomsky R, Langr F, Vortel V 1969 Immunohistochemical demonstration of gastrin in mammalian islets of Langerhans. Nature 223:618.
17. Larsson LI, Rehfeld JF, Sundler F, Håkanson R 1976 Pancreatic gastrin in foetal and neonatal rats. Nature 262:609.
18. Larsson LI 1980 Gastrointestinal cells producing endocrine, neurocrine and paracrine messengers. Clinics in Gastroenterology 9:485.
19. Oyama H, Kameda Y, Endoh M, Nagase Y, Matsuki M, Kakita K, Tenku A, Nishida S, Horino M 1984 Somatostatin-like immunoreactivity in mammalian thyroid glands: contents and partial characterization. Endocrinology 114:1028.
20. Lundberg JM, Hökfelt T 1983 Coexistence of peptides and classical neurotransmitters. Trends Neurosci 6:325.
21. Pearse AGE 1981 The diffuse neuroendocrine system: falsification and verification of a concept. In: Grossman MI, Braizier MAB, Lechago J (eds) Cellular Basis of Chemical Messengers in the Digestive System. UCLA Forum in Med Sci Nr 23, Academic Press, New York, p 13.
22. Le Douarin NM, Fontaine-Perus J 1981 The neural crest and the digestive tract: developmental relationships. In: Bloom SR, Polak JM (eds) Gut Hormones, Churchill Livingstone, Edinburgh, p 107.
23. Pictet RL, Rall LB, Phelps P, Rutter WJ 1976 The neural crest and the origin of the insulin-producing and other gastrointestinal hormone-producing cells. Science 191:191.

24. Larsson LI, Goltermann N, De Magistris L, Rehfeld JF, Schwartz TW 1979 Somatostatin cell processes as pathways for paracrine secretion. Science 205: 1393.
25. Larsson LI 1980 Peptide secretory pathways in the gastrointestinal tract: cytochemical contributions to regulatory physiology of the gut. Am J Physiol 239:G237.
26. Larsson LI 1984 Evidence for anterograde transport of secretory granules in processes of gastric paracrine (somatostatin) cells. Histochemistry 80:323.
27. Saffouri B, Weir GC, Bitar KN, Makhlouf GM 1980 Gastrin and somatostatin secretion by perfused rat stomach: functional linkage of antral peptides. Am J Physiol 238:G495.
28. Richelsen B, Rehfeld JF, Larsson LI 1983 Antral gland cell column: a method for studying release of gastric hormones. Am J Physiol 245:G463.
29. Saffouri B, Weir GC, Bitar KN, Makhlouf GM 1979 Stimulation of gastrin secretion from the perfused rat stomach by somatostatin antiserum. Life Sci 25:1749.
30. Chiba T, Kadowaki S, Taminato T, Chihara K, Seino Y, Matsuhara S, Fujita T 1981 Effect of antisomatostatin γ-globulin on gastrin release in rats. Gastroenterology 81:321.
31. Wolfe MM, Reel GM, McGuigan JE 1983 Inhibition of gastrin release by secretin is mediated by somatostatin in cultured rat antral mucosa. J Clin Invest 72:1586.
32. Sasagawa T, Kobayashi S, Fujita T 1974 Electron microscopic studies on the endocrine cells of the human gut and pancreas. In: Fujita T (ed) Gastroenteropancreatic Endocrine System - A Cell-biological Approach. Thieme, Stuttgart, p 17.
33. Schusdziarra V, Harris V, Conlon JM, Arimura A, Unger RH 1978 Pancreatic and gastric somatostatin release in response to intragastric and intraduodenal nutrients and HCl in the dog. J Clin Invest 62:509
34. Holst JJ, Knudsen S, Jensen SL, Nielsen OV, Poulsen SS Paracrine somatostatin and GRP-nerves in control of antral gastrin release. Program of the Somatostatin Symposium, Montreal, June 1984, # 14 (Abstract).
35. McIntosh CHS, Pederson RA, Koop H, Brown JC 1981 Gastric inhibitory polypeptide stimulated secretion of somatostatin-like immunoreactivity from the stomach? inhibition by acetylcholine or vagal stimulation. Can J Physiol Parmacol 59:468.
36. Uvnäs-Wallensten K 1980 Luminal secretion of gut peptides. Clinics in Gastroenterology 9:545.
37. Larsson LI 1981 Somatostatin cells. In: Bloom SR, Polak JM (eds) Gut Hormones. Churchill Livingstone, Edinburgh, p 350.
38. Patel YC, Wheatley T, Ning C 1981 Multiple forms of immunoreactive somatostatin: comparison of distribution in neural and nonneural tissues and portal plasma of the rat. Endocrinology 109:1943.

39. Brown M, Rivier J, Vale W 1981 Somatostatin-28: selective action on the pancreatic B cell and brain. Endocrinology 108:2391.
40. Mandarino L, Stenner D, Blanchard W, Nissen S, Gerich J, Ling N, Brazeau P, Bohlen P, Esch F, Guillemin R 1981 Selective effects of somatostatin-14, -25 and -28 on in vitro insulin and glucagon secretion. Nature 291:76.
41. Orci L, Unger RH 1975 Functional subdivision of islets of Langerhans and possible role of D cells. Lancet II:1243.
42. Fujita T, Yanotori Y, Murakami T 1976 Insulo-acinar axis, its vascular basis and its functional and morphological changes caused by CCK-PZ and caerulein. In: Fujita T (ed) Endocrine Gut and Pancreas. Elsevier, Amsterdam, p 347.
43. Bonner-Weir S, Orci L 1982 New perspectives on the microvasculature of the islets of Langerhans in the rat. Diabetes 31:883.
44. Kawai K, Ipp E, Orci L, Perrelet A, Unger RH 1982 Circulating somatostatin acts on the islets of Langerhans by way of a somatostatin-poor compartment. Science 218:477.
45. Kameda Y, Oyama H, Endoh M, Horino M 1982 Somatostatin immunoreactive C cells in thyroid glands from various mammalian species. Anat Rec 204:161.
46. Alumets J, Håkanson R, Lundqvist G, Sundler F, Thorell J 1980 Ontogeny and ultrastructure of somatostatin and calcitonin cells in the thyroid gland of the rat. Cell Tissue Res 206:193.
47. Kameda Y, Oyama H, Horino M 1984 Ontogeny of immunoreactive somatostatin in thyroid C cells from dogs and guinea pigs. Anat Rec 208:89.
48. Deschenes RJ, Lorenz LJ, Haun RS, Roos BA, Collier KJ, Dixon JE 1984 Cloning and sequence analysis of a cDNA encoding rat preprocholecystokinin. Proc Natl Acad Sci (USA) 81:726.
49. Larsson LI, Mørch-Jørgensen L 1978 Ultrastructural and cytochemical studies on the cytodifferentiation of duodenal endocrine cells. Cell Tissue Res 194:79.
50. Larsson LI 1977 Ontogeny of peptide-producing nerves and endocrine cells of the gastro-duodeno-pancreatic region. Histochemistry 54:133.
51. Rorstad OP, Brownstein MJ, Martin JB 1979 Immunoreactive and biologically active somatostatin-like material in rat retina. Proc Natl Acad Sci (USA) 76:3019.
52. Eriksen EF, Larsson LI 1981 Neuropeptides in the retina: evidence for differential topographical localization. Peptides 2:153.

22

PANCREATIC SOMATOSTATIN

GORDON C. WEIR AND SUSAN BONNER-WEIR

Department of Internal Medicine
Medical College of Virginia
Richmond, Virginia 23298

ABSTRACT

This is a review of pancreatic somatostatin which is limited in its scope and therefore focuses upon some selected issues. Throughout the entire review the same basic questions recur: Why do islets contain somatostatin? What is the physiological role of somatostatin and what does this peptide have to do with diabetes? Clear answers to these questions do not emerge, but a number of hunches are explored. The review provides a very brief look at somatostatin secretion, a discussion of the potential interactions which islet D cells might have with other islet cell types, consideration of how knowledge of islet anatomy may help us understand the D cell, and finally some comments about what happens to the D cell in diabetes and fasting.

INTRODUCTION

Although it has been known for over a decade that islet D cells contain somatostatin, we have a very poor understanding of the physiological or pathophysiological function of this peptide, which is such a potent inhibitor of insulin and glucagon secretion. Because the islet contribution to the somatostatin levels found in the portal vein and peripheral vascular plasma is dwarfed by that from the gastrointestinal tract- at least in mammals- it seems that islet somatostatin is unlikely to have a significant endocrine function. The best guess therefore is that islet somatostatin influences other islet cells through some kind of local secretion mechanism, with the A and PP cells being the most likely to be affected. There are reasons for thinking that B cells are normally little influenced by intraislet somatostatin and these will be discussed. Because of the rigorous evolutionary conservation of the structure of somatostatin, it must be assumed that this peptide is vital for survival, but the most logical locations for such a key role would be the central nervous sytem or the gastrointestinal tract. Perhaps islet D cells are vestigial in mammals and have a more important role in fish and birds where they constitute a larger proportion of the islet cell population (1, 2), but to make such an assumption would be unadventuresome and counterproductive.

Brief Overview of Islet Somatostatin Secretion

A great deal of information has been generated in the past few years about the control of islet somatostatin secretion and it is not the purpose of this short review to provide a comprehensive assessment of this area. Unfortunately, no exhaustive recent reviews are currently available and therefore the truly curious will have to wade through the literature. Table 1 is superficial and simplistic, with some discrepancies in the literature being ignored, but it does provide a rough picture of how various agents influence islet secretion. It is noteworthy that the increases and decreases of insulin secretion are identical to those of somatostatin secretion, except in the case of acetylcholine.

Table 1. Summary of How Various Agents Affect Insulin, Somatostatin and Glucagon Secretion

	Insulin	Somatostatin	Glucagon
Glucose	↑	↑	↓
Amino acids	↑	↑	↑
FFA	↑	↑ (?)	↓
Gastrin	↑	↑	↑
CCK	↑	↑	↑
GIP	↑	↑	↑
Secretin	↑	↑	↓
Bombesin	↑	↑	0
VIP	↑	↑	↑
Alpha adrenergic	↓	↓	↑
Beta adrenergic	↑	↑	↑
Acetylcholine	↑	↓	↑
Tolbutamide	↑	↑	↑↓
Insulin	↓	↓	↓
Somatostatin	↓	↓	↓
Glucagon	↑	↑	↓

Possible Interactions Between Islet Cells

Before homing in on the interactions which are likely to occur between islet cells, it should be useful to discuss those interactions which are possible. At the onset it should be stated that this short review will have a mammalian bias because most of our knowledge about somatostatin has been obtained in this class. Furthermore, pancreatic polypeptide will be largely ignored, mainly because we know so little about its physiological role. Although now well known, readers can be reminded that the islets of the dorsal lobe of the pancreas consist mainly of A, B, and D cells, whereas the islets of the smaller ventral lobe are made up of mostly B, D, and PP cells (3). With regard to possible interactions it seems that the major secretory product of any particular cell type is capable of affecting the secretion of all of the other cell types. One must become increasingly cautious about such statements, however, because of the large number of fragments resulting from processing of prepropeptides, which are currently being discovered. Some of these are bound to have important biological functions, with somatostatin-28 being a good example. In any event somatostatin can inhibit glucagon and insulin secretion. Glucagon is capable of stimulating insulin and somatostatin secretion, and insulin can inhibit glucagon secretion (4). The effects of insulin upon somatostatin secretion are less clear, but there is increasing evidence that in mammals, inhibition occurs (5, 6) even though stimulation is found in chickens (7). Things become even more complex because insulin can inhibit the B cell (8), somatostatin seems capable of inhibiting the D cell (9), and glucagon may be able to inhibit the A cell (10). The influence of the autonomic nervous system adds another layer of complexity, but this aspect has been reviewed elsewhere (11-13) and will not be dealt with here. Another interesting area which will be largely ignored in this review is the concept of the insular-acinar axis (4, 14). Because it has been shown that both somatostatin and insulin can influence pancreatic exocrine function, and because capillaries from islets can drain directly into acinar tissue, it is attractive to postulate that islets somehow regulate acinar function. The importance of this mechanism has not yet been defined and we must be cautious in our speculations because there is some evidence that at least some pancreatic exocrine tissue is supplied by blood which does not first go through islets (15).

Anatomical Considerations

Although the possible interactions are bewildering in their scope, the likely interactions seem limited by islet anatomy. One of the most important concepts is that of compartmentalization such that some islet cells must be anatomically shielded from other islet secretory products. This concept is based upon the finding that very small amounts of somatostatin and glucagon introduced into the arteries supplying the pancreas can have profound effects (10, 16-18). Thus, there appears to be an arterial compartment which contains very little somatostatin and glucagon, and a separate venous compartment which contains large amounts of these peptides after they have been secreted. We have explored the hypothesis that this compartmentalization results from polarization of islet cells. It was found previously that cultured isolated B cells can have a polarized appearance as might be expected from an epithelial cell, such that a basolateral portion of the cell adheres to the culture plate and an apical portion containing granules faces the media (19). We have since found that for analysis with electron microscopy, the polarization of B cells can be better appreciated after degranulation with glyburide treatment (20). This approach was coupled with an analysis of vascular pattern as determined by examination of consecutive adjacent sections of islets, and B cells could be seen which had residual granules facing a presumed venous-sided capillary, with another side of the cell facing an arterial-sided capillary. It therefore appears that in vivo B cells have basolateral and apical portions, and in fact B cells face two separate vessels. We can therefore speculate that the basolateral portion is the arterial or "sensing" side, and that the apical portion is the secretory side of the cell. Thus the sensing side of a cell may never come in contact with that cell's secretory product. One might guess that a similar polarity exists for A, D, and PP cells, but this remains to be demonstrated.

Compartmentalization within islets could also be achieved with a particular arrangement of the vasculature. Studies have been carried out in rat islets using the combined approach of corrosion casts with methyl merthacrylate and serial reconstructions with vessels marked with India ink injections (15). The B cell core was distinguished from the non-B cell mantle with immunohistochemical methodology. It was found that afferent arterioles enter islets through a gap in the mantle and then branch into capillaries within the B cell core. These capillaries then traverse the core and only coalesce after passing through the mantle. If interaction between islet cells can be caused by the blood borne transport of a peptide from one part of an islet to another, guesses can be made about which interactions could take place. It can be expected therefore that at least some mantle cells are bathed with high concentrations of insulin, unless there was a specialized group of capillaries which goes directly to the mantle without coming into contact with the apical secretory side of B cells. Such a possibility seems unlikely, in part because it has not yet been possible to show that very small amounts of exogenous insulin can influence A and D cell secretion; these small amounts of exogenous insulin presumably blend with and become lost in larger amounts of endogenous insulin. It seems virtually inconceivable that somatostatin or glucagon from the mantle could get to the B cell core via the vasculature. These vasculature studies do not, however, rule out paracrine interactions whereby peptides are transported from one cell to another through interstitial spaces. There is currently no information available about the direction of interstitial fluid flow within islets or how this flow might be channeled by tight junctions. If Starling's hypothesis about fluid leaving arterioles and being taken up by venules holds, there would be reason to think that interstitial fluid should flow from the B cell core to the non-B cell mantle. It may well be, however, that B cells on the periphery of the core, at least, are influenced by somatostatin and/or glucagon through a paracrine mechanism. The D cell seems to be a particularly attractive candidate for such a role because some morphologists feel that D cells tend to lie at the junction between A and B cells (21), and in addition, D cells often are seen to have dendritic-like processes (22) which could extend at least partially into the B cell core.

Another way in which D cells could communicate with other islet cell types is through gap junctions as it is now known that these specialized junctions can be found between islet cells of different types (23, 24). It can probably be assumed that D cells always have these connections with the A, B, or PP cells which happen to lie next to them, and that electric charge and small molecules are continually being passed from one cell to another. We know almost nothing about the functions of islet gap junctions, but the major islet secretory products cannot be expected to pass from one cell to another because the intracellular channels are too small (4). Some experimental data are now appearing which indicate that cell-free communication is not a very important process in short-term hormone release (25, 26), and perhaps these junctions will turn out to be important for growth, differentiation, or some sort of cell maintenance (blatant speculation).

Does Intraislet Somatostatin Influence Insulin Secretion?

The possibility that islet somatostatin might regulate insulin secretion is a very important question, particularly because B cells in diabetes could be adversely affected. The volume of B cells is markedly reduced in juvenile-onset (Type I) diabetes and even modestly reduced in maturity-onset (Type II) diabetes (27), and thus in both situations a greater proportion of B cells would be closer to the somatostatin-containing D cells. Unfortunately, few data are currently available which provide insight into this possibility. Our laboratory has been studying insulin secretion in a newly-described rat model of Type II diabetes where it has been found that in the presence of low glucose concentrations insulin secretion is actually increased even though the B cell mass is reduced to about 50% of normal (28-30). Thus, in this situation at least, local somatostatin cannot be exerting a very deleterious suppressive effect upon the residual B cells.

Within normal islets there is little reason to think that intraislet somatostatin has a substantial influence upon B cells. Because of the anatomical considerations which have already been discussed, it is difficult to see how very much islet somatostatin from the mantle could reach the B cell core. It does seem possible, however, that circulating somatostatin, most of which originates from the gastrointestinal tract, could have a suppressive effect, particularly because such small concentrations of both somatostatin-14 and -28 have been shown to inhibit secretion (17, 31). Studies have been carried out in which isolated islets incubated with somatostatin antiserum have been found to have enhanced insulin secretion (32, 33). Unfortunately, incubating isolated islets is in many ways unphysiological, particularly because their vasculature and neural input have been disrupted. Thus it is not surprising that insulin secretion is enhanced when the somatostatin which has been secreted into the incubation buffer is neutralized by the addition of antiserum. Therefore these findings seem to have limited relevance to actual in vivo events.

It is very difficult to design studies which provide evidence to either prove or disprove the hypothesis that islet cells communicate through local secretion or some other mechanism. An approach which is attractive conceptually is to disperse islet cells, purify them into homogeneous populations, and then see how their function compares with the same cell types which are contained in intact islets. Our laboratory and several others have carried out such studies and a lot has been learned about how to work with dispersed cells, but it is very difficult to draw conclusions about in vivo events from these in vitro experiments. Great progress has been made in purifying specific cell types using flow cytometry, elutriation, and density gradients (25, 34, 35). Unfortunately, acutely dispersed islet cells are not useful for secretion studies because they are so unresponsive, presumably because of the trauma of the dispersion process; however, after being allowed to recover in tissue culture conditions, their responsiveness improves (25). The secretion of cultured purified B cells has been studied with these cells being perifused after being immobilized on Bio Gel P2 beads and it has been concluded that single cells secrete less well than intact islets, suggesting that cell-cell communication is important for the maintenance of normal short-term release profiles (35). One should be very careful, however, about accepting these results at face value because there is no assurance that these isolated unprotected cells are not damaged by the perifusion procedure, whereas it can be expected that cells buried within intact islets would be far less vulnerable. We have used a different approach and have studied only those cells which have attached to the bottom of culture dishes, making the assumption that the discarded cells, which were floating and unattached, were unhealthy. It was found that these attached cells, which were almost entirely B cells and almost entirely single, were able to respond to glucose and arginine as well as B cells contained within intact islets which were cultured in an identical fashion (19, 25). Even though we are well aware of the risks of trying to relate these results to the function of in vivo islets, the data are compatible with the concept that B cells can function normally in the absence of cell-cell contacts and A or D cells. Obviously, much more work needs to be done with these and other approaches before this hypothesis can be accepted.

In trying to build the argument that islet D cells are unlikely to influence B cell function, one cannot ignore the work supporting the concept that local glucagon secretion, also originating from the islet mantle, might enhance B cell function. The best work supporting this idea has exploited the fact that dorsal islets contain B and A cells, whereas ventral islets contain B cells, but very few A cells. When islets are isolated from these separate portions of the pancreas, it is found that dorsal islets secrete more insulin than ventral islets (36). Even though these experiments can be criticized because of the unphysiological nature of incubating isolated islets, similar results have been found using perfused dorsal and ventral portions of the pancreas (37, 38). The enhanced insulin release from the perfused dorsal portion of the pancreas could be explained by a stimulatory effect of local glucagon secretion, but there could be many other reasons for such a result.

Another series of experiments concerned with the possibility that islet somatostatin might influence B cell function conclude that somatostatin receptors are delivered to the B cell plasma membrane by secretory granules. It is suggested that when insulin is being actively secreted there are more somatostatin receptors on the B cell surface and therefore these cells are more sensitive to the influence of somatostatin (39). This novel hypothesis introduces a new mechanism through which paracrine effects by somatostatin might be regulated. Even though this hypothesis is of interest, we favor the concept that insulin secretion occurs independently of intraislet somatostatin and glucagon secretion, even though, as has been mentioned before, circulating somatostatin from the gastrointestinal tract may well influence B cell function. Clearly much more work is needed before any of the hypotheses can be taken too seriously.

Does Intraislet Somatostatin Influence Glucagon Secretion?

Certainly, the juxtaposition of A and D cells, with their potential negative feedback loop mediated by glucagon and somatostatin, makes the possibility of a paracrine interaction between the two cell types attractive, but no definitive proof for such a relationship has emerged. The finding that such small concentrations of glucagon and somatostatin can influence these mantle cells tells us that at least some functional and presumably anatomical segregation exists between these two cell types. With all of the information which is now currently available about islet secretion, one might have expected that paracrine effects would have revealed themselves by now, and perhaps the evidence is there, with us not being smart enough to see it. What we seem to be left with are a variety of experiments which are consistent with the paracrine hypothesis and some of these will be discussed.

One of the most perplexing questions is how glucose affects islet secretion, and this is, of course, very important for those who are trying to understand diabetes mellitus. The basic facts which require explanation are that glucose stimulates insulin and somatostatin secretion, and inhibits glucagon secretion. One possibility is that glucose has direct effects upon each of these cell types and that there is no interaction between the different cell types. It seems reasonably safe to conclude that glucose directly stimulates B cells, but even this tenet is not absolute. The real uncertainty lies with the question of whether glucose has direct effects upon the A and D cells. It is of interest that gastric A and D cells do not appear to respond to changes in glucose concentration (40, 41). A popular hypothesis has been that glucose-induced glucagon suppression is mediated by local insulin secretion, and this has been analyzed in detail in an earlier review (4). Probably the earliest work which gave this hypothesis credibility was the finding that in situations where B cells were destroyed, such as Type I diabetes and streptozotocin and alloxan diabetes, the A cells are blind to changes in glucose concentration (4). This hypothesis is dependent upon the assumption that local insulin secretion can inhibit the A cell and some of the strongest evidence supporting this concept comes from the work of Asplin et al. (42). They were able to show that insulin infusions in normal man led to enhanced arginine-stimulated glucagon secretion, whereas in subjects with Type I diabetes the insulin infusions suppressed the glucagon responses. This result does not seem to be a peculiarity of the in vivo conditions because similar findings have been obtained using the isolated perfused canine pancreas technique (38, 43). An attractive explanation for these findings was that the infusion of exogenous insulin had suppressed endogenous insulin, as was shown by the fall in C-peptide levels, and that this released the A cells from the inhibitory effects of the intraislet insulin, resulting in the enhanced response to arginine. In the diabetic subjects with no endogenous insulin secretion, the exogenous insulin infusions were then able to suppress the arginine-stimulated secretion of glucagon. One can raise the question as to whether the differences could somehow be explained by paracrine somatostatin secretion, but this would require that the somatostatin secretion, or effects, were different in the two types of subjects, a possibility which has not yet been excluded.

The importance of local insulin secretion in the glucose suppression of glucagon secretion has been brought into question by several recent observations. One way to explain the glucagon rise seen after insulin-induced hypoglycemia has been to say that it was caused by the fall in endogenous local insulin secretion, and therefore it made sense that subjects with Type I diabetes would not have such a glucagon rise (44). A recent study has shown, however, that individuals with recently diagnosed Type I diabetes with no detectable C-peptide, had normal glucagon rises in responses to hypoglycemia (45). These findings place one in the position of guessing that the glucagon rises might have been caused by: 1) a direct effect of hypoglycemia, 2) a reduction in local somatostatin secretion, 3) some as yet unidentified mechanism, such as the autonomic nervous system (46), or 4) an effect from a very small number of B cells. Other recent experiments (47, 48) indicate that when glucose levels are normalized in alloxan-diabetic dogs, glucagon suppressibility is restored, even though in one of these (48) a definite small rise of insulin secretion could be discerned. The finding that somatostatin responsiveness to glucose is also restored (48, 49) provides a potential explanation for the A cell suppression. In spite of these provocative challenges, the concept that intraislet insulin regulates the A cell is far from dead. In fact, another recent study has found that infusion of insulin antiserum into the perfused rat pancreas causes an abrupt marked increase of glucagon secretion (50).

There are a number of other pieces of information which may provide clues about local interactions:

1) It now seems clear that the same dose of tolbutamide can have either stimulatory or inhibitory effects upon glucagon secretion, with the direction of change being dependent upon the concentration of glucose. The inhibitory effect is seen at a low glucose concentration and the relative increases in insulin and somatostatin are greater under these conditions, suggesting that the glucagon suppression could have been caused by either or both peptides, with the primary effect of tolbutamide upon the A cell being stimulatory (51, 52).

2) Investigators have looked closely at the timing of islet hormone release in the hope that the secretion of one peptide might precede the stimulation or suppression of a particular cell type, but these efforts have almost always been disappointing. A provocative result has, however, been seen in a study by Ipp et al. in which the infusion of morphine into the perfused canine pancreas led to the rapid suppression of somatostatin secretion which was followed two minutes later by increases of glucagon and insulin secretion (53). Such a finding is consistent with the possibility that somatostatin exerts a tonic suppressive influence upon both A and B cells.

3) Hopes have also been raised that somatostatin analogs might have specific effects upon either A or B cells and therefore uncover a paracrine or some other intraislet interaction. Indeed the somatostatin receptors on A and B cells do appear to differ, but unfortunately, thus far, the available analogs have not proved to be specific enough (54). An interesting result has, however, been obtained by Taborsky, who found in an in vivo study that the somatostatin analog [D-Ala^5-DTrp^8] S-14, which can inhibit the D cell, causes increases in insulin and glucagon secretion (55). This finding needs to be confirmed in an in vitro preparation such as the isolated perfused pancreas to rule out some indirect effect of the analog, which could have been caused by a gut hormone or some kind of activation of the autonomic nervous sytem.

4) Passive immunization has been another attractive approach, but when antiserum has been used in perfused pancreas studies, the results have usually been negative. These negative results are not surprising because it should not be expected that enough antiserum could reach critical interstitial spaces in high enough concentration to neutralize the high concentrations of peptide which are presumed to be present. When anti-somatostatin serum has been added to incubating isolated islets, increases of insulin and glucagon secretion have been seen (32, 33), but as has been discussed earlier, the unphysiological nature of this approach makes it difficult to accept the relevance of these findings to in vivo events. It has been found, however, that the infusion of somatostatin antiserum into the perfused chicken pancreas caused a large release of glucagon and a smaller release of insulin (56). These experiments must also be interpreted cautiously because the perfusion conditions could have led to an unphysiological opening of interstitial spaces, or perhaps the unique anatomy of the chicken pancreas permits local secretion in vasculature channels which makes passive immunization possible.

5) Studies with dispersed cells have been carried out in our laboratory, as has already been discussed, and it was found that cultured dispersed A cells secrete considerably more glucagon than A cells which are contained in similarly cultured islets (19, 25). These results are also consistent with the hypothesis that the A cells of intact islets are tonically inhibited by somatostatin secretion from adjacent D cells, but the relevance of these in vitro studies to in vivo islet function remains to be proven.

The several studies described above have been chosen from a large literature because they seem to provide the most provocative clues to the paracrine interactions which could take place, but in each case we have provided caveats about taking these results at face value, and indeed with more thought and space, many more criticisms could undoubtedly have been raised. As we continue to pick away at this difficult problem, we must always subject our findings to the toughest possible scrutiny.

Does Intraislet Glucagon Influence Somatostatin Secretion?

Even though it is attractive to think of there being a paracrine negative feedback loop between A and D cells, it is entirely possible that there is no loop, and that the only functional link is the somatostatin inhibition of glucagon secretion. There is very little evidence that intraislet glucagon stimulates D cell secretion, and there is some reason to think that such an effect may be weak, if present at all. For instance, epinephrine, acetylcholine, morphine, and β-endorphin all stimulate glucagon secretion and inhibit somatostatin secretion (11, 12, 53). These findings suggest that either these agents are very potent inhibitors of D cell secretion or that the intraislet glucagon effects are minimal. It would be of interest to know how much exogenous glucagon it would take to stimulate D cells while they are being suppressed by some of these agents, but we are unaware of any studies examining this question. One could use the same kind of arguments to suggest that the effects of somatostatin on the A cell may be weak because amino acids and several gut hormones are potent stimuli of both glucagon and somatostatin secretion, but at least in this case we know that relatively large concentrations of somatostatin cannot completely suppress stimulated glucagon secretion (54, 57). An additional point is that glucose suppresses glucagon secretion and stimulates somatostatin secretion, and this too raises questions about the potency of intraislet glucagon. Certainly there are stronger reasons for believing that intraislet somatostatin has a paracrine influence upon glucagon secretion than the reverse possibility.

Islet Somatostatin, Diabetes, and Obesity

The finding that somatostatin was present in islets was a startling discovery over ten years ago and has continued to fascinate students trying to understand the pathogenesis of diabetes. It has finally become clear that both glucagon and insulin are largely responsible for the metabolic derangements of diabetes, and therefore it is tantalizing that islets contain a peptide in substantial amounts which is a potent inhibitor of both A and B cells. We now know a lot about the secretion and morphology of pancreatic D cells in experimental diabetes, but in spite of this, we have almost no idea about how islet somatostatin is involved in the pathogenesis of any form of diabetes.

It did not take investigators long, once the somatostatin radioimmunoassay was developed, to find that in streptozotocin and alloxan diabetes there was an increase in the islet and pancreatic content of somatostatin (58, 59), and that this was accompanied by an increase in islet D cell volume (59, 60). In addition, the content of gastric somatostatin was increased, even though that of the CNS was not (59). Studies carried out in isolated perfused pancreases have shown that both basal and amino acid-stimulated somatostatin secretion are increased in rats with chemical diabetes (61). It has also been found that concentrations of somatostatin are elevated in peripheral and portal vein plasma of streptozotocin rats (62), and in the peripheral plasma of alloxan diabetic dogs (63), but it is very important to remember that most of the somatostatin found in plasma is thought to originate from the gastrointestinal tract and not the pancreas (62, 64). It seems likely that these D cell changes are secondary to insulin deficiency because after pancreatic transplantation into streptozotocin diabetic rats the increased somatostatin release from the perfused pancreas is normalized (65). An additional interesting point is that glucose-induced somatostatin release is not found in isolated islets from streptozotocin diabetic rats or from the perfused pancreas of alloxan-diabetic dogs, but responsiveness is returned after a period of in vivo insulin treatment (48, 49).

The streptozotocin and alloxan models of diabetes have been those most widely used for studies of D cell function, and therefore before going on to discuss other models of diabetes it seems worthwhile to pause briefly to see what insights might be found in the above data. One of the simplest explanations for some of the findings is that D cells are normally suppressed by either peripheral or intraislet insulin, and that when B cells are destroyed, D cells can grow and secrete more somatostatin. The best available data in mammals indicates that insulin can suppress stimulated somatostatin secretion (5, 6), even though this effect has been quite difficult for many laboratories to demonstrate, but this information does provide additional support for the concept of chronic insulin suppression. It is not clear in these models whether each individual D cell is secreting more, or whether the increased secretion can be solely explained on the basis of the increase in D cell mass. Because there is an actual decrease in the secretion of pancreatic glucagon in rats with chemical diabetes, as determined by perfused pancreas studies (66, 67), it seems hard to imagine that the D cell changes are the result of local A cell function, even though it is conceivable that the D cells are somehow responding to the increased circulating glucagon levels. Because in man it is generally assumed that the increased plasma glucagon levels seen in diabetes are coming from the pancreas, it is surprising that rats with chemical diabetes, which also have increased plasma glucagon levels, turn out to have reduced secretion of pancreatic glucagon. Presumably glucagon from the gut is responsible for the increased plasma levels in these rats. With regard to the possible importance of the increased secretion of islet somatostatin, one must wonder whether it could have an adverse effect on the very small number of residual B cells, even though reasons have already been given for thinking that this may not be true, but it is particularly tempting to speculate that the reduced A cell secretion is related to the increased D cell mass.

It is of considerable interest that in Type II human diabetes, both B and A cells are usually unresponsive to acute changes in glucose concentration; in Type I diabetes, A cells are usually blind to glucose; and in chemical diabetes in animals, there is evidence for blindness of A, B, and D cells (29, 68, 69). Our laboratory has generated an array of data supporting the concept that the chronic exposure of B cells to only modestly elevated glucose levels leads to a situation of "overwork", which is manifest by gross alteration in insulin secretion, the most striking characteristic being blindness to both acute increases and decreases in glucose concentration (30). For those attracted to the concept that the B cell is the islet glucose sensor, and that somehow the delivery of insulin to the islet mantle accounts for the responsiveness of A and D cells to glucose, the question must be raised as to whether blindness of B cells is the cause of the blindness of the other cell types. This explanation is made less attractive by recent reports stating that normalization of the glucose level in alloxan diabetic dogs restores the glucose responsiveness of both A and D cells (47, 48). Perhaps it will turn out that all three cell types independently respond to chronic hyperglycemia by becoming glucose blind, with a similar mechanism causing these changes in each cell type.

Interesting changes in the D cells are also found in other animal models of diabetes. For instance, the BB rat is a model of Type I diabetes, with insulin deficiency being caused by autoimmune destruction of islet tissue. Plasma samples obtained from the portal vein and the inferior vena cava are elevated and yet the pancreatic content of somatostatin is reduced (64). One group has found that somatostatin secetion from the perfused pancreas is reduced and lowered still further after insulin treatment of the rats (70, 71), whereas another group has reported increased secretion from the perfused pancreas of BB rats (72). The reason for the discrepancy is unclear, but the animals with the increased secretion were younger and may have sustained less immune D cell damage. It is of interest that the A and D cells of BB rats are damaged by a presumed immune mechanism, whereas in human Type I diabetes there is as yet no good evidence for such damage, even though circulating antibodies are found which react with islet non-B cells (73). There is another, less thoroughly characterized, model of islet immune injury, the non-obese diabetic (NOD) mouse which has been reported to have increased pancreatic somatostatin content (74), but these values were obtained only 3-15 days after the onset of glycosuria and perhaps a different result would have been obtained if the course of the disease had been longer.

The genetic obesity-hyperglycemia syndromes in mice have been studied in some detail and there are some discrepancies which leave some of us mildly confused. The most thorough study to date has been carried out by Berelowitz et al. (75), and they concluded that the pancreatic content of somatostatin was more strongly infuenced by genetic background than by the mutant genes. The C57BL/6J ob/ob and db/db mice had somewhat similar serum glucose and insulin values between the ages of 6 and 24 weeks, and during this period had a content of pancreatic somatostatin which did not differ from that found in control mice. In contrast the C57BL/KsJ ob/ob and db/db mice had more severe hyperglycemia, and serum insulin levels which dropped considerably during the period between 10 and 24 weeks, but nonetheless which remained higher than those found in the control mice. However, coincident with the fall in serum insulin there was an increase in the content of pancreatic somatostatin which was clearly greater than that found in the controls. In some ways this rise of pancreatic somatostatin is reminiscent of that seen in the hypoinsulinemic streptozotocin-diabetic model, but it needs to be noted that these C57BL/KsJ mice never had absolute hypoinsulinemia, even though it can be argued that they had relative hypoinsulinemia. There seems to be no easy explanation for the changes which have been described. It is of interest, however, that in spite of an impressive increase in the ratio of B to D cell volume (76), the pancreatic content of somatostatin is well maintained, even though other workers have reported both decreases and increases (77, 78). One could speculate that in these mice there is a neural or some other stimulus to islet growth and that the increase in the D cell mass is held in check by a suppressive effect of increased islet insulin secretion; an effect which weakens as insulin levels fall in the C57BL/KsJ animals. It is a pity that we do not know more about the secretion of pancreatic somatostatin in these difficult-to-study mice.

Other rodent models of obesity have been studied and rats with lesions of the ventromedial hypothalamus have been found to have increased pancreatic somatostatin content and enhanced somatostatin secretion from the perfused pancreas (79, 80). Very similar findings have been reported in the obese Zucker fa/fa rat (80), and one can guess that there is a similar, as yet unidentified, stimulus to islet growth in both models. For the sake of completeness, it should also be mentioned that in the diabetic Chinese hamster it has been found that pancreatic somatostatin content and D cell volume are reduced (81), but the pathogenesis of these changes remains obscure.

Because of the similarities between diabetes and fasting, it is interesting to note that rats fasted for 72 hours are found to have increased pancreatic somatostatin content (82). Because markedly reduced insulin secretion occurs during fasting it is possible that the mechanisms responsible for the change are the same as those taking place in the streptozotocin-diabetic rats.

As was suggested at the beginning of this section we have learned a lot about pancreatic somatostatin content and secretion in animal models of diabetes and obesity, but we have virtually no idea about how this islet somatostatin might contribute to the pathogenesis of these conditions. This level of ignorance is almost matched by our foggy understanding in the normal state about the influence of islet somatostatin upon the function of other islet cell types. Clearly we need new approaches and more experiments to unravel these puzzles. It would be very useful to have a specific toxin for D cells and there was optimism that cysteamine might serve this function (83, 84), but we must be concerned that this agent is not as specific as was originally hoped (85). An ideal tool would be a somatostatin analog which is a pure antagonist and hopefully such a peptide will eventually be developed. We must not allow ourselves to become discouraged at this early stage of investigation.

ACKNOWLEDGMENT

The authors thank Ellis Samols, who has been a source of inspiration and new ideas, and Jessie Reynolds, who has provided unfailing secretarial assistance. The work from our laboratory, which has been referred to, has been supported by grant AM-20349 from the National Institutes of Health and by a grant from the Juvenile Diabetes Foundation.

REFERENCES

1. Weir GC, Goltsos PC, Steinberg EP, Patel YC 1976 High concentration of somatostatin immunoreactivity in chicken pancreas. Diabetologia 12:129.
2. Ronner P, Scarpa A 1982 Isolated perfused Brockmann body as a model for studying pancreatic endocrine secretion. Am J Physiol 243:352.
3. Orci L, Baetens D, Ravazzola M, Stefan Y, Malaisse-Lagae F 1976 Pancreatic polypeptide and glucagon: non-random distribution in pancreatic islets. Life Sci 19:1811.
4. Samols E, Weir G, Bonner-Weir S 1983 Intraislet insulin-glucagon-somatostatin relationships. In: Lefebvre P (ed) Handbook of Experimental Pharmacology 66/II. Springer-Verlag, Berlin.
5. Gerber PPG, Trimble ER, Wolheim CB, Renold AE 1981 Effect of insulin on glucose- and arginine-stimulated somatostatin secretion from the isolated perfused rat pancreas. Endocrinology 109:279.
6. Kawai K, Unger RH 1983 Opposing actions of glucagon and insulin on splanchnic D cell function. J Clin Invest 71:721.

7. Honey RN, Weir GC 1979 Insulin stimulates somatostatin and inhibits glucagon secretion from the perfused chicken pancreas-duodenum. Life Sci 24:1747.
8. Iversen J, Miles DW 1971 Evidence for a feedback inhibition of insulin on insulin secretion in the isolated perfused canine pancreas. Diabetes 20:1.
9. Ipp E, Rivier J, Dobbs RE, Brown M, Vale W, Unger RH 1979 Somatostatin analogs inhibit somatostatin release. Endocrinology 104:1270.
10. Kawai K, Unger RH 1982 Inhibition of glucagon secretion by exogenous glucagon in the isolated perfused dog pancreas. Diabetes 31:512.
11. Samols E, Weir GC 1979 Adrenergic modulation of pancreatic A, B, and D cells: alpha-adrenergic suppression and beta-adrenergic stimulation of somatostatin secretion, alpha-adrenergic stimulation of glucagon secretion in the perfused dog pancreas. J Clin Invest 63:230.
12. Samols E, Stagner JI, Weir GC 1981 Autonomic function and control of pancreatic somatostatin. Diabetologia 20:388.
13. Palmer JP, Porte D 1981 Control of glucagon secretion: the central nervous system. In: Unger RH, Orci L (eds) Glucagon: Physiology, Pathophysiology and Morphology of the Pancreatic A-cells. Elsevier, New York, p 135.
14. Saito A, Williams JA, Kanno T 1980 Potentiation of cholecystokinin-induced exocrine secretion by both exogenous and endogenous insulin in isolated and perfused rat pancreata. J Clin Invest 65:777.
15. Bonner-Weir S, Orci L 1982 New perspectives on the microvasculature of the islets of Langerhans in the rat. Diabetes 31:883.
16. Samols E, Harrison J 1976 Remarkable potency of somatostatin as a glucagon suppressant. Metabolism 25 (suppl. 1):1495.
17. Kawai K, Orci L, Ipp E, Perrelet A, Unger RH 1982 Circulating somatostatin acts on the islets of Langerhans via a somatostatin-poor compartment. Science 218:477.
18. Weir GC, Samols E, Day JA, Patel YC 1978 Glucose and glucagon stimulate secretion of somatostatin from the perfused canine pancreas. Metabolism 27:1223.
19. Weir GC, Halban PA, Meda P, Wollheim B, Orci L, Renold AE 1984 Dispersed adult rat pancreatic islet cells in culture: A, B, and D cell function. Metabolism 33:447.
20. Bonner-Weir S 1984 Morphological evidence for B-cell polarity within the islet of Langerhans in the rat. Diabetes 33: (suppl. 1):81A.
21. Fujita T 1967 D cell, the third endocrine element of the pancreatic islet. Arch Histol Jap 29:1.
22. Leiter EH, Gapp DA, Eppig JJ, Coleman DL 1979 Ultrastructure and morphometric studies of delta cells in pancreatic islets from C57BL/KsJ diabetes mice. Diabetes 17:297.

23. Orci L, Malaisse-Lagae F, Ravazzola M, Rouiller D, Renold AE, Perrelet A, Unger R 1975 A morphological basis for intercellular communication between α- and β-cells in the endocrine pancreas. J Clin Invest 56:1066.
24. Meda P, Perelet A, Orci L 1980 Gap junctions and B cell function. Horm Metab Res 10 (suppl.):157.
25. Fletcher DJ, Grogan W, Barras E, Weir GC 1983 Hormone release by islet B cell-enriched and A and D cell-enriched populations prepared by flow cytometry. Endocrinology 113:1791.
26. Meda P, Sorenson R, Sheridan JD 1983 Perturbation of B-cell coupling in diabetic rat islets. Diabetes 32 (suppl. 1):41A.
27. Saito K, Yaginuma N, Takahashi T 1979 Differential volumetry of A, B, and D cells in the pancreatic islets of diabetic and non-diabetic subjects. Tohoku J Exp Med 129:273.
28. Bonner-Weir S, Trent DF, Honey RN, Weir GC 1981 Responses of neonatal rat islets to streptozotocin: Limited B-cell regeneration and hyperglycemia. Diabetes 30:64.
29. Weir GC, Clore ET, Zmachinski CJ, Bonner-Weir S 1981 Islet secretion in a new experimental model for non-insulin dependent diabetes. Diabetes 30:590.
30. Leahy JL, Weir GC 1984 Blindness to glucose in an experimental model of NIDDM: Inappropriate insulin and glucagon responses to glucose reduction. Clin Res 32:521A.
31. Mandarino L, Stenner D, Blanchard W, Nissen S, Gerich J, Ling N, Brazeau P, Böhlen P, Esch F, Guillemin R 1981 Selective effects of somatostatin-14, -25, and -28 on in vitro insulin and glucagon secretion. Nature 291:76.
32. Taniguchi H, Utsumi M, Hasegawa M, Kobayashi T, Watanabe Y, Murakami K, Seki M, Tsutsu A, Makimura H, Sakoda M, Baba S 1977 Physiological role of somatostatin: Insulin release from rat islets treated by somatostatin antiserum. Diabetes 26:700.
33. Itoh M, Mandarino L, Gerich JE 1980 Antisomatostatin gamma globulin augments secretion of both insulin and glucagon in vitro: Evidence for a physiological role for endogenous somatostatin in the regulation of pancreatic A and B cell function. Diabetes 29:693.
34. Pipeleers DG, Pipeleers-Marichal MA 1981 A method for the purification of single A, B and D cells and for the isolation of coupled cells from isolated rat islets. Diabetologia 20:654.
35. Pipeleers D, Veld P, Maes E, VanDeWinkel M 1982 Glucose-induced insulin release depends on functional cooperation between islet cells. Proc Natl Acad Sci (USA) 79:7322.
36. Trimble ER, Halban PA, Wollheim CB, Renold AE 1982 Functional differences between rat islets of ventral and dorsal pancreatic origin. J Clin Invest 69:405.
37. Samols E, Stagner J 1983 Dynamic differences in insulin secretion by the canine splenic and uncinate lobes. Diabetes 32 (suppl.):41A.

38. Leclerq-Meyer V, Marchand J, Malaisse WJ 1983 Insulin and glucagon release by the perfused ventral and dorsal parts of the rat pancreas. Diabetologia 25:175.
39. Sussman KE, Draznin B, Leitner JW, Mehler PS 1982 The endocrine secretion granule revisited-postulating new functions. Metabolism 31:959.
40. Lefebvre PJ, Luyckx S 1978 Glucose and insulin in the regulation of glucagon release from the isolated perfused dog stomach. Endocrinology 103:1579.
41. Goto Y, Note S, Berelowitz M, Frohman LA 1983 Somatostatin secretion from the isolated perfused rat pancreas or stomach. In: Mngola EN (ed) Diabetes. Excerpta Medica, Amsterdam.
42. Asplin CM, Paquette TL, Palmer JP 1981 In vivo inhibition of glucagon secretion by paracrine beta cell activity in man. J Clin Invest 68:314.
43. Stagner J, Samols E 1982 Differential glucagon and insulin release from the isolated lobes of the in vitro canine pancreas. Diabetes 31 (suppl. 2):39A.
44. Gerich J, Langlois M, Noacco C, Karam J, Forsham P 1973 Lack of glucagon response to hypoglycemia in diabetes: evidence for an intrinsic pancreatic alpha-cell defect. Science 182:171.
45. Bolli G, De Feo P, Perriello G, De Cosmo S, Compagnucci P, Santeusanio F, Brunetti P, Unger RH 1984 Mechanisms of glucagon secretion during insulin-induced hypoglycemia in man. Role of the beta cell and arterial hyperinsulinemia. J Clin Invest 73:917.
46. Hisatomi A, Maruyama H, Stake A, Vasko M, Orci L, Grodsky GM, Unger RH 1984 Mechanisms of the glucagon (IRG) response to hypoglycemia and its loss in diabetes. Diabetes 33 (suppl. 1): 79A.
47. Starke A, McGarry JD, Unger RH 1984 Evidence for direct glucose response by alpha cells and its attenuation by hyperglycemia. Diabetes 33 (suppl. 1):80A.
48. Hermansen K, Schmitz O, Orskov H 1984 Reversal of D and A cell insensitivity to glucose in alloxan diabetic dogs by treatment with the artificial beta cell (Biostator). Diabetes 33 (suppl. 1):81A.
49. Trimble ER, Gerber PPG, Renold AE 1981 Abnormalities of pancreatic somatostatin secretion corrected by in vivo insulin treatment of streptozotocin-diabetic rats. Diabetes 30:365.
50. Maruyama H, Hisatomi A, Orci L, Grodsky GM, Unger RH 1984 Insulin within islets is a physiologic glucagon release inhibitor. J Clin Invest 74:2296.
51. Samols E, Weir GC, Ramseur R, Day JA, Patel YC 1978 Modulation of pancreatic somatostatin by adrenergic and cholinergic agonism and by hyper- and hypoglycemic sulfonamides. Metabolism 27 (suppl. 1):1219.

52. Efendic S, Enzmann F, Nylen A, Uvnäs-Wallensten K, Luft R 1980 Sulphonylurea (Glibenclamide) enhances somatostatin and inhibits glucagon release induced by arginine. Acta Physiol Scand 108:231.
53. Ipp E, Dobbs RE, Unger RH 1978 Morphine and β-endorphin influence the secretion of the endocrine pancreas. Nature 276:190.
54. Weir GC, Schwarz JA, Mathe CJ 1980 Inhibition of glucagon and insulin secretion from the perfused rat pancreas by a B cell-selective somatostatin analog. Metabolism 29:68.
55. Taborsky G 1983 Evidence of a paracrine role for pancreatic somatostatin in vivo. Am J Physiol 245:E598.
56. Honey RN, Arimura A, Weir GC 1981 Somatostatin neutralization stimulates glucagon and insulin secretion from the avian pancreas. Endocrinology 109:1971.
57. Gerich J, Lovinger R, Grodsky G 1975 Inhibition by somatostatin of glucagon and insulin release from the perfused rat pancreas in response to arginine, isoproterenol and theophylline: Evidence for a preferential effect on glucagon secretion. Endocrinology 96:749.
58. Patel YC, Weir GC 1976 Increased somatostatin content of islets from streptozotocin-diabetic rats. Clin Endocrinol 5:191.
59. Patel YC, Cameron DP, Bankier A, Malaisse-Lagae F, Ravazzola M, Studer P, Orci L 1978 Changes in somatostatin concentration in pancreas and other tissues of streptozotocin diabetic rats. Endocrinology 103:917.
60. McEvoy RC, Hegre OD 1977 Morphometric quantitation of the pancreatic insulin-, glucagon-, and somatostatin-positive cell populations in normal and alloxan diabetic rats. Diabetes 26:1140.
61. Hara H, Patton G, Gerich J 1979 Increased somatostatin release from pancreases of alloxan diabetic rats perfused in vitro. Life Sci 24:625.
62. Patel YC, Wheatley T, Zingg HH 1980 Increased blood somatostatin concentration in streptozotocin diabetic rats. Life Sci 27:1563.
63. Schusdziarra V, Dobbs RE, Harris V, Unger RH 1977 Immunoreactive somatostatin levels in plasma of normal and alloxan diabetic dogs. FEBS Lett 81:69.
64. Patel YC, Wheatley T, Malaisse-Lagae F, Orci L 1980 Elevated portal and peripheral blood concentration of immunoreactive somatostatin in spontaneously diabetic (BBL) Wistar rats: suppression with insulin. Diabetes 29:757.
65. Kadowaki S, Taminato T, Chiba T, Goto Y, Nozawa M, Seino Y, Matsukura S, Fujita T 1980 Reversal of the enhanced somatostatin release from the isolated, perfused diabetic rat pancreas after the amelioration of diabetes by whole pancreas transplantation. Diabetes 29:742.

66. Pagliara AS, Stillings SN, Haymond MW, Hover BA, Matschinsky FM 1975 Insulin and glucose as modulators of the amino acid-induced glucagon release in the isolated pancreas of alloxan and streptozotocin diabetic rats. J Clin Invest 55:244.
67. Weir GC, Atkins RF, Martin DB 1976 Glucagon secretion from the perfused rat pancreas following acute and chronic streptozotocin. Metabolism 25:1519.
68. Weir GC, Knowlton SD, Atkins RF, McKennan KX, Martin DB 1976 Glucagon secretion from the perfused pancreas of streptozotocin-treated rats. Diabetes 25:275.
69. Hermansen K, Orskov H, Christensen SE 1979 Streptozotocin diabetes: A glucoreceptor dysfunction affecting D cells as well as B and A cells. Diabetologia 17:385.
70. Patel YC, Ruggere D, Malaisse-Lagae F, Orci L 1983 Alterations in somatostatin and other islet functions in the spontaneously diabetic BB Wistar rat: Biochemical and morphological characterization. Metabolism 32 (suppl. 1):28.
71. Ruggere MD, Patel YC 1984 Somatostatin, glucagon, and insulin secetion from perfused pancreas of BB rats. Am J Physiol 247: E221.
72. Boden G, Naji A, Barker CF, June V, Matschinsky FM 1983 Effect of spontaneous diabetes on hormone release in BB/Phi rats: Comparison between the isolated perfused pancreas/stomach/duodenum/spleen and the isolated perfused pancreas. Endocrinology 112:1777.
73. Bottazzo GF, Doniach D 1978 Islet-cell antibodies in diabetes mellitus. Evidence of an autoantigen common to all cells in the islets of Langerhans. Ric Clin Lab 8:29.
74. Matsushima Y, Makino H, Kanatsuka A, Osegawa M, Kumagai A, Nishimura M, Tochino Y, Makino S 1982 Pancreatic somatostatin contents in spontaneously diabetic KK and non-obese diabetic (NOD) mice. Horm Metab Res 14:292.
75. Berelowitz M, Coleman DL, Frohman LA 1980 Temporal relationship of tissue somatostatin-like immunoreactivity to metabolic changes in genetically obese and diabetic mice. Diabetes 29:717.
76. Baetens D, Stefan Y, Ravazzola M, Malaisee-Lagae F, Coleman DL, Orci L 1978 Alteration of islet cell populations in spontaneously diabetic mice. Diabetes 27:1.
77. Patel YC, Orci L, Bankier A, Cameron DP 1976 Decreased pancreatic somatostatin concentration in spontaneously diabetic mice. Endocrinology 99:1415.
78. Makino H, Matsushima Y, Kanatsuka A, Yamamoto M, Kumagai A, Nishimura M 1979 Changes in pancreatic somatostatin content in spontaneously diabetic mice, as determined by radioimmunoassay and immunohistochemical methods. Endocrinology 104:243.
79. Seino Y, Seino S, Takemura J, Tsuda K, Nishi S, Ishida H, Seno M, Usami M, Ikeda M, Imura H 1984 Changes in insulin, somatostatin, and glucagon secretion during the development of obesity in ventromedial hypothalamic-lesioned rats. Endocrinology 114:457.

80. Seino S, Seino Y, Takemura J, Tsuda K, Kuzuya H, Ishikawa K, Shimazu T, Imura H 1981 Somatostatin, insulin, and glucagon secretion from isolated perfused pancreas of obese rats. Am J Physiol 241:E146.
81. Petersson B, Elde R, Efendic S, Hökfelt T, Johansson O, Luft R, Cerasi E, Hellerstrom C 1977 Somatostatin in the pancreas, stomach and hypothalamus of the diabetic Chinese hamster. Diabetologia 13:463.
82. Trent DF, Schwalke MA, Weir GC 1984 Pancreatic and gut hormones during fasting: insulin, glucagon, somatostatin. Hormone Res 19:70.
83. Sorenson R, Grouse LH, Elde RP 1983 Cysteamine blocks somatostatin secretion without altering the course of insulin or glucagon release. A new model for the study of islet function. Diabetes 32:377.
84. Kanatsuka A, Makino H, Osegawa M, Kasanuki J, Suzuki T, Yoshida S, Horie H 1984 Is somatostatin a true local inhibitory regulator of insulin secretion? Diabetes 33:510.
85. Fujita Y, Amemiya H, Matoba K, Yajima Y, Yamamoto N 1984 Is cysteamine a specific depletor of pancreatic somatostatin? Diabetes 33(Suppl. 1):152A.

23

ROLE OF SOMATOSTATIN IN NUTRIENT REGULATION

V. SCHUSDZIARRA

Department of Internal Medicine I
University of Ulm
7900 Ulm/Donau, Steinhovelstrasse 9, Germany

INTRODUCTION

Somatostatin-immunoreactive material has been found in D cells of the stomach, small intestine and pancreas (1-6); additionally, it is present in vagal nerve fibres and in neurons of the myenteric and submucosal plexus of the intestinal tract (7-9). Within the gastro-intestinal tract and pancreas, an accumulation of D cells has been demonstrated in the fundic and antral area of the stomach and in the islets of Langerhans, whereas a more scattered distribution has been shown in the small and large intestine (10-12). This localization of somatostatin in organs which are exclusively responsible for adequate digestion, absorption and disposal of ingested nutrients raises the possibility that somatostatin might participate in the regulation of nutrient entry from the gastrointestinal tract into the circulation. Thus, somatostatin-containing D cells are in contact with nutrients at all stages of nutrient assimilation.

Such an integrative role of somatostatin is favoured by its topographical distribution. The accumulation of somatostatin-containing D cells at various levels within the gastrointestinal tract and pancreas provides the ideal morphological background for a regulatory function in digestive and absorptive, as well as metabolic, events. Locally released somatostatin could affect the cells positioned in close vicinity to the D cells in the antrum, fundus or islets of Langerhans, respectively. In addition to such a paracrine action, somatostatin could affect target cells following its secretion from nerve terminals of the autonomic nervous system. On the other hand, morphological and functional studies have provided evidence for Unger's concept of an endocrine role of somatostatin (13). Thus, D cells from the various organs could, via their contribution to the arterial plasma somatostatin levels, participate in the regulation of remote target organs.

Evidence for a potential paracrine role of somatostatin has recently been obtained by employing somatostatin analogs which are biologically active but do not crossreact with somatostatin antisera, thus permitting simultaneous measurements of somatostatin secretion (14). On the other hand, morphological findings of D cells in close proximity to the vascular system and exocytosis of secretory granules into the capillary system of the islets suggests that D cells release their secretory products not only into the interstitial space but also into the circulation (15, 16).

A role of somatostatin in the regulation of nutrient flux makes it almost mandatory to demonstrate the release of somatostatin from gastric, intestinal or pancreatic D cells in response to ingested nutrients. For an integrative function of somatostatin, arterial hormone levels should increase and such an increment should be able to elicit biological actions on exocrine, endocrine or motor functions of those organs normally involved in the processes of nutrient assimilation. Additionally, it would be reasonable to assume a regulation of somatostatin secretion not only by ingested, but also by absorbed and circulating, nutrients. This review will focus on, firstly, the release of somatostatin into the circulation during the ingestion of nutrients followed by an increase of peripheral plasma somatostatin levels; secondly, the regulatory mechanisms that participate in the modulation of postprandial somatostatin secretion such as neural and hormonal factors and circulating nutrients; thirdly, the biological action of circulating somatostatin providing evidence for its hormonal role; and fourthly, the alteration of somatostatin secretion and action in obesity.

Release of Somatostatin

Basal plasma somatostatin-like immunoreactivity (SLI) levels in the peripheral circulation are the result of its secretion from the splanchnic organs. In dogs, basal gastric and pancreatic vein SLI levels were found to be the highest followed by portal vein, arterial and inferior vena cava SLI concentrations. Similar results have been obtained in rats with regard to portal vein-arterial and arterio-venous gradients and to a certain extent in humans (17-20).

The ingestion of a mixed meal elicits a significant increase in peripheral vein plasma SLI levels as shown initially in dogs (15, 17, 18, 21, 22) and subsequently in humans (20, 23-25). This rise of peripheral plasma SLI levels is the result of an increased somatostatin secretion from the pancreas and stomach, whereas the contribution of intestinal D cells is uncertain (17, 26-28). In rats, a postprandial increase of SLI levels has been observed in the portal vein (19) but not in peripheral plasma (29). In dogs and humans, peripheral vein plasma SLI levels increased in response to all three basic nutrients - fat, carbohydrates and protein - the greatest somatostatin response was observed in response to protein or fat-rich meals (17, 25).

The augmentation of somatostatin secretion occurs during the gastric and intestinal (26, 30) but not cephalic (31) phase of a meal. Furthermore, gastrointestinal distention by the volume load of a meal has no effect on somatostatin secretion in dogs suggesting that the nutrient content is of major importance for the activation of D cells in the postprandial state (Fig. 1) (17, 32).

Another potent stimulus of gastric and pancreatic somatostatin secretion is acid. Acidification of a test meal elicits a marked increase of somatostatin release in dogs (17, 30), whereas preliminary data in humans indicate that acid may not be of similar importance (33).

In rats, acidification of the intragastric contents does not elicit increased somatostatin secretion *in vitro* from the isolated perfused stomach (34). A similar effect can be observed *in vivo* as shown in Fig. 2 indicating species differences with regard to the effect of acid on D cell function.

Modulation of postprandial somatostatin secretion

1. Neural mechanisms. Postprandial somatostatin secretion is influenced by the vagus, at least in dogs. Truncal vagotomy reduces

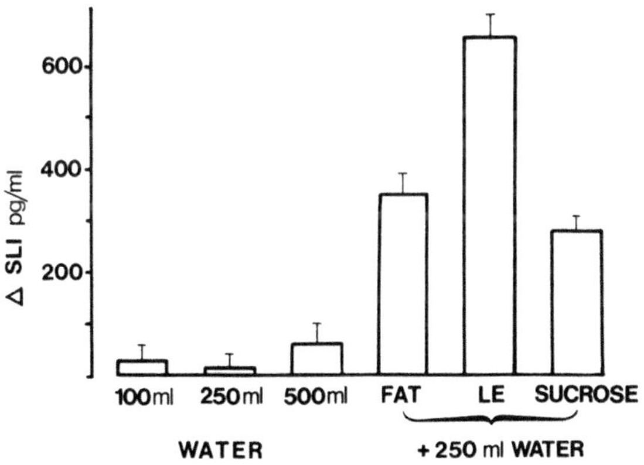

Fig. 1. Incremental peripheral vein plasma somatostatin-like immunoreactivity (SLI) in response to the intragastric instillation of 100, 250 or 500 ml water, respectively. In the same group of 8 conscious dogs 50 g fat (corn oil), liver extract (LE) or sucrose dissolved in or mixed with 250 ml water was given intragastrically (mean ± SE).

somatostatin levels during the gastric phase but elicits an increase during the intestinal phase of a meal (26, 30). Vagal stimulation, on the other hand, elicits species-dependent stimulatory or inhibitory effects, respectively. In dogs, electrical stimulation of the vagus augments somatostatin secretion, whereas in pigs and rats the same manoeuver results in an inhibition (35-41).

Cholinergic mechanisms participate in the stimulation of postprandial somatostatin release in dogs and man (30, 42, 43). The alteration of D cell function by cholinergic mechanisms is species-dependent, similar to vagal actions. Thus, the infusion of acetylcholine stimulates gastric and pancreatic D cells in dogs, whereas in pigs and rats somatostatin release is inhibited (36, 44-50). With regard to the interaction between cholinergic mechanisms and gastric D cells it should be noted that major differences can be observed with a change of the intragastric pH. In dogs, a neutral test meal activates mainly stimulatory cholinergic mechanisms, whereas acidification of the gastric contents to pH 2 demonstrates the existence of inhibitory muscarinic cholinergic mechanisms. Blockade of this cholinergic effect by atropine unmasks stimulatory non-cholinergic mechanisms which activate fundic D cells at low intragastric pH

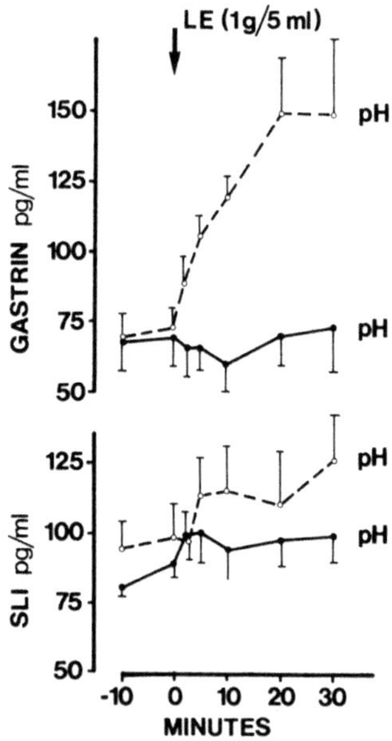

Fig. 2. Portal vein somatostatin-like immunoreactivity (SLI) and gastrin levels in response to intragastrically instilled liver extract (LE) at pH 7 (N = 6) or pH 2 (N = 6) in anesthetized rats (mean ± SE). Acidification of the test meal does not augment the SLI response as shown previously in dogs (30) but abolishes the gastrin response.

(30). In rats, acetylcholine inhibits gastric somatostatin secretion. This effect is completely abolished by an intraluminal pH 2 (34-36, 48).

Adrenergic mechanisms stimulate postprandial somatostatin release in dogs (51), whereas in humans they are probably of minor importance (43).

2. Intestinal hormones. The intraduodenal instillation of acid, a manoeuver known to provoke the release of the intestinal hormones CCK, GIP and secretin, stimulates pancreatic and gastric somatostatin release and raises arterial and peripheral vein somatostatin levels (17). The infusion of CCK-octapeptide, secretin and GIP stimulate gastric and pancreatic somatostatin release and augment peripheral vein SLI levels (52). Gastrin-17 had no effect in this study while in another study, when infused at higher doses, somatostatin release was stimulated (53). A mixture of these hormones at low doses together with a background infusion of amino acids elicited an increase of peripheral SLI levels supporting the concept that intestinal hormones participate in the regulation of postprandial somatostatin secretion. Recent studies with low doses of CCK and secretin have revealed evidence not only for stimulatory but also inhibitory interactions between gut hormones. This phenomenon will be discussed further below together with the effects of circulating nutrients.

3. Endogenous opioids. The role of endogenous opioids in postprandial somatostatin release has been studied in dogs and humans. In dogs, the addition of the opiate receptor antagonist naloxone to fat, protein or carboydrate test meals reduced the rise of postprandial somatostatin levels indicating that endogenous opioids stimulate D cell activity (32). However, this effect depends on the composition of the test meal, especially with regard to its carbohydrate content. The addition of carbohydrates, either orally or intravenously, to a fat or protein meal abolishes this inhibitory effect of naloxone and results even in stimulatory action of naloxone. This indicates that in the presence of carbohydrates, together with fat or protein, endogenous opiates have either an inhibitory or no effect on D cell function (54). The main regulatory factor seems to be the elevated level of circulating glucose. Similar results have been observed for postprandial SLI release in humans (55).

The effect of naloxone on postprandial somatostatin release is in part due to an interaction between gut hormones and endogenous opiates. As shown in Fig. 3 the stimulatory effect of a low dose infusion of CCK-4 or CCK-8 on somatostatin release is blocked by naloxone, suggesting that CCK stimulates endogenous opioids which in turn activate D cells. In addition to the regulatory function of the endogenous opioids, nutrient-derived material with opiate

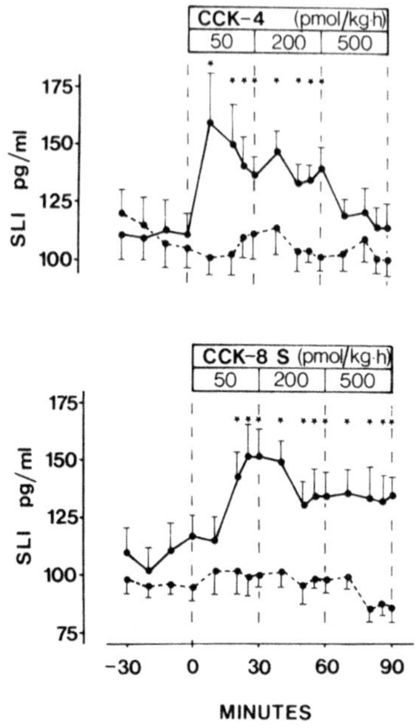

Fig. 3. Effect of intravenously infused CCK-4 (upper panel) or CCK-8S (sulfated, lower panel) upon peripheral vein plasma somatostatin-like immunoreactivity (SLI) without (solid line) or with (broken line) the opiate receptor antagonist naloxone (650 nmol/kg.h) in 6 conscious dogs (mean ± SE). * indicates significant difference of $p < 0.05$ or less between experiments with or without naloxone.

activity can modulate postprandial somatostatin secretion. β-casomorphins are peptides derived from β-casein of bovine milk and the addition of β-casomorphins or bovine milk to a protein-carbohydrate meal augments postprandial somatostatin release in dogs (56). This suggests that not only endogenous opioids but also nutrient-derived exorphins can modulate D cell function.

4. Histamine and prostaglandins. The infusion of the histamine H_2-receptor agonist impromidine stimulates, whereas the addition of the H_2-receptor blocker cimetidine reduces, postprandial somatostatin release in dogs (57, 58). Preliminary studies indicate that H_2-receptors might participate in the postprandial somatostatin response in man (33); however, further studies with adequate control of gastric acidity are necessary to support this concept.

Prostaglandins and somatostatin are present in the stomach and pancreas and both have numerous inhibitory and also some stimulatory effects upon gastric and pancreatic functions in common.

Prostaglandin infusions stimulate gastric and pancreatic somatostatin release in vitro and in vivo and the reduction of endogenous prostaglandins by indomethacin attenuates the postprandial somatostatin response (59-62). The more complex interaction between endogenous prostaglandins, somatostatin, gastrin and gastric acid secretion has been summarized recently (31) and a substantial species difference between dogs and rats has to be considered in this context (59, 63).

5. Pancreatic hormones. The islets of Langerhans contain four major endocrine cell types which are responsible for the secretion of insulin, glucagon, somatostatin and pancreatic polypeptide (64). The close proximity of these cells and the existence of tight gap junctions within the islet suggests complex interactions between these four hormones. The secretory pattern depends on the composition of the ingested foodstuff and each of the three basic nutrients elicits a typical secretory response as shown in Fig. 4. It has been reported that glucagon stimulates D cell function (65), whereas the effect of pancreatic polypeptide on somatostatin release is rather controversial (66, 67). Somatostatin itself has an inhibitory action on D cell activity (68). The major regulatory factor of the endocrine pancreas for D cell function is probably insulin. Although some authors were unable to demonstrate an effect of insulin on pancreatic somatostatin release in vitro (69-72) other studies were consistent with a somatostatin suppressing action of insulin (73-75).

In vivo, alloxan diabetic dogs have a hypersomatostatinemia which depends on the degree of insulin deficiency (21, 76) and which might be favoured by elevated levels of free fatty acids and β-hydroxybutyrate (77, 78).

In normal dogs, intravenously infused insulin elicits an inhibitory effect on postprandial gastric and pancreatic somatostatin release (79). In man, insulin infusion elicits an inhibitory effect on somatostatin release provided that the stimulatory effect of increased gastric acid secretion is excluded (80, 81).

6. Circulating nutrients. Following the digestion and absorption of a meal, nutrients increase in the circulation. In vitro studies have shown that glucose and amino acids stimulate somatostatin release from the isolated perfused canine and rat pancreas (82-86). Glucose has no effect on somatostatin release from the isolated rat stomach (unpublished observation). In vivo pancreatic, but not gastric, somatostatin release is augmented by amino acids and by a high dose of glucose (26, 76). Free fatty acids stimulate both pancreatic and gastric somatostatin release, whereas triglycerides have no effect (77, 87).

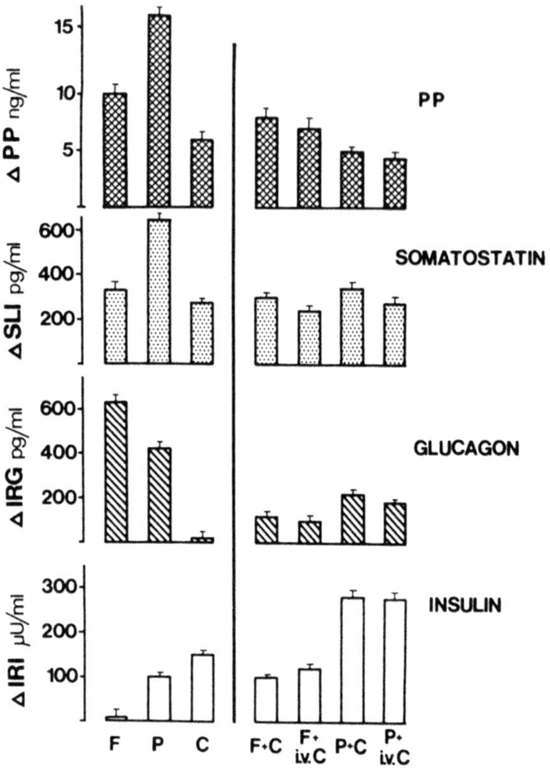

Fig. 4. Incremental levels of peripheral plasma insulin, glucagon, somatostatin and pancreatic polypeptide in eight conscious dogs following the intragastric instillation of fat (F, 50 g corn oil), protein (P, 50 g liver extract) or carbohydrate (C, 50 g sucrose) dissolved in or mixed with 250 ml water. In addition to combined fat/carbohydrate (F + C) or protein/carbohydrate (P + C) test meals carbohydrates were administered intravenously (iv C) as a glucose infusion (0.2 g/min) during fat or protein meals.

The elevation of circulating glucose levels by iv glucose during a fat meal elicits a slight but significant reduction of the somatostatin response (Fig. 4). Such an inhibitory effect of elevated glucose is even more pronounced during the ingestion of a protein meal (Fig. 4). These data suggest that the reduction of somatostatin levels after mixed carbohydrate/fat or carbohydrate/protein meals (Fig. 4) is mainly due to the absorbed and circulating glucose levels. Similarly, a physiological increase of glucose levels reduces somatostatin levels during iv prestimulation with acetylcholine and CCK indicating that the effect of glucose is not mediated by altered intestinal passage, gastric emptying or absorption of foodstuff (88).

Considering the inhibitory effect of insulin on somatostatin release, it is reasonable to assume that these effects of physiologically elevated glucose levels are mediated via the parallel augmentation of insulin secretion. It should be noted, though, that the slight reduction of the somatostatin response during the addition of carbohydrates to a fat meal is not related to the substantial increase of the insulin response when compared to fat alone (Fig. 4). During a protein meal, the decrease of somatostatin and the increase of insulin is fairly identical when carbohydrates are added. This indicates that the effect of glucose cannot entirely be explained by alterations of insulin secretion and other, as yet unknown, factors have to be considered.

The effect of intestinal hormones on D cell function is also modified by circulating nutrients. As shown in Fig. 5, the octapeptide of cholecystokinin (CCK-8) stimulates somatostatin release during a background infusion of saline. When glucose or amino acids are administered intravenously the somatostatin response to CCK is attenuated.

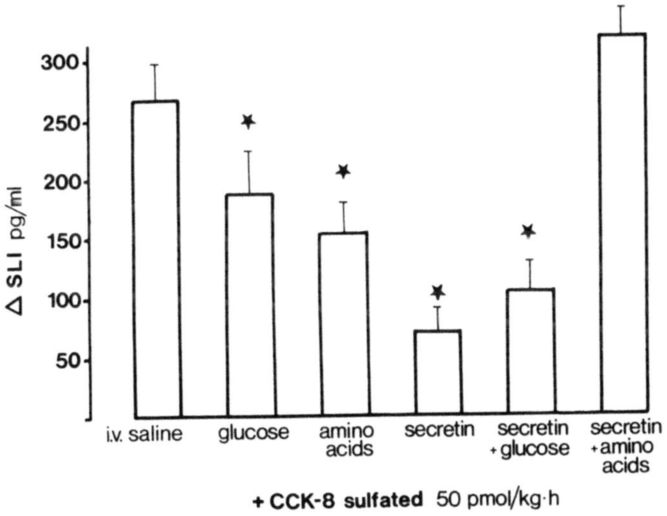

Fig. 5. Incremental peripheral vein plasma somatostatin-like immunoreactivity (SLI) in response to intravenously infused CCK-8 in a group of 6 conscious dogs. In addition to CCK-8 the dogs received an iv infusion of saline, glucose (0.2 g/min), amino acids (Aminoplasmal) or secretin (0.03 CU/kg.h), respectively. * indicates significant difference of $p < 0.05$ or less versus the saline control experiments.

The combination of CCK with secretin (0.03 CU/kg.h) virtually abolishes the increase of plasma somatostatin. The addition of glucose to these two hormones does not result in a substantial alteration of this inhibitory effect of secretin; however, the iv infusion of amino acids restores the somatostatin response to control values. These data demonstrate the existence of inhibitory interactions between intestinal hormones with regard to somatostatin release and they also indicate a modulatory role of circulating nutrients for the effect of intestinal hormones.

Physiological Effects of Somatostatin

The infusion of somatostatin at high pharmacological doses has been shown to have an inhibitory effect upon virtually all gastrointestinal and pancreatic exocrine and endocrine functions (see 89-92 for review). The infusion of synthetic somatostatin-14 at physiological rates, giving a rise of plasma somatostatin levels comparable to that observed after the ingestion of a meal, elicits inhibitory effects on several gastrointestinal functions as summarized in Table I. These data support the concept that somatostatin is a true endocrine factor (13) which acts via the circulation at least on some target organs, not excluding a local or paracrine effect on other target tissues. The existence of these two different mechanisms of action of somatostatin is supported by in vitro and in vivo studies (14, 93). Whether these are completely separate mechanisms or whether they act in an additive or potentiating manner is entirely unclear at the moment. It might be speculated, however, that the local release of somatostatin provides the necessary basic inhibitory tone so that even small increments of circulating somatostatin can reach the threshold level that is necessary to obtain the inhibitory effect at the target cell (29). Since the respective target cell is challenged with substantially different concentrations of the peptide by one or the other pathway, tight junctions might represent a possibility to separate the different somatostatin pools (93) which would also enable the "somatostatin-receptor" to maintain an adequate sensitivity.

Studies employing an antisomatostatin serum for the neutralization of endogenous circulating somatostatin demonstrate an augmentation of basal growth hormone and enteroglucagon levels and an elevation of postprandial levels of gastrin, insulin and pancreatic polypeptide but not GIP, glucagon and motilin (94, 95). Additionally, the rise of postprandial triglyceride levels is accelerated in the state of acute hyposomatostatinemia which indicates a role of somatostatin in nutrient entry from the gastrointestinal tract into the circulation (87, 95).

These data demonstrate that somatostatin inhibits some but not all gastrointestinal functions simultaneously. Apart from this selectivity, the functions that are under the influence of circulating

Table 1 . Effect of Physiological Infusion Rates of Synthetic Somatostatin-14 on Gastrointestinal and Pancreatic Exocrine and Endocrine Functions

Schusdziarra et al., 1979 (87)	2.5 ng/kg.min	Triglyceride and xylose uptake	dog
Vaysse et al., 1981 (96)	4.5 ng/kg.min	Pancreatic volume, bicarbonate and enzyme secretion	dog
Uvnas-Wallensten et al., 1981 (97)	4.0 ng/kg.min	Gastric acid secretion	dog
Aizawa et al., 1981 (98)	1.5 ng/kg.min	Delay of gastric interdigestive contractions	dog
Nakabayashi et al., 1981 (99)	2.5 ng/kg.min	Triglyceride absorption	dog
Johansson et al., 1981 (100, 101)	0.7 ng/kg.min	Gall bladder emptying Pancreatic enzyme secretion Glucose absorption Gastric emptying	man
Zyznar et al., 1981 (102)	0.5 ng/kg.min	Insulin Glucagon	man
Feurle et al., 1982 (103)	1.5 ng/kg.min 15.0 ng/kg.min	Insulin PP	dog
Schusdziarra et al., 1982 (29)	1.0 ng/kg.min 15.0 ng/kg.min	Insulin Gastrin	rat
Souquet et al., 1983 (104)	2.0 ng/kg.min	Basal insulin, glucagon	man
Colturi et al., 1983 (105)	2.0 ng/kg.min	Acid and gastrin secretion	man

somatostatin are not completely blocked. The secretory and/or motor activities are rather attenuated by somatostatin thereby preventing an exaggerated and overshooting response. An increase of somatostatin levels does not imply a decrease of all other endocrine and/or exocrine functions that are controlled by somatostatin; and an increase of somatostatin release together with an increase of other exocrine and endocrine functions is absolutely compatible with this "shock-absorber" function of somatostatin.

Somatostatin and Obesity

The effect of somatostatin on several functions within the gastrointestinal tract that are mainly concerned with the assimilation of nutrients suggests that disturbances of somatostatin release and/or function might, at least in part, be responsible for the development of a pathological state of nutrition such as obesity. It has been proposed that hyperinsulinism and obesity might be due, at least in part, to hyposomatostatinemia (13). This concept is supported by certain animal models such as obese mice (106-108). On the other hand, elevated somatostatin secretion has been demonstrated in association with hyperinsulinism and obesity in the obese Zucker rat and in the VMH-lesioned rat (109-113). Such a state of increased somatostatin release in obese rats has been observed not only *in vitro* but also *in vivo* (114).

Somatostatin content and/or secretion from the pancreas and stomach after a period of prolonged starvation has been reported to be increased or decreased (115-119) indicating that alterations of somatostatin secretion might be secondary to changes in food consumption; thus, adequate studies in pair-fed animals will have to be performed. In this context it is noteworthy that pair-feeding does not necessarily reduce hyperinsulinism in genetically obese rats (120).

The effect of infused somatostatin-14 with regard to inhibition of postprandial insulin secretion is increased in obese Zucker rats compared to their lean littermates (121). Similar effects were observed in a group of obese humans. The infusions of somatostatin-14 at doses of 0.5 and 1.0 ng/kg.min significantly inhibited basal insulin levels and postprandial insulin, gastrin and pancreatic polypeptide levels in the obese, whereas neither basal nor stimulated hormone levels were altered in a group of lean controls (122). The postprandial somatostatin response in the obese subjects was significantly attenuated compared to the lean control group. In another study, however, basal and stimulated somatostatin levels were not different between obese and lean subjects (123). These differences can be due to several factors such as liquid or solid test meals or the relative amount of fat, carbohydrate and protein in the test meals employed.

In conclusion, there is evidence that somatostatin is a true endocrine substance or hormone which has a regulatory role in nutrient homeostasis. The endocrine role of somatostatin does not necessarily exclude its potential local effects. Whether an alteration of the tissue somatostatin content or plasma somatostatin levels in obesity indicates that somatostatin plays a role as a pathogenetic factor remains to be established. The possibility that the observed changes of somatostatin are rather secondary to alterations of other functions such as hyperinsulinism should be considered, but even so, hyposomatostatinemia might facilitate the assimilation of nutrients.

REFERENCES

1. Hökfelt T, Efendic S, Hellerström C, Johansson O, Luft R, Arimura A 1975 Cellular localization of somatostatin in endocrine-like cells and neurons of the rat with special references to the A-cells of the pancreatic islets and to the hypothalamus. Acta Endocrinol 80 (Suppl 200):5.
2. Orci L, Baetens D, Dubois MP, Rufener C 1975 Evidence for the D-cell of the pancreas secreting somatostatin. Horm Metab Res 7:400.
3. Polak JM, Grimelius L, Pearse AGE, Bloom SR, Arimura A 1975 Growth hormone release inhibiting hormone in gastrointestinal and pancreatic D-cells. Lancet 1:1220.
4. Luft R, Efendic S, Hokfelt T, Johansson O, Arimura A 1974 Immunohistochemical evidence for the localization of somatostatin-like immunoreactivity in a cell population of the pancreatic islets. Med Biol 52:428.
5. Dubois MP 1975 Immunoreactive somatostatin is present in discrete cells of the endocrine pancreas. Proc Natl Acad Sci (USA) 72:1340.
6. Pelletier G, Leclerc R, Arimura A, Schally AV 1975 Immunohistochemical localization of somatostatin in the rat pancreas. J Histochem Cytochem 23:699.
7. Hökfelt T, Elfvin LG, Elde E, Schultzberg M, Goldstein M, Luft R 1977 Occurrence of somatostatin-like immunoreactivity in some peripheral sympathetic noradrenergic neurons. Proc Natl Acad Sci (USA) 74:3587.
8. Hökfelt T, Johansson O, Ljungdahl A, Lundberg JM, Schultzberg M 1980 Peptidergic neurons. Nature 284:515.
9. Uvnas-Wallensten K, Efendic S, Luft R 1978 Occurrence of somatostatin-like immunoreactivity in the vagal nerves. Acta Physiol Scand 103:907.
10. Arimura A, Sato H, Dupont A, Nishi N, Schally AV 1975 Somatostatin: Abundance of immunoreactive hormone in rat stomach and pancreas. Science 89:1007.
11. Kronheim S, Berelowitz M, Pimstone BC 1976 Radioimmunoassay for growth hormone release inhibiting hormone: method and qualitative tissue distribution. Clin Endocrinol 5:619.
12. Alumets J, Sundler F, Hakanson R 1977 Distribution, ontogeny and ultrastructure of somatostatin immunoreactive cells in the pancreas and gut. Cell Tiss Res 185:465.
13. Unger RH, Ipp E, Schusdziarra V, Orci L 1977 Hypothesis: Physiologic role of pancreatic somatostatin and the contribution of D-cell disorder to diabetes mellitus. Life Sci 20:2081.
14. Taborsky GJ Jr, GJ 1983 Evidence of a paracrine role for pancreatic somatostatin in vivo. Am J Physiol 245:E598.

15. Schusdziarra V, Ipp E, Harris V, Dobbs RE, Raskin P, Orci L, Unger RH 1978 Studies of the physiology and pathophysiology of the pancreatic D-cell. Metabolism 27 (Suppl 1):1227.
16. Grube D, Bohn R 1983 The microanatomy of human islets of Langerhans with special reference to somatostatin cells. Arch Histol Jap 46:327.
17. Schusdziarra V, Harris V, Conlon JM, Arimura A, Unger RH 1978 Pancreatic and gastric somatostatin release in response to intragastric and intraduodenal nutrients and HCl in the dog. J Clin Invest 62:509.
18. Schusdziarra V, Zyznar E, Rouiller D, Harris V, Unger RH 1980 Free somatostatin in the circulation: Amounts and molecular sizes of somatostatin-like immunoreactivity in portal, aortic and vena caval plasma of fasting and meal-stimulated dogs. Endocrinology 107:1572.
19. Berelowitz M, Kronheim S, Pimstone B, Shapiro B 1978 Somatostatin-like immunoreactivity in rat blood. J Clin Invest 61:1410.
20. Vinik AJ, Shapiro B, Glaser B, Wagner L 1981 Circulating somatostatin in primates. In: Bloom SR, Polak JM (eds) Gut Hormones. Churchill Livingstone, Edinburgh, p 371.
21. Schusdziarra V, Rouiller D, Harris V, Conlon JM, Unger RH 1978 The response of plasma somatostatin-like immunoreactivity to nutrients in normal and alloxan diabetic dogs. Endocrinology 103:2264.
22. Chayvialle JA, Myata M, Rayford PL, Thompson JC 1980 Effects of test meal, intragastric nutrients, and intraduodenal bile on plasma concentrations of immunoreactive somatostatin and vasoactive intestinal peptide in dogs. Gastroenterology 79:844.
23. Wass JAH, Penman E, Dryburgh JR, Tsiolakis D, Goldberg PL, Dawson AM, Besser GM, Rees LH 1980 Circulating somatostatin after food and glucose in man. Clin Endocrinol 12:569.
24. Vinik AJ, Levitt NS, Pimstone B, Wagner L 1981 Peripheral plasma somatostatin-like immunoreactive responses to insulin hypoglycemia and a mixed meal in healthy subjects and in non-insulin-dependent maturity-onset diabetics. J Clin Endocrinol Metab 52:330.
25. Penman E, Wass JAH, Medbak S, Morgan L, Lewis JM, Besser GM, Rees LH 1981 Response of circulating immunoreactive somatostatin to nutritional stimuli in normal subjects. Gastroenterology 81:692.
26. Schusdziarra V, Rouiller D, Pietri A, Harris V, Zyznar E, Conlon JM, Unger RH 1979 Pancreatic and gastric release of somatostatin-like immunoreactivity during the intestinal phase of meal. Am J Physiol 273:555.
27. Rouiller D, Schusdziarra V, Conlon JM, Harris V, Unger RH 1979 Release of somatostatin-like immunoreactivity from the lower gut. Gastroenterology 77:700.

28. Schusdziarra V, Dangel G, Henrichs I, Klier M, Pfeiffer EF 1982 Rate dependent stimulation of insulin and glucagon but not gastrin and somatostatin release during the intestinal phase of a meal. Horm Metab Res 14:169.
29. Schusdziarra V, Bender H, Torres A, Pfeiffer EF 1982 Dose-dependent inhibitory and non-inhibitory action of somatostatin on insulin release in rats. Regul Peptides 4:147.
30. Schusdziarra V, Rouiller D, Harris V, Unger RH 1979 Gastric and pancreatic release of somatostatin-like immunoreactivity during the gastric phase of meal. Effects of truncal vagotomy and atropine in the anesthetized dog. Diabetes 28:658.
31. Schusdziarra V 1983 Somatostatin - physiological and pathophysiological aspects. Scand J Gastroenterol 18 (Suppl 82): 69.
32. Schusdziarra V, Rewes B, Lenz N, Maier V, Pfeiffer EF 1983 Evidence for a role of endogenous opiates in postprandial somatostatin release. Regul Peptides 6:355.
33. Lucey MR, Fairclough PD, Wass JAH, Penman E, Besser GM, Rees LH 1983 Is gastric acid a factor in post-prandial plasma somatostatin release in man? Gastroenterology 84:61.
34. Schusdziarra V, Bender H, Pfeffer A, Pfeiffer EF 1984 Modulation of acetylcholine-induced secretion of gastric bombesin-like immunoreactivity by cholinergic and histamine H_2-receptors, somatostatin and intragastric pH. Regul Peptides 8:189.
35. McIntosh C, Pederson R, Muller M, Brown J 1981 Autonomic nervous control of the gastric somatostatin secretion from the perfused rat stomach. Life Sci 29:1477.
36. McIntosh C, Pederson RA, Koop H, Brown JC 1981 Gastric inhibitory polypeptide stimulated secretion of somatostatin-like immunoreactivity from the stomach, inhibition by acetylcholine or vagal stimulation. Can J Physiol Pharmacol 59:468.
37. Chiba T, Kadowaki S, Taminato T, Kodama H, Chihara K, Seino Y, Fujita T 1983 Effects of acetylcholine and vagal stimulation on somatostatin and gastrin release from isolated perfused rat stomach. Regul Peptides (Suppl 2):S2.
38. Lefebvre PJ, Luyckx AS 1980 Extrapancreatic glucagon: experimental studies using the isolated perfused dog stomach. In: Andreani D, Lefebvre PJ, Marks V (eds) Current Views on Hypoglycemia and Glucagon. Academic Press, London, p 27.
39. Uvnas-Wallensten K, Efendic S, Roovete A, Johansson C 1980 Decreased release of somatostatin into the portal vein following electrical vagal stimulation in the cat. Acta Physiol Scand 109:393.
40. Guzman S, Chayvialle JA, Banks WA, Rayford PL, Thompson JC 1979 Effect of vagal stimulation on pancreatic secretion and blood levels of gastrin, cholecystokinin, secretin, vasoactive intestinal peptide and somatostatin. Surgery 86:329.
41. Holst JJ 1982 Neural control of the pancreas. In: Bloom SR, Polak JM, Lindenlaub E (eds) Systemic Role of Regulatory Peptides. Schattauer, Stuttgart, p 171.

42. Schusdziarra V, Stapelfeldt W, Klier M, Pfeiffer EF 1981 Effect of acetylcholine upon the release of pancreatic and gastric somatostatin-like immunoreactivity treated dogs. Hepato-Gastroenterol 29:153.
43. Lucey MR, Wass JAH, Fairclough PD, Penman E, Rees LH 1983 Autonomic control of postprandial plasma somatostatin release in man. Gastroenterology 84:61.
44. Holst JJ, Jensen SL, Knuhtsen S, Nielsen OV 1983 Autonomic nervous control of pancreatic somatostatin secretion. Am J Physiol 245:E542.
45. Samols E, Weir GC, Ramseur R, Day JA, Patel YC 1978 Modulation of pancreatic somatostatin by adrenergic and cholinergic agonism and by hyper- and hypoglycemic sulfonamides. Metabolism 27 (Suppl 1): 1219.
46. Hermansen K, Christensen SE, Orskov H 1977 Characterization of somatostatin release from the pancreas. The role of calcium and acetylcholine. Diabetologia 16:261.
47. Wasada T, Dobbs RE, Harris V, Unger RH 1981 Effect of 2-deoxy-D-glucose on plasma somatostatin levels in conscious dogs. Endocrinology 108:1222.
48. Schusdziarra V, Bender H, Pfeiffer EF 1983 Release of bombesin-like immunoreactivity from the isolated perfused rat stomach. Regul Peptides 7:21.
49. Kaneto A, Kawazum S, Sato H, Kaneko T, Yanaihara C, Yanaihara N, Kosaka K 1981 Effect of the vagal and splanchnic nerve stimulation on the release of somatostatin, pancreatic polypeptide, glucagon and insulin. Biomed Res 2:166.
50. Kaneto A, Sato H, Kaneko T, Yanaihara C, Yanaihara N, Kosaka K 1981 Stimulation of somatostatin, pancreatic polypeptide, glucagon and insulin secretion by acetylcholine infused intrapancreatically in dogs. Biomed Res 2:57.
51. Schusdziarra V, Rouiller D, Harris V, Dey R, Unger RH 1980 Plasma somatostatin-like immunoreactivity in chemically sympathectomized dogs. Horm Metab Res 12:656.
52. Rouiller D, Schusdziarra V, Harris V, Unger RH 1980 Release of pancreatic and gastric somatostatin-like immunoreactivity in response to the octapeptide of cholecystokinin, secretin, gastric inhibitory polypeptide and gastrin-17 in dogs. Endocrinology 107:524.
53. Guzman S, Lonovics J, Chayvialle JA, Hejtmancik KE, Rayford PL, Thompson JC 1980 Effects of gastrin on circulating levels of somatostatin, pancreatic polypeptide and vasoactive intestinal peptide in dogs. Endocrinology 107:231.
54. Schusdziarra V, Rewes B, Lenz N, Maier V, Pfeiffer EF 1983 Carbohydrates modulate opiate receptor mediated mechanisms during postprandial endocrine function. Regul Peptides 7:243.
55. Schusdziarra V, Holland A, Maier V, Pfeiffer EF 1984 Effect of naloxone on pancreatic and gastric endocrine function in response to carbohydrate and fat-rich test meals. Peptides 5:65.

56. Schusdziarra V, Schick R, de la Fuente A, Holland A, Brantl V, Pfeiffer EF 1983 Effect of β-casomorphins on somatostatin release in dogs. Endocrinology 6:1948.
57. Schusdziarra V, Rouiller D, Harris V, Unger RH 1981 Role of histamine H_2-receptors in gastric and pancreatic release of somatostatin-like immunoreactivity during the gastric phase of a meal. Regul Peptides 2:353.
58. Schusdziarra V, Stapelfeldt W, Klier M, Maier V, Pfeiffer EF 1982 Effect of histamine H_2-receptor stimulation on post-prandial pancreatic and gastric endocrine function in dogs. Res Exp Med 181:253.
59. Schusdziarra V, Rouiller D, Jaffe BM, Harris V, Unger RH 1980 Effect of exogenous and endogenous prostaglandin E upon gastric endocrine function in dogs. Endocrinology 106:1620.
60. Saffouri B, Weir GC, Bitar KN, Makhlouf GM 1980 Gastrin and somatostatin secretion by perfused rat stomach: functional linkage of antral peptides. Am J Physiol 238:495.
61. Schusdziarra V, Rouiller D, Harris V, Wasada T, Unger RH 1981 Effect of prostaglandin E_2 upon release of pancreatic somatostatin-like immunoreactivity. Life Sci 28:2099.
62. Takemura J, Seino Y, Nishi S, Ishida H, Sakita M, Taminato T, Chiba T, Imura H 1983 Effects of prostaglandin E_2 and D_2 on gastric somatostatin and gastric secretion. Regul Peptides 6:379.
63. Schusdziarra V, Bender H, Pfeffer A, Kaminska D, Pfeiffer EF 1984 Effect of indomethacin on bombesin-like immunoreactivity, somatostatin and gastrin secretion from rat stomach, submitted for publication.
64. Pelletier G 1977 Identification of four cell types in the human endocrine pancreas by immunoelectron microscopy. Diabetes 26:749.
65. Schatz H, Kullek U 1980 Studies on the local (paracrine) actions of glucagon, somatostatin and insulin in isolated islets or rat pancreas. Febs Lett 122:207.
66. Trimble ER, Berthoud HR, Siegel EG, Jeanrenaud B, Renold AR 1981 Importance of cholinergic innervation of the pancreas for glucose tolerance in the rat. Am J Physiol 241:337.
67. Arimura A, Meyers CA, Case WL, Murphy WA, Schally AV 1979 Suppression of somatostatin levels in the hepatic portal and systemic plasma of the rat by synthetic human pancreatic polypeptide. Biochem Biophys Res Commun 89:913.
68. Ipp E, Rivier J, Dobbs RE, Brown M, Vale W, Unger RH 1979 Somatostatin analogs inhibit somatostatin release. Endocrinology 104:1270.
69. Patel YC, Weir GC 1976 Increased somatostatin content of islets from streptozotocin diabetic rats. Clin Endocrinol 5:191.
70. Kadowaki S, Taminato T, Chiba T, Nori K, Abe H, Goto Y, Seino Y, Matsukara S, Nozawa M, Fujita T 1979 Somatostatin release from isolated perfused rat pancreas. Possible role of endogenous somatostatin on insulin release. Diabetes 28:600.

71. Patel YC, Amherdt M, Orci L 1979 Somatostatin secretion from monolayer cultures of neonatal rat pancreas. Endocrinology 104:676.
72. Weir GC, Samols E, Loo S, Patel YC, Gabbay KH 1979 Somatostatin and pancreatic polypeptide secretion. Effects of glucagon, insulin and arginine. Diabetes 28:35.
73. Gerber PG, Trimble ER, Wollheim GC, Renold AE 1981 Effect of insulin on glucose and arginine-stimulated somatostatin secretion from isolated perfused rat pancreas. Endocrinology 109:279.
74. Rothman J, Ignarro LJ 1978 Effect of anti-insulin serum on pancreatic somatostatin release. Clin Res 26:775A.
75. Wass JAH, Penman E, Medbak S, Dawson AM, Tsiolakis D, Marks V, Besser GM, Rees LH 1980 Immunoreactive somatostatin changes during insulin-induced hypoglycemia and operative stress in man. Clin Endocrinol 12:269.
76. Schusdziarra V, Dobbs RE, Harris V, Unger RH 1977 Immunoreactive somatostatin levels in plasma of normal and alloxan diabetic dogs. Febs Lett 81:69.
77. Wasada T, Howard B, Dobbs R, Unger RH 1980 Evidence for a role of free fatty acids in the regulation of somatostatin secretion in normal and alloxan diabetic dogs. J Clin Invest 66:511.
78. Hermansen K 1982 Stimulatory effect of β-hydroxybutyrate on the release of somatostatin from the isolated pancreas of normal and streptozotocin-diabetic dogs. Diabetes 31:270.
79. Rouiller D, Schusdziarra V, Unger RH 1981 Insulin inhibits somatostatin-like immunoreactivity release stimulated by intragastric HCl. Diabetes 30:735.
80. Glaser B, Vinik AJ, Valtysson G, Zoghlin G 1981 Truncal vagotomy abolishes the somatostatin response to insulin-induced hypoglycemia in man. J Clin Endocrinol Metab 52:823.
81. Webb S, Levy I, Wass JAH, Lorens A, Penman E, Casamitjama R, Wu P, Gaya J, Martinez MJ, Rivera F 1983 Insulin induced somatostatin secretion in man is mediated by gastric acid. Regul Peptides (Suppl 2):S11.
82. Patton GS, Ipp E, Dobbs RE, Vale W, Orci L, Unger RH 1976 Response of pancreatic-immunoreactive somatostatin to arginine. Life Sci 19:1957.
83. Schauder P, McIntosh C, Arends G, Arnold R, Frerichs H, Creutzfeldt W 1976 Somatostatin and insulin release from isolated rat pancreatic islets stimulated by glucose. Febs Lett 68:255.
84. Schauder P, McIntosh C, Arends J, Arnold R, Frerichs H, Creutzfeldt W 1977 Somatostatin and insulin release from isolated rat pancreatic islets in responses to D-glucose, L-leucine, o-ketoisocaproic acid or D-glyceraldehyde: evidence for a regulatory role of adenosine 3'-5' cyclic monophosphate. Biochem Biophys Res Commun 75:630.

85. Schauder P, McIntosh C, Panten V, Arends J, Frerichs H, Creutzfeldt W 1977 Dynamics of somatostatin release from isolated rat pancreatic islets. Febs Lett 81:355.
86. Ipp E, Dobbs RE, Arimura A, Vale W, Harris V, Unger RH 1977 Release of immunoreactive somatostatin from the pancreas in response to glucose, amino acids, pancreozymin-cholecystokinin and tolbutamide. J Clin Invest 60:760.
87. Schusdziarra V, Harris V, Arimura A, Unger RH 1979 Evidence for a role of splanchnic somatostatin in the homeostasis of ingested nutrients. Endocrinology 104:1705.
88. Schusdziarra V, Stapelfeldt W, Klier M, Maier V, Pfeiffer EF 1981 Effect of physiological increments of blood glucose on plasma somatostatin and pancreatic polypeptide levels in dogs. Regul Peptides 2:211.
89. Schusdziarra V 1980 Somatostatin - a regulatory modulator connecting nutrient entry and metabolism. Horm Metab Res 12:563.
90. McIntosh C, Arnold R 1978 The radioimmunoassay and physiology of somatostatin in the pancreas and gastrointestinal tract. Zschr Gastroenterol 16:330.
91. Patel YC, Zingg HH, Fitzpatrick D, Srikant CB 1981 Somatostatin: some aspects of its physiology and pathophysiology. In: Bloom SR, Polak JM (eds) Gut Hormones, Churchill Livingstone, p 339.
92. Arimura A, Fishback JB 1981 Somatostatin: Regulation of secretion. Neuroendocrinology 33:246.
93. Kawai K, Ipp E, Orci L, Perrelet A, Unger RH 1982 Circulating somatostatin acts on the islets of Langerhans by way of somatostatin-poor compartment. Science 218:477.
94. Schusdziarra V, Rouiller D, Arimura A, Unger RH 1979 Anti-somatostatin serum increases levels of hormones from the pituitary and gut but not from the pancreas. Endocrinology 103:1956.
95. Schusdziarra V, Zyznar E, Rouiller D, Boden G, Brown JC, Arimura A, Unger RH 1980 Splanchnic somatostatin: A hormonal regulator of nutrient homeostasis. Science 207:530.
96. Vaysse N, Chayvialle JA, Pradayrol L, Esteve JR, Susimi C, Lapuelle J, Descos F, Ribet A 1981 Somatostatin 28: Comparison with somatostatin-14 for plasma kinetics and low-dose effects on the exocrine pancreas in dogs. Gastroenterology 81:700.
97. Uvnas-Wallensten K, Efendic S, Johansson C, Sjodin L, Cranwell PD 1981 Effect of intra-antral and intrabulbar pH on somatostatin-like immunoreactivity in peripheral venous blood of conscious dogs. The possible function of somatostatin as an inhibitory hormone of gastric acid secretion and its possible identity with bulbogastrone and antral chalone. Acta Physiol Scand 111:397.

98. Aizawa I, Itoh Z, Harris V, Unger RH 1981 Plasma somatostatin-like immunoreactivity during the interdigestive period in the dog. J Clin Invest 68:206.
99. Nakabayashi H, Sagara H, Usukura N, Yoshimitsu K, Imamura T, Seta T, Yanase E, Kawato M, Hiraiwa Y, Sakato S, Takeda R 1981 Effect of somatostatin on flow rate and triglyceride levels of thoracic duct lymph in normal and vagotomized dogs. Diabetes 30:440.
100. Johansson C, Kollberg B, Efendic S, Uvnas-Wallensten K 1981 Effects of graded doses of somatostatin on gallbladder emptying and pancreatic enzyme putput after oral glucose in man. Digestion 22:24.
101. Johansson C, Visen O, Efendic S, Uvnas-Wallensten K 1981 Effect on gastrointestinal propagation and absorption of oral glucose in man. Digestion 22:126.
102. Zyznar E, Pietri A, Harris V, Unger RH 1981 Evidence for the hormonal status of somatostatin in man. Diabetes 30:883.
103. Feurle GE, Spoleanschi P, Stander M, Klempa I 1982 Dose-response study of somatostatin meal-stimulated levels of pancreatic polypolypeptide and insulin in the dog. Digestion 23:119.
104. Souquet JC, Rambliere R, Riou JP, Beylot M, Cohen R, Mornex R, Chayvialle JA 1983 Hormonal and metabolic effects of near physiological increase of plasma immunoreactive somatostatin-14. J Clin Endocrinol Metab 56:1076.
105. Colturi TJ, Unger RH, Peters M, Feldman M 1983 Physiologic role for circulating somatostatin in gastric secretion in man. Gastroenterology 84:60.
106. Patel YC, Orci L, Bankier A, Cameron DP 1976 Decreased pancreatic somatostatin concentration in spontaneously diabetic mice. Endocrinology 99:1415.
107. Patel YC, Cameron DP, Stefan YC, Malaisse-Lagae F, Orci L 1977 Somatostatin: Widespread abnormality in tissues of spontaneously diabetic mice. Science 198:930.
108. Berelowitz M, Coleman DL, Frohman LA 1980 Temporal relationship of tissue somatostatin-like immunoreactivity to metabolic changes in genetically obese and diabetic mice. Diabetes 29:717.
109. Trimble ER, Herberg L, Renold AE 1980 Hypersecretion of pancreatic somatostatin in the obese Zucker rat. Diabetes 29:889.
110. Goto Y, Carpenter RG, Berelowitz M, Frohman LA 1980 Effect of ventromedial hypothalamic lesions on the secretion of somatostatin, insulin, and glucagon by the perfused rat pancreas. Metabolism 29:986.
111. Seino Y, Seino S, Katemura J, Tsuda K, Nishi S, Ishida H, Seno M, Usami M, Ikeda M, Imura H 1984 Changes in insulin, somatostatin, and glucagon secretion during the development of obesity in ventromedial hypothalamic-lesioned rats. Endocrinology 114:457.

112. Seino S, Seino Y, Takemura J, Tsuda K, Kuzya H, Ishikawa K, Shimazu T, Imura H 1981 Somatostatin, insulin and glucagon secretion from isolated perfused pancreas of obese rats. Am J Physiol 241:E146.
113. Seino S, Seino Y, Sakurai H, Takemura J, Kuzuya H, Imura H, Ishikawa K, Shimazu T, Usami M, Ideda M 1981 The effect of ventromedial hypothalamic nuclei destruction on somatostatin and insulin release from the isolated perfused rat pancreas. Life Sci 28:2231.
114. Sheppard MC, Shapiro B, Hudson A, Pimstone BL 1980 Tissue and serum somatostatin-like immunoreactivity in lean and obese Zucker rats. Horm Metab Res 12:236.
115. Boden G, Baile CA, McLaughlin CL, Matschinsky FM 1981 Effects of starvation and obesity on somatostatin, insulin and glucagon release from an isolated perfused organ system. Am J Physiol 241:E215.
116. Tsuda K, Seino Y, Seino S, Takemura J, Kuzuya H, Chiba T, Imura H 1981 Effect of starvation on gastric somatostatin release. Life Sci 29:27.
117. Koop H, Schwab E, Arnold R, Creutzfeld W 1982 Effect of food deprivation on rat gastric somatostatin and gastric release. Gastroenterology 82:871.
118. Voyles NR, Awoke S, Wade A, Bhathena SJ, Smith SS, Recant L 1982 Starvation increases gatrointestinal somatostatin in normal and obese Zucker rats: A possible regulatory mechanism. Horm Metab Res 14:392.
119. Tanigawa K, Kuzuya H, Seino Y, Seino S, Tsuda K, Sakurai H, Imura H 1982 Effect of starvation on somatostatin content of pancreas and gatrointestinal tract of the guinea pig. Horm Metab Res 14:245.
120. Martin RJ, Gahagan J 1977 Serum hormone levels and tissue metabolism in pair-fed lean and obese Zucker rats. Horm Metab Res 9:181.
121. Bender H, Schusdziarra V, Pfeiffer EF 1984 Increased sensitivity to somatostatin in obese Zucker rats. Clin Physiol Biochem. (in press).
122. Schusdziarra V, Lawecki J, Ditschuneit HH, Lukas B 1984 Hyposomatostatinemia and increased sensitivity to synthetic somatostatin in obesity. Acta Endocrinol 105 (Suppl 264):27.
123. Sasaki H, Nagulesparan M, Dubois A, Vesquez B, Johnson GC, Sievers ML, Unger RH 1983 Hyperinsulinemia in obesity: Lack of relation to gastric emptying of glucose solution or to plasma somatostatin levels. Metab Clin Exp 32:701.

24

REGULATION AND ACTIONS OF GASTROINTESTINAL SOMATOSTATIN

GARY L. PITTENGER, AARON I. VINIK, ANDREA A. HELDSINGER AND SUSAN SEINO

Department of Surgery and Internal Medicine
University of Michigan Medical School
Ann Arbor, Michigan 48109

Somatostatin (SS), first isolated from ovine hypothalami (1), is also present in large amounts in the gut in several species including man (2-5), providing the second largest store of tissue SS in the body. In the gut the peptide is found in neural structures in the deep submucosa and muscularis and muscularis mucosae (6), as well as in endocrine cells located in the mucosal layer and the epithelia of gut segments (7, 8). The SS containing nerve terminals are spread diffusely along the gatrointestinal tract; the endocrine cells are found concentrated in the fundus and antrum of the stomach, the pancreas, and spread diffusely throughout the rest of gastrointestinal tract (2, 6, 7). The functional correlate of this distribution has not been established. It does appear that circulating SS originates predominantly from the stomach, which may prove to be the primary source for the systemic hormonal form of the peptide (9). Percutaneous transhepatic venous sampling in humans for estimation of SS-like immunoreactivity (SS-LI) levels reveals the highest concentrations in the gastroepiploic vein and the gastrocolic trunk without a positive gradient in the splenic or mesenteric veins (10). Thus, the stomach is likely to be the major source of circulating SS and it is unlikely that the pancreas, small, or large bowel contribute in any measure.

Larsson has characterized the types of SS cell in the gut (11), and Fujita has identified a variety of peptide containing structures ranging from typical endocrine cells to neuroendocrine cells with projections resembling axons and neural structures (12). Therefore, SS may be a hormone, a neuroendocrine transducer, or a neurotransmitter within the gut. We therefore examined the distribution of SS in the different layers of the proximal, mid, and distal gut, which presumably harbor the different elements. Within the tissue layers the distribution of SS changes markedly (13, 14), progressing distally from the stomach (Table 1). In the antrum, 41% of the tissue SS is located in the mucosal epithelium, with the remainder in the submucosa and muscle layers, clearly compatible with either endocrine or neural function. Similarly, 45% of the tissue SS in the proximal small intestine is in the mucosal epithelial layer. In the distal small bowel, however, 87% of the tissue SS is found in the epithelial layer, while only a small portion of the peptide lies in the deeper layers of the gut. Here SS probably functions as a hormone or paracrine effector. In the colon this is reversed; the epithelial layer contains no detectable SS. In the colon all SS lies in the deep mucosa and muscle layer, and from this observation a neural or neuroendocrine function can be expected.

There is growing evidence that there are several SS genes, and that the prohormone may be processed differently in endocrine and neural tissues (15-17). Furthermore, it seems that the dominant form in most endocrine cells is somatostastin-28 (SS-28) and that somatostatin-14 (SS-14) is the prime candidate for a neurotransmitter function (18). For this reason, the variation in the types of SS found in relation to the level of the gastrointestinal tract was examined. SS from all layers of the antrum (epithelium, mucosa, muscle) in chromatographic studies corresponds with tetradecapeptide SS. The antrum is unique in that SS-14 is released from both endocrine and neural layers. Thus, the identification of the molecular

Table 1. Mean ± SE (and Range) SS-LI Content (pg/mg extracted protein) in the Rat Gastrointestinal Tract, n = 6

	Epithelial cells	Submucosal Scrapings	Muscle
Gastric antrum	1400 ± 400 (680-2570)	1540 ± 830 (390-4130)	510 ± 140 (210-750)
Proximal small intestine	39 ± 26 (0.07-140)	7 ± 2 (3-13)	40 ± 1 (1.6-78)
Distal small intestine	279 ± 106 (0.1-639)	5 ± 2 (0.6-11)	36 ± 8 (16-56)
Colon	1.75 (1.75)	75 ± 2 (22-148)	323 ± 70 (224-582)

(Vinik et al., Endocrinology, 1981)

species does not help to distinguish the cell of origin in the antrum. In contrast, SS extracted from the epithelial and mucosal layers of the small bowel consists principally of a high molecular weight form. In the muscle layer of the small bowel, two-thirds of the SS is the tetradecapeptide, and one-third the larger form. In the epithelial layer of the colon, what little SS there is, is the larger form.

The mucosal layer contains an approximately equal mix of tetradecapeptide and large SS, whereas the muscle layer contains principally tetradecapeptide SS. The anticipated differences in molecular species do exist, and they are not limited to single tissue layers. It must be concluded that if SS-14 is the neuro-transmitter and SS-28 the endocrine effector, then both forms of activity reside in the small and large gut.

The different molecular forms may be derived from processing of different gene products. Ensinck et al. (19) have described differential processing mechanisms for SS in the SS secreting cells. While both neural and epithelial endocrine cells contain prosomatostatin (20), the processing of the prohormone in endocrine cells is through SS-28, whereas the processing to SS-14 in neural cells follows a path which does not include this larger peptide (21). Thus the distribution of the different forms of SS in the gastrointestinal tract parallels the processing mechanisms of the cell types identified within the layers. What remains to be determined is whether this relates to gene expression or cellular mechanisms of post-translational processing and the intimate functions of the secreted products.

Regulation of the Release of Somatostatin

There are two types of gastric endocrine cells. The deeper or "closed" cells do not have any of the plasma membrane exposed to the lumen of the gastrointestinal tract. These are found in the fundus and the antrum (12). The other type, the "open" cell, does have a portion of the plasma membrane exposed to the lumen of the gut, and these cells are found exclusively in the antrum in the stomach (22). These morphologic characteristics appear to have implications for the origin of stimuli for the regulation of the release of SS from gastric tissues, and the directional flow of secreted SS.

Studies of the release of SS from the stomach have provided conflicting results. In the rat, whole stomach perfusion studies have implied that release from the stomach is almost entirely into the circulation (23). Preliminary studies with the isolated whole rat stomach model in our hands have shown release into the circulation (Fig. 1). *In vivo* studies with the cat show that large amounts of SS are released into the lumen of the stomach (24-26). In humans, significant amounts of SS are released into the lumen (27). These

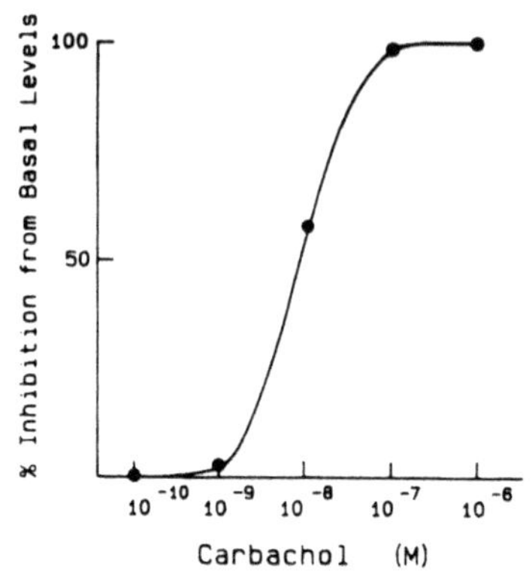

Fig. 1. In the isolated whole stomach of the rat, SS-LI is released into the circulation. Carbachol inhibits SS-LI release in a dose-dependent manner.

confusing results may reflect not only species differences in regulation of SS release, but also differences in the control mechanism of release from the antrum and from the fundus of the stomach, that cannot be distinguished by whole organ perfusion or *in vivo* techniques.

The regulation of the release of SS from the gastric antrum containing a mixed population of open and closed cells is unique. In studies of the isolated antrum, the release of SS is predominantly into the lumen (28-30). Gastric antral SS secretion is exquisitely sensitive to luminal stimuli. The most potent luminal regulator of SS release is H^+ (28, 29). As seen in Fig. 2, when the luminal pH is low, SS is released copiously into the lumen. As the luminal pH rises, SS release drops until at pH 6 and above no further effect can be seen. The gastrin response over the same pH range argues against the release of SS being due to tissue damage, as gastrin release is lowest at the same pH levels that SS release is highest (Fig. 2).

While various cations can release SS from the gut, osmolarity *per se* does not seem to be an important factor (30). Along with H^+, Ca^{2+} is an important regulator of the gastric D cell (Fig. 3). This is not unexpected, as Ca^{2+} acts as a second messenger in stimulus-secretion coupling in a number of gut endocrine systems, including gastrin (31), insulin (32), and glucagon (33). At low luminal pH, when SS release is intensely stimulated, Ca^{2+} is a potent enhancer of release. At high luminal pH, when SS secretion is low, Ca^{2+} acts as a weak primary stimulus. However, Ca^{2+} also has a unique inhibitory role in the release of SS from antral mucosa. A23187, a Ca^{2+} ionophore that increases the permeability of cell membranes to Ca^{2+}, has no effect on the release of SS. La^{3+}, which displaces membrane-

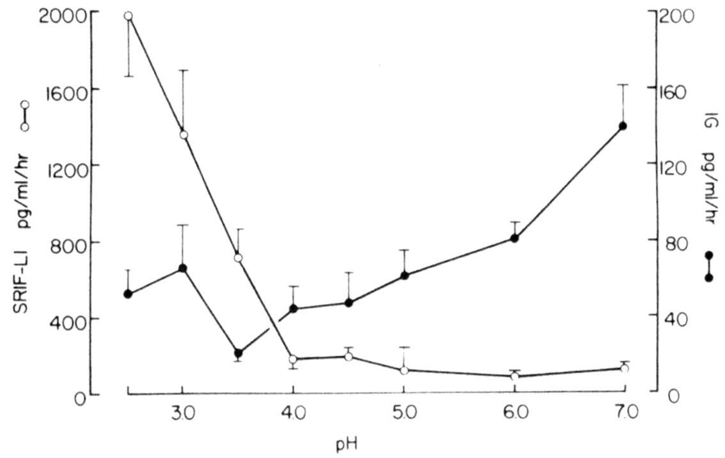

Fig. 2. The release of SS-LI (shown as SRIF-LI) and immunoreactive gastrin (IG) from isolated canine antral mucosa is pH dependent. SS-LI release is high at low luminal pH and falls rapidly as the pH increases. Gastrin release is weakly stimulated at low pH, falls as pH increases to about 3.5, and rises with further increase in pH.

bound Ca^{2+} flux, is a good stimulus for the release of SS from antral tissue (Fig. 4). The inhibitory role of Ca^{2+} in the release of SS is rapidly apparent when Ca^{2+} is completely removed by exposure to 10^{-3} M EGTA (Fig. 4). The release of SS by the gastric antrum, especially at a neutral pH, i.e., in the unstimulated condition, by depletion of Ca^{2+} is sometimes as great as that in response to the physiologic stimulus, low luminal pH. Thus, while under some conditions, Ca^{2+} does act as a second messenger to release SS through stimulus-secretion coupling, it also exerts an inhibitory influence on the release of SS from gastric mucosa. The role of Ca^{2+} in SS release is further amplified by the sensitivity of the antrum to various neurohumoral agents. Somatostatin release

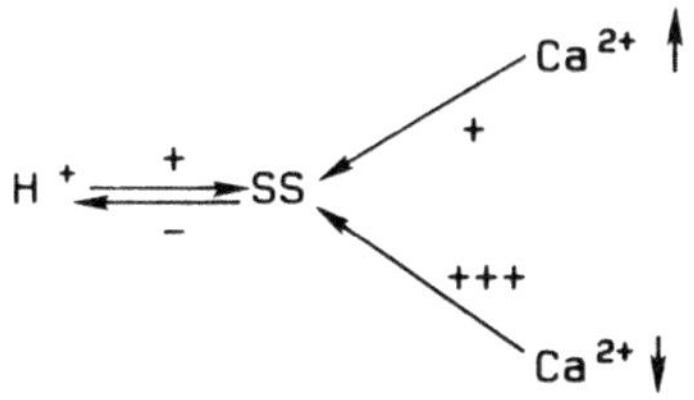

Fig. 3. The release of SS is part of an inhibitory feedback loop with acid secretion. SS is also stimulated by both high and extremely low Ca^{2+} concentrations.

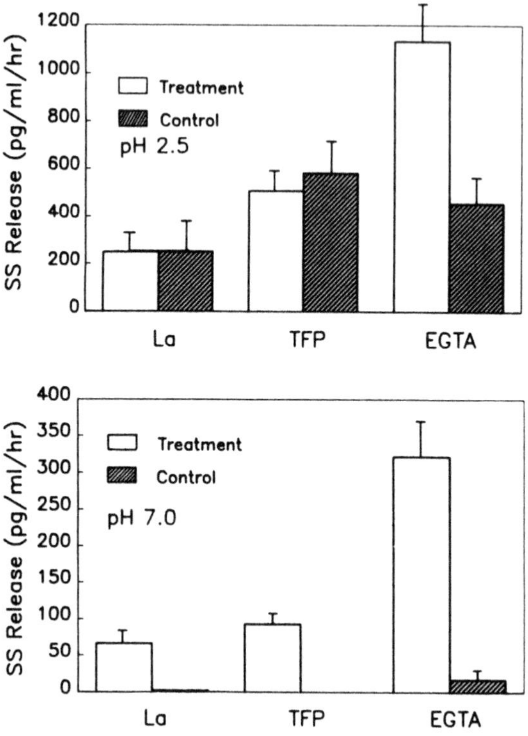

Fig. 4. The release of SS at low luminal pH is stimulated by EGTA, but not affected by La^{3+} or TFP. At high luminal pH all three antagonists of Ca^{2+} action stimulate the release of SS from isolated canine antral mucosa.

appears to be regulated by inhibitory cholinergic (34-36) (Fig. 1) and by stimulatory adrenergic neuromodulation (37-39). Since both forms of neurotransmitter action appear to be dependent upon Ca^{2+}, this further amplifies the role of Ca^{2+} in regulating SS release.

The adenylate cyclase-cAMP messenger system plays a more limited role in the release of SS from gastrointestinal tissues. Exposure of antral tissue to dibutyryl adenosine-3',5'-monophosphate (dbcAMP), a stable cyclic-AMP analog, did not stimulate SS release. Likewise, inhibition of phosphodiesterase activity with iso-butyl-methylxanthine was unable to stimulate release of SS from antral tissue. Thus the cAMP system appears to be less important for the regulation of the SS secreting cells.

In contrast, Ca^{2+}/calmodulin appears to be important in regulation of the release of SS. Inhibition of Ca^{2+}/calmodulin with the phenothiazine, trifluoperazine (TFP), which binds to and inactivates the Ca^{2+}/calmodulin complex, paradoxically stimulates SS release (Fig. 4). TFP is a markedly hydrophobic compound, however, and may also act at the plasma membrane level to inactivate the newly discovered phospholipid-dependent Ca^{2+}-sensitive protein kinase (C-kinase) (40). Whatever the mechanism, it does seem that Ca^{2+} is essential to regulation of SS secretion, and that SS may have important functions in regulating overall Ca^{2+} balance. For this reason, it became essential to examine the role of Ca^{2+} in SS action.

Somatostatin as a Regulator of Gut Function

Along with the familiar pathways of peptidergic regulation (endocrine and neuroendocrine), SS released by the gut may act by two other recently described modes. Paracrine action, first proposed in 1953 by Feyrter (41), involves release of the peptide by the endocrine cell into the intercellular space, whence the peptide acts on adjacent cells. Many of the D cells in the mucosa of the gut have dendritic-like processes extending from the cell body and terminating on or near cells unknown to be regulated by SS (10). The SS released from these cell extensions likely exerts a paracrine regulatory function on the cells adjacent to the site of release. This could provide the capacity for direct, local control or for endocrine, exocrine, and neural functions of the gut.

The other important mode of regulation of gut function by SS is from the luminal surface of the tissue, as a "lumone" (42). The effects of SS administered into the lumen of the gut include inhibition of gastric acid secretion (43), inhibition of gastrin release both into the lumen and into the circulation, and inhibition of pepsin output (44). Whatever the mode of delivery, as a neurotransmitter, endocrine or paracrine effector, or lumone, SS is an important regulator of gastrointestinal functions.

The mechanism of action of SS on these target cells is still unclear. As yet there is no conclusive evidence supporting the presence of SS receptors on any target cell type so far examined in the gut. Until such a moiety can be confirmed, it must be assumed that SS regulates gastric function by means other than receptor binding, at least to the target tissues expressing responsiveness to SS. This implies the presence of at least one mediator of SS action and one possibility, the prostaglandins, has been implicated (45). The apparent binding of SS to a phosphatase in gastric tissue (46) has not yet been duplicated in another laboratory, as far as we are aware.

In vivo, SS has been shown to inhibit gastric acid secretion, both by inhibiting gastrin secretion (47), and by a more direct action not involving gastrin (48). The mechanism of SS action has not been resolved. The cytochemical bioassay using guinea pig parietal tissue (49) is an extremely sensitive technique for examining regulation of acid secretion. Using this system, gastrin is found to be the most potent stimulus for acid secretion (50), while histamine is the most efficacious (51). Cholinergic stimuli, e.g. carbachol, are also effective in physiologic diseases (52, 53).

The mechanism of action of histamine appears to involve both an H_1 and H_2 receptor activation of adenylate cyclase (54) and an increase in cellular cAMP (52). Somatostatin does not inhibit basal acid secretion, nor the effects of small, submaximal doses of histamine. It does, however, inhibit the effects of maximally effective and supramaximal doses of histamine (Fig. 5). Although this suggests that SS may inhibit the cAMP-mediated acid secretion, SS is ineffective in mitigating the effects of dbcAMP, the stable cAMP analog. It could presumably act by decreasing cAMP generation, or alternatively, by attenuating another pathway involved in histamine action. At high doses histamine activates a Ca^{2+}/calmodulin pathway and this action can be inhibited by antagonists of calmodulin (52). It is therefore possible that the action of SS resides in the Ca^{2+}/calmodulin pathway of histamine action. That possibility is further supported by the observation that SS entirely abolishes the action of carbachol (Fig. 5), whose action is entirely dependent upon Ca^{2+} (52). These observations on the inhibitory actions of SS further amplify the role of SS as a Ca^{2+}-dependent hormone.

While examining the role of SS in the action of gastrin, somewhat surprising results were obtained. Somatostatin-14 in doses less than 10^{-6} M completely inhibited the actions of gastrin in a noncompetitive manner. Doses of SS-14 higher than 10^{-14} M proved to have intrinsic agonistic activity at the same time that the action of gastrin was abolished (55).

Since the inhibitory action of SS showed such sensitivity to Ca^{2+}, the agonist action of the peptide was examined with agents modulating Ca^{2+}. The agonistic activity of SS on parietal cells is modulated by Ca^{2+} (Fig. 6). The site of action was examined using antagonists of Ca^{2+} and Ca^{2+}/calmodulin. Removal of extracellular Ca^{2+} with EGTA and the administration of $LaCl_3$, which blocks Ca^{2+} influx and efflux, completely abolished the agonist property of SS. Inhibition of calcium-binding proteins (probably both calmodulin and C-kinase) with pimozide and trifluoperazine resulted in a significant reduction in SS stimulation of the parietal cell. Thus Ca^{2+} is important not only for the release of SS from gut tissues, but also for the action of SS on target tissues.

In contrast to agents that act to prevent Ca^{2+} mediated cellular events, receptor blockers for two known parietal cell agonists were not successful in abolishing the agonist activity of SS. Cimetidine, an H_2 receptor blocker, could only reduce the response to SS by about 40%. The cholinergic receptor blocker, atropine, was even

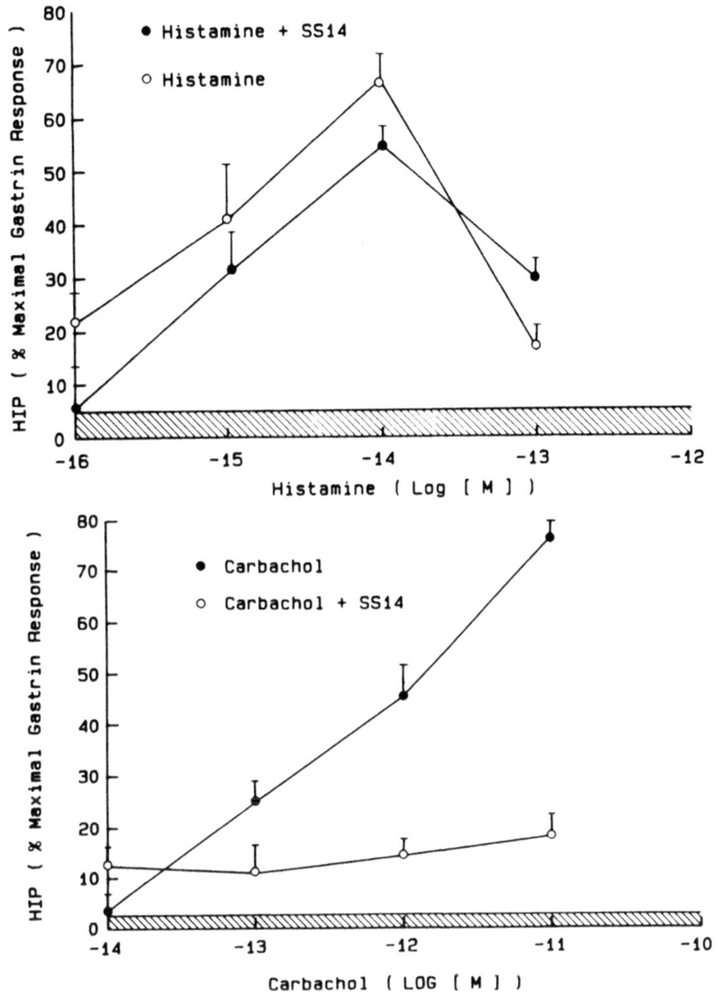

Fig. 5. In the cytochemical bioassay, SS is a partial antagonist of the stimulation of hydroxyl ion production (HIP) by histamine, but completely inhibits the stimulation of HIP by carbachol.

less effective, demonstrating no ability to reduce SS stimulation of parietal cell function. Thus, the agonistic property of SS could at best be only partially through effects on intermediate cells such as mast cell or cholinergic neurons.

Figure 7 presents the current hypothetical model for the various actions of SS on a gut target cell, the parietal cell. Somatostatin may act indirectly by stimulating the degranulation of mast

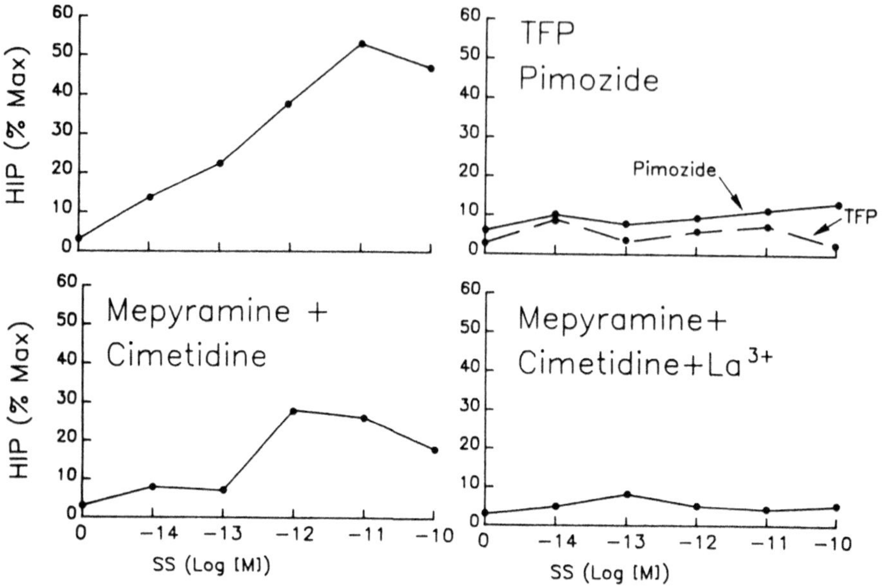

Fig. 6. TFP (10^{-4}M) and pimozide (10^{-4}M) completely inhibit the HIP dose respone to SS. Mepyramine (10^{-6}M), an H_1 receptor blocker, and cimetidine (10^{-5}M), an H_2 receptor blocker, administered together partially antagonize the HIP response to increasing doses of SS. Adding $LaCl_3$ (10^{-6} M) along with meptramine and cimetidine completely blocks the HIP stimulation by SS.

cells (56), releasing histamine, which then acts on the parietal cell as an agonist. It could simply potentiate histamine action at the target cell itself. Somatostatin may also act indirectly to inhibit the parietal cell by promoting the release of prostaglandins from the tissue (57). Alternatively, the peptide may act directly by altering the Ca^{2+} equilibrium, both inside and outside the parietal cell. The cellular mechanism may depend upon Ca^{2+}/calmodulin or other as yet unidentified kinase systems. Yet another pathway for direct activity is an alteration of the phosphatase activity within the tissue, and a number of studies examining phosphorylation of membrane proteins are being carried out in several laboratories. Thus, the regulation of gut function by SS is complex, SS being both an agonist and antagonist of gut function; both actions appear to be intimately related to the Ca^{2+} balance within the tissue.

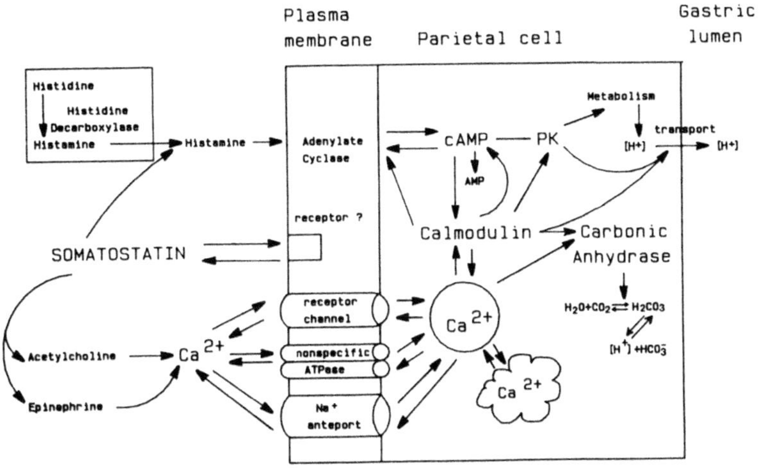

Fig. 7. Our current model of the possible mode of action of SS on the parietal cell (oxyntic cell) includes direct action through a SS receptor on the plasma membrane, an indirect action through degranulation of local mast cells releasing histamine, and several Ca^{2+}-dependent actions on the plasma membrane.

CONCLUSION

As more becomes known about the release and functions of SS in the gastrointestinal tract, the importance of Ca^{2+} equilibrium becomes more evident. The regulation of the release of SS from tissues in the gut is unique. Particularly in the stomach, SS release is exquisitely sensitive to such luminal factors as pH and Ca^{2+}. In addition, the regulatory action of SS in the gut are Ca^{2+}-dependent. Of particular note, Ca^{2+} has been shown to overcome the inhibition of insulin secretion by SS (58). Furthermore, SS has been shown to inhibit gut transport of Ca^{2+} (59). It is our speculation that gut SS may play an essential role in Ca^{2+} balance and aside from parathyroid hormone, vitamin D, and calcitonin, it may represent a major modulator of Ca^{2+} homeokinesis.

ACKNOWLEDGMENT

These studies were supported by a grant from the Kroc Foundation and National Institutes of Health grants R01-AM27077-02 and 5M01-RR00042-24 and the Michigan Diabetes Research Training Center grant 5-PGO-AM20572.

The authors would like to thank Mary Harper for her careful editorial review of the manuscript, Anita Burck and Kathy Simpson for their skillful preparation of the graphics, and Cathy Pfaus for expert preparation of the manuscript.

REFERENCES

1. Brazeau P, Vale W, Burgus R, Ling N, Butcher M, Rivier J, Guillemin R 1973 Hypothalamic peptide that inhibits the secretion of immunoreactive pituitary growth hormone. Science 179:1779.
2. Arimura A, Sato H, Dupont A, Nishi N, Schally AV 1975 Somatostatin: abundance of immunoreactive hormone in rat stomach and pancreas. Science 189:1007.
3. Kronheim S, Berelowitz M, Pimstone BL 1976 A radioimmunoassay for growth hormone release-inhibiting hormone: method and quantitative tissue distribution. Clin Endocrinol (Oxf) 5:619.
4. McIntosh C, Arnold R, Bothe E, Becker H, Kobberling J, Creutzfeldt W 1979 Gastrointestinal somatostatin: extraction and radioimmunoassay in different species. Gut 19:655.
5. Canese MG, Bussolati G 1977 Immuno-electron-cytochemical localization on the somatostatin cells in the human antral mucosa. J Histochem Cytochem 25:1111.
6. Hökfelt T, Elfrin LG, Elde R 1977 Occurrence of somatostatin immuoreactivity in some peripheral sympathetic noradrenergic neurons. Proc Natl Acad Sci (USA) 74:3587.
7. Polak JM, Grimelius L, Pearse AGE, Bloom SR 1975 Growth-hormone release inhibiting hormone in gastrointestinal and pancreatic D cells. Lancet 1:1220.
8. Alumets J, Sundler F, Häkanson R 1977 Distribution, ontogeny and ultrastructure of somatostatin immunoreactive cells in the pancreas and gut. Cell Tissue Res 185:465.
9. Vinik AI, Shapiro B, Glaser B, Wagner L 1981 Circulating somatostatin in primates. In: Bloom SR, Polak JM (eds) Gut Hormones. Churchill Livingstone, Edinburgh, p 371.
10. Glaser B, Valtysson G, Fajans SS, Vinik AI, Cho K, Thompson N 1981 Gastrointestinal/pancreatic hormone concentrations in the portal venous system of nine patients with organic hyperinsulinemia. Metabolism 39;10:1001.
11. Larson LI, Golterman H, DeMagistris L, Rehfeld JF, Schwartz TZ 1979 Somatostatin cell processes as pathways for paracrine secretion. Science 205:1393.
12. Fujita T, Kobayashi S 1977 Structure and function of gut endocrine cells. Int Rev Cytol (Suppl) 6:187.
13. Vinik AI, Gaginella TS, O'Dorisio TM 1980 Quantification and characterization of somatostatin-like immunoreactivity in isolated cells, mucosa and muscle of intestine of the rat. Gastroenterology 78:1285.
14. Vinik AI, Gaginella TS, O'Dorisio TM, Shapiro B, Wagner L 1981 The distribution and characterization of somatostatin-like immunoreactivity in epithelial cells, submucosa, and muscle of the rat stomach and intestine. Endocrinology 109:1921.
15. Warren TG, Shields D 1982 Cell-free biosynthesis of somatostatin precursors: evidence for multiple forms of preprosomatostatin. Proc Natl Acad Sci (USA) 79:3729.

16. Gomez S, Morel A, Nicolas P, Cohen P 1983 Regional distribution of the Mr 15,000 somatostatin precursor, somatostatin-28 and somatostatin-14 in the rat brain suggests a differential intracellular processing of the high molecular weight species. Biochem Biophys Res Commun 112:297.
17. Noe BD, Spiess J 1983 Evidence for biosynthesis and differential post-translational proteolytic processing of different (pre)prosomatostatins in pancreatic islets. J Biol Chem 258:1121.
18. Patel YC, Wheatley T, Ning C 1981 Multiple forms of immunoreactive somatostatin: comparison of distribution in neural and non-neural tissues and portal plasma of the rat. Endocrinology 109:1943.
19. Baskin DG, Ensinck JW 1983 Immunocytochemical evidence that somatostatin-28 is a terminal peptide in rat intestinal mucosa. Diabetes 32 (Suppl 1):167 (Abstract).
20. Lauber ML, Camier M, Cohen P 1979 Higher molecular weight forms of immunoreactive somatostatin in mouse hypothalamic extracts: evidence of processing in vitro. Proc Natl Acad Sci (USA) 76:6004.
21. Patel YC 1983 A high molecular weight form of somatostatin-28 (1-12)-like immunoreactive substance without somatostatin-14 immunoreactivity in the pancreas, Evidence that somatostatin-14 synthesis can occur independently of somatostatin-28. J Clin Invest 72:2137.
22. Larsson LI 1980 Peptide secretory pathways in the GI tract: cytochemical contributions to regulatory physiology of the gut. Am J Physiol 239:G237.
23. Saffouri B, Weir GC, Bitar KN, Makhlouf GM 1980 Gastrin and somatostatin secretion by perfused rat stomach: functional linkage of antral peptides. Am J Physiol (Gastrointest Liver Physiol) 1:G495.
24. Uvnas Wallensten K, Efendic S, Johannson C, Sjodin L, Cranwell P 1980 Effect of intraluminal pH on the release of somatostatin and gastrin into antral, bulbar, and ileal pouches of conscious dogs. Acta Physiol Scand 110:391.
25. Alino SF, Garcia D, Uvnas-Mosberg K 1982 Evidence of a cholinergic, pH dependent, vagally mediated release of antral somatostatin. Acta Physiol Scand 515 (Suppl):21.
26. Aino SF, Garcia D, Uvnas-Mosberg K 1983 On the interaction between intragastric pH and electrical vagal stimulation in causing gastric acid secretion and intraluminal release of gastrin and somatostatin in anesthetized rats. Acta Physiol Scand 117:491.
27. Wisen O, Uvnas-Wallensten K, Efendic S, Johansson C 1980 Release of gastrin and somatostatin into the gastric lumen of healthy subjects and patients with duodenal ulcer and achlorhydria. Acta Physiol Scand 108:297.

28. Fink AS, Hedenbro JL, Vinik AI, Unger RH, Fiddian-Green RG 1980 A reciprocal relationship between the release of immunoreactive gastrin and somatostatin-like immunoreactivity from canine antral mucosa in vitro. Curr Surg 37:63.
29. Vinik AI, Pittenger G, Wagner L, Fiddian-Green RG 1981 Factors regulating the release of immunoreactive somatostatin from isolated canine antral mucosa. In: Millar RP (ed) Neuropeptides, Biochemical and Physiological Studies. Churchill Livingston, Edinburgh, p 315.
30. Pittenger G, Vinik AI, Fiddian-Green RG, Wagner L 1984 A dual role of calcium in release of somatostatin from canine gastric antral mucosa. Am J Physiol 246 (Endocrinol Metab 9):E361.
31. Fiddian-Green RG, Pittenger G, Kothary P, Vinik AI 1983 Role of calcium in the stimulus-secretion coupling of antral gastrin release. Endocrinology 112:753.
32. Grodsky GM, Bennett LL 1966 Cation requirements for insulin secretion in the isolated perfused pancreas. Diabetes 15:910.
33. Gerich JE, Frankel BJ, Fanska R, West L, Forsham PH, Grodsky GM 1974 Calcium dependency of glucagon secretion from the in vitro perfused rat pancreas. Endocrinology 94:1381.
34. McIntosh C, Pederson R, Muller M, Brown J 1981 Autonomic nervous control of the gastric somatostatin secretion from the perfused rat stomach. Life Sci 29:1477.
35. Chiba T, Kadowaki S, Taminato T, Kodama H, Chihara K, Seino Y, Fujita T 1983 Effects of acetylcholine and vagal stimulation of somatostatin and gastrin release from isolated perfused rat stomach. Regul Peptides (Suppl 2):S2.
36. Uvnas-Wallensten K, Efendic S, Roovete A, Johannson C 1980 Decreased release of somatostatin into the portal vein following electrical vagal stimulation in the cat. Acta Physiol Scand 109:393.
37. Koop H, Behrens I, McIntosh CHS, Pederson RA, Arnold R, Creutzfeldt W 1980 Adrenergic modulation of gastric somatostatin release in rats. FEBS Lett 118:248.
38. Goto Y, Berelowitz M, Frohman LA 1981 Effect of catecholamines on somatostatin secretion by isolated perfused rat stomach. Am J Physiol 240:E274.
39. Koop H, Behrens I, Bothe E, Koschwitz, McIntosh CHS, Pederson RA, Arnold R, Creutzfeldt W 1983 Adrenergic control of rat gastric somatostatin and gastrin release. Scand J Gastroenterol 18:65.
40. Takai Y, Kishimoto A, Inoue M, Nishizuka Y 1977 Studies on a cyclic nucleotide-independent protein kinase and its proenzyme in mammalian tissues, I. Purification and characterization of an active enzyme from bovine cerebellum. J Biol Chem 252:7603.
41. Feyrter F 1983 Uber die peripheren endocrinen (parakrinen), Drusen des Menschen Vienna/Dusseldorf, Verlag, Mandinch, p 27.
42. Vinik AI 1978 Regulation of gastrin release from oriented sheets of human antral mucosa in vitro. In Bloom SR (ed) Gut Hormones. Churchill Livingstone, Edinburgh, p 156.

43. Fiddian-Green RG, Pittenger G, Kothary P, Vinik AI 1980 Effect of luminal somatostatin on acid secretion and gastrin release. Scand J Gastroenterol 15:305.
44. Gomez-Pan A, Reed JD, Albinus M, Shaw B, Hall R, Besser GM, Coy DH, Kastin AJ, Schally AV 1975 Direct inhibition of gastric acid and pepsin secretion by growth-hormone release-inhibiting hormone in cats. Lancet 1:888.
45. Takemura J, Seino Y, Nishi S, Ishida H, Sakita M, Taminato T, Chiba T, Imura H 1983 Effects of prostaglandin E2 and D2 on gastric somatostatin and gastrin secretion. Regul Peptides 6:379.
46. Reyl F, Lewin MJM 1981 Somatostatin is a potent activator of phosphoprotein phosphatase in the digestive tract. Biochem Biophys Acta 675:297.
47. LeRoith D, Vinik AI, Epstein S, Baron P, Olkenitzky MN, Pimstone BL 1985 Somatostatin and serum gastrin in normal subjects and in patients with pernicious anemia, chronic liver disease and renal disease. S Afr Med J 49:1601.
48. Barros D'Sa AA, Bloom SR, Baron JH 1975 Direct inhibition of gastric acid secretion by growth-hormone release-inhibiting hormone in dogs. Lancet 1:886.
49. Hansson HPJ 1967 Histochemical demonstration of carbonic anhydrase. Hitochemie 11:112.
50. Heldsinger AA, Vinik AI 1984 Action of gastrin in guinea pig oxyntic cells. Studies using quantification cytochemistry. J Clin Invest 74:124.
51. Klaff LJ, Vinik AI, Heldsinger AA 1981 Comparison of potency of acid secretagogues in the activation of carbonic anhydrase (CA) in guinea pig parietal cells. In: Millar RP (ed) Neuropeptides, Biochemical and Physiologic Studies. Churchill Livingstone, Edinburgh, 35:336.
52. Walker W, Vinik AI, Heldsinger AA, Kaveh R 1983 The role of calcium and calmodulin in activation of the oxyntic cell by histamine and carbamylcholine in the guinea pig. J Clin Invest 72:955.
53. Vinik AI, Heldsinger AA 1984 Cytochemical quantification of physiologic regulation of oxyntic cell carbonic anhydrase. Ann NY Acad Sci 429:592.
54. Vinik AI, Heldsinger A, Skoglund ML 1983 Evidence for histamine H_1 and H_2 receptors in guinea pig oxyntic cells. J Pharmacol Exp Ther 22:115.
55. Vinik AI, Shapiro B, Pienta K, Heldsinger A 1981 Somatostatin is an agonist and noncompetitive antagonist of gastrin in oxyntic cell function. Endocrinology 109:1117.
56. Theoharides T, Douglas WW 1978 Somatostatin induces histamine secretion from rat peritoneal mast cells. Endocrinology 102:1637.

57. Lingunsky M, Goto Y, Debas H, Yamada T 1983 Prostaglandins mediate inhibition of gastric acid by somatostatin in the rat. Science 219:301.
58. Curry DL, Bennett LL 1974 Reversal of somatostatin inhibition of insulin secretion by calcium. Biochem Biophys Res Commun 60:1015.
59. Scholz D, Schwille P 1978 Somatostatin and intestinal calcium absorption in man. Metabolism 27 (Suppl 1):1349.

25

INTESTINAL SOMATOSTATIN FUNCTION

KIERTISIN DHARMSATHAPHORN

Department of Medicine
University of California
San Diego Medical Center
San Diego, California 92103

ABSTRACT

Somatostatin is present throughout the intestine, both in D cells at the luminal surface and in neural elements. It inhibits the release or action of many gut hormones known to regulate gastrointestinal function and undoubtedly has a wide range of actions. In the intestine, available information indicates that somatostatin may have an important regulatory role for water and electrolyte absorption and secretion. The peptide affects both the epithelial transport function and the intestinal motility function. The outcome associated with administration of somatostatin is inhibition of water and electrolyte secretion. Somatostatin has been shown to effectively reduce stool output in diarrheal syndromes associated with endocrine tumor and other conditions. Clinical application of somatostatin in diarrhea still awaits development of an orally active and/or gut-specific analog. Some preliminary results indicate that this may be possible in the future.

INTRODUCTION

Somatostatin, a 14 amino acid peptide (S-14 or SRIF) with growth hormone release inhibition properties, was initially isolated from sheep hypothalami (1). Later, the peptide was isolated or detected in hypothalamic tissues and other organs of all mammalian species, as well as in other lower animals; different molecular forms of somatostatin have been recognized. In man, somatostatin is widely distributed. Somatostatin-like immunoreactivity is abundant in the central nervous system, the peripheral nervous system, and the gastrointestinal tract. In the gastrointestinal tract, somatostatin affects many functions of the digestive system. Its effects on gastric function have been summarized by Dr. Vinik in Chapter 24. In this chapter, which summarizes intestinal functions, emphasis will be given to the effect of somatostatin on intestinal water and electrolyte absorption. The effect of somatostatin on gut motility will be discussed only briefly since knowledge concerning normal gut motility mechanisms and its regulation still remains to be elucidated. Undoubtedly, in the future when the motility mechanism is better understood, discussion of absorption and secretion will have to take into account this important aspect, which is considered to be an integral contribution of gut water and electrolyte balance mechanisms.

Localization of Somatostatin in the Intestine

Somatostatin-containing cells, the D cells, are widely distributed in the gastrointestinal mucosa, with the highest number found in the upper intestine. These cells are located in the region of the crypt of Lieberkuhn and have microvilli in contact with gut lumen (2-4). Beneath the epithelial cells of the intestine, somatostatin has been detected and found to be widely distributed in the neural structure, e.g. the submucosal plexus, myenteric plexus, and vagus nerve (3-6). In the lamina propria, an area immediately beneath the epithelial cells, there is a rich supply of somatostatin (3). The localization of somatostatin-like immunoreactivity suggests that somatostatin may be released locally in the intestine to serve certain paracrine or neurocrine functions in addition to a classical endocrine function.

Intestinal Somatostatin Function

Somatostatin undoubtedly has a wide spectrum of functions in the gut. This can be judged from the fact that it inhibits the release and/or function of a wide variety of peptide hormones and neurotransmitters which are released in the intestine in response to food or other stimuli. Examples include gastrin, secretin, cholecystokinin, vasoactive intestinal polypeptide, gastric inhibitory polypeptide, motilin, pancreatic polypeptide, and enteroglucagon (7-12). In the crypt region of the gut wall, which secretes these peptides, somatostatin is in a position to come in contact with other endocrine cells (13). Furthermore, the finding that somatostatin-like immunoreactivity in portal blood is higher than in peripheral venous circulation, and its response to stimuli, also suggest possible systemic endocrine functions of somatostatin related to the gastrointestinal tract (14-16). Although somatostatin is likely to have a wide range of paracrine or neurocrine functions in regulating or modulating the action of these hormones, its specific physiological role still remains to be defined. The physiological studies of somatostatin related to the small intestine emphasize two aspects: 1) antimotility functions and 2) antisecretory functions. The results of studies designed to determine the effects of somatostatin on calcium and nutrient absorption are not conclusive and are difficult to evaluate; therefore, they will not be discussed here.

Intestinal Motility

Regarding antimotility funtions, somatostatin clearly delays gastrointestinal transit as judged by x-ray studies (17-18). The mechanisms by which somatostatin delays gastrointestinal transit have not been defined. This is mainly because gastrointestinal transit and its regulatory mechanisms are relatively complex and lack simple model systems which will conveniently allow characterization of the mechanisms. It is also likely that the mechanism of action of somatostatin related to smooth muscle functions may be a complex one and is a reflection of the inhibitory action of somatostatin on many other hormonal functions. A study using isolated myenteric plexus/longitudinal muscle of the guinea pig ileum provided interesting findings which suggest that somatostatin inhibits the release of acetylcholine (19, 20). Besides acetylcholine, a number of other hormones mentioned above, including cholecystokinin and motilin, are likely to have important regulatory roles in gut motility function. The antimotility mechanism of somatostatin may be defined when the physiological basis of gut motility related to gastrointestinal transit is better delineated (21, 22).

Intestinal Water and Electrolyte Transport

The remaining discussion will deal with the antisecretory function of somatostatin which, in contrast to the antimotility function, can be studied in a simple isolated gut model system. The antisecretory function of somatostatin has been observed in the small and large intestine of a variety of animal models, including man. In the rat small intestine, somatostatin inhibits PGE_1- and theophylline-induced water and electrolyte secretion, while having little or no effect by itself on the basal state (23) (Fig. 1). Similar effects have been observed in the rat colon (24, 25). Both PGE_1 and theophylline cause secretion by increasing cellular cAMP. This increase in cAMP level was not inhibited by somatostatin while intestinal secretion stimulated by cAMP was inhibited (Fig. 2). Our studies suggest that somatostatin blocks an intermediate step in the secretory processes beyond the step of cAMP production. The same antisecretory effect is observed in the rabbit and dog intestine (26-28). In man, somatostatin was also found to inhibit water secretion, particularly that caused by the overproduction of peptide hormones or neurotransmitters, while at the basal state it had little or no significant effect (29-32). The effectiveness of somatostatin has been demonstrated in patients suffering from severe watery diarrhea due to carcinoid syndrome (29, 30) (Fig. 3) and VIPoma (31). A patient with severe diarrhea associated with colonic pseudoobstruction, and some patients with Crohn's disease and short

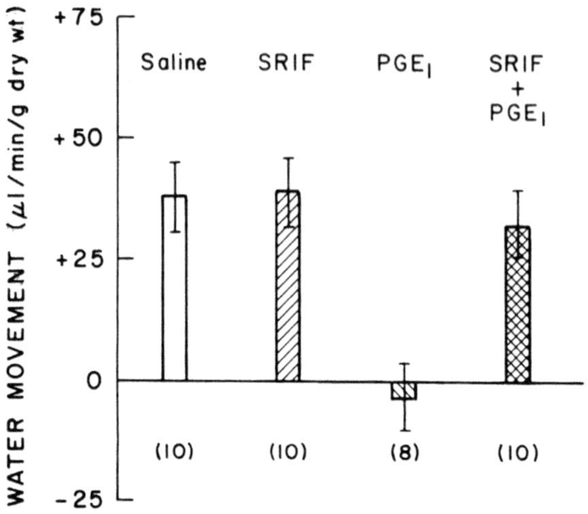

Fig. 1. The effect of somatostatin-14 (SRIF) on prostaglandin E_1-induced net water absorption in the rat jejunum. Water absorption was determined over 45-min intervals, utilizing jejunal perfusion. Basal absorption was determined before somatostatin (10 µg/kg/min) or prostaglandin (5 µg/kg/min) infusions. PGE_1 abolished net water absorption and caused a small net secretion. Pretreatment with somatostatin (SRIF + PGE_1) inhibited the response to PGE_1. (Adapted from Gastroenterology 78:1554, 1980).

bowel syndrome also responded well to somatostatin (33, 34). The fact that somatostatin appears to inhibit the hypersecretory state, while it has little or no effect by itself, suggests that somatostatin has antisecretory properties, i.e. it inhibits or interferes with the secretory process once it has been turned on, rather than stimulating an absorptive process, which is independent and unrelated to the secretory mechanism.

In our recent study utilizing a human colonic epithelial cell line, we have also observed the antisecretory effect of somatostatin (35) (Fig. 4). Somatostatin partially reversed VIP-, PGE_1-, and A23187-induced short circuit current, which in our system correlates with chloride secretion (36, 37). The mechanisms by which somatostatin reverses or inhibits the secretory process in the intestine have yet to be determined. The fact that somatostatin affects both cAMP- and Ca^{++}-mediated secretion without altering the cAMP level suggets that somatostatin is blocking an intermediate step in the secretory process common to both cAMP- and CA^{++}-mediated secretion. This may well be at the very distal step in the secretory process, i.e. at the level of electrolyte transport pathways. The chloride secretory pathways have been shown to be intimately

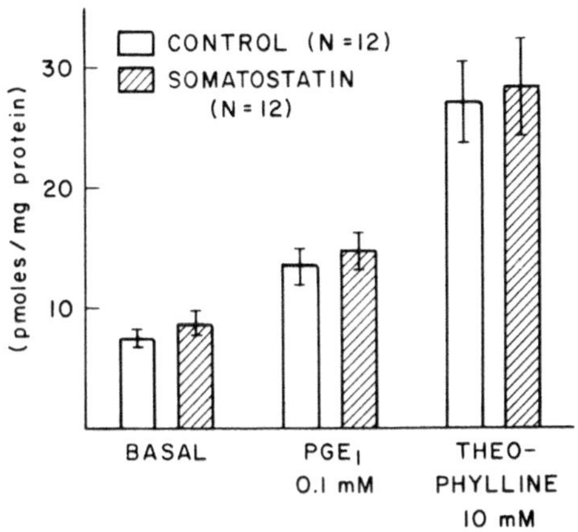

Fig. 2. The effect of somatostatin on mucosal cyclic AMP content in rat jejunal mucosa. Somatostatin has no effect on PGE_1 and theophylline-induced increases in mucosal cAMP levels. (Adapted from Gastroenterology 78:1554, 1980.)

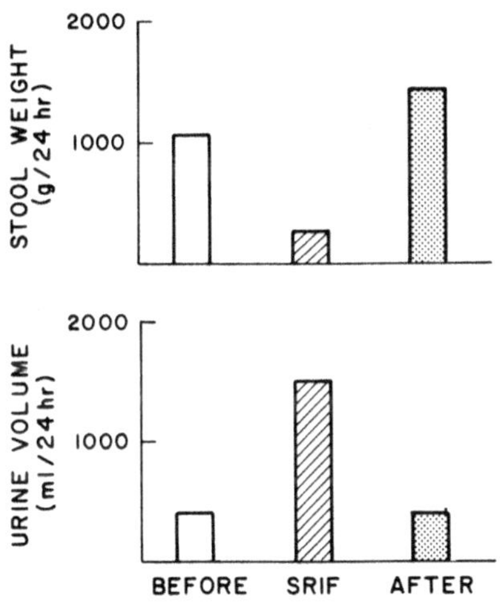

Fig. 3. The effect of somatostatin-14 (SRIF) infusion (4 μg/min) on fecal and urinary excretion in a patient with the carcinoid syndrome and diarrhea. Stool weight decreased significantly on the day that somatostatin was infused and diarrhea recurred with discontinuation of somatostatin infusion. Daily urine volume reflected stool output. (Adapted from Ann Intern Med 92:68, 1980.)

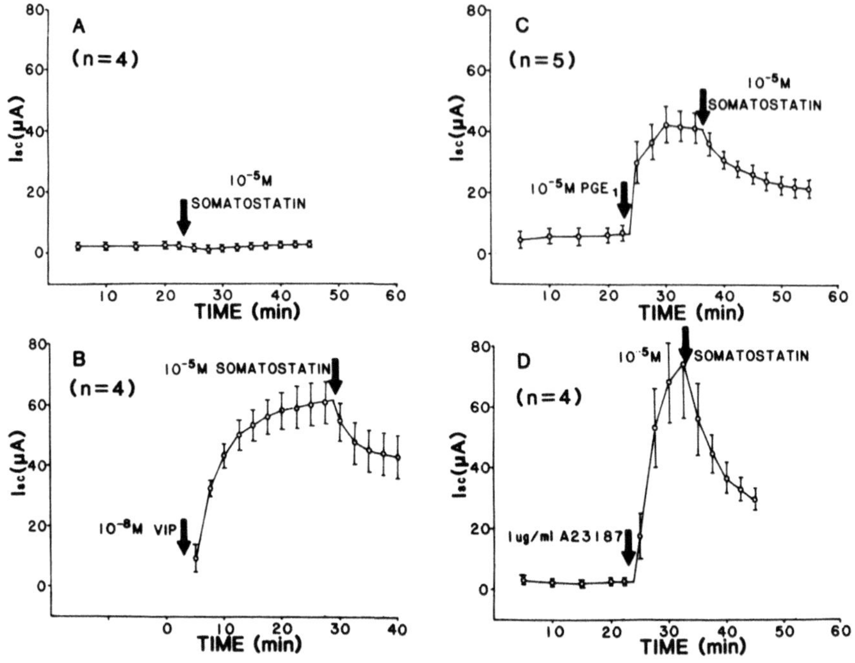

Fig. 4. The effect of somatostatin on short circuit current (Isc). Somatostatin had little or no effect by itself. Somatostatin partially reversed the Isc (which reflects net Cl^- secretion) induced by VIP, PGE_1, and A23187. (Adapted from Am J Physiol 246:G204, 1984).

involved in the secretory process, and somatostatin may well interfere with the regulation of one of the chloride secretory pathways. Whether this regulation of gut epithelial cells occurs at the protein kinase level, cytosolic calcium level, or another level is not known at this time. Cultured epithelial cell lines may serve as a useful model system for the study of the mechanism of action of somatostatin in the intestine.

Clinical Applications of Somatostatin in Digestive Diseases

The fact that somatostatin has been shown to be quite effective in controlling diarrhea in patients with endocrine tumors and in certain hypersecretory states suggests the potential use of somatostatin as an antidiarrheal agent. However, the use of somatostatin in clinical medicine is limited by two major drawbacks. One is the need for continuous intravenous infusion or intramuscular injection. Another major consideration is the wide range of side effects due to the fact that somatostatin can affect many other organ systems. The elevation of blood sugar levels and associated steatorrhea are potentially troublesome (29, 34).

Regarding the route of administration, synthesis of somatostatin analogs, which are smaller and more stable, may allow the drug to be administered orally and make the medication practical. The intestine can absorb a small amount of peptide hormones intact, although little is known about polypeptide absorption and the structural requirement that may facilitate it. Ongoing clinical trials of oral peptides, e.g. enkephalin analog, may provide new information and a future basis for oral application of the peptide with antisecretory properties. Cyclic hexapeptide analogs of somatostatin have been administered orally in animals with encouraging results (38).

Regarding the systemic side effects, it may be possible to eliminate many of the adverse effects, provided that gut receptors for somatostatin are different from other receptors. In this case, gut specific somatostatin analogs may have little or no systemic action. The findings that structural requirements for somatostatin's action in various organ systems may be different suggest the possibility of developing a gut selective analog (39-44). In collaboration with Dr. Jean Rivier, Dr. Wylie Vale, and Dr. Marvin Brown, we have tested a series of somatostatin analogs for intestinal action (45). In this study, each amino acid in the somatostatin molecule was systematically substituted, deleted, or altered. The potency of each analog was determined by measuring ion transport in the rabbit ileum and rat colon using the modified Ussing chamber technique. Results were then compared to the non-enteric effect of somatostatin, including inhibition of the stimulated release of growth hormone from cultured rat anterior pituitary cells and inhibition of arginine stimulated insulin and glucagon release in the rat *in vivo* (see Table 1). We found that substitution with L-alanine, or deletion of amino acids at Phe^{6}, Phe^{7}, Trp^{8}, and Lys^{9} of the somatostatin molecule, or deletion of Thr^{10}, reduced the ion transport properties as well as the inhibition of growth hormone, insulin, and glucagon release to near zero. This indicates that Phe^{6} Phe^{7}, Trp^{8}, and Lys^{9} are necessary for somatostatin receptor binding, while Thr^{10} serves as an essential spacer. More importantly, we have observed that substitution or deletion of Phe^{11} and substitution with alanine or D-isomer at Lys^{4} resulted in compounds with intestinal ion transport properties, which demonstrated little or no inhibition of insulin or glucagon release. Therefore, Phe^{11} and Lys^{4} do not appear to be critical for biologic activities in the rabbit ileum and rat colon, as they are for some other endocrine effects. Alteration of either one of these amino acids may result in a gut-specific analog in the rat and rabbit. Whether the results can be extended to man still remains to be tested. These results suggest that somatostatin receptor subtypes in the gut may be different from others and that it may be possible to design a gut-

Table 1. Relative Potency of Somatostatin Analog

Analog	Release inhibition of:			Ion transport	
	Growth hormone	Insulin	Glucagon	Rat colon	Rabbit ileum
Somatostatin (S-14)	100	100	100	100	100
[D-Lys^4] -S-14	22	1	1	100	139
[Ala^4] -S-14	60	12	12	---	94
[Ala^{11}]-S-14	3	<10	<10	27	52
des-Phe^{11} -S-14	2	< 1	< 1	9	34

Ion transport potencies were obtained from the rat colon and rabbit ileum *in vitro* utilizing the Ussing chamber technique. Inhibition of the stimulated release of growth hormone was obtained from cultured rat anterior ptiuitary cells *in vitro* and inhibition of arginine-stimulated insulin and glucagon release from the rat *in vivo*. (Adapted from J Clin Invest 71:840, 1983.)

specific analog of somatostatin which has antisecretory functions, while having fewer side effects. Hopefully, further development of somatostatin analogs and future clinical trials may make the clinical use of somatostatin a realistic objective.

ACKNOWLEDGMENT

This study was supported by grant AM 28305 from the National Institutes of Health. Dr. K. Dharmsathaphorn is the recipient of an NIH Research Career Development Award AM 1146 and an American Gastrooenterological Association/Glaxo Research Scholar Award. We would like to thank Ms. Vicky Huebner who typed and edited the manuscript.

REFERENCES

1. Brazeau P, Vale W, Burgus R, Ling N, Butcher M, Rivier J, Guillemin R 1973 Hypothalamic polypeptide that inhibits the secretion of immunoreactive pituitary growth hormone. Science 179:77.
2. Polak JM, Pearse AGE, Grimelius L, Bloom SR, Arimura A 1977 Growth hormone release-inhibiting hormone in gastrointestinal and pancreatic D cells. The Lancet 1:1220.
3. Ferri G-L, Adrian TE, Ghatei MA, O'Shaughnessy DJ, Probert L, Lee YC, Buchan AMJ, Polak JM, Bloom SR 1983 Tissue localization and relative distribution of regulatory peptides in separated layers from the human bowel. Gastroenterology 84:777.

4. Penman E, Wass JAH, Butler MG, Penny ES, Price J, Wu P, Rees LH 1983 Distribution and characterization of immunoreactive somatostatin in human gastrointestinal tract. Regul Peptides 7:53.
5. Hökfelt T, Schultzberg M, Johansson O, Ljungdahl A, Elfvin L, Elde R, Terenius L, Nilsson G, Said S, Goldstein M 1978 Central and peripheral peptide producing neurons. In: Bloom SR (ed) Gut Hormones. Churchill Livingstone, Edinburgh, p 423.
6. Uvnas-Wallensten K, Efendic S, Luft R 1978 The occurrence of somatostatin-like immunoreactivity in the vagal nerves. Acta Physiol Scand 102:248.
7. Konturek SJ, Tasler J, Cieszkowski M, Coy DH, Schally AV 1976 Effect of growth hormone release-inhibiting hormone on gastric secretion, mucosal blood flow and serum gastrin. Gastroenterology 70:737.
8. Boden G, Sivitz MC, Owen OE, Essa-Koumar N, Landor JH 1975 Somatostatin suppresses secretin and pancreatic exocrine secretion. Science 190:163.
9. Konturek SJ, Tasler J, Obtulowicz W, Coy DH, Schally AV 1976 Effect of growth hormone-release inhibiting hormone on hormones stimulating exocrine pancreatic secretion. J Clin Invest 58:1.
10. Mitznegg P, Bloom SR, Domschke W, Domschke S, Wunsch E, Demling L 1977 Pharmacokinetics of motilin in man. Gastroenterology 72:413.
11. Kayasseh L, Haecki WH, Gyr K, Stadler GA, Rittman WW, Halter F, Girard J 1978 The endogenous release of pancreatic polypeptide by acid and meal in dogs. Scand J Gastroenterol 13:385.
12. Gerich JE, Patton GS 1978 Somatostatin. Physiology and clinical applications. Med Clin N Am 62:375.
13. Larsson LI, Goltermann N, DeMagistris L, Rehfeld JF, Schwartz TW 1979 Somatostatin cell processes as pathways for paracrine secretion. Science 205:1393.
14. Schusdziarra V, Harris V, Conlon JM, Arimura A, Unger R 1978 Pancreatic and gastric somatostatin release in response to intragastric and intraduodenal nutrients and HCl in the dog. J Clin Invest 62:509.
15. Penman E, Wass JAH, Medbak S, Morgan L, Lewis JM, Besser GM, Rees LH 1981 Response of circulating immunoreactive somatostatin to nutritional stimuli in normal subjects. Gastroenterology 81:692.
16. Rouiller D, Schusdziarra V, Conlon JM, Harris V, Unger RH 1979 Release of somatostatin-like immunoreactivity from the lower gut. Gastroenterology 77:700.
17. Efendic S, Mattsson O 1978 Effect of somatostatin on intestinal motility. Acta Radiol Diagn (Stockh) 19:343.
18. Johansson C, Efendic S, Wisen O, Uvnas-Wallensten K, Luft R 1978 Effects of short-term somatostatin infusion on the gastric and intestinal propulsion in humans. Scand J Gastroenterol 13:481.

19. Guillemin R 1976 Somatostatin inhibits the release of acetylcholine induced electrically in the myenteric plexus. Endocrinology 99:1653.
20. Teitelbaum DH, O'Dorisio TM, Perkins WE, Gaginella TS 1984 Somatostatin modulation of peptide-induced acetylcholine release in guinea pig ileum. Am J Physiol 246:G509.
21. Thor P, Krol R, Konturek SJ, Coy DH, Schally AV 1978 Effect of somatostatin on myoelectrical activity of small bowel. Am J Physiol 235:E249.
22. Peeters TL, Janssens J, Vantrappen GR 1983 Somatostatin and the interdigestive migrating motor complex in man. Regul Peptides 5:209.
23. Dharmsathaphorn K, Sherwin RS, Dobbins JW 1980 Somatostatin inhibits fluid secretion in the rat jejunum. Gastroenterology 78:1554.
24. Carter RF, Bitar KN, Zfass AM, Makhlouf GM 1978 Inhibition of VIP-stimulated intestinal secretion and cyclic AMP production by somatostatin in the rat. Gastroenterology 74:726.
25. Dharmsathaphorn K, Racusen L, Dobbins JW 1980 Effect of somatostatin on ion transport in the rat colon. J Clin Invest 66:813.
26. Dharmsathaphorn K, Binder HJ, Dobbins JW, Leo L 1980 Somatostatin stimulates sodium and chloride absorption in the rabbit ileum. Gastroenterology 78:1559.
27. Guandalini S, Kachur JF, Smith PL, Miller RJ, Field M 1980 In vitro effects of somatostatin on ion transport in rabbit intestine. Am J Physiol 238:G67.
28. Barbezat GO, Reasbeck PG 1981 Somatostatin inhibition of glucagon-stimulated jejunal secretion in the dog. Gastroenterology 81:471.
29. Dharmsathaphorn K, Sherwin RS, Cataland S, Jaffe B, Dobbins J 1980 Somatostatin inhibits diarrhea in the carcinoid syndrome. Ann Intern Med 92:68.
30. Davis GR, Camp RC, Raskin P, Krejs GJ 1980 Effect of somatostatin infusion on jejunal water and electrolyte transport in a patient with secretory diarrhea due to malignant carcinoid syndrome. Gastroenterology 78:346.
31. Ruskone A, Rene E, Chayvialle JA, Bonin N, Pignal F, Kremer M, Bonfils S, Rambaud JC 1982 Effect of somatostatin on diarrhea and on small intestinal water and electrolyte transport in a patient with pancreatic cholera. Dig Dis & Sci 27:459.
32. Krejs GJ, Browne R, Raskin P 1980 Effect of intravenous somatostatin on jejunal absorption of glucose, amino acids, water, and electrolytes. Gastroenterology 78:26.
33. Mulvihill S, Passaro E Jr, Debas H, Yamada T 1984 Severe diarrhea after colonic pseudo-obstruction: treatment with somatostatin. N Engl J Med 310:467.
34. Dharmsathaphorn K, Gorelick FS, Sherwin RS, Cataland S, Dobbins JW 1982 Somatostatin decreases diarrhea in patients with the short-bowel syndrome. J Clin Gastroenterol 4:521.

35. Dharmsathaphorn K, McRoberts JA, Mandel KG, Tisdale LD, Masui H 1984 A human colonic tumor cell line that maintains vectorial electrolyte transport. Am J Physiol 246:G204.
36. Cartwright C, McRoberts J, Mandel K, Masui H, Dharmsathaphorn K 1984 Stimulation of Cl^- secretion in a human colonic epithelial cell line. Clin Res 32:279A (Abstract).
37. Cartwright C, Mandel K, Weymer A, Dharmsathaphorn K 1984 Synergism between cyclic-AMP and calcium mediated secretion in a human colonic epithelial cell line. Gastroenterology 86:1042 (Abstract).
38. Veber DF, Freidinger RM, Schwenk Perlow D, Paleveda WJ Jr, Holly FW, Strachan RG, Nutt RF, Arison BH, Homnick C, Randall WC, Glitzer MS, Saperstein R, Hirschmann R 1981 A potent cyclic hexapeptide analogue of somatostatin. Nature 292:58.
39. Murphy WA, Meyers CA, Coy DH 1981 Potent, highly selective inhibition of growth hormone secretion by position 4 somatostatin analogs. Endocrinology 109:491.
40. Meyers CA, Coy DH, Murphy W, Redding TW, Arimura A, Schally AV 1980 [Phe^4] Somatostatin: a potent, selective inhibitor of growth hormone release. Proc Natl Acad Sci (USA) 77:577.
41. Sarantakis D, McKinley WA, Jaunakais I, Clark D, Grant NH 1976 Structure activity studies on somatostatin. Clin Endocrinol 5:275.
42. Brown M, Rivier J, Vale W 1977 Somatostatin: analogs with selected biological activities. Science 196:1467.
43. Vale W, Rivier C, Brown M 1978 Biologic and immunologic activities and applications of somatostatin analogs. Metab Clin Exp 27:1391.
44. Brown M, Rivier J, Vale W 1979 Somatostatin: central nervous system actions on glucoregulation. Endocrinology 104:1709.
45. Rosenthal LE, Yamashiro DJ, Rivier J, Vale W, Brown M, Dharmsathaphorn K 1983 Structure-activity relationships of somatostatin analogs in the rabbit ileum and the rat colon. J Clin Invest 71:840.

26

SOMATOSTATIN-PRODUCING TUMORS

MICHAEL BERELOWITZ

Division of Endocrinology and Metabolism
University of Cincinnati College of Medicine
Cincinnati, Ohio 45267

INTRODUCTION

As peptide hormones have been identified with increasing frequency over the past years, so too, have tumors of endocrine or non-endocrine tissue that contain them. Traditionally, such tumors have been classified by their histochemical characteristics or morphological appearance however, more recently, it has been suggested that they should rather be classified according to their secretory products. The secretory products of endocrine tumor cells can usually be identified immunohistochemically. Such studies have indicated that tumors frequently contain several cell types and that different peptides can occur within the same cell. It is usual, however, that one cell type predominates and that the biological manifestations of a tumor are due to hypersecretion of a single peptide. Endocrine tumors which produce somatostatin have origins as diverse as those of the tissues that normally synthesize the peptide. Tumors containing somatostatin as a primary product (somatostatinomas) have been described in the pancreas and duodenum while a variety of endocrine and non-endocrine tumors have been shown to contain somatostatin-producing cells.

Pathological Spectrum of Somatostatin-Producing Tumors

A. Somatostatinoma: somatostatin as a primary tumor product

i) Pancreatic somatostatinoma. Somatostatin is normally present in D cells of the pancreatic islets, and tumors of the D cells have been described that contain and secrete high concentrations of the peptide. Such tumors are not common and to date only 21 patients have been described in the world literature (1-22). The primary tumor in these patients was located more frequently in the head of the pancreas than in the body or tail and at the time of resection was invariably large in size (ranging from 1.5 to 10 cm in diameter). Histology revealed a picture typical of islet-cell tumor with solid nests and cords of cells penetrated by a fibrovascular stroma. Most tumors demonstrated evidence of malignancy (usually of low grade) with local infiltration and metastases to the liver and draining lymph nodes. Immunohistochemical staining for somatostatin was invariably present in most if not all cells of primary and metastatic tumor. Staining for other peptides most frequently revealed cells containing calcitonin (5, 6, 8, 10), adrenocorticotropin (ACTH) (3, 10) and other islet peptides (including insulin, glucagon and pancreatic polypeptide). D cell secretory granules of varying density and size have usually been seen in tumor cells on electron microscopy. Primary and metastatic tumor extracts contained concentrations of immunoreactive somatostatin 100-1000 times that in normal pancreas.

ii) Duodenal somatostatinoma. A novel psammomatous variant of duodenal carcinoid tumor that appears to derive from somatostatin containing D cells has recently been described in 13 patients (23-34). Such tumors have generally been located in the second part of the duodenum in the periampullary region. Usually identified as a nodule in the duodenal mucosa, the tumors have been associated with superficial ulceration, local infiltration and metastatic involvement of regional lymph nodes and the liver. Histologically, the tumors have a carcinoid appearance with insular and trabecular patterns: a characteristic feature in most tumors has been the presence of laminated calcified basophilic structures resembling psammoma bodies most frequently located in grandular lumena. Immunohistochemical staining indicated that the tumors consist almost exclusively of somatostatin-containing cells. Calcitonin immunoreactivity was present in a few cells in one tumor (23) but no other peptide products have been identified. Neurone-specific enolase staining was positive in somatostatin-containing cells (32, 34) when studied. Electron microscopy revealed the presence of large nodules formed of microfilaments in the cytoplasm of tumor cells with D cell secretory granules. Extracts of primary and metastatic tumor tissue contained somatostatin at 10-20 times the concentration present in normal tissue.

iii) Jejunal somatostatinoma. A single case report described a somatostatin-containing carcinoid tumor in the jejunal wall, 15 cm from the ligament of Treitz that was associated with spread to regional lymph nodes (35).

B. Somatostatin-containing tumors: somatostatin as a secondary tumor product

Usually identified by immunocytochemical screening, a variety of tumors have been shown to contain a varying proportion of somatostatin-positive cells. Such tumors include:

i) Carcinoid tumors: In a study of 18 midgut carcinoid tumors, 6 were found to contain somatostatin-positive cells on immunohistochemical staining but they never constituted the majority (36). Carcinoid tumors originating in other locations also contain somatostatin including thymic and bronchial tumors (37).

ii) Medullary carcinoma of the thyroid: Somatostatin is normally present in a sub-population of C cells of the human thyroid. Thus, it is not surprising that somatostatin is present in malignant C cells in primary and metastatic medullary carcinoma of the thyroid (38-42). Somewhat surprising is the fact that somatostatin-containing cells have not been identified in areas of C cell hyperplasia (38, 42), a pre-malignant phase of the tumor. Together with calcitonin that was invariably present, ACTH was also frequently identified in tumor cells. Extracts of tumor tissue contained somatostatin at 10-1000 times the concentration found in normal tissue.

iii) Phaeochromocytoma: Normal human adrenal medulla contains somatostatin that is present in a small percentage of cells. Studies of phaeochromocytoma tissue (32, 43-52), both adrenal and extra-adrenal, reveal somatostatin-positive cells in varying proportions. Some tumors demonstrated only isolated somatostatin-positive cells (43, 52) while others contained somatostatin in up to one third of tumor cells (48). Similar and parallel variations were found in somatostatin extracted from tumor tissue. Other peptides frequently present in phaeochromocytoma tissue included met-enkephalins and vasoactive intestinal polypeptide.

iv) Small-cell carcinoma of the lung: Extracts of squamous carcinoma of the lung and normal lung tissue contain no detectable immunoreactive somatostatin. By contrast the peptide is present in high concentrations in one third of small-cell carcinomas (37, 40, 53, 54). An association was noted between ACTH production and somatostatin in two of the reports (37, 54).

v) Retinoblastoma: Somatostatin immunoreactivity is present in amacrine and ganglion cells of the normal human retina. In 4 retinoblastomas, somatostatin-containing cells were scattered throughout the tumor tissue (55).

vi) Other gastro-entero-pancreatic tumors: Somatostatin-positive cells are an invariable finding in endocrine tumors of the pancreas and gut. Seldom obtrusive in number they are usually identified by immunohistochemical screening or measurement of tumor extracts (56).

Biochemical Characterization of Tumoral Somatostatin

A. Tissue somatostatin content

Immunoreactive somatostatin concentration was highest in pancreatic somatostatinoma tissue (1-5000 μg/g tissue) with lesser concentrations in duodenal somatostatinoma (0.05 - 6.4 μg/g), medullary carcinoma of the thyroid (0.02 - 9.2 μg/g) and phaeochromocytoma (0.01 - 5.5 μg/g).

B. Chromatographic characterization of tumor somatostatin

In general tumoral somatostatin demonstrated molecular heterogeneity on gel, thin-layer, ion-exchange or polyacrylamide-gel electrophoresis. Three peaks of immunoreactivity were usually demonstrable that corresponded to the 10-15K somatostatin precursor, a form coeluting with somatostatin-28, and one coeluting with somatostatin-14. The proportion of these forms varied between tumors suggesting differences in efficiency of post-translational processing. Occasional tumors contained somatostatin-14 as a major form (11, 12, 39, 40, 46, 49); by contrast one tumor contained only large molecular weight forms (31).

C. Structural characterization of tumor somatostatin

Amino acid analysis of somatostatin-14-like immunoreactivity purified from two tumors revealed a composition identical to that of somatostatin-14 (20, 46).

Somatostatin RNA was purified from a pancreatic somatostatinoma (16) and the human somatostatin 1 gene cDNA cloned and sequenced. From the gene structure the amino acid sequence of preprosomatostatin was deduced and found to contain somatostatin-28 with somatostatin-14 at the C-terminus.

From these findings it is apparent that somatostatin-containing tumors synthesize authentic somatostatin precursor peptides that are processed with variable efficiency to produce molecules that have chromatographic characteristics similar to those of biologically active somatostatin-28 and -14. In a small number of studies this has been confirmed by demonstrating *in vitro* somatostatin biological activity of partially purified tumoral somatostatin (1, 7, 41, 46, 49).

Circulating Plasma Somatostatin Associated with Somatostatin-Producing Tumors

Considerable differences still exist between various investigators in extraction techniques, antiserum recognition and normal values as they apply to human plasma somatostatin measurement. These technical differences make comparisons between studies difficult, although certain conclusions can be drawn.

A. Pancreatic somatostatinoma

Circulating plasma somatostatin levels in peripheral plasma are elevated 8-40 times control in most reported cases (1, 5-7, 12, 15, 17-19, 21) although much higher elevations have been described (in some cases up to 500 times normal control) (11, 13, 14). In contrast, a minority of patients have exhibited normal or only slightly elevated peripheral plasma somatostatin levels (8, 19).

In a few cases selective venous sampling has been performed that indicated elevated hepatic-portal vein somatostatin levels (5) with a 10-fold arterio-venous gradient across the pancreatic bed (12).

Chromatographic characterization of circulating somatostatin has revealed molecular heterogeneity with a pattern similar to the tumor of origin (5-7, 11, 12, 14, 15, 17).

B. Duodenal somatostatinoma

Peripheal venous plasma somatostatin has only been studied in three cases and normal to slightly elevated levels were found (23, 31, 33). Plasma levels rose late in the course of one patient associated with deterioration in liver function (31).

C. Medullary carcinoma of the thyroid

In cases of medullary carcinoma of the thyroid peripheral venous plasma somatostatin levels appear to correlate with disease extent. Thus basal levels are elevated 10-24 fold in 4 of 9 patients (39-41) with a decrease in serum levels following successful surgery (41) and an increase in levels following development of metastatic disease (41).

D. Phaeochromocytoma

A lesser (2-3 fold) elevation of peripheral plasma somatostatin levels has been described in patients with phaeochromocytoma (44, 48-50). Selective venous sampling in one patient revealed a step-up in levels associated with tumor venous effluent (50).

Clinical Presentation and Characteristics of Somatostatin-Producing Tumors

It has long been known that somatostatin infusion results in widespread inhibitory effects on endocrine and exocrine secretions and on a variety of gastrointestinal functions. On the basis of such studies, a series of clinical associations could be predicted that would be associated with high circulating levels of endogenous somatostatin. These associations, features that comprise the somatostatinoma syndrome, have now been described in certain patients with somatostatin-producing tumors although not in all cases.

A. Somatostatin-producing tumors associated with the clinical somatostatinoma syndrome

As originally defined (57), the somatostatinoma syndrome consists of i) insulin sensitive, non-ketosis prone diabetes mellitus (due to growth hormone, insulin and glucagon inhibition), ii) steatorrhoea (due to inhibition of gastrointestinal endocrine and exocrine secretions) and iii) cholelithiasis (due to inhibition of gall bladder contractility). The full syndrome has only been described in patients with pancreatic somatostatinoma and then only in 6 of 21 subjects (1, 6-8, 15, 21). Diabetes mellitus plus gall bladder disease coexisted in 3 patients (2, 18, 22) while another 3 patients had diabetes mellitus and steatorrhoea (5, 10, 13). An additional patient with small-cell carcinoma of the bronchus (54) presented with features of the syndrome (diabetes mellitus and steatorrhoea) together with Cushing's syndrome due to ectopic ACTH production.

Patients with pancreatic somatostatinoma who demonstrated clinical features of the somatostatinoma syndrome had a marked female predominance (10:2) and a wide age range (30-70 yr) at the time of presentation, characteristics similar to patients without clinical features of somatostatin excess. A similar lack of correlation existed between serum somatostatin levels and clinical features in patients with pancreatic tumors.

The lack of clinical evidence of somatostatin excess in patients with non-pancreatic somatostatin-producing tumors could relate to lower levels of somatostatin production and/or secretion or, perhaps, to greater production of higher molecular weight non-biologically active forms.

B. Somatostatin-Producing Tumors Unassociated with Clinical Somatostinoma Syndrome

i) Duodenal somatostatinoma. By contrast with pancreatic tumors, patients with duodenal somatostatin-producing tumors were largely males (9:4) aged 26-79 yr. Three patients had neurofibromatosis (29, 32, 34), and two had associated phaeochromocytomas (32,

34). Patients presented with abdominal, especially epigastric, discomfort or pain (23, 24, 29, 30), obstructive jaundice (30, 31, 33) and a history of peptic ulcer disease (29, 34).

ii) Other somatostatin producing tumors. These were unassociated with distinguishing clinical features or evidence of somatostatin over-production. Features were those of the primary tumor and the presence of somatostatin in tumor tissue was an incidental pathological finding.

C. Other clinical endocrine syndromes associated with somatostatin-producing tumors

One patient with a pancreatic somatostatinoma presented with ectopic ACTH syndrome (3). ACTH and somatostatin were both demonstrated in tumor cells immunohistochemically but no data were available regarding tumoral somatostatin secretion.

Two patients with pancreatic somatostatinomas presented with hypoglycemia (11, 19) in the presence of elevated (11) or normal (19) serum insulin levels. In both cases insulin was present in tumor cells and may have been co-produced.

Endocrine and Gastroenterological Evaluation in Patients with Somatostatin-Producing Tumors

A. Pituitary hormones

Normal (2, 10, 11) or low (6, 18) basal growth hormone levels with reduced responsiveness to arginine stimulation (2, 6, 11, 15, 18) or insulin-induced hypoglycemia (6) were demonstrated in patients with pancreatic somatostatinoma. Other pituitary hormone levels and responsiveness to stimuli were normal.

B. Pancreatic hormones

Fasting serum insulin and C-peptide levels were normal in patients with pancreatic somatostatinoma except in a patient with hypoglycemia (11). In patients with impaired glucose tolerance or frank diabetes mellitus, poor insulin or C-peptide responses to oral glucose (2, 5, 15, 18), arginine (2, 10, 15, 18), a mixed meal (6, 18), or sulphonylureas (18, 19) were seen.

Serum glucagon levels in pancreatic somatostatinoma patients were reported as normal under basal conditions (6, 7, 11) with poor responses to arginine (2, 6, 7, 15, 18), and insulin-induced hypoglycemia (7).

C. Gut hormones

Gastrin levels were normal basally (6, 8, 11) with normal responses to a meal (6, 8).

D. Gastric acid secretion

In most patients with pancreatic somatostatinoma who were evaluated, basal acid secretion was low (1, 5, 6, 18, 21) with decreased responses to pentagastrin stimulation (1, 5, 6, 18, 21). Two patients however had normal results (2, 10).

E. Pancreatic exocrine function

Pancreatic insufficiency was documented in all three cases in which testing was reported (5, 6, 18).

F. GI function studies

Rapid whole gut transit time (5) and delayed gastric emptying (6) have been reported together with delayed postprandial nutrient absorption (5, 6, 18).

Dynamic Tests of Somatostatin Secretion

Serum somatostatin responsiveness to a variety of agents has been studied in patients with pancreatic somatostatinoma. Oral glucose (6, 7, 15, 18), arginine infusion (6, 15, 18), mixed meal (6, 18) and insulin-induced hypoglycemia (7) have given mixed results. Sulphonylureas, especially tolbutamide, have consistently stimulated somatostatin release (7, 8, 19, 23) and may provide a means of diagnosing pancreatic somatostatinoma.

Tumor Localization Procedures

Pancreatic somatostatinomas have been demonstrated by a variety of techniques including barium meal (1, 5, 6), ultrasonography (5, 6, 12, 21), abdominal CT Scan (8, 12, 15, 21, 22), and angiography (2, 6, 8, 13, 19, 22).

Duodenal somatostatinomas have been localized on upper GI series (23, 24, 29, 30), endoscopy (23, 24, 33) and abdominal CT scan (29, 30, 31).

Therapy and Outcome

Whenever possible, surgical resection of somatostatin-producing tumor tissue has been attempted. Pancreatic somatostatinoma was generally treated by Whipple's procedure or pancreatectomy. Duodenal somatostatinoma was similarly treated by Whipple's procedure or duodenectomy. In addition chemotherapy, usually streptozotocin, was administered in a number of cases.

The prognosis in patients with pancreatic somatostatinoma has not proven good. Eight of 21 patients in the literature have died immediately to nine months following surgery. The remaining patients recovered with remission from clinical features of somatostatinoma. Patients with duodenal somatostatinoma had a somewhat better prognosis with one tumor-related death described 7 months postoperatively.

Experimental Models of Somatostatin-Producing Tumors

Tumoral somatostatin excess has been produced in animals through transplantable islet cell tumors in the NEDH (58) and Lewis (59) rat and transplantable medullary carcinoma of the thyroid in the WAG/Rij rat (60-63). Somatostatin secretion is particularly high in WAG/Rij rats with transplantable medullary thyroid cancer and these animals demonstrate impaired insulin and growth hormone responsiveness to stimuli (60). Both tumoral and plasma somatostatin were heterogeneous in this model (60, 61) with chromatographic patterns similar to those seen in human cases of somatostatinoma. The mRNA encoding somatostatin in tumor tissue from these rats has been cloned and characterized and the structure of rat preprosomatostatin identified (63).

In vitro studies using somatostatin-producing cell lines obtained from human small cell carcinoma of the lung have provided greater insights into the mechanisms of tumoral somatostatin biosynthesis (53).

Experimental models of tumoral somatostastin biosynthesis, secretion and biological effects should provide greater understanding of somatostatin-producing tumors and the somatostatinoma syndrome in man.

REFERENCES

1. Larsson LI, Hirsch MA, Holst JJ, Ingemansson S, Kuhl C, Lindkaer Jensen S, Lundqvist G, Rehfeld JF, Schwartz TW 1977 Pancreatic somatostatinoma: Clinical features and physiological implications. Lancet i:666.
2. Ganda OP, Weir GC, Soeldner JS, Legg MA, Chick WL, Patel YC, Ebeid AM, Gabbay KH, Reichlin S 1977 "Somatostatinoma": A somatostatin-containing tumor of the endocrine pancreas. New Eng J Med 296:963.
3. Kovacs K, Horvath E, Ezrin C, Sepp H, Elkan I 1977 Immunoreactive somatostatin in pancreatic islet-cell carcinoma accompanied by ectopic A.C.T.H. syndrome. Lancet i:1365.

4. Ganda OP, Soeldner JT 1977 "Somatostatinoma": Follow-up studies. New Eng J Med 297:1352.
5. Galmiche JP, Colin R, DuBois PM, Chayvialle JA, Descos D, Paulin C, Geffroy Y 1978 Calcitonin secretion by a pancreatic somatostatinoma. New Eng J Med 299:1252.
6. Krejs GJ, Orci L, Conlon JM, Ravazzola M, Davis GR, Raskin P, Collins SM, McCarthy DM, Baetens D, Rubenstein A, Aldor TAM, Unger RH 1979 Somatostatinoma syndrome: Biochemical, morphologic and clinical features. New Eng J Med 301:285.
7. Pipeleers D, Somers G, Gepts W, De Nutte N, De Vroede M 1979 Plasma pancreatic hormone levels in a case of somatostatinoma: Diagnostic and therapeutic implications. J Clin Endocrinol Metab 49:572.
8. Gerlock AJ, Muhletaler CA, Halter S, Goncharenko V 1979 Pancreatic somatostatinoma: Histologic, clinical, and angiographic features. AJR 133:939.
9. Galmiche JP, Chayvialle JA, Dubois PM, David L, Descos F, Paulin C, Ducastelle T, Colin R, Geffroy Y 1980 Calcitonin-producing pancreatic somatostatinoma. Gastroenterology 78:1577.
10. Asa SL, Kovacs K, Killinger DW, Marcon N, Platts M 1980 Pancreatic islet cell carcinoma producing gastrin, ACTH, α-endorphin, somatostatin and calcitonin. Amer J Gastroenterol 74:30.
11. Wright J, Abolfathi A, Penman E, Marks V 1980 Pancreatic somatostatinoma presenting with hypoglycaemia. Clin Endocrinol 12:603.
12. Penman E, Lowry PJ, Wass JAH, Marks V, Dawson AM, Besser GM, Rees LH 1980 Molecular forms of somatostatin in normal subjects and in patients with pancreatic somatostatinoma. Clin Endocrinol 12:611.
13. Lowry SF, Burt ME, Brennan MF 1981 Glucose turnover and gluconeogenesis in a patient with somatostatinoma. Surgery 89:309.
14. Conlon JM, McCarthy D, Krejs G, Unger RH 1981 Characterization of somatostatin-like components in the tumors and plasma of a patient with a somatostatinoma. J Clin Endocrinol Metab 52:66.
15. Axelrod L, Bush MA, Hirsch HJ, Loo SWH 1981 Malignant somatostatinoma: Clinical features and metabolic studies. J Clin Endocrinol Metab 52:886.
16. Shen L-P, Pictet RL, Rutter WJ 1982 Human somatostatin I: Sequence of the cDNA. Proc Natl Acad Sci 79:4575.
17. Patel YC, Ganda OP, Benoit R 1983 Pancreatic somatostatinoma: Abundance of somatostatin-28(1-12)-like immunoreactivity in tumor and plasma. J Clin Endocrinol Metab 57:1048.
18. Schusdziarra V, Grube D, Seifert H, Galle J, Etzrodt H, Beischer W, Haferkamp O, Pfeiffer EF 1983 Somatostatinoma syndrome. Clinical, morphological and metabolic features and therapeutic aspects. Klinische Wochenschrift 61:681.

19. Pipeleers D, Couturier E, Gepts W, Reynders J, Somers G 1983 Five cases of somatostatinoma: Clinical heterogeneity and diagnostic usefulness of basal and tolbutamide-induced hypersomatostatinemia. J Clin Endocrinol Metab 56:1236.
20. Bohlen P, Brazeau P, Esch F, Ling N, Wehrenberg WB, Guillemin R 1983 Human growth hormone releasing factor and somatostatin from two pancreatic tumors: isolation and characterization. Regul Peptides 6:343.
21. Kelly TR 1983 Pancreatic somatostatinoma. Am J Surg 146:671.
22. Sakazaki S, Umeyama K, Nakagawa H, Hashimoto H, Kamino K, Mitsuhashi T, Yamaguchi K 1983 Pancreatic somatostinoma. Am J Surg 146:674.
23. Stacpoole PW, Kasselberg AG, Berelowitz M, Chey WY 1983 Somatostatinoma syndrome: does a clinical entity exist? Acta Endocrinol 102:80.
24. Kaneko H, Yanaihara N, Ito S, Kusumoto Y, Fujita T, Ishikawa S, Sumida T, Sekiya M 1979 Somatostatinoma of the duodenum. Cancer 44:2273.
25. Ito S, Yamada Y, Iwanaga T, Kaneko H, Shibata A 1982 Somatostatin-28 like immunoreactivity in normal and tumour issue from duodenum and pancreas. Acta Endocrinol 101:421.
26. Kaneko H, Toshima M, Kobayashi H, Kitazawa M, Ito S, Iwanaga T, Kusumoto Y, Fujita T, Nitta H 1983 Duodenal somatostatinoma: Immunohistopathology and review of literature. Acta Pathol Jpn 33:153.
27. Kaneko H, Toshima M, Kobayashi H, Kitazawa M 1983 Ultrastructural characteristics of duodenal somatostatinomas: I. Somatostatinoma cells and Schwann-like cells. Acta Pathol Jpn 33:347.
28. Kaneko H, Sumida T, Toshima M, Kobayashi H, Kitazawa M 1983 Ultrastructural characteristics of duodenal somatostatinomas: II. Granules and vesicles. Acta Pathol Jpn 33:359.
29. Dayal Y, Nunnemacher G, Doos WG, DeLellis RA, O'Brien MJ, Wolfe HJ 1983 Psammomatous somatostatinomas of the duodenum. Am J Surg Pathol 7:653.
30. Marcial MA, Pinkus GS, Skarin A, Hinrichs HR, Warhol MJ 1983 Ampullary somatostatinoma: Psammomatous variant of gastrointestinal carcinoid tumor - an immunohistochemical and ultrastructural study. Report of a case and review of the literature. Am J Clin Pathol 80:755.
31. Somers G, Pipeleers-Marichal M, Gepts W, Pipeleers D 1983 A case of duodenal somatostatinoma: Diagnostic usefulness of calcium - pentagastrin test. Gastroenterology 85:1192.
32. Cantor AM, Rigby CC, Beck PR, Mangion D 1982 Neurofibromatosis, phaeochromocytoma, and somatostatinoma. Br Med J 285:1618.
33. Jensen SL, Christiansen LA, Oxholm A-M, Holst JJ 1984 Duodenal somatostatinoma. Br J Surg 71:159.
34. Griffiths DFR, Jasani B, Newman GR, Williams ED, Williams GT 1984 Glandular duodenal carcinoid - a somatostatin rich tumour with neuroendocrine associations. J Clin Pathol 37:163.

35. Alumets J, Ekelund G, Hakanson R, Ljungberg O, Ljungqvist U, Sundler F, Tibblin S 1978 Jejunal endocrine tumour composed of somatostatin and gastrin cells and associated with duodenal ulcer disease. Virchows Arch A Path Anat and Histol 378:17.
36. Lundqvist M, Wilander E 1981 Somatostatin-like immunoreactivity in mid-gut carcinoids. Acta Path Microbiol Scand, Sect A, 89:335.
37. Penman E, Wass JAH, Besser GM, Rees LH 1980 Somatostatin secretion by lung and thymic tumours. Clin Endocrinol 13:613.
38. Deftos LJ, Bone HG, Parthemore JG, Burton DW 1980 Immunohistological studies of medullary thyroid carcinoma and C cell hyperplasia. J Clin Endocrinol Metab 51:857.
39. Saito H, Saito S 1980 Clinical significance of plasma somatostatin determination in medullary carcinoma of thyroid. Lancet i:1191.
40. Roos BA, Lindall AW, Ells J, Elde R, Lambert PW, Birnbaum RS 1981 Increased plasma and tumor somatostatin-like immunoreactivity in medullary thyroid carcinoma and small cell lung cancer. J Clin Endocrinol Metab 52:187.
41. Saito S, Saito H, Matsumura M, Ishimaru K, Sano T 1981 Molecular heterogeneity and biological activity of immunoreactive somatostatin in medullary carcinoma of the thyroid. J Clin Endocrinol Metab 53:1117.
42. Charpin C, Andrac L, Monier-Faugere MC, Hassoun J, Cannoni M, Vagneur JP, Toga M 1982 Calcitonin, somatostatin and ACTH immunoreactive cells in a case of familial bilateral thyroid medullary carcinoma. Cancer 50:1806.
43. Lundberg JM, Hamberger B, Schultzberg M, Hokfelt T, Granberg P-O, Efendic S, Terenius L, Goldstein M, Luft R 1979 Enkephalin- and somatostatin-like immunoreactivities in human adrenal medulla and phaeochromocytoma. Proc Natl Acad Sci (USA) 76:4079.
44. Bernard P, Lebras J, Pradel J, Viguier AC, Curet P, Grellet J 1980 Exploration angiographique d'un cas d'apudome surrenalien a triple composante hormonale. J Radiol 61:121.
45. Faurel JP, Bernard P, Saigot TH, Bousquet O, Sarrazin A 1982 Pheochromocytome secretant du vaso-active intestinal peptide et de la somatostatine: Une observation. Nouv Presse Med 11:1483.
46. Corder R, Sykes JEC, Lowry PJ 1982 Characterization of the somatostastin-like immunoreactivity extracted from an adrenal medullary tumour. Bioscience Reports 2:147.
47. Corder R, Lowry PJ 1982 Large-molecular-weight somatostatin in human adrenal medullary tissue. Bioscience Reports 2:397.
48. Saito H, Saito S, Sano T, Kagawa N, Hizawa K, Tatara K 1982 Immunoreactive somatostatin in catecholamine-producing extra-adrenal paraganglioma. Cancer 50:560.
49. Berelowitz M, Szabo M, Barowsky HW, Arbel ER, Frohman LA 1983 Somatostatin-like immunoactivity and biological activity is present in a human phaeochromocytoma. J Clin Endocrinol Metab 56:134.

50. Sano T, Saito H, Inaba H, Hizawa K, Saito S, Yamanoi A, Mizunuma Y, Matsumura M, Yuasa M, Hiraishi K 1983 Immunoreactive somatostatin and vasoactive intestinal polypeptide in adrenal phaeochromocytoma: An immunochemical and ultrastructural study. Cancer 52:282.
51. Wu P, Penman E, Coy DH, Rees LH 1983 Evidence for direct production of somatostatin-14 from a larger precursor than somatostatin-28 in a phaeochromocytoma. Regul Peptides 5:219.
52. Hassoun J, Monges G, Giraud P, Henry JF, Charpin C, Payan H, Toga M 1984 Immunohistochemical study of Phaeochromocytomas: An investigation of methionine-enkephalin, vasoactive intestinal peptide, somatostatin, corticotropin β-endorphin, and calcitonin in 16 tumors. Am J Pathol 114:56.
53. Szabo M, Berelowitz M, Pettengill OS, Sorenson GD, Frohman LA 1980 Ectopic production of somatostatin-like immuno- and bioactivity by cultured human pulmonary small cell carcinoma. J Clin Endocrinol Metab 51:978.
54. Ghose RR, Gupta SK 1981 Oat cell carcinoma of bronchus presenting with somatostatinoma syndrome. Thorax 36:550.
55. Sano T, Saito H, Saito S, Kagawa N, Hizawa K 1981 Somatostatin immunoreactive cells in human retina and retinoblastoma. Biomed Res 2:709.
56. Bloom SR, Polak JM, Welbourn RB 1979 Pancreatic apudomas. World J Surg 3:587.
57. Unger RH 1977 Somatostatinoma. New Eng J Med 296:998.
58. Chick WL, Warren S, Chute RN, Like AA, Lauris V, Kitchen KC 1977 A transplantable insulinoma in the rat. Proc Natl Acad Sci (USA) 74:628.
59. Chick WL, Appel MC, Weir GC, Like AA, Lauris V, Porter JG, Chute RN 1980 Serially transplantable chemically induced rat islet cell tumor. Endocrinology 107:954.
60. Berelowitz M, Cibelius M, Szabo M, Frohman LA, Epstein S, Bell NH 1980 Somatostatin-like immunoreactivity in a transplantable medullary carcinoma of rat thyroid: Partial chromatographic and biological characterization. Endocrinology 107:1418.
61. Birnbaum RS, Muszynski M, Roos BA 1980 Tumor and plasma somatostatin-like immunoreactivity in transplantable rat medullary thyroid carcinoma. Cancer Res 40:4192.
62. Goodman RH, Jacobs JW, Dee PC, Habener JF 1982 Somatostatin-28 encoded in a cloned cDNA obtained from a rat medullary thyroid carcinoma. J Biol Chem 257:1156.
63. Funckes CL, Minth CD, Deschenes R, Magazin M, Tavianini MA, Sheets M, Collier K, Weith HL, Aron DC, Roos BA, Dixon JE 1982 Cloning and characterization of a mRNA-encoding rat preprosomatostatin. J Biol Chem 258:8781.

PERIPHERAL SOMATOSTATIN

PANEL DISCUSSION

MODERATOR: J. ENSINCK

DR. J. ENSINCK (Seattle): We have just heard Dr. Larrson pointing out that the peripheral somatostatin-containing cell is represented morphologically by either D cells, as found in the islets and in the gastrointestinal mucosa, or by nerve cells located in the muscle layers. He has emphasized the need to reconcile the ubiquitous distribution of these cells with the putative role of somatostatin as a modulator of cellular activity. Dr. Weir, in addressing the question of the local interactions between A, B, and D cells in the pancreatic islets, has allowed that a case can be made for the paracrine control of somatostatin on A cells, and possibly adjacent B cells in the peripheral part of the islet. However, he has pointed out that the limits imposed by the vascular supply make it unlikely that locally produced somatostatin could influence the central core of the B cells. On the other hand, Dr. Schusdziarra has provided a great deal of evidence that somatostatin is released into the circulation, presumably mostly from the gastrointestinal tract, thereby supporting the possibility that somatostatin as a hormone may act on distant target cells. Dr. Vinik has provided intriguing information characterizing agonistic vs antagonistic activities on the oxyntic hydrogen-secreting cell of the stomach and the paradoxical responses of somatostatin secretion to ambient calcium levels. Dr. Dharmsathophorn has shown inhibition of ion and water movement across intestinal cells. These perturbations are in keeping with physiological functions for somatostatin in the intestinal tract. And lastly, you have just heard Dr. Berelowitz talk on the origin and clinical manifestations associated with excess circulating somatostatin-related peptides from somatostatinomas, and, when present, they are in keeping with the evidence that the pancreas and the gastrointestinal tract are the major organs of somatostatin action. In the overall context of this afternoon's program, therefore, there is a continuing perplexing issue that still confronts us in the reconciliation of the paracrine vs endocrine functions of somatostatin-related peptides. In order to fuel further discussion on this topic, I would like to develop some additional concepts quickly. On the first slide (Fig. 1) are schematically depicted the somatostatin-containing cells in the GI tract and the pancreas on the left, and the products of posttranslational processing of prosomatostatin in these cells. As we heard yesterday, despite some differences in opinion, it seems probable that in the islet D cell, in peripheral nerves, and therefore presumably in the gastrointestinal neurons, somatostatin-14 is the predominant terminal product. In contrast, the fate of pro-S is seemingly different in the epithelial cells. Dr. Patel, Dr. Weir, Dr. Vinik and Dr. Berelowitz have all previously reported that the mucosa is laden with somatostatin-28, and my colleagues, Dr. Francis, Dr. Baskin and I have evidence that somatostatin-28 is not further processed to any major extent in the epithelial cells. Moreover, as pointed out by Dr. Larsson, the juxtaposition of the epithelial cell between the gastrointestinal lumen and vascular space implies that it serves a different function than in the adjacent neurons. That this may be the case is suggested by data on the next slide (Fig. 2) in which we have measured peripheral plasma levels of somatostatin-28 in man before and after eating. As first observed by Polonsky in man, and confirmed in this slide (Fig. 2), and also reported by Holst in the perfused pig intestine at this meeting, circulating somatostatin-28 rises after food intake. In contrast, we have found that there is virtually no change in the levels of somatostatin-14 or in this instance, somatostatin-12 (des Ala^1 Gly^2 S-14 - resulting from

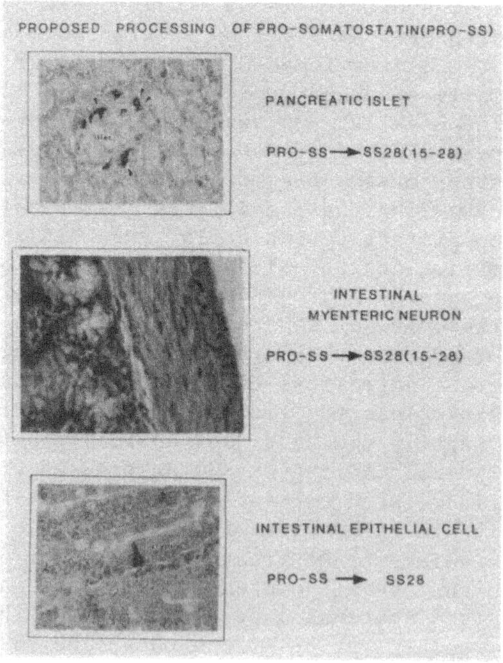

Fig. 1.

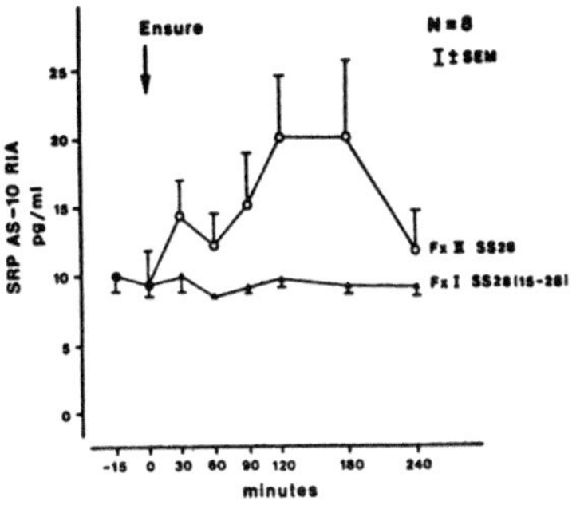

Fig. 2. Levels of SS28 and SS28(15-28) in plasma from healthy young men before and after the intake of Ensure.

degradation of the N-terminus of somatostatin-14), implying that it is not stimulated during nutrient absorption. Therefore, it seems plausible that the intestinal epithelial cell, by releasing S-28 as a traditional hormone during substrate absorption, may signal other cells at distant sites where somatostatin-14 released from GI neurons and D cells in the pancreas may act locally. In this setting, therefore, I would address questions to Dr. Weir and to Dr. Schusdziarra. Dr. Schusdziarra, would you comment on the measurement of S-28 and S-14 in your dogs or normal volunteers as well as obese individuals?

DR. V. SCHUSDZIARRA (Ulm, FRG): In the dogs we have never found somatostatin-28 in substantial quantities although there are some other reports by Dr. Chayvialle's group from France, who found some somatostatin-28 in dog plasma. In humans we find both somatostatin-14 and somatostatin-28, in almost equal amounts in the postprandial situation.

DR. J. ENSINCK: Are there any changes or differences you know of in obese individuals?

DR. V. SCHUSDZIARRA: I don't know, but I think Dr. Wass and Dr. Penman have some similar data finding S-28 and S-14 in extracted plasma. So there's not much of a difference.

DR. J. ENSINCK: Dr. Weir, in view of the concept of compartmentalization, would you comment on the notion that arterial delivery of somatostatin-28 might exert a modulating effect on the central B cell core?

DR. G. WEIR (Richmond): Well, I see no reason why it couldn't. Certainly, a number of people have shown that very small amounts of somatostatin will inhibit insulin secretion and the levels which you found in blood are certainly very close to that. After a meal, it would make sense that those somatostatin levels would rise to a point where they could have some inhibitory effect. Obviously, it is not enormous because insulin rises are quite prominent after meals.

DR. J. ENSINCK: Are there any questions from the floor that specifically address these issues and others that have been raised throughout the afternoon?

DR. S. SZABO (Boston): Dr. Larsson you mentioned the coincidence of calcitonin and somatostatin staining in several cells. But is this a species-specific item because if I am correct, this is not the case in the cat. Would you comment on whether or not this is a coincidence or might there be some relationship between calcium or calcitonin and somatostatin?

DR. L. LARSSON (Copenhagen): Yes I think the thyroidal somatostatin story is probably the most complicated one of all because it's really in that location that we find the largest species differences. In the cat it is absolutely absent as far as we can detect by immunocytochemistry, but of course there is a lower limit of detection in immunocytochemistry, so we can't say for sure that there aren't 10 or 100 molecules present in a cell. Compared to the other species, however, it is very striking in the cat where instead we find large amounts of somatostatin-like immunoreactivity in the parathyroid gland. I would not dare to speculate at this time about any physiological relevance of this particular finding. The data have been shown to emphasize that there are very vast species differences and that we have to be very careful in comparing data from one type of species to another. I think that this also applies to some degree to the islet cells and the gastrointestinal somatostatin cells.

DR. S. SZABO: Question to Dr. Vinik: The stimulatory role of somatostatin on gastric secretion is really very interesting, especially since it occurs at extremely low doses. If I am correct, all of your studies were performed *in vitro*. Are there any *in vivo* data which would show that somatostatin indeed stimulates acid secretion under certain conditions?

DR. A. VINIK (Ann Arbor): I haven't seen any data which suggest that, under the conditions that have been studied, somatostatin has proved to be a stimulator. Most of the studies that have examined acid secretion have, in fact, examined that at levels of somatostatin which would be astronomic, compared with those which could be regarded as physiological. I think that these studies need to be done.

DR. B. FRANCIS (Seattle): Dr. Berelowitz, your talk about somatostatinomas was very interesting and provided a very good review of what we have seen in somatostatinomas. There seems to be a very obvious difference between pancreatic somatostatinomas and the duodenal somatostatinomas and the absence of a lot of somatostatinomas that, for instance, have a neural origin. My question is: are we in fact seeing a different embryological development of a cell that, in fact, is not the same as what Dr. Pearse and Dr. Polak have for many years tried to lump together as apudomas? Are we seeing cells, instead, that come from a completely different embryological source which we don't know yet, and provide a syndrome of endocrine-secreting tumors that would give us a hint to the embryological development of these tumors?

DR. M. BERELOWITZ (Cincinatti): You don't ask hard questions do you? Basically, I think that the whole concept of apudomas is one that I am not going to get into at all; I will leave that to Dr. Derek LeRoith sitting at the back there smiling like crazy. But what I would say is that clearly there are differences that exist between these tumors. For instance, what would define an islet cell tumor histologically, pathologically and clinically and what would define a carcinoid histologically, clinically and biochemically? I don't know if anybody knows what the origin of these tumors is in terms of the final original cell. Is it the EC cell for the carcinoid, or the D cell for the pancreatic somatostatinoma, or why the pancreatic somatostatinoma should make more and more biologically active material and why it should have characteristic clinical features. I don't know that anybody knows these things. There are pieces of evidence that I tried to point out based on certain commonalities which are tying to tell us something. The fact that duodenal carcinoid is seen with phaeochromocytoma, is seen with neurofibromas, is seen with calcitonin secretion, and that calcitonin secretion with medullary cancers of the thyroid is associated with somatostatin, may be giving us hints about commonalities of origin but I am not in a position to be able to speculate about any of these issues. It's certainly interesting though.

DR. B. FRANCIS: There are also some further data that were presented many many years ago by a researcher by the name of Van Andrews from South Africa, who showed that the cells from the somites of chicks, at the level where the pancreas should migrate, do not in fact migrate into the pancreas. So, I think that a lot of these cells that we have sort of lumped together as apudomas in these tumors may not be, and may have a different embryological development.

DR. M. BERELOWITZ: I am very happy to stay clear of that subject.

DR. G. TABORSKY (Seattle): I think I would just like to make a comment on your last few slides. I think there is a tendency to view the role of somatostatin with regard to the islet as either an endocrine one or a paracrine one. I think that, in fact, it may be both. I think there is fair evidence now that very low concentrations of somatostatin can have an endocrine function to inhibit primarily insulin secretion, and my own and some other data seem to suggest that the paracrine action of somatostatin on the islet, if present, is predominantly on glucagon. So, I think that they are not mutually exclusive and would like to emphasize that both are possible.

DR. J. ENSINCK: I agree. I think the issue of whether or not insulin secretion is inhibited by somatostatin-28 has to be placed in the context of whether or not the peripheral cells in Susan Bonner-Weir's model may in fact be influenced by the circulating peptide. I think that Gordon Weir would agree that this concept is a possibility. Based on the vascular supply, the central B cell mass would have difficulty in being regulated through a paracrine effect from pancreatic-derived somatostatin.

DR. G. TABORSKY: I think that particular comment also depends largely on the species in which you look, as Dr. Larsson pointed out. The rat islet, although it is commonly shown at these meetings, is not representative of all species and I would urge some caution in this interpretation and the general application of the rat islet as a model for either human or dog.

DR. J. HOLST (Copenhagen): I have a comment and a question. The comment is about acid secretion at low concentrations of somatostatin. We just completed a study in which we found that an elevation of somatostatin, as small as 5 pmol/l, very significantly inhibited acid secretion in man. So, it is really a very potent inhibitor of acid secretion. This inhibition took place without any influence whatsoever on gastrin concentrations. Now, the question is to Gordon Weir. From my review of the literature on the cytoarchitecture of the islets and particularly their relation to the microvasculature, I think the only constant feature is the variability. Now that you have come up with a very elegant presentation of what could be the solution to all these problems, I would like to ask you, did you look at other species?

DR. G. WEIR: I sure wish my wife was here to hold my hand. No, she hasn't, and nobody else has either. These studies were done in rats and it is true that there are a lot of differences but there are some things which are consistent also, in that the A and D cells are almost always together and the B cells are almost always together. So even though the human is somewhat different from the rat, there are, I think, more similarities than differences. Now when you get to such things as horses and whatnot, where the A and D cells may be in the center of the islet, then it is going to be fascinating to take a look to see where exactly that arterial tree goes. Does it plunge into the B cells first or does it plunge into some other part?

DR. A. VINIK: Jens, I think that is a very interesting observation of yours on the very low level, say 5 pmol of somatostatin. You will recall that I showed that subthreshold doses, i.e. doses of somatostatin below the agonist concentrations of somatostatin, are inhibitory for the stimuli. That is they inhibit histamine and they inhibit carbachol-stimulated acid secretion. If the amount of somatostatin that you are giving, when you give 5 pmol, approximates the fmol range that I am using in the *in vitro* tissue, that is what I would expect it to do. If you can exclude the presence of the other agonists you would then detect the agonist role of somatostatin. So it has given us a model for studying the mechanism of action of somatostatin. One thing, in addition, is that when we use fentomolar concentrations of somatostatin intralumenally, we are able to show that acid secretion is inhibited.

DR. KLIVER (FRG): I have a question for Dr. Berelowitz about the somatostatinoma syndrome. It is well known that somatostatin is able to reduce the TSH response after TRH application, but I have never heard that patients with somatostatinomas were suffering from hypothyroidism. So my question is what about the thyroid hormones? Are they normal or are they subnormal in these patients?

DR. M. BERELOWITZ: In the patients that have been studied, normal responsiveness has been reported. The only way that I could explain that, is that there has never been a consistent change in TSH in any situation where we suspect there may be elevated somatostatin, except possibly in children treated with growth hormone for growth failure. That is the only place where there is even a vague suggestion that there may be abnormalities, and my explanation for that would be, first of all, I think that while somatostatin inhibits TSH, I don't believe that somatostatin plays a major role in the regulation of TSH. I think that most of the regulation of TSH is occurring at the pituitary level directly by thyroid hormone. And the second thing is that you always have to take into consideration the fact that TRH is acting there and that any change in somatostatin could easily be matched by a corresponding change in TRH. And why shouldn't that occur with growth hormone? I can't give you a conclusive answer.

DR. Y.C. PATEL (Montreal): I am a little bit more optimistic than Gordon Weir was about the evidence for a functional role of the D cells within the islet. I think that the kinds of *in vitro* antibody neutralization experiments, that say Jack Gerich did, together with some recent data using cysteamine, have clearly shown that neutralization of released somatostatin or depletion of intracellular somatostatin certainly has a pronounced stimulatory effect on glucagon secretion. I think you referred to some of those data yourself. But also when you disperse the islet cells and grow them in monolayer, and particularly if you grow the monolayer within a matrix of collagen as Lelio Orci has done, the islet cells do come together maintaining the same precise adult type islet cell relationships, with the glucagon cells and the somatostatin cells together. They do recognize each other and join up exactly as you see them in vivo. Concerning insulin, again the cysteamine data do show that removal of islet somatostatin has a stimulatory effect on insulin regulation. Morphology, to some extent, argues against a direct B and and D cell interaction, but I would like to ask Dr. Larsson what he thinks. I have heard it referred to many times, about his feeling that the same cytoplasmic processes that he described for the gastric D cells also apply to the islet D cells, but I have never actually seen the data. How strongly do you feel about that?

DR. L. LARSSON: Extremely strongly. They do exist within the islets. Again I am sorry to have to be so dreary all the time, but there are species differences. There are definitely processes in the rat islets; in the guinea pig islets, they are enormous and there you have quite another anatomy where the processes sort of make a network over all of the islet and where it would be very hard for B cells to escape from coming into contact with somatostatin processes. So perhaps the guinea pig islet would be a much better model than the rat islet where, as Orci reported many years ago, the D cells are restricted to the mantle area and to the glucagon area, but even there you can see processes going in towards the center of the islet. One of the interesting things is that that type of arrangement seems to be preserved even when you make a monolayer culture of neonatal rat pancreas where you can see long, fine somatostatin cell processes. I think we have in the gut a very simple situation because the gastrin cells and the somatostatin cells are spaced apart by many, if I may say, uninteresting cells, and in that way it is possible to show a connection with double staining. It is much more difficult to demonstrate this as clearly in the islets because you always have this entire three dimensional architecture to consider, so perhaps the question should be re-examined in primary monolayer cultures of the pancreas where you think you have the same type of architecture.

DR. G. WEIR: Yogesh, I do not want to be a wet blanket, but I think that we have to look extremely hard at our data. With regard to the passive immunization approaches, I think that is a particular case in point. When one studies isolated islets or monolayer cultures, the system is unphysiologic in that both the vasculature and the nervous system have been disrupted. When you have tissue like that sitting in a bath, obviously, somatostatin is going to be secreted and that somatostatin is going to have access to the A cells and the

B cells. So to put antiserum in and find that insulin or glucagon secretion increases, I don't think means anything as to what happens in vivo. I just think that with those studies and with so many other similar studies we really have to be very tough in interpreting them.

DR. Y.C. PATEL: Yes, I agree that the immunoneutralization experiments with isolated islets have certain problems that you have mentioned but at the same time they provide some fundamental insights which I am not ready to dismiss. If you accept that usually the anatomical relationships between the islet cells are preserved in isolated islets and that antibodies penetrate the isolated islets because they have been "opened up" with trypsin digestion, then essentially what you are considering in these experiments is the secretory capability of the A and B cells without the effects of somatostatin. We know that under these circumstances, certainly the A cells hypersecrete, and there is now supporting data from several laboratories. Furthermore, your own data on the separate cell types suggest that the enriched A cell fractions hypersecrete glucagon. Now if you accept that there is normally a special anatomial relationship between the A and D cells, then I think all these observations add up to the fact that the A cell removed from the influence of the D cell has a higher secretion of glucagon, which clearly implies an inhibitory modulating role of D cells on A cells.

DR. J. GERICH (Rochester): I would like to make a few comments about what Gordon said. Granted that when we studied isolated islets and incubated them with and without anti-somatostatin serum we found when we added the anti-somatostatin serum we got increases in both insulin and glucagon release. Now, as Gordon Weir points out, one problem with that finding is that you may artificially get a build up of somatostatin levels in the flask that ordinarily would not be available to the A and B cells and these would exert an inhibitory effect, and then when you add the antiserum you prevent this. I am not so sure that this is a very strong objection because, when you actually measure how much somatostatin does build up in the flasks it is about a doubling or tripling, at most, of the levels that I think would be within a physiologic range that you might expect to build up within the interstitial fluid of the islet. So I would still say that that type of experiment, plus the cysteamine experiments, provide substantial evidence for some type of paracrine effect. Now, what's just been touched on here is how does one get differential control of insulin and glucagon secretion via somatostatin. It would seem to me that if you block the secretion of both hormones you are going to neutralize your effect and that physiologically there must be some way to get differential control. A few years ago Dr. Mandarino, in my laboratory, compared the effects of S-28 and S-14 in the perfused rat pancreas and he found that S-14 was a much more potent inhibitor of glucagon release than insulin release and the opposite was the case for S-28. Now since the islet contains predominantly S-14, you might postulate that S-14 subserves a paracrine effect and predominantly affects glucagon whereas perhaps S-28, which is released into the circulation after meals, may serve a hormonal effect and predominantly act on insulin secretion. Now, I wonder what is the teleologic reason for having an inhibitor of insulin secretion after a meal and perhaps this is a safeguard against hypoglycemia resulting after a meal. We know that there is greater insulin secretion after a meal than after iv glucose. Perhaps we prevent hypoglycemia from occurring by having somatostatin-28 feed back on insulin secretion and maybe Dr. Schusdziarra, or you Gordon, would like to comment on this.

DR. G. WEIR: I think it is very interesting and a very nice hypothesis. Maybe Dr. Schusdziarra could shed some light on this.

DR. V. SCHUSDZIARRA: I would go even further. Considering the teleological aspect, it may be necessary to prevent exaggerated insulin secretion in order not to have downregulation of insulin receptors. Several years ago Olefsky showed that when you have an elevation of insulin by 30 μU/ml, which is not very much but if you have that consistently for 3-4 hours, you can already demonstrate downregulation of insulin receptors. You might have some initial step for the development of insulin insensitivity and the hyperinsulinemia, so I think it is reasonable to assume that there should be some sort of regulation. I don't think that it is necessarily a clear-cut inhibition by having an increase in somatostatin. What you try to avoid is having some exaggerated insulin secretion in some sort of a shock absorber function that somatostatin might have.

DR. J. GERICH: Since antiserum is now available that is specific for the S-28 molecule and since we are talking about a potential hormonal role for it, perhaps I might suggest some experiments to people who have this antiserum where you would specifically neutralize the 28 molecule after meals and see what happens.

DR. PALMER (Houston): I have just a comment really for Dr. Berelowitz. He mentioned at the end of his talk that he had a small cell carcinoma cell line. From our work on somatostatin secretion by D cells, I might mention that there is also one other cell line which is derived from medullary carcinoma cells by Susan Lyong which we have recently shown to secrete very large quantities of somatostatin. These cells are also responsive to glucocorticoids; for example, in the regulation of the synthesis and secretion, so this is another cell model. Interestingly, it is also one of the better models for a developing carcinoma because there is always hyperplasia preceding the development of carcinoma in these cells. So they are interesting for a couple of reasons.

DR. M.D. RUGGERE (Montreal): I just would like to comment on Dr. Gerich's last statement. If someone used somatostatin specific antibody for S-28 and attached the antibody to the N-terminal half of the molecule they might not necessarily neutralize the bioactivity if the cyclized ring portion remains available for receptor binding. So we have to make sure that such an antibody would or would not interfere with receptor binding of S-28. I think that everyone should carefully look at their specific S-28 antibodies to see if they are capable of neutralizing the biological activity of S-28 before proceeding with antibody neutralizing experiments.

DR. J. ENSINCK: If there are no further questions or answers, Dr. Patel would like to address the audience. Before he takes the podium, may I express to him and to Dr. Gloria Tannenbaum, and members of their Local Organizing Committee, the gratitude of those of us who have been privileged to attend this superbly organized symposium in which we have all benefited from interactions and interesting information. Thank you, Dr. Patel, Dr. Tannenbaum.

SUMMARY AND CONCLUSIONS

SUMMARY AND CONCLUSIONS

YOGESH C. PATEL

We have now come to the end of two days of exhaustive review of some of the key developments in the somatostatin field over the last decade. The vigorous panel discussions have generated many new ideas and the individual experts have focused on some of the future directions in their respective areas. My task now is to recapitulate, to fill in some of the gaps, and to give you my perception of the field as I have seen it evolve over the last ten years and where I see it heading over the coming years.

Table I lists what I consider to be the most significant landmarks in somatostatin research to date. The events are in approximate chronological order. The discovery of somatostatin-14 in 1973 in Guillemin's laboratory gave birth to the field and was rapidly followed by the realization that the peptide possessed multiple biological actions and was widely distributed in neuroendocrine cells in many regions of the body. The development of specific antisera to somatostatin and the application of these antibodies in passive immunization experiments provided proof of a physiological role of somatostatin in GH and TSH regulation. The demonstration of release of somatostatin from nerve endings in response to depolarization afforded the first direct glimpse of its possible role as a neurotransmitter substance. The identification of specific membrane receptors for somatostatin initiated the most meaningful studies of the mechanism of action of the peptide. Morphological data, coupled with the use of in vivo and in vitro immunoneutralization experiments, gave an early indication of an important physiological role of somatostatin on nutrient absorption and on islet cell function. The discovery in 1980 of somatostatin-28, as a second biologically active molecular form was a signal achievement which ushered in the biosynthesis era which has dominated the field since. This period saw the elucidation of the structure of 5 separate preprosomatostatin molecules in fish and mammalian cells, the identification and structural characterization

Table I. Landmarks in Somatostatin Research

1) The isolation of somatostatin-14.
2) Demonstration of multiple biological actions.
3) Demonstration of wide anatomical distribution of somatostatin cells.
4) Elucidation of a physiological role in GH/TSH regulation.
5) Demonstration of somatostatin release from nerve endings following depolarization.
6) Identification of specific membrane receptors.
7) Demonstration of a physiological role on nutrient absorption and on islet cell function.
8) Discovery of somatostatin-28.
9) Elucidation of the structure of preprosomatostatins.
10) Identification of multiple genes for somatostatin.
11) Discovery of Somatostatin-28$_{[1-12]}$ and related molecular forms.
12) Transfer and expression of somatostatin gene in heterologous tissues.

of multiple genes for somatostatin, the discovery of somatostatin-28$_{[1-12]}$ and related molecular forms, and culminated in the elegant experiments described by Drs. Goodman and Shields at this meeting, of the transfer and expression of somatostatin genes in heterologous tissues. Thus, over the last 10 years, the originally proposed, somewhat narrow view of somatostatin-14 as a specific regulator of pituitary GH secretion, has been expanded to the concept of somatostatin-14 as one, and perhaps the most important member of a family of somatostatin-like peptides, widely distributed in neural and nonneural tissues, and subserving important physiological functions both locally as a neurotransmitter, neuromodulator, paracrine regulator, or "lumone" and systemically as a true hormone. The development of these concepts early in the somatostatin field, in many ways, served as a prototype for the understanding of the other neuropeptide systems that followed. Today we should stop thinking of somatostatin as somatostatin-14 or a hypothalamic hormone, or an islet hormone, or a gut hormone, or any other such single entity but consider it as a diffuse system of regulatory cells.

Future developments in the biosynthesis area will, I believe, continue to be heavily dominated by the molecular biologists. I see a lot of growth and excitement in this area as we learn about the regulation of somatostatin gene expression with increasing use of gene transfer and deletion type experiments. These approaches promise fundamental insights into the function of the pro-segment of somatostatin and particularly the structural requirements necessary for recognition by processing enzymes. There should be identification of other somatostatin genes and elucidation of the factors and molecular mechanisms involved in the regulation of somatostatin biosynthesis. The diversity of the somatostatin genes will now undoubtedly focus special attention on comparative animal studies of the evolution of somatostatin genes and of the nature and function of somatostatin in invertebrate species. Other growth areas should be the characterization of some of the newer molecular forms (e.g. glycosylated catfish somatostatin-22, anglerfish somatostatin-28, mammalian somatostatin-28 [1-12]-like forms), their biosynthetic relationships, biological actions, secretion, and possible separate physiological functions. Further characterization of the somatostatin family of peptides will no doubt reveal other instances of nonproteolytic posttranslational modifications of the kind described at this meeting by Drs. Dixon and Spiess (e.g. glycosylation and hydroxylation). Finally, there will be continuing attempts to purify and characterize the somatostatin-14 and somatostatin-28 converting enzymes, with the prospect of an early breakthrough in our understanding of the regulation of the proteolytic procesing of prosomatostatin and of differential, tissue-specific processing so characteristic of mammalian somatostatin cells.

Like the biosynthesis field, the area on the mechanism of action of somatostatin and somatostatin analogs is a rapidly expanding one, which should see a number of significant future developments such as elucidation of receptor heterogeneity, and in particular, resolution of the question of whether there are separate receptors for the various somatostatin peptides. We should hear a lot about the regulation of receptor function, and on solubilization and structural studies of the somatostatin receptor unit. Beyond the receptor, it is expected that there will be further elucidation of the mechanisms involved in receptor-effector coupling and other post-receptor events. This applies particularly to the question of whether the somatostatin receptor in normal tissues is coupled to adenylcyclase and the guanine nucleotide binding proteins, as demonstrated so well now for tumor cells. I expect that there will be a major effort to characterize some of the intracellular actions of somatostatin such as those on DNA replication and cell proliferation, the cytoskeleton, and calcium flux. One of the most significant developments would be the availability of potent and selective pharmacological antagonists for somatostatin. As you have heard at this meeting, the search for suitable long acting and selective analogs has been a long, frustrating, and expensive undertaking. These analogs are badly needed, and perhaps the encouraging clinical results with compounds such as SMS 201-995 presented at this meeting, will put new heart, and hopefully, new money into somatostatin analog research by the pharmaceutical companies.

In contrast to the two previous areas, elucidation of brain somatostatin function poses formidable problems. Nonetheless, it was really heartening to see at this meeting how quick some of the recent progress has been. As Wylie Vale pointed out, we have now clearly made the transition from simple descriptive studies to functional mechanisms in the brain. Some of the immediate growth areas, as I visualize them, are: (1) the elucidation of the neuropharmacological, neuropeptide, and other control mechanisms involved in the regulation of somatostatin secretion from nerve cells in different regions of the brain; (2) the elucidation of a physiological relationship between hypothalamic somatostatin and growth hormone, growth factors and GRF; (3) further studies to clarify the existence and functional significance of autoregulation by somatostatin nerve cells; (4) continuing neuroanatomical studies to delineate central and peripheral somatostatinergic pathways; (5) elucidation of the role of brain somatostatin on the autonomic nervous system-mediated visceral functions such as acid output, adrenal medullary secretion, and gut motility which are known to be profoundly affected by centrally administered somatostatin; (6) clarification of the precise role of somatostatin in the pathophysiology of disease states such as Alzheimer's disease and Huntington's chorea.

Studies of islet somatostatin function will continue to focus on the delineation of the paracrine relationships between the D and other islet cells. In these efforts, the use of antagonists and of agents such as cysteamine and pure populations of islet cells should be of considerable value. Little is currently known about the function of somatostatin in the largest somatostatin-producing organ in the body, the gut. The issues here are as complex as those for the brain, and whilst some of the big answers to questions such as the physiological role of somatostatin on motility and on the numerous digestive and absorptive events may take time to come, much of the fundamental work still needs to be tackled. This includes the development of suitable in vitro systems for studying the biosynthesis and secretion of somatostatin. The characterization of somatostatin receptors in the gastrointestinal tract has not been accomplished. Finally, with all the somatostatin in the gastrointestinal tract, there must be disease states other than tumors associated with somatostatin dysfunction, waiting to be identified.

As we move off in different directions and pick away slowly at these numerous individual challenges, we must not lose sight of the fact that despite its many faces, somatostatin is above all a regulatory system exerting perhaps a common general function over its varied target cells. In the present rudimentary state of our knowledge, this function can be perhaps best illustrated by the A and D cells of the islets of Langerhans, which share a very special anatomical relationship, as reviewed just a short while ago by Gordon Weir and Lars Larsson. These two cells are naturally associated in vivo, but even in vitro, they clearly seem to recognize each other and show the ability to come together in culture after dispersal. And yet the A cell secretes more in the absence of its D cell partner. It's as if the D cells are the <u>necessary</u> brakes for the A cells. To my mind, when we understand such inhibitory control we will truly begin to understand somatostatin.

The last ten years have witnessed an explosive growth in this field. Well over a thousand papers on somatostatin have already been published. The uniqueness of somatostatin as a model system has attracted researchers from diverse fields. Unfortunately, the inability to find quick answers has dampened the initial enthusiasm of workers in some areas. I hope that this meeting has served to rekindle everyone's interest and that you remain as optimistic about the research potential of the somatostatin system as I am.

AUTHOR INDEX

SUBJECT INDEX

GPSR Compliance

The European Union's (EU) General Product Safety Regulation (GPSR) is a set of rules that requires consumer products to be safe and our obligations to ensure this.

If you have any concerns about our products, you can contact us on ProductSafety@springernature.com

In case Publisher is established outside the EU, the EU authorized representative is:

Springer Nature Customer Service Center GmbH
Europaplatz 3
69115 Heidelberg, Germany

Batch number: 10838062

Printed by Printforce, the Netherlands